Delmar's Integrative
Herb Guide for Nurses

Delmar's Integrative Herb Guide for Nurses

BY
MARTHA LIBSTER, MS, RN

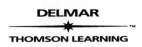

Australia   Canada   Mexico   Singapore   Spain   United Kingdom   United States

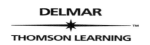

DELMAR

THOMSON LEARNING

Delmar's Integrative Herb Guide for Nurses
by Martha Libster

Health Care Publishing Director:
William Brottmiller

Product Development Manager:
Marion S. Waldman

Product Development Editor:
Jill Rembetski

Executive Marketing Manager:
Dawn F. Gerrain

Channel Manager:
Gretta Oliver

Technology Project Specialist:
Joe Saba

Editorial Assistant:
Robin Irons

Art/Design Coordinator:
Connie Lundberg-Watkins

Production Coordinator:
Nina Lontrato

Project Editor:
David Buddle

Library of Congress Cataloging-in-Publication Data
Libster, Martha.
    Delmar's integrative herb guide for nurses / by Martha Libster.
    p. cm.
    Includes bibliographical references and index.
    ISBN 0-7668-2710-0
    1. Herbs—Therapeutic use.
2. Nursing. I. Title: Integrative herb guide for nurses.

    RM666.H33 L634 2001
615'.321—dc21
                    2001047256

Notice to the Reader

Dedication

My deepest love and gratitude . . .

To my childhood friends, Robin and Carolyn, who taught me to play with
       bullfrogs and salamanders and to eat sassafras.
To my friend Mindy, who grazes with me now.
To my sister Sara, for feeding me marigolds when I was but one year old.
To my brother John, for exuding his love of the green and the game.
To Grandpa Art, who taught me how to heal with aloe.
To Gramma Sally, who taught me how to care for gardenias.
To Mimi, who gave me the Thomson genes and a love for beauty.
To Granddaddy Edward William, who knew a perfect rose when he saw it.
To my mom and dad, Connie and Bill, for encouraging my connection
       with nature.
To all of my teachers, including those of the plant kingdom, for their inspiration.
And most especially, to my husband Harold and my puppy Sheeva, for always
       keeping me rooted.

". . . while pursuing the humblest occupations, such as planting or cutting flowers, I had perceived, as a chink of light through a door opened quickly, a greater plan of things than our programme for the year, a larger world than that surrounding us, and one universal pattern of things, in which all existence has its place. . . . I have felt peace descend on me while I have handled plants, so that a rhythm and harmony of being has been brought about. That harmony is the beginning of health. . . ."

Elaine Penwardin, *It's the Plants That Matter* (1967)

Contents

Chapter 3   Plants and Paradigms

Chapter 4   Carefulness and Conservation

Chapter 5   Nursing Care and Plants: Back to the Roots

Chapter 6   Plant Profiles   111

Chapter 7   Comfort and Pain Relief   133

Foreword

Years ago, when Martha Libster approached me for advice, I was delighted. I wanted nurses and physicians to write herbals for nurses and physicians in lingo they understand and believe. As I recall, I told her that I knew the herbs and she knew the clinic. Let's get them together—nurse, herb, and clinic. It's done. Nice work, Martha! You have compiled the right amount of useful experience and information on most of the important herbs in common use in America.

Delmar's Integrative Herb Guide for Nurses brings to nurses, and more important, perhaps, their patients, a nurse's view of plant medicine as a practical and timely choice in the care of at least some patients. (No one medicine is best for all patients!) It also acquaints nurses with plant therapies, reminding them of their historical connection with plant healing in patient care and providing the readers with a fundamental introductory understanding of herbal therapies and their potential integration with nursing practice.

This book stresses the importance of good relationships with the environment and plants, an essential part of our environment. Prominent nurse theorists, including Florence Nightingale, have focused on the importance of the environment in patient care. Getting to know plants firsthand, through gardening, nature walks, and so on, makes you believe in the power of the "green pharmacy." And believing is half of healing. I have long maintained that I want the best medicine for myself and my family, be it natural or synthetic. Since Martha started this labor of love, many herbs (e.g., saw palmetto and St. John's wort) have proven themselves as good as their more expensive pharmaceutical counterparts, with fewer side effects. Herbs increasingly are being recognized as safe and gentle medicines, which our genes have long experienced.

I think American medicine will be improved by an infusion of rational herbalism and phytomedicine into modern allopathy. I even predict a hybrid vigor from this marriage of the best of disparate disciplines.

—James A. Duke, PhD, Economic Botanist, USDA (retired), author of
The Green Pharmacy

Preface

Nurses and their patients have used herbs in healing for centuries. Historically, caregivers, including nurses, have been taught by family members and community healers how to use flowers, leaves, seeds, and roots in comforting others. This trend continues today as herbalism is rapidly evolving as a science and a healing art. Indeed, it is changing so quickly that today's nurse might wonder where she or he can learn about herbal therapies when the subject is no longer taught as a regular part of nursing school curriculum. Patients have questions about plant use as they continue their cultural traditions of using plants for self-care. Many nurses also want to continue the time-honored tradition of using herbs in their practice. Although numerous books on the subject of healing plants are available, no single book on herbs speaks to the unique educational needs of the practicing nurse.

Delmar's Integrative Herb Guide for Nurses fills this need by providing a context for the use of herbal remedies that reflects a nursing model of care. It introduces nurses to the science and art of plant use in healing in a way that is understandable and immediately applicable to practice. The focus of this herb guide is for the nurse to learn about using an integrative approach to the therapeutic use of plants. An integrative approach with herbs means that although herbs may not necessarily be used in patient care, nurses and patients consider the modality as an option alongside conventional, biomedical practices and other healing modalities. If patients then choose to use herbs, they work with their health practitioners to create a plan for the appropriate holistic blend of herbal and biomedical therapies.

This text provides an opportunity for the reader to explore this integrative approach to understanding human-plant relationships while using plants in healing. The integrative approach is demonstrated in this book by its inclusion of information from the different paradigms associated with the use of herbs, such as biomedical research, cultural traditions, and nursing history. It also includes examples from my extensive clinical experience with herbs.

Why I Wrote This Book Now

I wrote this book for two reasons: (1) I have read and referenced numerous herbal texts over the years, none of which fully addressed my questions as a professional nurse and herb practitioner. (2) It is my belief that plant therapies have been, and continue to be, an integral part of caregiving and self-care practices, which is why 80% of the world's population still uses herbs despite the advances in biomedicine.

While some herbal care information has been recorded in older nursing textbooks, before the institutionalization of nursing in the late 1800s, caregivers rarely documented their work with plant therapies, except perhaps in diaries and recipe books. There are few, if any, current books on the subject of herbalism and nursing practice. This book has been written with the intent of recapturing and reclaiming nurses' history of plant use in caregiving. It also has been written to share my many years of reflection on what nurses can add to the practice of herbalism. Because nurses walk between the worlds of biomedicine and the patients they serve who are using herbal remedies, they must have an understanding of herbs. Many people like to go with a guide when they go on herb walks through nature's pharmacy. *Delmar's Integrative Herb Guide for Nurses* has been written to serve as that guide.

Organization

Although many herbals are created for reference purposes, *Delmar's Integrative Herb Guide for Nurses* has been written to facilitate its use as a daily reference and a textbook. Chapters 7 through 18 contain the profiles of fifty-eight herbs and can be used as a reference. The herbs profiled in this book were chosen specifically because of their familiarity to nurses and their potential for use in nursing practice and research. Chapters 1 through 6, 19, and 20 include supporting text that provides the reader with a foundational understanding of topics in herbalism, such as basic botany, medicine making, different paradigms for understanding herb use, how to talk with patients about their use of herbs in self-care, and suggestions for the safe use of herbs.

SPECIAL FEATURES:

This text contains the following special features:
- Profiles of fifty-eight herbs relevant to nursing practice
- Herb information organized by health patterns nurses encounter in daily practice for easier referencing
- Data provided from biomedical, nursing, and botanical literature, and traditional healing resources
- Color insert that includes full color botanical illustrations of each herb
- Recommendations for addressing the safe use of herbs in patient care
- Specific questions and interventions for nurses to use when discussing herb use with patients
- Reader opportunities to nurture the nurse-plant relationship using recipes for self-care found in each herb profile
- Sample curriculum for herb education for nurses
- Guidelines for patient interaction for each of the fifty-eight herbs profiled
- Index cross-referenced for botanical and common names of plants as well as health patterns

How to Use This Book

Because *Delmar's Integrative Herb Guide for Nurses* has been written as a reference as well as a text, it is possible for a reader to open the book anywhere and learn about the therapeutic uses of plants; however, the reader will gain so much more from reading the herb profiles in chapters 7 through 18 if the book is read in its entirety first before using it as a reference. This book guides the reader into the world of healing plants (see chapter 1), provides a foundation for their use through a brief historical explanation (see chapter 2), and then discusses the different paradigms surrounding herb use (see chapter 3). The guide then provides suggestions for the safe use of herbs (see chapter 4) and how to make herbal remedies that could be used in nursing care (see chapter 5). Chapter 6 describes how to use the herb profiles in chapters 7 through 18, explaining each of the sections used in the herb profiles in detail, and including fascinating information on ten different cultural uses of herbs. Chapters 19 and 20 guide the reader to the next steps to be considered after reading the *Integrative Herb Guide*, such as resources for further learning, how to report herb research to the public, nine questions and interventions to use when talking with patients about using herbs, and guidelines for the nurse to use when preparing to use herbs in practice. Readers will find these chapters vital to implementing what is learned from reading the fifty-eight herb profiles.

The references for *Delmar's Integrative Herb Guide for Nurses* are listed in the back of the book. There are two reference lists. The "General Reference List" includes the references that appear frequently throughout the fifty-eight herb profiles. The remaining references are organized by chapter and by herb profile (chapters 7 through 18). A glossary is also included in the back of *Delmar's Integrative Herb Guide for Nurses*.

Audience

Although written for nurses at all levels of practice, the public, other health care professionals, nursing students, students of herbalism, and nurse educators can benefit from reading *Delmar's Integrative Herb Guide for Nurses*.

FOR THE EDUCATOR:

Please note the sample 32-week curriculum in chapter 19 that references each chapter of *Delmar's Integrative Herb Guide for Nurses* so that it can be used to assist in preparing an introductory course in nature care (the use of herbs in caregiving).

FOR HEALTH CARE PROFESSIONALS:

Please note the section in chapter 20, Talking with Patients About Herbs, and its subsection, 9 Questions and Interventions. I have used these questions as a basis for numerous lectures for health care professionals and have had feedback that they are very helpful.

FOR STUDENTS AND THE PUBLIC:

You will find this book full of the information you need when using herbs in self-care. At the end of each herb profile, you also will find a section called Nurturing the Nurse-Plant Relationship, which includes recipes for self-care with herbs. Don't let the heading keep you from exploring these opportunities for wonderful experiences with plants.

Supplement

Delmar's Integrative Herb Guide for Nurses CD-ROM is available as a companion to the text. This browser-based CD runs on both Windows and Macintosh operating systems and includes a searchable database of all of the herbal profiles included in the book, as well as seventeen video clips that provide step-by-step instruction on how to prepare and use a variety of herbal remedies, such as teas, herbal oils, tinctures, and creating a healing environment with herbs.

Your Herb Stories Welcome

Delmar's Integrative Herb Guide for Nurses is a work in progress. If you have any stories about the clinical use of herbs in nursing practice in your country, please let me know. Contact the author by e-mail: martha@integrativeassociates.com or fax 303-280-3111.

Acknowledgments

I wish to thank the following people with all my heart for their invaluable guidance and inspiration in the creation of this herb guide: Barb Fine; Cheri Richards; Al Leung; Magdalena Abramova; Keith Miller; Roberta Lee; Dennis Worthen and the fine staff of the Lloyd Library; Helen Sweet; Rise Smythe-Freed; the librarians at the W.H.O. in Geneva, Switzerland; Sandra Jeanne Fucci; Roger Wicke; Jim Duke; Marlaine Smith; Roshani Tobias; Jane McCabe; Marion Waldman for her vision; Robin Irons for her support and ingenuity; and a most special thanks to my editor and friend, Jill Rembetski, whose patience, support, and honesty knows no limits. I am in your debt.

Delmar's Integrative Herb Guide for Nurses was written with the support of a talented interdisciplinary team of experts from the fields of nursing, herbalism and herb education, ethnobotany, medical geography, pharmacy, and medicine. I am eternally grateful for the support of the following review board members and contributors.

Review Board

Sue C. DeLaune, MN, RNC
President, SDeLaune Consulting
Adjunct Faculty, William Carey College School of Nursing
New Orleans, LA

Trish Flaster
CEO/President
Botanical Liaisons
Boulder, CO

Mindy Green, MSc
Director of Education
Herb Research Foundation
Boulder, CO

Marlaine C. Smith, RN, PhD
Associate Professor and Director
Center for Integrative Caring Practice
University of Colorado Health Sciences Center School of Nursing

Contributors

Nanette Judd, RN, MPH, PhD
Faculty at the University of Hawaii School of Medicine
Honolulu, HI
Contributor on Hawaiian information

Ruby J. Martinez, RN, PhD, CS
University of Colorado Health Sciences Center School of Nursing
Contributor on lifestyle choices introduction and tobacco

Jane M. McCabe, RN, MSN, OCN
Oncology Clinical Nurse Specialist
Contributor on restoration chapter

Dana Murphy-Parker, MS, RN, CNS
Professor of Nursing
Arizona Western College
Yuma, AZ
Contributor on lifestyle choices introduction and marijuana

Matthias Seidel, MD
Filderklinik
Filderstadt, Germany
Contributor on anthroposophical medicine and mistletoe

Roshani Tobias, RN
Clinical Herbalist
Faculty, North Carolina School of Natural Healing
Contributor on Western herbalism and sleep and rest

Teresa Vigil, LPN
Director, Los Dónes
San Luis, CO
Contributor on Hispanic information

About the Author

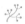

Martha Libster is the director of Integrative Associates, LLC, a consultation and education firm. She has extensive experience in the integration of conventional nursing practice and complementary therapies such as herbal therapies, reflexology, jin shin jyutsu, and electromagnetic therapies. She has practiced in a wide variety of healthcare settings, including six years (1989–1994) in a holistic health facility where she was the coordinator of herb programs. As coordinator, she managed the growth, harvesting, processing, and utilization of over 100 plants and plant therapies. She also served as the Natural Health Care Hotline director for the Herb Research Foundation in Colorado in 1995.

Ms. Libster is a certified practitioner and consultant in traditional Chinese and Western herbal medicine. She teaches throughout the country on the use of plant therapies in healing practice to both health professionals and the public in addition to teaching numerous nursing, wellness, and health-related subjects. She holds bachelor degrees in dance education/movement therapy from New York University and in nursing from Mount St. Mary's College, and a master's degree in psychiatric nursing from the University of Colorado Health Sciences Center. She is presently working on her doctoral dissertation entitled, *Herbal Diplomats: The Use of Plant Therapies by 19th Century American "Nurses,"* through the School of Humanities—Medical History at Oxford Brookes University in England. She is the author of *Demonstrating Care: The Art of Integrative Nursing* (Delmar).

Introduction

The colors of flowers, the aromatic fragrances of barks and leaves, the pungent power of a pepper, and the tangy taste of lemons are just a few of the experiences people encounter when they connect with the sensual beauty of the world of plants. Think for a moment with which plants *you* connect. Do you wake up to a cup of coffee or a pot of tea each day? Do you like mustard as a condiment, curried foods, or onions in your omelet? Do roses raise your spirits? Did your parents use herbal remedies to help you feel better when you were sick as a child, and if so which ones were your favorites? As a part of the Earth environment, plants are present in many aspects of everyday life. Plants and herbal remedies are often part of peoples' memories.

Before the advent of manufactured, synthetic drugs, herbs were a major source of the remedies used in healing and comforting. Herbs are still used today, and there is a growing interest among health practitioners in recapturing the knowledge of healing plants. Numerous books have been written on the use of healing plants, with pharmacists, physicians, and herbalists serving as the focal users of these texts. Yet recently, few, if any, specific texts have been written for the professional nurse on the use of medicinal plants. It certainly is not because nurses have no interest in healing plants! Quite to the contrary, nurses, midwives, housewives, and other caregivers from the simplest home, to the estate, to the hospital, to the battlefield, have been well versed in the use of plant therapies, an herbal folk wisdom that has continued to exist even with the development of exciting, technologically based remedies and therapies.

Nurses, like other community healers, have at times throughout history even been considered *experts* on herbal therapies. St. Hildegarde of Bingen (1098–1178 A.D.), for example, used healing plants in her caring work, and she also wrote extensively about it (Flanagan, 1996). Some nurses choose to continue this historic tradition today in their service to humanity. Why nurses might be interested in pursuing the integration of herbal remedies into their care of patients is the subject of this book. Because you have picked up this book, you may be wondering yourself just how you can do it. It may be difficult to imagine how herbs can be integrated into a practice that in the twenty-first century has become technologically advanced and, in so many ways, distanced from a health care culture that once routinely turned to healing plants.

Herbs are being rediscovered by nurses at a time when the present health care culture is experiencing tremendous change economically and philosophically. Whether a nurse practices in the countryside of an indigent third world country or in an inner city hospital, the challenges are great. The idea of change, of learning about herbs and thinking about integrating them into practice, for example, could cause anyone to become stressed at the very thought. Yet the idea of working with plants has the potential of being very different. Herbs are not just another protocol, technique, or modality. The science and art of working with healing plants offers an opportunity for caregivers to connect with and learn about nature and the Earth environment. And often with just the first interaction with plant remedies, caregivers find that the sensual, healing experience herbs provide patients can have potent healing effects on a caregiver as well.

With all the potential for healing, nurses may still be skeptical about approaching the possibility of integrating herbs into nursing care. Change of any kind is rarely welcomed, but that is often because it is perceived as a threat to the way things are in the present moment. People are especially threatened by change when they believe that they are going to have to *give up* some way of doing their work or living their life. People forget that change also can occur as a result of *adding on* to the repertoire of the way they do things. When considering herbs as part of caring practice, remember that herbs cannot replace or take anything away from the way nursing is practiced today. Herbs are an opportunity for adding on to, expanding, and including in nursing care what Florence Nightingale stressed in her vision of nursing, a recognition and integration of the environment in practice.

That is why this book is titled *Integrative Herb Guide for Nurses.* It offers an opportunity for considering how to *integrate* or *add* herbs to caring practice in some way. The concept of integration neither means replacement nor does it necessarily mean inclusion. *Integrative nursing practice* means that at the very least, a healing modality, in this case the use of herbs, is considered as an option alongside conventional, often technologically oriented, caring practices when the health care, decision-making process occurs as part of the healing relationship between nurse and patient. Nurses need to be able to find ways to integrate both conventional/biomedical and traditional time-honored practices, such as the use of herbs, into their practice because that is what patients often already do as part of cultural practice and belief.

This integrative herb guide provides traditional and cultural information about a plant, what it is called, how it is used, and what beliefs and rituals may surround that plant's use in a particular community. Nurses need to understand the folk or vernacular (the people's) uses of plant therapies because their work is with people. Nurses often hear from patients that they use plants the way their families and communities have for centuries. Herb use is tightly woven into the fabric of communities as a form of self-expression of the individuals in a community. It must be regarded as a valued part of the lifestyle of a person and their community.

Nurses also need the knowledge of plants that is gained through biomedical research and clinical practice. In addition to working closely with people, nurses are also part of the biomedical world. This world provides tremendous insight into the inner working of plants and their constituents. Nurses need biomedical in addition to traditional information because they provide care for patients who use biomedical therapies.

It is also common that patients use both plant and conventional biomedical therapies. Patients make choices about their health care that use the best of both worlds—the wisdom and knowledge from tradition as well as newer data and technology. Nurses too are able to have the best of both worlds. They too can find ways to integrate all that they learn about herbs from biomedicine and tradition. Herbal remedies have been researched and used from both biomedical and traditional worldviews. The nurse's challenge is to find a way to use the knowledge acquired over time about particular healing plants to put the patient in the "best condition possible for nature to work upon him" (Nightingale, 1969, p. 110). This book is meant to facilitate the process of integration by providing research, information, and stories about plants from multiple perspectives.

Humans have explored the use of plants in healing for centuries. The way people use plants develops over time and encompasses more than just the knowledge of the plant; there is a deeper *wisdom* that evolves from a healing plant's use over time. This wisdom is often conveyed or passed down as part of oral history from generation to generation. It is this plant wisdom that people often follow. *Merriam-Webster's Collegiate Dictionary* (1999) defines wisdom as "accumulated philosophic or scientific learning; ability to discern inner qualities and relationships; insight; good sense." Wisdom is a virtue, a strength that is expressed in many ways. Wisdom is a deep inner knowing and discernment that can lead to great works of art, exploration, and invention. Integration of the wisdom associated with centuries of plant use in healing entails understanding herbs not only from a biomedical perspective but also from the perspective of relationship, insight, and good sense.

Knowledge and then wisdom evolve over time with experience and education. Nurses too have their own personal and professional experiences with the use of herbs that are brought to their pursuit of greater understanding of healing plants. As you read, you may find yourself slipping into a memory, perhaps of your favorite coffee place or the time you received a rose from an admirer. I encourage you to take note of that plant memory and maybe even keep a journal of your plant stories and experiences. Your knowledge and wisdom of plants is rooted in *your* experience.

With all the many wonderful innovative healing modalities, nurses and their patients consider herbs simply because they are everywhere. As part of the evolving Earth environment, they are familiar. Herbs, a ready source of healing and comfort, grow outside your back door and you may not even know it. And your patients may not know it either. People need to know what they can use from their own environments to help themselves and their families. They need to learn the wise use of healing herbs. Wisdom, as defined by Merriam-Webster, involves relationship. The process of learning the wise use of healing plants begins with the development of a relationship with plants.

Nurses historically have had a relationship with healing plants. Before the development of pharmaceutical drugs, nurses and other caregivers used remedies made of plant materials. It is only more recently, over the course of approximately sixty years, that modern nursing has come to depend on pharmaceuticals and has all but eliminated the use of plants in healing and caring practice. Just as a nurse must enter the world of the patient to understand who that patient is and what their needs for healing and care really are, the nurse must enter the world of the plant to truly understand and gain insight and wisdom into the appropriate use of the plant in the healing of the individual patient. It is my hope that what is learned in this book will inspire your creativity and your interest in the world of plants and what they have to offer the sick, the uncomfortable, and the weary. May what you learn here serve as a bridge between you and your patients, many of whom have strong and lasting relationships with herbs. So fix that cup of tea or coffee, take a sip, and enter the world of healing plants.

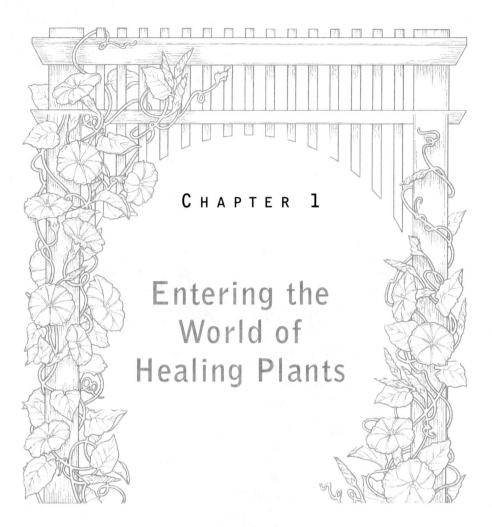

CHAPTER 1

Entering the World of Healing Plants

THE GARDENS, FORESTS, MOUNTAINS, DESERTS, and even the oceans and rivers are alive. Part of that which makes them alive is the plant life that grows in, on, and around them. If you think for a moment about your experience of nature, you might recall a fragrance, a color, a shape, a taste, or a texture associated with that experience. Interacting with nature is a very sensual experience. Each experience is vividly stored away in the memory of environment, surroundings, or home. Human beings have shared the planet with plants for a long time. We have memories of interactions with plants. Plants can leave a lasting impression.

1

I remember during my childhood in New England walking to school along a street lined with maple trees *(Acer saccharinum)*. I remember the maples growing bigger and bigger each year, enduring numerous seasons, and turning beautiful colors—red, yellow, and orange—in the fall. The colors were so vivid it was as if the tree were calling out to me to find out what makes it so. Every year people would stick metal buckets with a tap into the tree to collect the sap. I marveled how the liquid oozing from the tree looked like water but somehow ended up on the breakfast table as rich, brown sweet syrup. One day I decided to taste the sap right out of the tree. So I stuck my little finger right near the spout where it dripped out of the tree and waited for the next drop. As it formed on my finger I remember thinking, "I hope it's okay to eat this without it being cooked." I had a vision of the huge vats of bubbling sap turning into maple syrup at the sugar house in the next town. I knew about the processing but had never had the sap in its raw form. Then I remembered seeing my mom stick her finger in a bucket once and knew that it was okay. My finger went into my mouth without hesitation and what followed was an indescribable taste. The sap of the maple was nectar and a taste that I would always associate with home. I also remember laughing when my grandmother from the Midwest sent us a recipe that people in Ohio used to "make maple syrup" from corn syrup and chemical flavorings. If you have the real syrup why would you ever want a synthetic? Well, maybe because there isn't enough syrup to go around for everyone who wants it.

Plants create powerful experiences and memories. We also can learn important lessons about nature and our world from interacting with plants. Plants are also a rich source for the lessons of the powerful healing forces of nature. Not only is maple syrup from the maple tree one of the sweetest delicacies I know, but also, because of my relationship and experience with the tree, it is a source of healing. It is a point of connection with the joys of my own childhood that I carry into my work with children and families.

Many people have stories of healing that include a unique member of the plant kingdom. According to the World Health Organization (WHO), 80% of the world's population continues to use their traditional methods of healing, including the use of medicinal plants (Farnsworth, Akerele, Bingel, Soejarto, & Guo, 1985). This is important information for nurses. As both plant therapies and biomedicine evolve in the twenty-first century, nurses will be called upon more than ever to explore ways of helping people integrate their traditional healing methods and the gifts of biomedicine into their lives. With the current advances in communication and technology, people all over the world potentially have greater access to the blessings of Western biomedicine. But as statistics demonstrate, few people, even those who live in countries where biomedical technology is prevalent and accessible, want to rely solely on or utilize only biomedicine. There is a growing realization among nurses, physicians, pharmacists, herbalists, and traditional healers around the world that people are using an integrative approach to their health care and that as society has become technologically advanced, traditional healing modalities such as the use of herbs have never disappeared.

WHO created the Traditional Medicine Programme over 20 years ago to assist nations around the world in this process of integration. How people and practitioners integrate their traditional healing ways, such as the therapeutic use of plants, with conventional biomedical therapies is very diverse. When a nurse decides to learn more about integrating healing plants into health care, she or he might wonder where to go for help. Although historically nursing programs have taught the use of plants as part of nursing care, conventional nursing programs have followed the trend in biomedicine to move away from teaching the use of herbs. To begin recapturing the art and science of plant use in nursing, nurses must reconnect with plants by first entering the world of plants, experiencing them, and getting to know them. Like a child exploring the drippings of a maple tree for the first time, approaching reconnection with the plant world can stimulate the feelings of joyful curiosity and wonder that often provide a foundation for fruitful scientific exploration and creative (integrative) endeavor.

The Relationship of People and Plants

Growing up in the theatre, I learned the power of illusion, the greatest illusion of all being the ease with which actors, dancers, and musicians perform their work when in reality weeks, months, and even years often go into a finished work of art. When a successful performance is over, an audience leaves with feelings of joy and often of connection with a character or story that resonates with them. Such is the work of the artist. The ballerina makes her exquisite turns look effortless after years of classes, rehearsals, and bleeding feet and an aching body. Sports figures do the same for their audiences. The soccer player makes his continual running and scoring look effortless. Plants are very much like the artist or the athlete. They too make their work seem effortless. A rose, for example, is so beautiful in its simplicity. Yet the geometric configuration of its petals, the chemicals that make up its fragrance, and the variation in color from bush to bush are actually complex.

Just as the artist, dancer, and soccer player please their audiences with a work that, although seemingly effortless to create, has in reality taken months and sometimes years to perfect, so too is it with plants and plant medicines. Plant medicines contain the essence of the "work" of the plant. They contain chemical compounds, nutrients, and other more esoteric properties that affect people's healing. Medicinal plants can affect changes in the physical body and in the human mind, emotions, and spirit.

Plant or herbal medicines are often referred to as "crude" medicine. Plant remedies can be used in a form close to the natural state, as the word "crude" denotes. Yet, they are not necessarily simple in that natural state. Plants and plant medicine may appear simple and in certain health systems may be used in a simple fashion, such as in a tea, but they are actually quite complex. Throughout this book are numerous examples of how this natural complexity can be of great benefit to the person taking the remedy. As people begin to enter the world of healing plants through study and use, they find that there is much detail that can be learned about healing plants—when they grow, how they grow, what they look like, what chemical substances they contain, and how they can affect healing. Plants are as diverse as human beings.

As sometimes happens in human-to-human relationships, you may feel an immediate kinship with some plants. On the other hand, some plants may be as foreign to you as a stranger you meet in your hometown. More than 250,000 higher species of chemically distinct plants exist on the Earth. Of known plant species, about 35,000 to 70,000 species have been used at one time or another for medicinal purposes by a particular culture. It is estimated that only 15% of all angiosperm, or flower-bearing plants, have been biomedically examined. Only a small portion of the plant kingdom has had their internal compounds identified for a known physiologic action or had their healing properties examined by rigorous study with double-blind, placebo-controlled trials (Farnsworth & Soejarto, 1991, p. 26). A whole new world is waiting to be explored from this perspective.

INDIVIDUAL AND INTERNATIONAL RELATIONS:

Although a healing plant may not have been explored biomedically, it may have been explored by people through use or interaction. This plant-human relationship can be personal and individual. For example, a woman might use her favorite fragrance, lemon verbena, because her deceased mother whom she loved very much also wore the same fragrance. By wearing lemon verbena she is able to carry an aromatic remembrance of her mother with her while she heals her feelings of loss. The plant-human relationship also occurs as part of group, community, or ethnic history and tradition.

For example, the Scottish people's relationship with the thistle is so developed that the plant is the national emblem for the country and is pictured on the country's coins (Figure 1-1). In the summer of 1999, Queen Elizabeth of England performed a ceremony in St. Giles Cathedral during which she knighted a man into the Order of the Thistle, claimed to be the most ancient of the orders and introduced by James V in 1540. The thistle was again at the heart of this event. The worldwide

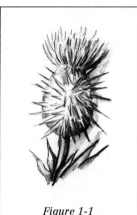

Figure 1-1
Scottish thistle.

recognition of Bulgarian rose oil as the best rose oil for perfuming is another example of a community-wide relationship with a plant. "The fragrance of rose has inspired poets and lovers throughout the ages. Although originally distilled in Asia Minor, today Bulgaria is the world's largest producer, making the most valued rose oil" (Keville & Green, 1995).

Many aspects of various cultures including economy, socialization, spiritual practice, and health care have developed around certain plants. For example, *Camellia sinensis*, the leaves of which are harvested for black and green tea, is an institution in Japan and China. The tea ceremony in Japan, originally choreographed years ago and recognized as a national treasure, is still performed to this day. It is believed that some of Japan's highest ideals are demonstrated in the four basic principles of the ceremony—harmony, respect, purity, and tranquility. Tea also was the focus of at least one major historical event, the American Revolutionary War, which was launched with the dumping of barrels of English tea into Boston Harbor in protest of taxation without representation by the King of England. What a powerful plant the *Camellia* is!

These human-plant relationships are just a few examples of the influence plants have had on the evolution of human beings. Plants provide remedies for so many human needs. They provide the lumber and materials to make shelter. Plant materials are used to make protective clothing and food and medicines, and they are even used in religious rituals. Plants can affect all aspects of human life, including those times when healing is sought. Plant life is so common that people may not be aware of their dependence upon plants for food and medicine until they get sick and have a great need for the plant. Perhaps it could even be said that some people take plants and plant products for granted. If one does not live off the land and gather plants for food or warmth or medicine, it can be quite easy to forget where coal, morphine, or rice comes from. In a technologically advanced, industrialized world, a plant user can get completely cut off from the provider.

People may never see any of the vegetables they eat growing in a garden or field. They may have no knowledge of the "work" of the cabbage or the carrot that appears in the supermarket as if by magic. They may have no idea what plants have been collected to create the medicine they take to extend their lives. With this severance from the source of plant products, the relationship between the plant and the person changes. People no longer experience what it is like to lose a crop and be grateful the next season when there is an abundant harvest. When the plant-human relationship is not valued and nurtured, the human plant users can become just that—users. This disconnection between human and plant kingdoms can lead to exploitation of plant resources.

"For thousands of years, since the beginnings of the Neolithic domestication, the human being has tended to assume a dominating and exploitative attitude toward nature . . . this anthropocentric attitude assumes that nature is an unlimited repository of resources, to be exploited for our benefit" (Metzner, 1999, p. 175).

Our relationship with plants is the foundation for how we use plants for healing purposes. Think what it would mean to find a cure for diseases such as cancer or acquired immunodeficiency syndrome (AIDS) that would save many lives. What if the cure were found to be a particular root or the bark of a plant, but the immediate need for the cure and the amount needed was calculated as being capable of destroying an entire population of this curing plant within one year after harvest? Should the plant be sacrificed to save *human* lives? The relationship of humans and plants today has an impact on future populations of people and plants. The decisions made today impact future decisions.

Some traditional healers say that our relationship with a plant is the reason we are or are not healed by the plant despite its active constituents and biochemical properties. In some cultures, a person is only healed by a plant medicine when the plant spirit appears to them in a dream and gives them guidance for healing. It is helpful to know about the botanical and chemical properties of a plant, or what can be called the inner workings of a plant, but just as a person is more than the inner workings of his or her red blood cells, for example, so is the plant more than its biochemical constituents. We learn more about a person by getting to know them. We can learn about plants and healing herbs in a similar way.

When we walk into a field and see the business of the ants around the anthill we wonder about the world of the ant. When we walk in the forest, we wonder about the lives of the magnificent birds that live in the towering trees high up above us. Entering the quiet world of a single plant also can have a similar effect. It can take us out of self-centeredness and remind us of our connection with the boundless beauty of nature. We come to realize that what we do to nature, we are doing to ourselves. "Our health is intimately connected to the health of our environment. The contemporary world view which sees a radical distinction between human as subject and world as object can obscure our recognition of how much we rely on nature for health and survival" (Burkhardt, 2000, p. 35).

Beginning to establish a relationship with nature is an opportunity for a sacred, healing, and learning experience. When exploring the world of healing plants you can find fascinating scientific data about the inner working of those plants, and you also can find traditional stories of beautiful plants and the sacred teachings and rituals about those plants that have existed for centuries.

Many indigenous peoples (people who are native to the area in which they live) have well-established beliefs that the natural world is the realm of the spirit and is sacred. Indigenous healers have tremendous respect for plants and their traditional plant remedies. Indigenous peoples have connections with plants and nature that many members of industrialized countries have lost. There is a growing interest in industrialized countries in healing the split or dissociation that has occurred between people and the natural world. "The entire culture of Western industrial society is dissociated from its ecological substratum. We have the knowledge of our impact on the environment . . . but we do not attend to it. Individuals feel unable to respond to the natural world appropriately because the political, economic, and educational institutions in which we are all involved have this dissociation built into them" (Metzner, 1999, p. 95).

As we enter the world of healing plants, we begin to establish a relationship with the plants, and we reestablish a connection or relationship with that natural part of ourselves. By observing, seeking to understand, and even emulating the mutual respect that exists in the relationship between indigenous or folk healers and healing plants, we can begin to heal the split or dissociation between people and nature. We can heal the split between nature and science. We can begin the process of reconnecting with the Earth, the world of healing plants, and the tremendous natural potential for greater health that plants have to offer the human world.

THE CHLOROPHYLL CONNECTION:

Although humans may have disconnected from the plant world, at the biologic level, the connection has not been severed. Biomedical science confirms what traditional healers know instinctively, that plants and humans are very similar and interdependent. The chlorophyll found in green plants and the oxygen-carrying molecule, hemoglobin, found in human red blood cells are nearly identical in atomic design (Figure 1-2). The most striking difference between the two is that the

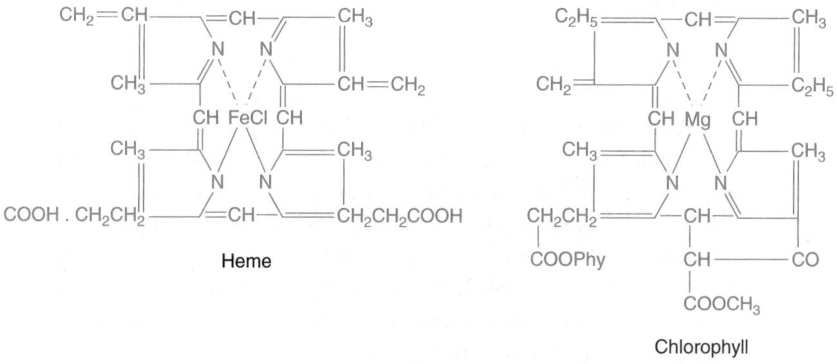

Figure 1-2
The chemical structures of heme and chlorophyll.

porphyrin ring of heme is built around iron (Fe), and the porphyrin ring of chlorophyll is built around magnesium (Mg). Although science has found that heme and chlorophyll are not interchangeable, their similarity in structure and respective functions still captures scientific interest.

Numerous studies have been done on the health benefits of chlorophyll in humans. Because many of these studies were performed before 1960 and there has been little research since, the research presented here is dated but relevant. It is not just a story that the cartoon character Popeye's claim to strength was related to his love of the green leafy vegetable, spinach *(Spinacia oleracea L.)*. Research for more than 60 years, although still unclear, has provided some data for how chlorophyll seems to help "build blood." Scientists such as Dr. Arthur Patek (1936) have found from studying patients with iron-deficiency anemia that when patients received iron and chlorophyll treatment together rather than separately, the number of red blood cells and blood hemoglobin level increased more quickly than with iron or chlorophyll alone. Some animal studies have led researchers to hypothesize that chlorophyll's ability to "build blood" is related to its tendency to stimulate bone marrow (Hughes and Latner, 1936). More recently, scientists have found that some porphyrins, the ringlike structures in heme and chlorophyll, stimulate the synthesis of the protein portion of the hemoglobin molecule, enhancing the body's ability to produce globin (Hammel-Dupont & Bessman, 1970).

The ability of chlorophyll to "build blood" has been researched for years, and health care practitioners, including nurses, have researched other healing benefits of chlorophyll. Because chlorophyll is insoluble in aqueous solutions, chlorophyllin, the copper-sodium salt, food-grade derivative of chlorophyll, is often used in human trials. Some animal studies with mice have shown that chlorophyll extracted directly from Indian spinach leaves or in commercially purified form demonstrates a strong chromosome-damaging activity (Sarkar, Sharma & Talukder, 1996). For this reason, the chlorophyll products on the market often contain chlorophyllin instead of chlorophyll.

Research has shown that chlorophyll or its derivatives have been successful in significantly decreasing symptoms of constipation and excessive flatus (Young & Beregi, 1980), decreasing urine and fecal odors related to incontinence (Dory, 1971; Young & Beregi, 1980), and decreasing the odors related to colostomy, ileostomy, and chronically infected skin ulcerations (Golden & Burke, 1956). It has a drying and deodorizing effect on wounds that has been shown to be superior to penicillin (Bowers, 1947). One chlorophyllin ointment, also containing urea and papain, has been shown to increase enzymatic debridement and decrease wound-healing time in patients with decubitus ulcers (Burke & Golden, 1958). Some small human trials have shown that chlorophyll can reduce symptoms of rhinitis, otitis externa, and otitis media in humans (Bowers, 1947). Intravenous chlorophyll *a* has been shown in human studies to rapidly reduce symptoms associated with pancreatitis (Yoshida, Yokono, & Oda, 1980).

So what has happened to the use of chlorophyll or chlorophyllin? Although these studies seem to indicate that biomedical health practitioners no longer suggest chlorophyll for their patients as they used to, complementary therapy practitioners do. Chlorophyllin continues to be sold in health food stores in liquid or capsule forms. People continue to attest to the health benefits of eating a diet that includes green leafy vegetables. Some practitioners recommend chlorophyll, often referred to as "liquid sunlight," in the form of wheat grass juice, blue-green algae, barley green, and alfalfa supplements.

Humans are completely dependent on plants for their very lives. Chlorophyll is involved in photosynthesis, a process that ultimately produces the oxygen fundamental to sustaining human life. The word "chlorophyll" is derived from the Greek *chloros,* meaning "green," and *phyll,* meaning "leaf." Chloroplasts are organelles found in the cytoplasm of the plant where light energy is actually transformed into food, the process of photosynthesis. When a green plant turns yellow it simply means that the leaf has lost chlorophyll.

During the first phase of photosynthesis, the chloroplast pigments in plants gather sunlight and, in a fraction of a second, split water molecules into hydrogen and oxygen atoms. The oxygen is released into the atmosphere through pores in the leaves and the stem of the plant for the respiratory process of animals, plants such as mushrooms, and humans. During the second phase of photosynthesis, carbon dioxide unites with the sugar ribulose diphosphate, and hydrogen from the first phase is added. Several types of sugars are produced. Numerous glucose molecules unite to form molecules of starch and cellulose. Starch is the principal food stored in plants and can be utilized later as an energy source, whereas cellulose is incorporated into the cell wall of the plant and usually is not decomposed.

The release of oxygen from plant photosynthesis and the absorption of carbon dioxide from the environment by plants is critical to human survival, yet how often do we think about this magical process that goes on in our presence all day long without a sound? Humans have never been able to duplicate the process of photosynthesis, which enables all cellular respiration. If it were not for plants and the exquisite process of photosynthesis, humans would have no food, clothing, shelter, or warmth and no air to breathe.

Although plants utilize the carbon dioxide released by humans in respiration, they are certainly not dependent upon humans for survival. The relationship between humans and plants could be characterized as one of benevolence on the part of plants. "The most striking thing about this relationship (between plants and humans) is that we need them but they don't need us. . . . Plant communities do just fine without people" (Cowan, 1995, p. 28). We do on occasion help plants. For example, we help seed them. As we walk through the woods, the seeds of a plant that may not be thriving cling to our clothes and then are dropped in a new location, thereby potentially giving the plant a better location for growth.

Biomedical science cannot fully explain why plants help as they do. Plants do not help human beings in the same ways. This is seen most clearly in the individual healing qualities possessed by various plants. Some plants soothe the skin; others irritate and stimulate the skin and circulation. Some plants cause the mind to hallucinate and some plants increase heart rate. Many cultural traditions recognize the powerful spirits or essences of plants as being the reason for the ways in which a plant helps humans. Plant science also has shown that chemical constituents found in certain plants are thought to be responsible for the actions of those plants. These scientific and spiritual qualities of the plant make up its *personality.*

Plant Personalities

Establishing a relationship and getting to know the personality of healing plants can be a foundation for the safe and effective use of plants as healing agents. Getting to know the personality of a plant is similar to getting to know a patient. The more health practitioners know about a particular patient, the better they are at providing care that addresses the individual needs of the patient. Addressing individual patient needs can potentially increase the ability to provide safe and effective care. For example, if a patient with a history of asthma visits an emergency room and is experiencing an upper respiratory infection, a practitioner might be more cautious with that patient because the practitioner doesn't know the patient at all. They have no relationship with the patient, and theoretically, asthmatics can be prone to attacks during or after respiratory infections. The practitioner might not hesitate to recommend a course of antibiotics. However, if the practitioner has known this same patient for five years and knows first hand that the patient has not had an asthma attack in years and has managed to work through one respiratory infection each year at about the same time, the practitioner might be less concerned and less inclined to prescribe antibiotics. It is easier to provide individualized care and have a better sense of the risk to the patient of a particular intervention when there is a relationship.

With plants, a more intimate understanding of a plant can lead to a more informed, knowledgeable use of that plant, especially when suggesting a plant remedy for others. This is why clinical herbalists are required to get to know the herbs they work with through tea tastings, herb walks, and visual inspection of dried whole plant. Some herbal practitioners harvest the plants and make their own remedies as well. The integration of evidence about a plant from a variety of sources, including biomedical data, folklore, cultural tradition, pattern of use, and personal experience, increases the likelihood of the appropriate use of a plant in healing.

One often overlooked source of evidence is found in the plant itself. A noted Swiss-German physician (1493–1541) named Paracelsus developed one system of understanding plant personality called the "doctrine of signatures." The doctrine of signatures states that each plant has been created with a signature, something in the way it looks or how it grows, that lets the user know the healing purpose of the plant. The doctrine of signatures encourages detailed observation of the plant's characteristics and the human-plant relationship. Each plant has a personality or unique qualities. An understanding of the personality of a plant's medicinal use can be gained through understanding the patterns of growth of the plant itself, determining the activities of the plant constituents, and clinically observing the interaction of the plant and a patient as manifested in stimulation of the different physical organs and energy systems of the body. The doctrine of signatures is discussed further in chapter 2.

BOTANY:

Botany, or the properties and life phenomena exhibited by a plant (Merriam-Webster, 1999), is an entire field of study devoted to understanding plant personalities. The purpose of this section is to provide a brief overview of botany as part of the introduction to the world of healing plants. One of the first things nurses learn in the preparation to care for human beings is human anatomy and physiology, so it will not surprise nurses that, when beginning to learn about the use of plants in healing, botany is studied. A brief explanation of botanical science highlighting the following three areas of plant personality is presented: (1) growth patterns and plant designs, (2) plant constituents and active medicinal principles, and (3) the sensory experience of human-plant interactions.

Growth Patterns and Plant Designs

Latin names are important in botanical science for several reasons. First, botanical names often describe some aspect of the growth pattern of the plant. For example, the Latin name for red clover, *Trifolium pratense,* describes the plant as having *tri-,* or three, *folium,* or leaves, three leaves. Red clover has three leaves and its leaves each have three lobes. Second, Latin names provide a clarifying, common language for identification of plants and sharing that information from person to person. Both purposes lead to the overall human goal of being able to properly identify a plant as useful for human consumption either as food or medicine. A plant has only one Latin name, but it may have numerous common names that vary from culture to culture. The Latin name allows one to communicate about medicinal plants internationally because the plant name is standardized all around the world.

The Latin binomial nomenclature for plants is credited as the work of Carl Linnaeus, a Swedish botanist (1701–1778) who wanted to create a universal way of communicating about plants. In learning to recognize and identify plants, it is best to first practice identifying plants and their growth patterns by family, then genus, and then species. One example of a plant family is the *Rosaceae* or rose family. Strawberries, raspberries, and roses belong to this family. The family name is always capitalized. The genus is the first name of the plant and is always capitalized. The second name assigned a plant is the species, and it is written in lower case unless the second name is the name of a person, then it may be capitalized as well. Both genus and species names are italicized.

After genus and species, the variety of plant may be listed. For example, one species of the common herb thyme has the Latin name *Thymus serpyllum* and the white flower variety is called *Thymus serpyllum var. albus* (white). When referring to a group of plants with the same genus name, the genus name can be abbreviated to the first letter followed by a period after spelling out the genus name the first time. For example, *Thymus serpyllum* would appear as *T. serpyllum.* If a particular document discusses a group of plants with the same genus and different species then the name will appear as the genus followed by the abbreviation *"spp.,"* which means species plural. *"Spp."* also can be used when writing that many plants within a specific genus are applicable.

Plant Parts

• *Seeds.* Plants can be identified in various stages of development, although some are easier to identify at certain times rather than others. While the current classification system relates to flowers, plants are likely to be classified by their deoxyribonucleic acid (DNA) in the future. Plants can be identified by their seed (Figure 1-3). For example, compare an apple seed and a dill seed that you might have in your kitchen. Notice the differences in color, size, outer coating, and markings. Seeds are dormant and capable of germination. Seeds can survive environmental conditions that their parent plants could not. They are tiny packages of tremendous potential. When a seed germinates and begins the growth process, cotyledons, or seed leaves, are formed. The seeds of flowering plants contain either one or two cotyledons, identifying it as a dicot (two cotyledons) or a monocot (one cotyledon). Angiosperms, or flowering plants, which make up the largest group in the plant kingdom called a "division," are either monocots or dicots (Figure 1-4). The word "angiosperm" is from the Greek *angeion* (vessel) and *sperma* (seed), indicating that these plants have seeds that are formed inside vessels, or fruits, as they are more commonly known. Angiosperm are sophisticated life forms that supply most of the vegetables in the human diet and our supply of hardwood. Monocots include grasses, cereal grains, sugar cane, lilies, aloe, iris, and orchids. Dicots, the larger of the

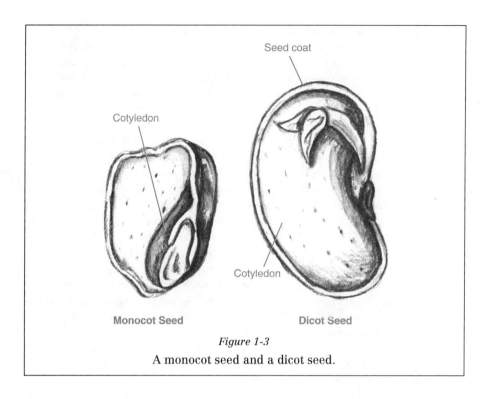

Figure 1-3

A monocot seed and a dicot seed.

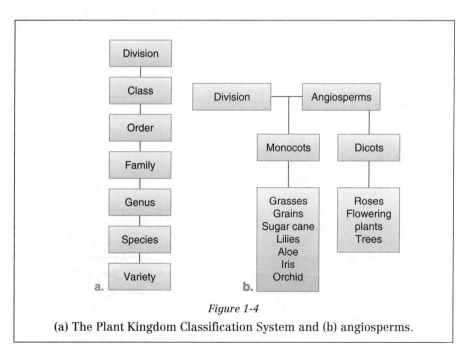

Figure 1-4

(a) The Plant Kingdom Classification System and (b) angiosperms.

two groups, include roses, other flowering plants, and trees of all sorts. The other major division of plants known as "Gymnosperms" (or naked seed division) produce seeds in cones, such as a pinecone. *Thuja occidentalis* and *Ginkgo biloba* are members of the Gymnosperm division.

The seed feeds itself by absorbing water; doubling in size; and breaking down starches, proteins, and fats present in the cotyledons and endosperm, a food storage structure of the seed, which it then sends to the embryo where new structures of a seedling can be formed. The seed sends out roots as it uses oxygen in the soil for the germination process. As the small leaves burst through the soil and are exposed to light, germination ends. The seedling is capable of photosynthesis and therefore is capable of feeding and sustaining itself, a process known as "autotrophic nutrition." Humans are heterotrophic organisms; that is, we rely on foods formed from other sources.

• *Roots.* Many gardeners often ignore the root systems of plants for the appeal of the plant's colorful blossoms and intricate leaves. But in herbalism, the roots of plants are very important because they often contain medicinal constituents (Figure 1-5). Some roots are edible, such as the root of *Angelica sinensis,* but many roots are not traditionally eaten whole or in a powder form in a capsule. They usually are decocted, extracted with water and heat, either because it is safer than eating the root or because the healing constituents are more available through decoction.

Roots serve three purposes for the survival of the plant.

1. Roots keep the plant anchored to the soil.
2. Roots store excess food for potential future needs of the plant.
3. Roots enable the plant to absorb water and minerals from the soil environment.

A plant usually has either a fibrous or a taproot system. Some plants have both. The fibrous system, such as is found in grasses, is composed of numerous thin-branched roots. A taproot has one or two longer, sparsely branched roots that go deeper into the soil. Carrots *(Daucus carota)* and horseradish root *(Armoracia rusticana)* are examples of taproots. These types of root systems can be huge. At the other extreme, cacti have very shallow fibrous root systems so that they can catch every drop of moisture possible that passes through their hard desert soil.

Roots are thought to be very strong medicine in some cultures. We witness their strength not only in their potent medicinal actions but also in the way they grow, often pushing their way through concrete and buildings. Each branch of root is an exact replica of the root that created it. The constituents of the food found in the roots of plants are discussed further in the section about plant constituents. Roots are often harvested in the autumn when the energy and nutrients of the plant have returned fully to the root rather than being in the stems, leaves, and flowers. Some plants' roots are best harvested

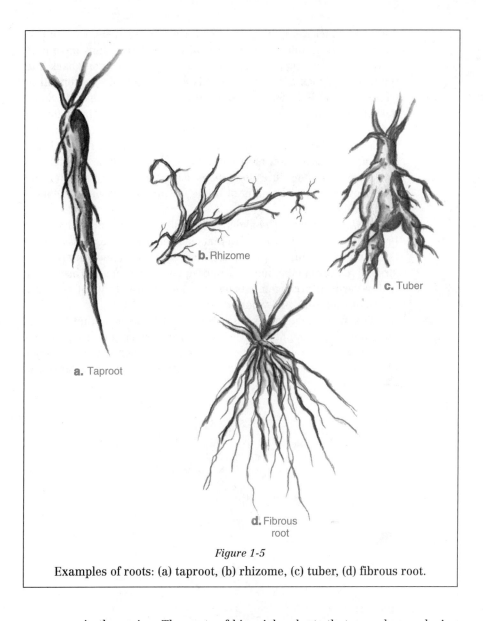

Figure 1-5

Examples of roots: (a) taproot, (b) rhizome, (c) tuber, (d) fibrous root.

in the spring. The roots of biennials, plants that grow leaves during the first years and then flower and bear fruit and die during the second year, are harvested in the autumn of the first year or spring of the second year. Allowing the plant to stay in the ground over the winter helps turn the starches in the root to sugars, making the harvest in the spring more flavorful.

During the second year, after the plant has achieved the full maturity of a summer season, the medicinal principles of the plant travel to the aerial or above-ground parts, leaving the root hollow and of little if any medicinal value. The roots of perennials, plants that come back year after year, enduring the seasons, can be collected in the autumn after the aerial parts of the plant have died back, demonstrating that the energy of the plant has gone back into the root. Burdock *(Arctium lappa)* is an example of a perennial in which the root is collected and dried the first year in the fall. Some herbalists prefer to collect the roots of certain plants the following spring after the herb has had a full winter of garnering its strength in the root. Many perennial plants are best harvested for medicine after at least two years of growth. Tubers and rhizomes, which are underground stems, are sometimes collected in or just after the flowering season of the plant or in the fall after the aerial parts have died back.

• ***Shoot System.*** The shoot system of a plant includes the stem, branches, and leaves. To ensure that each leaf receives necessary sunlight and air circulation, the plant stem sections called "internodes" stretch and spread the buds and subsequent leaves apart. Three basic leaf patterns or arrangements on the stem occur with plant growth—alternate, opposite, and whorled (Figures 1-6 and 1-7).

The stem functions as a support for the leaves so that they get adequate light for photosynthesis, with the exception of *Equisetum spp.* in which the stem is photosynthetic. In general, the difference between a tree and a shrub is that the tree has one main trunk to

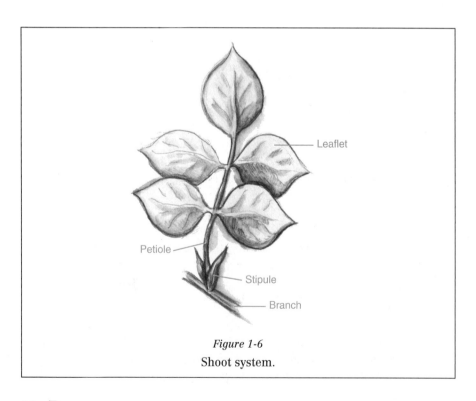

Figure 1-6
Shoot system.

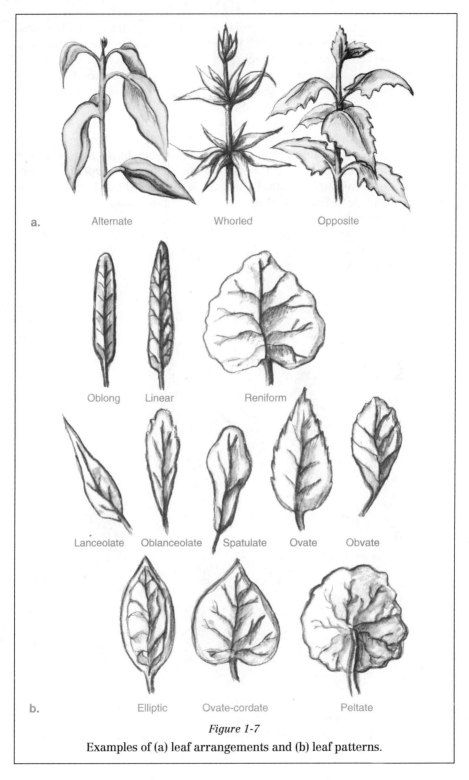

a.   Alternate   Whorled   Opposite

Oblong   Linear   Reniform

Lanceolate   Oblanceolate   Spatulate   Ovate   Obvate

b.   Elliptic   Ovate-cordate   Peltate

Figure 1-7

Examples of (a) leaf arrangements and (b) leaf patterns.

support its leaves, and shrubs are smaller with many woody stems. The bark of a tree or shrub is the place on the stem where it thickens and turns brown and rough.

The leaves of plants are truly miraculous. They are designed to capture light to be used in photosynthesis. The three parts of the leaf are (1) the leaflets; (2) the petiole, or small stem that attaches the leaflet to the branch; and (3) the stipule, the anchor for the petiole on the branch. Not all plants have stipules. The leaflets also have identifying patterns. Some leaflets are simple and some are compound (Figure 1-8). They can be pinnately compound, where the leaves are organized alongside a central axis such as the plants in the pea family *(Fabaceae)*. They can be palmately compound, where the multiple leaflets extend out from one central point like the fingers on the palm of a hand such as the maple *(Aceraceae)*. It is unknown how a plant design, including the leaf pattern, is actually created.

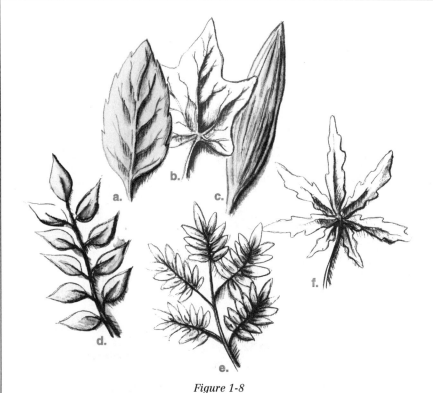

Figure 1-8
Some identifying patterns of leaflets: (a) pinnate venation, (b) palmate venation, (c) parallel venation, (d) pinnately compound, (e) bipinnately compound, and (f) palmately compound.

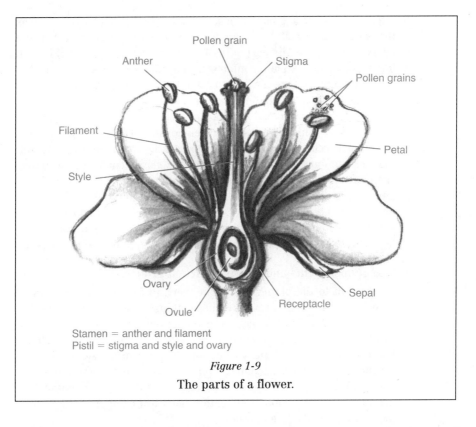

Pollen grain

Anther

Stigma

Pollen grains

Filament

Petal

Style

Ovary

Sepal

Receptacle

Ovule

Stamen = anther and filament
Pistil = stigma and style and ovary

Figure 1-9
The parts of a flower.

• ***Flowers.*** The intricacies of nature are found in the design of the flowers plants produce. Flower structures are created at the tip of the flower stalk or pedicel. The stem tip known as the "receptacle" bears the flower parts (Figure 1-9). Flowers are arranged within the bud in rings or whorls. The outer whorl is called the "calyx" and has several sepals. The words "calyx" and "sepal" are derived from the Greek, meaning "covering." This covering is usually shed or curls backward as the flower emerges from the bud. Together, the calyx and the corolla, layers of petals, are considered the perianth of a flower. The petals of a flower can be many different colors and can add to the data used to identify a plant. The flower color and shape often relate to the type of insect or animal with which the flower has a symbiotic relationship. Pollination among many plants occurs as a result of an insect recognizing a plant by its color, leaf or petal pattern or markings, and scent.

The male reproductive structures called "stamens" that emerge from the center of the petals are composed of long thin stalks called "filaments" and little bulbs on the end called "anthers." Pollen, which contains the sperm cells, develops in the anther. The female part of the plant is called the "pistil." At the tip of the pistil is a sticky surface called a "stigma" where the pollen attaches. The style is the long, stemlike attachment to the stigma, and it secures the pistil at the base, known as the "ovary." The pollen germinates and enters the style and then the ovary. The ovary is the part of the flower that has the potential to turn into fruit. Not every plant contains all reproductive parts.

The plant can use the scent of the flower to attract insects or animals that assist in pollination or to deter predators. Those animals and insects that are welcomed by a plant are rewarded with food (nectar), setting up an important symbiotic relationship. Plant growth patterns are often a result of some protective process between the plant and animals or the environment from which they both benefit. For example, cacti have spines to keep away predators and to act as condensers for any moisture that might be present in the atmosphere. Very few plants are camouflaged by their color, but many emit noxious odors or other chemical defenses that act against predators. These substances are known as "secondary products" or "metabolites" produced by the plant.

Plant Constituents and Active Medicinal Principles

In addition to the plant's metabolic work to extract energy from its food by the process of photosynthesis, it also makes starch, fats, cellulose, and proteins. Among the proteins the plant produces are enzymes that catalyze chemical activities that enable healthy cellular function within the plant. Various biochemical processes lead to the synthesis of several secondary plant metabolites that function as chemical defenses in the plant. These secondary plant metabolites are often the biochemical indicators used to distinguish one species or family of plant from another.

Understanding a plant's constituents also helps us understand its potential use in herbalism. It is important to note, however, that most expert clinical herbalists do not necessarily find that dissecting plants into their numerous constituents leads to a better understanding of a particular plant's healing action in an individual patient. Each and every healing plant has numerous plant constituents. Understanding plant constituents may guide practice to some degree, but whether or not a particular herb is appropriate for a patient is ultimately determined by many factors related to the total herb personality and the individual patient's needs, not just plant constituents. Some of the basic constituents of plants, such as acids, alkaloids, and volatile oils, are briefly described here.

Acids. One of the most common plant acids is called "tannic acid" or "tannins." Tannins bind with proteins causing water to leave the cell and constriction of tissues. This is referred to in herbalism as having an "astringent" effect. It is not surprising that plants with tannins often have a recognizable puckering and drying effect on the tissues such as the mucous membranes of the mouth. Some examples of tannin-rich plants are tea *(Camellia sinensis)* and raspberry leaf *(Rubus idaeus)*. Tannins are generally antiseptic, antioxidant, antiviral, coagulant, and anti-inflammatory. The tightening of tissues is referred to as a tonifying effect. *Oxalic acid* is also astringent and is sour tasting and can be found in rhubarb *(Rheum rhaponticum),* for example. Oxalic acid can be very irritating to the digestive tract and can combine with calcium in the bloodstream, forming insoluble calcium oxalate, which can deplete the body's calcium levels and also can lodge in the kidneys (McGuffin, Hobbs, Upton, & Goldberg, 1997). *Citric acids* are found in citrus and other fruits. *Formic acid* is the acid that enables stinging nettle *(Urtica doica)* to sting upon contact with a passerby. This acid loses its bite when the plant containing it is cooked.

Alkaloids. Alkaloids contain nitrogen and are bitter tasting, water-soluble, and usually basic in nature. The majority of plant alkaloids are known to have a narcotic, analgesic, or sedative effect on the central nervous system and have played an important role in the development of human medicine. *Valerian,* an herbal sedative, contains *terpenoid alkaloids.* Some alkaloids, like caffeine, are stimulants and can be addicting. One alkaloid often mentioned in the scientific and medical literature is the *pyrrolizidine alkaloid.* This alkaloid, found in plants like comfrey, is toxic to humans and may cause liver damage. Other common alkaloids are *quinolines* as are found in quinine and the *isoquinolines* from opium poppy *(Papaver somniferum)* that are found in morphine and codeine. Some of the most common alkaloids, *methylxanthines,* are caffeine, theophylline, and theobromine. The names of alkaloids can be recognized by their ending, "-ine."

Carbohydrates. Carbohydrates are aldehyde or ketone alcohols containing hydrogen, carbon, and oxygen in which the oxygen and hydrogen are usually in the same ratio as water (Tyler, Brady & Robbers, 1988). Carbohydrates are classified into two groups: sugars and polysaccharides. Sugars, such as fructose, are identified by their sweet taste. Plant polysaccharides include *mucilage,* the slimy moist substance found in plants such as aloe and psyllium; *inulin,* often found in the root of plants such as dandelion; *pectin,* a complex polysaccharide found in plants such as apple and citrus fruits; *gum,* thicker and stickier than mucilage and found in Agar for example; and *cellulose*, the polysaccharide from which wood is made.

Glycosides. Glycosides are involved in the regulatory, protective, and sanitary functions of the plant. Glycosides are made up of a sugar and an aglycone molecule. Most glycosides, with the exception of saponins, are inactive unless separated from the sugar. Mustard and other plants known for their skin-irritating property on humans are examples of *sulfur glycosides.* Peach and apricot pits contain *cyanhydric glycosides,* which occur widely in nature and contain nitrogen, hydrogen, and carbon. They react with cytochrome oxidase, an enzyme that links oxygen to individual cells and causes the cells to asphyxiate. Although the body has a way of dealing with very small amounts of cyanide by adding a sulfur molecule, excessive amounts of this glycoside are poisonous to the human body. Carbon-based *phenol glycosides,* the last group of glycosides, include *flavonoids*, the plant constituents found in many fruits and vegetables, well known for their antiviral, anti-inflammatory, and antioxidant qualities; *saponins,* recognizable by their ability to form foam in water, are found in plants such as potatoes *(Solanum tuberosum),* tomatoes *(Lycopersicon esculentum),* and soapwort *(Saponaria officinalis).* Although they are able to destroy the cell membrane of erythrocytes, they are not readily absorbed by the human digestive system, so they usually pass through the body. They also can be easily broken down when cooked. *Saponins* usually have anti-inflammatory or immunostimulating effects.

The *anthroquinone glycosides* found in plants such as senna, aloe, and rhubarb are digested by bile, absorbed by the small intestine, and excreted through the colon, thereby having a laxative effect; however, some plants, such as St. John's wort *(Hypericum perforatum),* that contain this glycoside are not laxatives because they are not fat soluble. *Cardiac glycosides* stimulate the contractions of the heart muscle and are found in plants such as *Digitalis.* All of these are considered dangerous and not to be used by the uneducated. *Coumarins* are phenol glycosides that are sweet smelling, like freshly cut hay, and may be found in plants in the parsley (Apiaceae) family. There are numerous types of coumarins in the plant world that fall under the general classifications of coumarins: hydroxycoumarins, methoxycoumarins, furanocoumarins, pyranocoumarins, and dicoumarols. Coumarin is not an anticoagulant per se (Bruneton, 1999, p. 270). Because dicoumarols destroy vitamin K, they are the type of coumarins that act as anticoagulants. Coumarin-type anticoagulant drugs were created based on a model of the coumarin that was found in fungal contamination of sweet clover (Bruneton, 1999, p. 271).

Essential or Volatile Oils. Volatile oils, also referred to as essential oils, are unstable and separate easily from the plant and evaporate into the air. They are the cause of the fragrance associated with the plant. Volatile oils are combinations of aromatic molecules of which there are thousands in existence in the plant world. For example, eucalyptol is an *oxide* found in the Eucalyptus tree. Oxides are a chemical classification within the larger group of plant constituents known as "essential oils." Other types of volatile oils include, but are not limited to, alcohols, aldehydes, esters, ethers, ketones, phenols, and terpenes.

Resins. *Resins,* like pine pitch and myrrh, are formed from oxidized volatile oils. They are sticky, not soluble in water, and are secreted from the plant when it is injured. Resins are often used medicinally as astringents and antiseptics.

Latex. *Latex* is the milklike or yellowish sap that oozes from plants such as dandelions. Latex is acrid and sometimes bitter as well. Latex, from the Latin word for fluid, contains small particles of rubber and historically has been the source of natural rubber. The presence of latex in a plant often is a signal that the plant is medicinal (Hutchinson, 1995). The presence of latex also can mean that the plant can be very irritating to the skin.

Acrid Substances. Plants with *acrid* substances include horseradish and mustard. The acrid substances in these and other plants are related to the glycosides in the plant. Acrid substances taste hot or pungent.

The Sensory Experience of Human-Plant Interactions

To understand the personality of the plant, we learn the growth pattern of the plant and about the plant's inner workings, or constituents. We also need to understand the plant's preferences and how it interacts with its environment, including humans. We quickly learn how to recognize stinging nettle *(Urtica doica)* when we are stung by it as we accidentally brush up against it when hiking in the mountains. Although painful, the sting of nettle has healing benefits. Nettle stings can help relieve the pain in arthritic joints. Whether or not a person wishes to ever encounter nettle again depends on the experience or relationship with the plant. If a person's only experience is the hurtful sting and they or loved ones have no need for the healing benefit, they may never go back to the plant. They may even avoid nettle. However, if the person finds the nettle helpful, they may learn what it looks like and where it grows so that it can be found whenever there is a need.

When people choose to learn about plant personalities, often because of a perceived need for the benefits of the plant, they eagerly observe the plant and its behavior, such as where the plant grows. People can use all of the human senses to learn about healing plants. We can taste the plant as long as it is not poisonous. We can see the pattern of growth and smell the fragrance it may emit. We can touch the plant's leaves and feel its edges and boundaries, how it defines itself in space. We also interact with the energy field of the plant, although we may not be aware of it. "Human beings and the environment are energy fields; they do not have energy fields . . . human and environmental fields are integral with one another" (Rogers, 1992, p. 30). Plants as part of the environment are also energy fields. This energy field can be sensed by our own bodies in much the same way we feel the presence or energy field of another human being. The energy field or life force of a plant can even be measured.

A book by Peter Tompkins and Christopher Bird (1973), called *The Secret Life of Plants,* outlines numerous studies of plants utilizing scientific instruments such as those that measure electrical voltage, demonstrating that plants exhibit a life force or energy field. Studies also demonstrate that plants specifically relate to their environment in ways such as adapting to human wishes, responding to music, and communicating with humans. They move very slowly, so they must be observed very closely in addition to being measured by instruments.

Scientists have found that many plants have special abilities. For example, "Plants are even sentient to orientation and to the future . . . a sunflower plant's, *(Silphium laciniatum),* leaves accurately indicate the points of a compass. Botanists at London's Kew Garden found that

Indian licorice, *(Arbrus precatorius),* is able to predict cyclones, hurricanes, tornadoes, earthquakes, and volcanic eruptions" (Tompkins & Bird, 1973, p. xiii).

Plant medicine healers teach that with plants, just as with humans, the *whole* is greater than the sum of the parts. Just as people are not only identified by their livers or some other organ or cell, and people with cancer have a greater identity and personality that is well beyond that of their cancer cells, whole plants found in their natural state are more than their plant constituents or their taste or their leaf patterns. One traditional plant healer recommends that after becoming familiar with a plant, a person, "begin to connect with it. Be still. Take your time. . . . Experience the world around you as the plant does . . . (and after a period of quiet with the plant) . . . approach the spirit of the plant and introduce yourself. Explain that you have come to learn, and ask if you may learn from this plant or use it in some way. If the reply is positive, then ask the spirit to teach you" (Cowan, 1995, p. 43).

This way of getting to learn about healing plants may seem very different or foreign to some. To others, as occurs with people of many cultures who hold plant life sacred, this suggested way of connecting with a plant may not seem unusual. In many cultures, the learning experience of the plant's personality includes the spirit of the plant. "Holy people the world over make distinctions about the body of the plant and its spirit . . . they say that it is the sacred *properties* of the plants that heal. The body of the plant helps but it is not the main factor in healing" (Buhner, 1996, p. 33). It is understood that the breath and rituals of the healer must activate the "medicine" in the plant. Nurses need to be aware that the traditional uses of healing herbs include spiritual philosophies and teachings such as these.

This guide provides an opportunity for nurses to begin considering all aspects of the science and art of healing herbs. The wisdom that emanates from the natural world is not only absorbed through the mind but is felt, tasted, seen, heard, touched, and smelt as one enters a relationship or connection with a plant. As you enter the world of plants remember to use all of your senses as you get to know the herbal remedies that come from these exquisite life forms called "plants."

CHAPTER 2

A History of Healing

Making Medicine

M ANY PEOPLE DIRECTLY EXPERIENCE THE WORLD OF PLANTS
every day, even though they may not be fully aware of it. For example, people who live in wood homes may never have had to grow or
cut a tree, but they can experience the benefit of a sturdy home made
from wood cut from the trunk of a tree. Many people wear clothes that
have been made from natural plant fibers such as cotton and linen.
Members of industrial societies rarely make their own clothes from purchased fabrics, let alone weave their own cloth. The industrial revolution has created an easier life for many people, but it also has created a
distance between people as consumers of plant products and the creative process related to the plant products they regularly use. Although
many people may not make their own cloth or cut the timber for their
homes, they do still make their own "medicine," often on a daily basis.
For example, many people enjoy making a stimulating cup of coffee
(Coffea arabica) or tea *(Camellia sinensis)* in the morning. They may or
may not know that the constituent known as caffeine found in coffee and
tea is a stimulant, but they do know that when they drink their beverage

of choice they often feel more mentally and physically alert. When they need an energy boost they know they have the option of making a cup of tea or coffee to help. They are making their own medicine— from a plant.

In addition to plant-derived caffeine, it has been estimated that between 35% and 50% of modern pharmaceutical drugs are derived from natural sources such as plants, and the majority of these products were originally used as traditional medicine or poison (Holmstedt & Bruhn, 1983). "A recent study led by Francesca Grifo, director for the Center for Biodiversity and Conservation at the American Museum of Natural History, puts the figure closer to 60%" (Taylor, 1996, p. 926). Although the pharmaceutical industries, like the lumber and textile industries, have taken over what used to be each person's responsibility and make most of the prescription and over-the-counter drugs on the market, people continue to make their own medicines from plants. Self-care with plant medicines is not a new or old practice; it is an ongoing process. Plant medicines have evolved over time and are, with the help of technology, not just available in whole plant and extract forms or salves. Many plant medicines are now sold in capsules, tablets, and sprays and may actually look like pharmaceutical drugs. One American writer states, "From early Colonial days until about 1900, health care was usually provided in the home by women who relied on botanical remedies, which at first they prepared, and later purchased as patent medicines" (Brown & Marcy, 1991, p. 339). It is cumbersome to make our own cloth, our own medicines, and our own homes. Many welcome the relief of not having to attend to what could be daily chores. Interestingly, with all the modern conveniences provided by the pharmaceutical industry, people still choose to make their own "medicine." They make that cup of coffee or tea in the morning and more!

People use plant remedies in their self-care practices, in part, because plant medicines are often more accessible and affordable. This does not mean that if drugs and surgery were more accessible and affordable that people would stop using the herbs. People use their own time-tested, native (or vernacular) healing methods that include the use of plant therapies because the plant medicines are perceived as beneficial. People often use both conventional or biomedical and vernacular healing practices at the same time. Ethnographic research has demonstrated that vernacular health belief systems, of which plant medicine is a part, "have among their central values concerns for appropriate and timely intervention and for seeking the proper specialist. . . . Combined use of conventional medicine and one or more vernacular strategies is extremely common. . . . The persistence of vernacular health belief systems is not restricted to the ignorant, the desperate, the remote, the deprived, or the unacculturated" (O'Connor, 1995, pp. 21, 26, 32). People most often make logical and careful decisions about their use of plant medicines, including how to integrate the use of biomedical and herbal modalities.

NURSES AND PLANT MEDICINES:

How do nurses fit into this picture of the evolution of plant medicines? What do nurses know about the plant medicines people use in vernacular healing practices? What do they know about the plants that often provide the matrix and/or material for the development of many of the drugs they administer? Some nurses, who have been in practice for a number of years, may remember a time when there was no unit-dosing system in the hospitals. Medications often had to be prepared and the dose measured out for the individual patient. This process could take hours during the course of a day. For safety reasons, and because nurses have so many tasks they do in the course of a day, hospital pharmacy departments began the unit-dosing system, leaving nurses with only the five rights to attend to: right patient, right time, right dose, right route, and right medication. Identifying the right medicine is done by carefully examining the label on the medication packaging.

Nurses and their patients rarely have knowledge of what goes into the making of the medicines they encounter. Nurses are taught the basics of pharmaceutical science with the goal that they safely administer medications under the direction of practitioners with prescriptive privileges. Nurses are not expected to know everything about the production, source, and chemical composition of the drugs they administer or discuss with patients. Historically, physicians often prepared, prescribed, and administered their own medications. Now there is a more collaborative system where pharmacists, physicians, and nurses all have varying responsibilities for the use of pharmaceutical drugs. Each practitioner and patient trusts the health care system and the education of the practitioners to support the development of medicines that are of excellent quality.

In herbal medicine, there is a similar desire for remedies that are of excellent quality. Traditional healers and conventional herbal practitioners often grow or wildcraft (harvest from the wild) the medicinal plants themselves. If they do not, the practitioner is mindful of the quality of their sources for plant materials. Practitioners make the medicine themselves or teach patients how to make the medicine for themselves. There is no unit dose because the dosages are, for the most part, individualized. The education of the practitioner includes being able to work with the plants directly in this way. People who work with medicinal plants are expected to understand the plant in much the same way, and perhaps even in more ways, than nurses are expected to understand pharmaceutical drugs. Nurses who work with plant medicines find that they often have more of a relationship with the medicine they administer or discuss with a patient than they do with pharmaceuticals, simply because they may grow the plant, harvest it, and prepare the medicine. The nurse can also have a direct connection with the source of medicine when working with plants.

Before the advent of modern pharmaceuticals, nurses administered the medicines of the time. For example, in the early 1900s, American nurses administered an "emulsion" of asafetida *(Ferula assafoetida),* a pungent gum resin, by mouth to infants and adults with colic or gas pains (Tracy, 1938, p. 367). They applied flaxseed *(Linum usitatissimum)* poultices to the chests of patients with pneumonia (Harmer, 1924, p. 206). Now, some nurses use and/or recommend plant remedies in ways described throughout this book. As nurses reflect on their present and future roles related to the use of plant medicines in providing health care, it is important for nurses to understand a little about the history of plants and their use as medicine.

WHEN FOOD BECOMES MEDICINE:

By definition, a medicine is "a substance or preparation used in treating disease; something that affects well-being" (Merriam-Webster, 1999). By definition, just about any substance on the planet could be a medicine, if it is used to treat disease or it affects someone's well-being in some way. Water, for example, is a substance that is used in treating disease. Water is used to prepare medicines and wash the bodies of the sick. Water also affects the well-being of a person. Without water, people cannot survive. Does this mean that water is medicine? It can indeed be used medicinally in the care and treatment of the ill. And some who have tasted the special mineral waters found in the western United States, for example, or at Lourdes in France, say that water itself can indeed be medicine. When does water become medicine and not just a fluid we need to drink every day to survive?

A substance becomes a medicine when people decide to call it medicine. What is called medicine is different for various cultures. Water becomes medicine at Lourdes because many people have seen the water heal the lame and the dying. The water is proclaimed to be healing. Water becoming medicine is a good example of how an everyday substance can become medicine. It can be named medicine because the substance itself is shown to heal, it is intentionally *used* for medicinal purposes and found to be healing, and it becomes a medicine because people assign healing properties to it. All substances have the potential to be medicine. All plants have the potential to be medicine. The age-old definition of a weed is "a plant for which no use has been discovered yet." Humans often do not value a plant until it has meaning for them. Assigning the title of "medicine" to a plant may be one of the highest human honors that can be bestowed on a plant. There are five types of plant use by humans:

1. Weeds—no use
2. Ornaments—aesthetic use
3. Foods—nourishing use
4. Medicine—care and cure use
5. Abused substance—excessive use

When a plant is given the label of "medicine," it then becomes an object of power. Plants that can heal are valued in societies because they have the potential to heal and extend life. The plant is no longer an ornament, a pretty object growing outside the backdoor. It is no longer a food used to nourish the body alone; it can be a commodity and a resource used to cure and heal. The plant becomes a source of revenue because it is valued for its healing properties. Countries that use plants as medicine often have regulatory bodies whose job it is to determine standards for the plant medicines. This subject is explored in greater detail in chapter 4. Determining standards includes being able to identify how a plant is used. It may be quite simple for a society to determine when a plant is considered a weed. Humans do not use a plant deemed a weed, and it is either ignored or destroyed. At the other end of the spectrum, plants that are abused such as opium poppy *(Papaver somniferum)* and marijuana *(Cannabis sativa)* are clearly able to be identified by members of a society. Such plants may be highly valued (and expensive) for their ability to create a certain effect on the body and mind, such as euphoria, but are considered plants of potential abuse because they may be linked to addictive behavior or excessive recreational use in humans. Plants used as ornaments and foods are clearly identifiable as well. Ivy *(Hedera sp. L.),* for example, is used as house plant, and raspberries *(Rubus idaeus L.)* are eaten for dessert.

The ability to discern when a plant is a medicine and not a food is often more difficult. Some plants are only used as foods or medicine, but some can serve both purposes. How a plant is used does not determine its categorization as a food or medicine because plant medicines can be eaten just as plants are used for food. How a plant looks or how much it costs cannot help determine whether it is a medicine or food. The difference between a plant used for food and a plant used for medicine lies in the *intent* of the user.

The Intent

When a plant becomes a medicine, valued for its ability to heal, it is used for care and cure. Potatoes *(Solanum tuberosum)* are one example. People in some countries eat potatoes as a staple food. Potatoes are sold as food and valued as food. Some people also know the medicinal value of potatoes. Herbalists may recommend the medicinal use of the potato, based on their recognition that part of the personality of the plant is demonstrated in the appearance of the root (the potato) and its numerous "eyes." Traditional healing for the human eye has often included putting potato on the outside of the eye. After peeling, the inner part of the potato can be used to heal styes that appear on the eyelid, for instance. "Potato" becomes "potato medicine" when it is used with the intent to care for and cure the eye. Potato can be part of a healthy diet and contribute to the healthy lifestyle of a person, but it is "medicine" when it is used for the care of a specific health concern.

Grapes *(Vitis vinifera)* are another example. Grapes would only be considered a weed by those who have the vines growing in their yard when they cannot identify the plant as grape. Red, purple, and green grapes are eaten as fruit. The leaves also are included in Greek and Middle Eastern cuisines. Grapes also have anti-inflammatory and pain-relieving properties because of constituents such as ferulic acid, salicylic acid, ascorbic acid, and quercetin. Traditionally grapes, fresh or dried (raisins), have been used in relieving discomfort related to arthritis and migraine. Grapes also are used in producing wine, which has a number of medicinal benefits. Wine was historically prescribed as *Spiritus fermentae.* Grapes, as wine, also can be used excessively. The grape in the form of wine is a good example of a plant that can be *used* medicinally in the same way it would be used as a food. Wine is taken by a patient as medicine in the same way it is taken as part of a meal. The difference is in the intent or purpose of the user.

A Brief Historical Perspective

The human intent to heal with plants has been traced back to the earliest days of our species' evolution. The remains of medicinal plants, the pollen grains of eight plants including *Ephedra sp.* have been discovered in the burial site of a Neanderthal man (Solecki, 1975). The intent to heal has never changed, but the way in which humans use and perceive medicinal plants has undergone many changes. The history of plant medicines includes people who used and developed plant medicines, and then wrote about them in herbals or formularies, including physicians such as Galen (131–200 A.D.) and Avicenna (980–1037 A.D.).

Other histories of the use of plants may be communicated orally and may never have been recorded let alone taught as part of medical or herbal curriculum. Herbal medicine has many histories because the ways in which different cultures have used plants as medicine are unique. One can learn the ways of different cultures and their healing methods to understand that the historical uses of plants as medicines have both similarities and differences around the globe. The focus of this brief historical account is more general in describing the parallel histories of the use of plant medicine by scientists and by the people of a culture. Scientists include physicians, pharmacists, and formally educated biomedical health practitioners. The people include the public, priests and shamans, traditional healers, midwives, village wise women, and housewives. Although scientists are people and people are scientific in their approach to using herbs, the terms as they are used here are related to the primary perspective of the individual in their exploration of plant medicines. "The term scientific has taken on an evaluative function, connoting 'better' and 'more reliable'. This evaluative usage has almost wholly supplanted the solely descriptive use of the term" (O'Connor, 1995, p. 14). Using the name "scientist" in reference to the group of biomedical practitioners is in no way meant to be evaluative. This is explained further.

There is a parallel, yet distinct, difference in the histories between scientists and people in relation to the development of plant medicine. The perception and intent of how plant medicines are used in healing are quite different between the two groups. Historically, scientists and people have maintained their distinct beliefs and practices regarding plants as medicine. Scientists have excluded and continue to exclude the people's plant knowledge, which has been gathered over the course of centuries of use from their biomedical work and writings. For example in Western Europe,

> The teachings of Galen marked the beginning of a sharp division between the professional physician on the one hand and the traditional healer on the other. In professional medicine, careful observation of a plant's specific action disappeared and was replaced by Galen's theoretical approach which assigned every plant to its proper station in an orderly scheme. . . . The amateur expected his plants to do their work gently and thoroughly, but not necessarily quickly: every countryman knows you can't hurry nature. . . . The professional doctor was confident he could hurry nature as much as he wished to (Griggs, 1991, p. 16).

The people's medicinal practice of using whole herbs, often singly, has often been called "simple" or crude medicine by the biomedical community. These terms were part of a campaign of discrediting the plant knowledge of the people. Some of the scientific leadership has been highly prejudicial in their remarks about the practices of the people. For example, Benjamin Rush, M.D., one of the founding fathers of the U. S. Constitution and a highly regarded physician of the 1700s, has been quoted as saying about the plant medicine practices of Native Americans, "We have no discoveries in the *material medica* to hope for from the Indians of North America . . . it would be a reproach to our schools of physic if modern physicians were not more successful than the Indians even in the treatment of their own disease" (Rush as reported in Vogel, 1970, p. 63). The competition on the part of some in the scientific community is exemplified in the following statement. In the United States, "the American Medical Association in alliance with the hospital and pharmaceutical industries vanquished the rival medical sects (that practiced botanical and homeopathic medicine) and destroyed the patent medicine industry, replacing its botanical medicines with the synthetic over-the-counter products of the 'ethical' pharmaceutical industry" (Brown & Marcy, 1991, p. 340). There has been a history of competition and lack of unity between scientists and people that some American historians describe as being due to the commodification of health care (Caplan, 1989).

As the rise of formally educated health practitioners continued throughout history, many of the practitioners treated only the wealthy; therefore, many poorer people were left to be treated by the herbalists and lay practitioners. For example, in China, during the government of Mao, it was recognized that the country did not have enough Western drugs or practitioners to provide health services for the entire population of the country. In 1929, the Chinese government outlawed the practice of traditional Chinese medicine (TCM) because the Kuomintang government had decided that TCM was "unscientific" (Griggs, 1991). Mao created a system of "barefoot doctors," traditional practitioners who had some training in Western medicine, to care for the people, primarily the poor rural populations. Many people do not consider the care provided by traditional practitioners to be of less value. In fact, the Chinese government values and markets its traditional system of health care to other countries; hence the steady flow of Western practitioners entering China for tours and education in traditional modalities such as acupuncture and herbalism. The socioeconomic drive to create a health care system for all Chinese people created an integrated system of traditional and conventional (Western) medicine that exists today. The need for more practitioners to provide health care services is still prevalent. As discussed in more detail in chapter 3, the World Health Organization (WHO) has created a program for supporting the integration of traditional healers, such as herbalists, into the health care system of its member states.

In some cases, the people have been just as competitive and exclusionary as the scientists. Many traditional healers have performed their services in private and do not share their wisdom and years of experience with the biomedical community. The difference, however, between the scientists' and the people's behaviors is that the people have often excluded or hidden from the biomedical world in an attempt to preserve their plant medicine traditions. As in China, the science and political leaders of many countries throughout history have attempted, and continue to attempt, to control and even outlaw the traditional use of medicinal plants by the people by labeling the practices unscientific, unproven, or potentially unsafe. Often these labels are applied without adequate study of the cultural practices. Because traditional healers in many cases have not been able to practice openly, the knowledge and wisdom associated with many traditional plant medicine practices is on the verge of extinction. The traditional healers who use and teach the use of indigenous plants have gradually disappeared. In Hawaii, for example, traditional healers, known as "kahuna" (or keepers of the secrets), were driven underground in the 1800s when licensing of health practitioners occurred as a result of Westerners coming to live on the islands. Today, access to traditional healers is still by word of mouth in Hawaii and the average age of traditional Hawaiian healers is 70 years of age (Judd, 1997).

History demonstrates some of the vast differences between traditional healers' and scientists' views of healing, health care, and medicinal use of plants. "In keeping with scientific tradition modern biomedicine has striven to separate itself from broader cultural concerns and influences (and has considered itself largely successful in the attempt)" (O'Connor, 1995, p. 22). Science continues to attempt to separate itself from the people. Regarding the use of plants, the values of the scientific world and the world of the people and their healers are quite different. Chapter 3, Plants and Paradigms, addresses the different value systems in depth.

Recently, there has been a growing awareness of an ability to integrate the values and practices of biomedicine and tradition in the use of plant medicines. It has been demonstrated in many countries that people often choose to combine the use of herbs and conventional biomedical practices in some way. An American study showed that, "Among the 44% of adults who said that they regularly take prescription medications, nearly 1 in 5 (18.4%) reported the concurrent use of at least 1 herbal product, a high-dose vitamin, or both" (Eisenberg et al., 1998, p. 1572).

Integration is happening in the science world as well. In Nigeria, nursing schools are teaching their students how to work with patients who are using both traditional and biomedicines (personal communication, Chika Grace Ugochukwu, June 29, 1999). There also have been some scientists throughout history who have managed to help to bridge the gap between the traditional healers/the people and the scientific/biomedical community. They are the herbalists, the ethnobotanists, and the pharmacognosists.

The Herbalist

The herbalist, now sometimes referred to interchangeably as either a clinical or medical herbalist, studies some of the same theories studied historically by the scientists. Physicians, for example, used a significant number of plant medicines in practice until the boom in synthetic reproduction of plant constituents found in the science of pharmacology became more prevalent. Chinese physicians studied the Pen Ts'ao of Shen Nung recorded in 2800 B.C. and today TCM practitioners continue to learn and use the ancient concepts of early Chinese plant medicine treatment. Herbalists study the concepts recorded in the writings of Greek and Roman physicians who were renowned for their knowledge of plant medicines. The teachings of Dioscorides, Hippocrates, and Galen, to name a few, are still discussed today in herbal education and historical texts. Medicinal plants have been used within a theoretic or scientific framework for centuries.

Herbalists study the humoral theory of physicians such as Hippocrates and Galen. "In Hippocratic teaching the healthy body was one in which the four 'humors' of blood, bile, phlegm, and choler were equally balanced. . . . Careful observation of a plant's specific action disappeared, and was replaced by Galen's theoretical approach which assigned every plant to its proper station in an orderly scheme" (Griggs, 1991, pp. 15–16). Herbalists study a system of plant use defined by renowned physicians such as Avicenna (980–1037) and, much later, Culpeper (1616–1654) who included the science of astrology in determining which plant was used for a particular patient. "The Arabs were experts in astrology, which they had developed to a precise science . . . both the patient and the medicinal plant were subject to astrological influences. . . . Culpeper consulted the motion of the planets when prescribing for his patients" (Griggs, 1991, pp. 25, 97). Many herbalists today study the science of astrology not only for the purpose of matching the plant with the patient but also for the purpose of understanding order in nature. Plants and stars are both believed to be linked to the natural order of the universe (Rossi, Mangrella, Loffreda, & Lampa, 1994). Historically, herbalists have understood the effects of astrology (the position of the stars, the moon, and the planets at the time of harvest or medicinal use) on the properties of herbs given to patients. There are also some herb manufacturers who integrate astrological principles when growing, harvesting, and creating their products.

Another historical theory that is learned by clinical herbalists is the Doctrine of Signatures often associated with the work of Paracelsus, a Swiss-German physician (1493–1541). The Doctrine of Signatures states that each plant has a signature, something in the way it looks or how it grows, that lets the user know the healing purpose of the plant. For example, the potatoes mentioned before have "eyes" and are therefore used in the healing of the eyes. Also, the shape of *Panax ginseng* root looks like the shape of the human body. This signature of the whole body suggests that ginseng's properties support the whole person. And indeed, ginseng is traditionally used to promote energy or "qi" in the whole body. The signature of violets is that they hide from the sun and love the shade; therefore, they have been found to be of benefit to the migraine sufferer whose individual "signature" or "pattern" is a sensitivity to light and the seeking of solace of a darkened room. In the Doctrine of Signatures, there is a matching of signatures or patterns of the patient with the plant.

Some may consider this theoretic system primitive. If they mean primitive in the sense that it is "relating to the earliest stage of development" (Merriam-Webster, 1999), this is not the case. If they mean that the Doctrine of Signatures is "of a people or a culture that is nonindustrial and often nonliterate and tribal" (Merriam-Webster, 1999), this is not really the case either. "Time-honored" would be a far better descriptor for theories such as the Doctrine of Signatures, or those theories used in Ayurveda (traditional medicine of India) and TCM that continue to be referenced by the clinical herbalist when deciding on the proper remedy for the individual. The Doctrine of Signatures and other theories used in plant medicine are part of an adaptive system of knowledge used by intelligent people. In the case of the Doctrine of Signatures, numerous health practitioners, especially in Germany and Switzerland, continue to develop their understanding of nature and how it may apply to the healing of human body in regard to the Doctrine of Signatures.

Paracelsus was an unusual physician in his time because he valued the medicinal plant knowledge of the country healers. He worked and studied with them. He also was very biomedically oriented in that he believed and taught that the action of a plant remedy, "did not depend upon its qualities such as moistness, but on its *specific* healing virtue, which was determined by its chemical properties" (Kremers & Urdang as cited in Griggs, 1991, p. 50). Paracelsus and other renowned teachers of plant medicine, such as American herbalist John Christopher, also maintained a strong conviction in the folk belief that medicinal plants grow where they are needed. All of these theories are taught today as part of herbal education.

At one point in my herbal education, I learned the aforementioned theory that medicinal plants grow where they are needed. The theory was demonstrated in a vivid experience I had working as a nurse on a postpartum labor and delivery unit. During the course of a number of weeks, several babies had been delivered by performing a fourth-degree episiotomy on the mothers. This really concerned me because the women were so uncomfortable after delivery. I was also concerned because I had, over the years, observed a number of deliveries with a midwife who massaged the perineum of her laboring mothers with St. John's wort *(Hypericum perforatum)* oil to help the cervix relax and widen more easily. Her experience was that the oil often prevented the need for any episiotomy, let alone such an extensive one.

As these women came into my care, I could not help but wish that our labor and delivery team might consider another approach such as that used by my colleague. One morning, I was parking my car behind the hospital (we parked near a field), and I looked up in the hazy sunlight to see a field of small, yellow flowers. Every year, I have wildcrafted St. John's wort flowers to make oil and tinctures for my family and friends. As you might imagine, when I went to investigate, I found that the yellow flowers were indeed St. John's wort. There was a huge field of the flowers growing literally outside the back door of the hospital. Never before had I seen such a demonstration of what I had learned early on as an herbalist. The medicines we need really do grow outside our back door.

I harvested what I needed for my remedies and left the rest. Unfortunately, the labor and delivery staff never did take advantage of the healing power of the St. John's wort. The flowers would have gone by before I could have gotten approval to even introduce the oil to the staff at the hospital. The plant was there though, ready and willing. Ironically, a few months later I heard a pharmacist say on a radio program about herbs that, "There is no good source for St. John's wort here in the United States." I wondered if people might interpret what he said to mean that St. John's wort does not grow in the United States. It actually grows quite well in many locations and is considered a noxious weed (a plant that moves into a location not allowing other plants to grow) in some states. And there certainly was a good source right outside the hospital where I worked.

Although some herbalists' roles in a community may be similar to that of a shaman or traditional healer, many herbalists study medicinal plants both from the perspective of the science of the time and the cultural traditions of the use of a particular medicinal plant. They often value and make decisions about which plant medicine they will use with a patient based on both viewpoints. For example, the *Materia Medica* of the traditional Chinese herbalist contains information not only about the energetic qualities of the herb, such as whether the herb moves "qi" or drains dampness, but also contains information about laboratory data, such as the antibacterial or antifungal activity of an herb and what type of organism is affected by its activity in vitro. Herbalists also have a medical language comprised of terms that physicians and nurses once used. Some of these terms are explained within this text in detail; for those that may only be mentioned, please refer to the glossary.

The Ethnobotanist

The second example of those who have been able to bridge the two worlds of tradition and science is the ethnobotanist. Ethnobotany is the study of the relationships between people and plants. Ethnobotanists research "the way people incorporate plants into their cultural traditions, religions, and cosmologies," which leads to a greater understanding of the people themselves (Balick & Cox, 1996, p. 4). Ethnobotanists often study indigenous peoples' use of medicinal plants. One of the oldest forms of ethnobotanical research is the search for new drugs among the plants used in traditional practices. In the United States, Canada, and western Europe, there is a "one in four chance that a medicine contains an active ingredient derived from a plant. . . . Pharmacognosist Norman Farnsworth, of the University of Illinois, estimates that 89 plant-derived drugs currently prescribed in the industrialized world were discovered by studying folk knowledge" (Balick & Cox, 1996, p. 25).

The two major goals of ethnobotany as an observational science are described as (1) "the possibility of finding new species valuable for agriculture or industry or of discovering and salvaging new chemicals from the wild floras of the world," and (2) "understanding the psychological aspects of the ways that aboriginal peoples interpret and treat their useful plants" (Schultes & von Reis, 1995, p. 12). Ethnobotanists are critical players in the conservation of plant biodiversity and indigenous plant wisdom.

Since early history, ethnobotanists of many cultures have recorded the plants used for healing purposes. Historical writings and recordings such as the Ebers papyrus of the Egyptians, the *Shen Nung* of the Chinese, and the *Caraka Samhita* (a Sanskrit medical text of India) have been results of the work of ethnobotanists of the day. Today, in addition to their observation and recording skills, ethnobotanists use the modern techniques and technology of the molecular biologist and the chemist to answer questions related to the behavior of plants, the human behavioral response to plants, and the relationship of people and plants. "Ethnobotany must be highly interdisciplinary, drawing from aspects of botany, anthropology, archeology, phytochemistry, pharmacology, medicine, history, religion, geography, and numerous other tangentially pertinent sciences and arts" (Schultes & von Reis, 1995, p. 12). Many of the drugs administered by nurses today, such as aspirin *(Filipendula ulmaria),* codeine *(Papaver somniferum),* quinine *(Cinchona pubescens),* and vincristine *(Catharanthus roseus)* exist as a result of the tremendous successes of ethnobotanical researchers who provide a bridge between the two worlds of science and the people.

The future of the ethnobotanist is not so much focused on the search for the drug that will be the next "magic bullet" as it is to explore "how a specific group of people perceives plants they use, how it interprets those perceptions, how those perceptions influence the activities of members of that society, and how those activities, in turn influence the ambient vegetation and the ecosystem upon which the society depends" (Schultes & von Reis, 1995, p. 44). Ethnobotanists go beyond simple observation in the charting of the various plants used in a particular culture. They go beyond the focus of searching for what man can take from the plant world in the form of drugs and look to the relationship of people and plants and how that relationship is expressed in the evolution of the whole ecosystem. Ethnobotanists are scientists who "walk" between both the scientific world and the world of the people and their healers, often serving as translators for both realms.

The Pharmacognosist

The pharmacognosist is the third scientist whose role often provides a bridge between the scientific world and that of the people. Pharmacognosy is defined by some as the science of "descriptive pharmacology dealing with crude drugs and simples" (Merriam-Webster, 1999). Some refer to pharmacognosy as the study of natural drugs and their constituents, where natural drugs refers to "products not made by chemical synthesis" (Leung & Foster, 1996, p. xxix). The difference between the two definitions is significant because it represents the changes that have occurred in the field over the past thirty years or so. The pharmacognosist traditionally educated in modern medical chemistry also learned ethnobotany, such as plant identification; traditional uses as potential indicators for modern use; and recognition and understanding of the importance of sources for plant products. The traditionally trained pharmacognosist is the bridge between science and the people in much the same way as the ethnobotanist.

Today, traditional pharmacognosy is virtually nonexistent and is rarely taught in university programs. Courses entitled "pharmacognosy" or "plant or natural product medicine" taught today focus on the plants as sources of modern drugs for which they attempt to identify and isolate a single active principle that represents the values of biomedicine. Plants often contain dozens of active principles, which can cause a scientist to wonder at the relevance of the data. The new pharmacognosist has no knowledge of the plants themselves and rarely can identify the medicinal plants studied. One traditionally educated pharmacognosist describes the role of the present day pharmacognosist as, "slave to their analytic techniques and equipment. They don't design experiments geared at how good an herb is, they design an approach or method of study to fit the analytic technique or equipment" (personal communication, A. Leung, November 14, 2000). The conventionally trained pharmacognosist distances himself from the traditional use of plant medicine and becomes a part of the world of "science." Traditionally trained pharmacognosists, however, with their knowledge of traditional uses of plant medicine and other ethnobotanical principles as well as modern medicinal chemistry do continue to serve as bridges between the two worlds of the people and science.

A HISTORY OF NURSING AND PLANT MEDICINE:

In their own way, nurses too have served and continue to serve as bridges between science and the people. Often as caregivers, nurses are called upon to bridge communication between patients and their health practitioners. Although professional nurses are educated in the biomedical world of the "scientist," they also learn to stay in touch with the health beliefs and practices of their patients, the "people." Nurses value connection and relationship with patients and therefore, by the nature and necessities of their practice, they have stayed connected with both worlds. Nurses not only have a history of caregiving that includes the conventional, technical skills, and theoretic underpinnings of the world of science, but also they have an even longer history of human caring and providing comfort in ways that are directly connected to the health beliefs and traditional practices of the people. In particular, nurses have a history with the use of plant medicines. American history includes several examples of nurses using their plant medicine skills.

As previously mentioned, until the proliferation of pharmaceutical drugs, American nursing texts routinely included the plant medicines of the day. Nurses were taught plant medicine theory as a matter of course. Virginia Henderson included information on plant use in her theory (which she called a definition) and practice texts, which have been used worldwide since the mid-1900s. For example, nurses were taught the health benefits of a "counterirritant" action on the skin that can be stimulated by some plants such as mustard and cayenne. The purpose of herbal counterirritant use was to deeply warm and stimulate circulation in a particular area of the body. "Counterirritation relieves the affection of the organ over which it is applied by reflex nerve relation between the skin and the organ, and by producing a change in the blood supply to the organ. The mental effect of substitution of a new and superficial pain also assists in the result" (Harmer & Henderson, 1955, p. 264).

Earlier in history, nurses were known to practice independently with the aid of plants as therapeutic modalities. Nurse-midwives routinely used plant therapies in their work with women. In the Pulitzer Prize–winning book *A Midwife's Tale: The Life of Martha Ballard Based on her Diary 1785-1812*, the American midwife grows, harvests, dries, and uses the medicinal herbs from her garden in her care of women. She used some of the same plant medicines as the physicians in the town, such as rhubarb and senna, but did not use the "dramatic therapies" such as the mercurial compound known as calomel that the physicians used (Ulrich, 1990, p. 56). Martha Ballard was held in high esteem in her town and practiced independently. She "summoned a physician twice in twenty-seven years" (Ulrich, 1990, p. 180) and she used plant medicines often in practice.

During the Civil War, a nurse named Mary Ann Bickerdyke from Ohio, whose source of nursing education is unknown, opened a private practice in physio-botanic medicine in the 1800s, during a time when almost 50% of the population of the state of Ohio was using therapies and remedies suggested by practitioners educated in the practices of the Thomsonian Medico-botanical movement (as reported by Haller, 1997). Another source reports that 4 million people out of a total population of 17 million inhabitants of the United States at that time used the herbs and therapies recommended by the Thomsonian botanical practitioners for self-care (Rothstein as reported in Ehrenreich & English, 1978).

In addition to being in private practice, Bickerdyke was also the staff herbalist at her local hospital. During the war, she served as a noncommissioned nurse of the Union army where she "established over 300 field hospitals and nursed casualties on nineteen battlefields. . . . A pragmatic herbalist, she replaced limited medicines with blackberry cordial for diarrhea, jimsonweed for pain, and bloodroot and wild cherry for stimulants" (Snodgrass, 1999, p. 26). Although she encountered opposition to her use of botanical medicines in the army hospitals, when she was in charge of the hospital, the "patients were bathed, put to bed in clean clothes on clean bedding, dosed with black root and goldenseal, sassafras tea and beet juice, and fed all the milk and fresh vegetables they would take. A surprisingly large number of them recovered" (Baker, 1952, p. 142). Nurse-herbalist Mary Ann Bickerdyke was known as the "cyclone in calico" and was honored many times for her tremendous service.

Before the creation of antibiotics and other pharmaceuticals, plant medicines were what nurses, physicians, and other healers all used in their practices. Plant therapies are not new to the world of science and technology. History clearly shows the influence plants have had in the development of healing practices of the people, professional health care providers, and health care systems of nations. Herbal medicine and the practice of using plants in healing is not a passing fad related to the emergence of complementary therapies. Many of the modalities now being called "complementary" have been used for centuries in many cultures. The use of herbs is an evolving science and art. It is a healing modality that continues to be used and explored by many health practitioners and the public, and the use of herbal medicines is not new to nursing practice.

Nurses have had a history of acting as bridges between the people and the scientists and are trusted and relied upon in society to fulfill their role. Nurses must formally reclaim their history with plant medicines. They can bring back the teaching of herbal therapies in nursing curricula. As the knowledge base grows again, nurses will be better able to integrate their understanding of plant therapies with their ability as translators between the people and the scientists. Nurses' understanding of plant therapies must be informed by an integrated view of both the science and art that is expressed in both the plant knowledge of the people and the scientists.

CHAPTER 3

Plants and Paradigms

Interdisciplinary Interest

HERBS CAN BE A PART OF EVERY HEALTH PRACTITIONER AND healer's practice. Plants are everywhere and the knowledge of their use is in every community. In some cases, herbs are used for similar conditions among different communities and then again, they also may be used for different reasons. A plant used for the treatment of cancer in one country might be used as a cure for warts in another. A plant revered as a spiritual icon in one country might be used as an intravenous injection for the treatment of cancer in another.

As is true for all evolving species, a vast wealth of knowledge and wisdom is emerging from the plant kingdom. Changes occur in the lives of plants just as they do in the lives of people. Plants are influenced by changes in their environment. People are part of that environment. As the interest people have in certain plants changes, the environment for those plants changes. Each time the healing potential of a plant is recognized, that plant's evolution is changed forever as a result of its relationship with human beings.

The interest in plants and their healing properties can be found in many healing disciplines. Health care providers and patients have a common interest in medicinal plants. The nature of that interest, the intent, however, can be quite different. For example a horticulturist and a farmer might be interested in the strawberry *(Fragaria spp. L.)* plant because of the delicious fruit it produces, and they seek to understand the plant better so that they can help it produce a higher yield of sweeter berries. A health care practitioner, in addition to enjoying the fruit of the strawberry, might be interested in the nutritional qualities of the fruit and the leaves, such as its antioxidant and vitamin C content, and how the plant affects the health and well-being of people.

An interest in healing plants often is sparked by an experience or interaction with a plant. The experience may be pleasant or it may be uncomfortable. For example, a group of people might hear of a story about how a man's prostate was "healed" when he took saw palmetto berries. One person who heard the story might think, "Oh my father has prostate problems, maybe the berries would help him feel better." Another person might think, "Oh that's poppycock! I've never heard of a berry healing a prostate." Another might think, "Well it helped him, but it probably won't help every man. I want to see some scientific studies that prove it works before I consider it." These reactions represent just a few of the numerous possible responses to an herbal remedy. These thought processes are perspectives that come from inner belief systems, cultural upbringing, education, and life experiences. These perspectives are often part of a larger paradigm or philosophy about life. A person's paradigm or worldview is important as an expression of one's sense of self. Therefore, the paradigm is never judged as "bad" or "good." It just is. Personal paradigms can change, but because they often are rooted deeply in belief patterns that have evolved over time, they rarely change quickly.

A person's paradigm or personal philosophy influences both the way one sees the world and is shaped by the way one experiences the world. A person's paradigm is important to understand when discussing plant therapies because the way people view their human world is often what they bring to and project onto the world of plants. Over the years, the differences in paradigm have contributed to the underlying disagreement among the scientists and the people regarding the focus of the use of healing plants. As stated previously, in general the people have a tendency to explore the plant as a whole, and the scientists' primary value is to understand and explore a plant's constituents or parts.

Nurses experience this paradigmatic tension each time they work to individualize the care of a patient. Patients do not like to be referred to as "the tumor in room 117." They do not like to be referred to as their "parts." The concept of personhood is a holistic concept. People are more than their tumor, or their broken arm, or their blood; they are more than their physical body. They are personality, mind, and spirit. For the purpose of understanding and progression of knowledge, scientists, including nurses, have researched and studied the "parts" of people. Studying the parts of something is a very natural process for the scientist. In the case of the patient with a tumor, however, if the practitioner studies the tumor, or the place in the body where the tumor is growing, and never puts the tumor and body part back into the whole "picture" of the person, the patient may feel dehumanized in the process. The understanding of both the part and the whole must be integrated when caring for the patient using any modality, including herbs.

Dehumanization of patients can occur as a result of interaction with health care providers who focus on the disease and curing the disease rather than the person with an illness that is experienced as part of his or her life. The personal account of life with cancer by Arthur Frank (1991) in his book, *At the Will of the Body,* includes a poignant description of his interaction with different paradigms of health and healing. He describes the impact of returning to his hospital room and finding a sign on his door that said "Lymphoma," a diagnosis that had not been confirmed or communicated to him. He writes that, "Medicine cannot enter into the experience [referring to the lived experience of illness]; it seeks only cure or management. It does offer relief to a body that is suffering" (p. 52).

Nurses are in a position where they can choose to draw on both the experience of the whole person and the science of the parts. Nurses interact with both the worldviews and paradigms of scientists and the people. Nurses walk between both worlds as part of their daily work. They understand the compassionate drive for producing a cure and the need of the person to be recognized as a whole being. When nurses prepare patients for surgery, they consider the requirements of biomedical science and the needs of the patient. For instance, they make sure that the patient understands the surgical procedure and that a patient's religious beliefs regarding sedation are respected. The patient may need time to pray before sedation, and the nurse makes sure that the patient's wishes are honored. This is one example of the daily interaction that occurs between the worldviews of science and the people.

Nurses, like the herbalist, pharmacognosist, and ethnobotanist, are quite adept at listening to and interacting with both worlds. Plant therapies provide an opportunity for growth in the integration of the understanding that comes from looking at the parts and the whole. Because nurses have a history both with the use of plant medicines and being able to bridge the worlds of science and the people, they have much to contribute when it comes to furthering the understanding of healing plants. This chapter describes different paradigms that nurses encounter as they explore the use of herbs.

Plants and the Biomedical Paradigm

Nurses are very familiar with the biomedical paradigm because many nurses work in the biomedical world every day. Nurses share in the visions and beliefs of biomedical practitioners such as physicians and pharmacists. The strengths of the biomedical worldview include valuing the cure, a persistent attempt to find the cause (diagnose), the disease in need of curing, and the deft use of technology to make discoveries on the cellular level. The cure is highly valued because it is equated with life and health. Research is one means of determining the efficacy of the cure. The biomedical paradigm includes a conviction regarding the benefits of good research in supporting clinical provision of safer and more efficacious health care. The gold standard of research is the randomized, double-blind, placebo-controlled trial because it is a form of inquiry that focuses on a very specific variable and seeks to isolate that variable so that its unique qualities can be recognized. Research questions are often answered through evaluation of quantifiable data. Nurses understand the value of quantifiable data and controls in clinical trials. They too perform such studies. How does the biomedical paradigm translate when addressing plant therapies? The following questions are some of the most commonly asked by the biomedical practitioner:

1. Are there any clinical trials on the use of this plant drug?
2. How safe is this herbal drug for human consumption?
3. How efficacious is this herbal drug in curing specific disease?
4. How should the herb be used? What is the dose?
5. What are the active ingredients/constituents in the crude herb drug, and can they be synthesized?
6. What are the risks of harmful interactions between herbs and the therapies prescribed such as drug therapies?

I often hear these questions from many nurses, physicians, and pharmacists. These questions stem from the underlying values of the biomedical paradigm. The problem often encountered by patients and traditional healers who use plants in healing when they reveal the use to biomedical practitioners is that if these questions cannot be answered, then the herb is considered suspect, even useless. There is a sense of ethnocentrism as the biomedical culture raises its values for herbs as the "gold standard" for understanding healing plants. The biomedical questions about herbs often are asked as if a duel were about to begin rather than a meeting of the minds! Perhaps nurses might want to consider reframing the questions as follows:

1. What type of research questions need to be asked about plant therapies and nursing care, and what methodologies will best answer these questions?
2. How is safe use determined in the use of plant medicines?

3. Do plants "cure disease," or do they act in other ways?
4. How are the plants used, how long have they been used by people and practitioners, and is dosing possible?
5. What are the healing properties, characteristics, and personality of the plant?
6. Herbs must "interact" with other therapies in some way. How can herbs and biomedical therapies be integrated, and how can I help the patient understand the benefits and risks associated with choosing a plan of care that includes herbs if they are indicated and the patient wishes to use them?

These are broader, plant-focused questions. Many plant science experts often ask these kinds of questions. Norman Farnsworth, Research Professor of Pharmacognosy at the University of Illinois, and colleagues (1985) have raised these kinds of questions in relation to the study of plants used in traditional medicine: "Is it desirable to put in effort to discover pure compounds in the hope of using them as drugs per se or is it preferable to go on using traditional preparations and make no attempt to identify the active principles?" (p. 967). Although they may value understanding the active principles of a plant, they first question the relevance and purpose of the information.

In general in the biomedical paradigm, each plant is considered a potential drug and the greatest value is placed on the plant's constituents rather than the plant as a whole. The underlying question might be summarized as "What makes this plant work?" The following sections discuss four ways herbs are often viewed by the practitioners within a biomedical paradigm.

PLANTS AS POTENTIAL DRUGS:

First of all, plants are viewed as potential drugs. Most pharmaceutical drugs have been developed from plants and their constituents.

> *In the developed world, the active constituents of medicinal plants are of major importance; plant extracts are of minor importance as drugs. It is known that ca. 119 drugs of known structure are still extracted from higher plants and are used globally in allopathic medicine . . . 10–15% of the 250,000 species of flowering plants on the planet have been used medicinally. However, only a fraction of these are of sufficient importance to be considered as candidates as registration as drugs in developing countries based on widespread and continuous use and with some type of experimental confirmation of their biological activities (Farnsworth, 1992, p. 87).*

Some of the prescription and over-the-counter drugs for which plants or their derivatives are used include caffeine, opium, tincture of benzoin, oatmeal, chlorophyll, reserpine, scopolamine, vincristine, morphine, ipecac, psyllium, digoxin, ephedrine, and theophylline. These and many more drugs have brought relief to people over the years, and they are the result of the hard work and vision of those with a biomedical worldview. The call continues to go forth for more research into herbal drugs because they are cheaper and most people and national health care programs are looking for cost savings.

The cost of a new prescription drug going through the research and development phases and the formal approval process set forth by the Food and Drug Administration in the United States is estimated to be between hundreds of thousands to millions of dollars, depending on such things as the number of phases of clinical trials to be undertaken and the drug being tested (personal communication, FDA Consumer Hotline, Denver, 2000). This is one of the most expensive drug approval systems in the world today. If drug companies were to put this kind of money into the development of plant drugs, they could only recoup their costs if they held exclusive rights or a patent on the herbal drug to sell it. However, plants are not patentable because they are common and used by many. Drug companies can "patent extraction techniques or they can modify some natural compound to make a semi-synthetic from a natural starting material . . . modern Americans like Europeans are coming to prefer a natural drug, while the drug companies prefer a synthetic they can protect" (Duke, 1984, p. 3). Although some pharmaceutical companies have begun to take a second look at plant medicines, there are still some very big issues with the approach of searching for the active compounds.

Medicinal plants have very complex chemical structures. Identifying one special active constituent that can create a certain health-giving action in the human body is not easy. It would be like saying that "an apple a day keeps the doctor away" only because of the fructose or the pectin in the fruit. Plant medicines can elude the biomedical mind, which often tries to find the one drug for the particular disease. It may be the ideal, but one plant researcher writes, "The bioavailability of these chemicals in an herbal formula or in an ingested herb is most likely very selective and dependent upon the physiological state of the individual consumer" (Leung & Foster, 1996, p. xii). It is speculated that this may account for why herbs such as ginseng have been used for so many centuries in China for so many different conditions, yet ginseng still has not been proven "effective" by modern science. Herbs deliver a smorgasbord of biochemical constituents to the body, and biomedical technology may not be able to address modalities, such as herbs, that potentially work in multiple pathways at one time. The researcher may pay top money for the research and development of an herb or herbal formula only to end up with more questions about a particular plant's biologic and medicinal activity.

Herbs have been shown to save money on the user side of the economic picture. One paper on the costs of herbal medicines to health maintenance organizations (HMOs) reported that if St. John's wort were given to depressed patient subscribers in the HMO instead of Prozac and were effective in only 25% of cases, the cost savings estimated to the HMO would be $250,000 (Kincheloe, 1997). The paradox is that although the research and approval of a pharmaceutical drug made from a plant may be valued and desired, the reality is that it is often economically impractical for drug companies to promote the very products those in the biomedical world may want.

RIGOROUS TESTING:

The second view of the biomedical paradigm is that plant medicines must be treated as drugs and submitted to the same rigorous testing and controls used for drugs. It is often implied that the potential for harm to a patient taking plant medicines is just as great as if they were using a pharmaceutical drug, and therefore, toxicity, dosing, and standardization should be established for all herbal drugs. Some scientists warn that herbs should not be used until such data are thoroughly collected and evaluated (Newall, Anderson, & Phillipson, 1996). Although this concern may arise out of an ethical duty to do no harm, no data support the view that herbs should be considered as potentially harmful as the potent pharmaceutical drugs that scientists have created for diseases that require strong medicines. The issues regarding the safe use of herbs are discussed in greater detail in chapter 4.

STANDARDIZATION:

The third biomedical view is that controlling the quality and quantity of plant constituents in a standardization process (such as European phytopharmaceuticals) provides for safer and more effective use of herbal remedies. In the biomedical paradigm, it is believed that standardization to a specific plant constituent makes the remedy more potent, more effective, and easier to use, at least for those who are more familiar with dosing pharmaceutical drugs than with traditional or clinical herbalist dosing strategies for a particular herb. Standardized herbal products have become "drugs of choice" in some countries. Standardization is discussed in more detail in chapter 4. It is important to know that in plant science, standardization based on one particular chemical constituent is not considered representative of the total activity of a medicinal plant. The selected components are meant to be biologic markers of product quality of total plant extractions (Leung & Foster, 1996), not medicinal effectiveness.

Standardization of chemical constituents may appear to be easier to study in clinical trials and often is touted by biomedical practitioners as an "evolution" in herbal medicine. Along with standardization comes a cleaner, smaller package. Processed standardized herbs are usually sold in capsule or tablet form, similar to pharmaceuticals. The consumer is spared the fuss of dealing with whole herb products and knowing how to prepare them for their healing applications. Taking a pill is easier and more enjoyable (i.e., no odd taste) for many consumers. Even though biomedical practitioners may feel they are providing a service to patients, some may question the so-called evolution in the use of herbal medicines just as they might other technologic advances.

Clinical science in botanical medicine was well developed among nineteenth century physicians in America and England. Doctors knew how to choose plant medicines for patients and knew their common dosages, which were individualized for the patient. The use of standardized plant extracts is now being promoted as "a professionalization of botanical medicine, an enhancement of nature by laboratory science creating a quasi-pharmaceutical for 'scientific' professional use" (Kenner, 1998, p. 55). The role of technology in general is being questioned among members adhering to the biomedical paradigm. "It is apparent that technology has indeed come between the patient and the doctor and that although scientific devices disgorge much information knowledge as to how to treat the patient properly may still be lacking" (Inglefinger, 1978, p. 945). Nurses must seriously consider any unstudied biomedical belief that a standardized herbal preparation is inherently better or safer for use than a remedy that is not standardized.

AN HERBAL REVOLUTION:

A revolution is defined as a "change in paradigm" (Merriam-Webster, 1999). If the change in paradigm were for biomedical practitioners to once again consider using herbs and also to work together with traditional healers and clinical herbalists, some would want to change and others would not.

The fourth view of the biomedical paradigm has to do with the two perceptions of what the herb revolution is about. The first, perhaps stemming from the historical issues between the scientists and the people, is that there needs to be a revolution on herbal medicines to expose dangerous nonbiomedical practitioners who use plant therapies in helping their patients. Some believe that those who heal with herbs are pretending to have medical skills—that they are "quacks." "Orthodox medicine does not reject medicines derived from herbs but it does reject quackery" (Penn, 1986, p. 898), possibly implying that biomedical practice with herbs is not subject to quackery.

Others of the biomedical paradigm understand that "herbal medicine differs from orthodox medicine not only in the form in which plants are administered but also in its underlying philosophy" (Houghton, 1995, p. 137) and the way herbal practitioners provide their service. They understand that quackery can exist in any group of professionals and that philosophical differences should be respected.

Secondly, some biomedical practitioners are revolutionary in that they realize that there are valid viewpoints other than those often held in biomedicine regarding the best means of studying the efficacy and safety of herbal medicines. Some biomedical practitioners suggest that "long and widespread use together with closely-detailed records of individual case histories" (Houghton, 1995, p. 137) be considered when examining an herb's safety and efficacy. Others recommend including experimental case studies as a way of studying efficacy of herbs. It also is thought to be important that biomedical practitioners broaden the scope of literature searches associated with herbal research to go beyond the available literature in Western publications or a MEDLINE database (McPartland & Pruitt, 2000). For example, Chinese medical journals include research on herbs that is sometimes excluded in the West because of differences in research methodology. These are just a few of the diverse biomedical responses to the ongoing herbal "revolution."

At the same time that herbs and the philosophy regarding their use is being questioned in the biomedical world, some are even questioning the beliefs regarding some of the oldest biomedical drugs. Aspirin, first introduced to the American public in 1899, is considered the most popular drug of all time. Aspirin, acetylsalicylic acid, was developed from the plant, *Filipendula ulmaria* also known as *Spiraea ulmaria* (Balick & Cox, 1996). It is among the top ten drugs prescribed in the United States (Lewis, 2000). A pioneer in biotechnology who has developed drug delivery systems for cancer and heart patients questions the recommendation of other biomedical colleagues who prescribe an aspirin a day. He writes that, "Taking an aspirin for the rest of your life can, in proper doses knock out bad eicosanoids [a family of biological substances including thromboxanes and prostaglandins] at a slightly faster rate than it knocks out good eicosanoids. But taking aspirin is a tricky game to play, sort of like lighting a cigarette with a stick of dynamite. . . . No one knows what the 'proper' dose of aspirin is, especially over a long period of time. . . . Long-term aspirin may be the biological equivalent of a loose cannon" (Sears, 1995, p. 161). Changes are happening in the biomedical paradigm in relation to drugs and especially with plant therapies. As interaction among disciplines increases, new questions about herbs and new ways of answering those questions emerge.

Nurses must not rely completely upon the values and standards of the biomedical paradigm, which work well for the biomedical world but do not seem best fitted to the use of plant therapies. There is a call for a new worldview even among those who may have held the biomedical paradigm for some time. Nurses must realize that, as changes occur, they must be observant of what aspects of their own biomedical paradigm inform their work with medicinal plants and which do not. This examining of one's own paradigm is part of reflective practice and also part of developing skills in integrative nursing.

Plants and the Traditional Paradigm

An old story in Chinese herbal medicine helps illustrate a traditional paradigm of the use of herbs. A group of herbal students was ready for their final exam. Their teacher told them to search eight miles out on all sides of the city and bring back samples of all the plants they could find that had absolutely no medicinal value. Within a few days all but one of the students had returned, each with a few plants. Finally on the fifth day, the last student returned looking very sad indeed, for he was empty handed. "Why so sad?" asked the teacher. "You are the only one qualified to pursue the herbal path."

Although this story is just one example of a traditional paradigm of the use of herbs, in general, the traditional paradigm is representative of the "people's" cultural beliefs about plant use. Because cultures and plant populations differ from country to country, the specifics of a particular traditional paradigm (or worldview) about plants differs from country to country. This chapter deals with the traditional use of herbs in the broad sense because it is beyond the scope of this book to examine each individual culture's traditional uses of herbs. The traditional use of herbs and herb use in the biomedical world, which is also a culture in its own right, are compared and contrasted.

Traditional medicine is defined by the World Health Organization (WHO, 1996) as "the ways of protecting and restoring health that existed before the arrival of modern medicine . . . approaches to health that belong to the traditions of a country and have been handed down from generation to generation" (1996, p. 1). Some traditional healing with plants has been passed by word of mouth as part of the folklore of a country. The oral tradition of passing on information about herbs includes a belief system and a philosophy as well as the details of the actual use of the healing plants. Some traditional systems such as traditional Chinese medicine (TCM), Kampo medicine in Japan, and Ayurveda in India are highly documented, theoretically based, and often researched. In addition to herbalists, WHO classifies acupuncturists, traditional birth attendants, and mental healers as traditional healers (WHO, 1996). Many countries have traditional healers who are indigenous peoples who use herbs as part of their healing practices. Balick and Cox (1996) define indigenous people as those "who follow traditional, nonindustrialized lifestyles in areas that they have occupied for generations" (p. 5). So a TCM practitioner in the United Kingdom, for example, although a practitioner of a traditional form of medicine, would not be considered an indigenous healer.

Indigenous healers are great resources on the plants growing in their regions. Their relationships with plants are strong and direct. Indigenous healers wildcraft or cultivate their own herbs, and use the plants directly. They retain their knowledge of use of plants. Many indigenous cultures "perceive the earth as existing not in the realm of the profane, but in the realm of the sacred, a worldview that distinguishes them from many Western traditions. Indigenous legends emphasize the need to protect the earth not because it is useful to humans but because it is sacred" (Balick & Cox, 1996, p. 182).

The traditional paradigm has some poignant differences from the biomedical paradigm. Whereas the main question of the biomedical paradigm might be "What makes this plant work?", the main question of the traditional paradigm might simply be "How can this plant be used for healing?" The need for understanding the components that make up the plant before deciding whether or not it can be used is not necessarily part of the traditional paradigm. "Typically, practitioners of traditional medicine view the biomedical search for a single, so-called active ingredient as an inappropriate application of their empirically and culturally grounded health knowledge" (Bodeker, 1995, p. 235). In traditional practice, herbs are often used synergistically in combination as opposed to the biomedical approach of targeting a single constituent.

In folkloric healing or domestic medicine types of traditional practice, herbs often have been used historically as single remedies, sometimes called "simples." In the twelfth century, European apothecaries or pharmacists were busy developing all sorts of new complex drugs from animals, vegetables, and minerals because they could not have "made the barest living by selling the simples that grew in their customers' gardens or flourished in the nearest patch of waste land" (Griggs, 1991, p.29). Today, many pharmacies are selling large amounts of herbal preparations to people who have no knowledge of the plant, let alone are able to grow it themselves. A simple today might be considered a capsule of a single herb. This is very different from the approach of those practicing from the domestic or folkloric view in which a single fresh herb might be used as a tea or topical application.

Traditional practitioners also have their own language for describing illness. Their paradigm does not include seeking to control nature, destroy pathogens, or eradicate diseases. Although the explanations about cause for illness and rationale for use of a particular herb may be very different than that of the biomedical paradigm, they are similarly scientifically based. Often the traditional practitioner uses logic and some form of pattern recognition when describing illness. They match the pattern of illness with an herb or herbs that bring about greater balance and health. Traditional medical knowledge is typically coded into household cooking practices, home remedies, and health prevention/maintenance beliefs and routines (Bodeker, 1995, p. 232). Many people who use traditional and folk medicines also use the remedies of biomedicine. Traditional health care alternatives abound in areas well served by conventional medical care, as a survey in any major metropolitan area in the United States would demonstrate.

People choose to use traditional healing methods for many reasons. Their decisions can be quite logical and are based on trust. People who have seen the effectiveness of plant remedies used by their families may suspect the newest treatment introduced by the biomedical practitioner. That is human nature, and it is also very logical. People also know from experience and from long historical use that plant medicines are gentler medicines and have not had the same adverse effects that pharmaceutical drugs do. Because many of the day-to-day health concerns are not life threatening, many people logically turn to lifestyle issues such as diet and home remedies (e.g., plant medicines) to effect changes that result in greater comfort and health. People have a sense of timing in their healing process. Although they often prefer to provide self-care and not rely on someone else for care, they also ask for help when it is needed. Ethnographic fieldwork has "repeatedly revealed that vernacular health belief systems have among their central values concerns for the appropriate and timely intervention and for seeking the proper specialist" (O'Connor, 1995, p. 21). These concerns are shared by those with a biomedical paradigm. The differences lie in the treatment that is deemed necessary and "where the search for relief ought to begin" (O'Connor, 1995, p. 21).

Some folk remedies from one culture can be misinterpreted as harm or abuse when acted upon in another culture (Hansen, 1997). For example, when I was a school nurse in a part of the United States that had taken in many Hmong people who wanted to emigrate, I had been given some education as to their beliefs. One day a child came to school with small burn marks along his spine. Some might have thought that the parents were abusing the small child by burning him with what looked like it might have been a cigarette, but the child had been burned on certain acupuncture meridian points to heal the cold sore on his lip. Although other treatments for cold sores are less physically harmful, the parents' intent was not to harm but to heal. It is important that the traditional paradigm be understood before passing judgments on healing practices, including the use of herbs.

The tension between the herbal practices of those of the traditional paradigm and those of the biomedical paradigm is often fanned by the interaction and sometimes, collision, of the two paradigms. In my experience, people respect and use their own herbal traditions and like to learn from other traditions, too. People like to learn about the herbal science of the biomedical world as well. They often seek information about all options from both paradigms, especially for chronic conditions; health promotion; and day-to-day discomfort, such as minor pain. Biomedical practitioners who understand as much as possible about their patients' belief systems and what their traditional use of plants is like can better develop a healing and helping relationship with their patients when they seek help from the biomedical world. Because of their extensive history of use and their prevalence in contemporary societies, plant therapies continue to be an ever-present part of the traditional health care practices of the people. As countries continue to address the struggle to provide health care for all, traditional healers are becoming more valuable each day. They are part of the integration process and have begun to provide primary health care. WHO training with those of the traditional paradigm to provide primary health care, "produced positive changes in healers, their clients, and modern health staff" (Hoff, 1992, p. 182). Nurses must consider that, in the near future, they will most likely find themselves providing their healing and caring service alongside traditional practitioners with varying health belief systems, if they are not already doing so.

Plants and the Nursing Paradigm

How can plants be used in caring for and comforting people? That is the question of the nursing paradigm. The biomedical paradigm includes the curing or taking away of disease; the traditional paradigm focuses on the balancing of symptoms. The focus of the nursing paradigm is caring and comfort. Caring is an expression of self and its expression is influenced by culture. Comfort too is related to feelings about self and is often related to cultural and subcultural norms. Plant use is influenced by cultural traditions and practices. How nurses view the use of plants as therapies, remedies, and medicines depends not only on their personal culture but also their professional culture.

For instance, nurses in China have included in their three-year curriculum the subject of "native medicine," TCM, and acupuncture. The nurses in the intensive care units in China are familiar with a "unique aspect of care . . . the use of a Chinese herbal medicine called *don-sen* for intravenous infusion" (Chang, 1983, p. 391). The herbal infusion is used in cases of myocardial infarction and is reported to have a positive effect on dilation of coronary arteries. Nurses whose education includes the use of plant therapies regard plants as part of their practice. Nurses practicing in countries such as China work in health care systems that have integrated the use of traditional and biomedical paradigms.

Historically, nurses have used plants in their caring for and comforting of patients. Although some nurses may have disregarded the use of plants in exchange for more technologic knowledge of the biomedical world, plants are still an active part of nursing practice. The primary reason plants are an active part of practice is because the people who are the focus of nursing work use plants actively in their own self-care practices.

Nurses are mindful of the cultural beliefs and practices of their patients. Nurses understand the reverence for nature and natural healing methods, including the use of plants, just as they understand the values of the biomedical paradigm. Nurses have the best of both worlds, so to speak. For example, nurses can learn from patients, as an ethnobotanist would learn in the field, about the traditional uses of plant therapies. Nurses also can have access to the most recent discoveries about the biochemistry of the plant's active constituents. The nurse is perfectly positioned to bring together knowledge of plants from both the biomedical and traditional paradigms. Merging of this knowledge is an example of the integrative nursing approach.

Integrative nursing has been defined as "the creation of evolving, healing relationships with patients. The nurse observes the patient's need for greater harmony and balance in their life and then addresses those needs by offering care that is a holistic blend of biomedical and caring modalities" (Libster, 2001, p. 26). In applying the integrative nursing approach to the use of plant therapies, nurses first seek to understand the patient's use of herbs for health and healing. Then the nurse creates ways of working with the patient that include using herbs as a caring modality or biomedical intervention. For example, the nurses in the intensive care unit in China have an integrated understanding of the traditional and biomedical use of some plants. They also have an understanding of intravenous therapy and the related nursing considerations. The Chinese nurses have the opportunity to create a holistic blend of caring, biomedical, and traditional modalities for healing the patient with myocardial infarction.

Another example is the research that nurses have done on the use of bran supplement with prune juice and applesauce for discomfort related to constipation in the elderly. Biomedicine has produced evidence that high intake of fiber can have a laxative effect in people. Plant substances such as bran, prune juice, and other high-fiber foods have been used traditionally by some people in self-care for constipation. In one study, the bran supplement was suggested for use along with the standard bowel management program used in the elderly residents of a health care facility. Nurses decided not only to use the traditional remedies but also to study their effects as well. The quasi-experimental study found that the inclusion of the bran supplement resulted in a significant reduction in overall use of laxatives among the elderly patients (Gibson, Opalka, Moore, Brady, & Mion, 1995).

Nurses research patients' self-care practices and folk remedies as well. One phenomenological study entitled "Understanding Ethnic Women's Experiences with Pharmacopeia" found that among women who used folk remedies such as herbs, foods, and over-the-counter medicines, the actual remedies were not as critical to the care of the person who was ill as the "meaning of the cultural memories inherent in acts of caring" (Davis, 1997, p. 425). This raises an important issue for caregivers. The demonstration of caring, how the herbs are prepared and applied, may be of vital importance to the overall effectiveness of the remedy, perhaps even more important than the biochemical constituents in the plant.

Plant therapies continue to be developed as part of nursing practice. In England and the United States, for example, aromatherapy, the use of the essential oils of aromatic plants, continues to be researched and used in clinical practice (Buckle, 1999; Burns, Blamey, Erdder, Lloyd, & Barnetson, 2000). Herbal essential oils are suggested for use in therapeutic massage and baths as inhalation therapy; in addition, they occasionally are recommended for oral use by patients. Herbs have been used extensively in midwifery practice in several countries (Belew, 1999; Bunce, 1987; Ehudin-Pagano, Paluzzi, Ivory, & McCartney, 1987; McFarlin, Gibson, O'Rear, & Harman, 1999). One nurse writes, "Herbal medicine is not a modern, faddish, late 20th century phenomena, but rather one which is established, culturally diverse and sophisticated" (Stapleton, 1995, p. 148).

Because of the nature of their work, community health nurses in particular are encouraged to integrate cultural concerns and activities into their care plans as a means of gaining trust and building healing relationships with patients. Some of the botanical home remedies used for common ailments found during an ethnographic study of the health culture of rural blacks in Virginia are onion syrup, lemon, catnip, ginger, cabbage leaf, potato, tobacco, mullein, flaxseed, and aloe (Roberson, 1987). Community health nurses often see the traditional uses of plant remedies first hand and are ideally positioned to integrate cultural and traditional considerations into their care plans.

"Over the past three decades, there has been a gradual conceptual shift from nursing as a biomedically driven discipline to a more socioculturally informed discipline. . . . Human beings, as defined in nursing, are integrated wholes and are not distinct from their culture, sociopolitical values, family, biology, genetics, physiology, and societal attributions" (Meleis, 1996, p. 4). It is a natural transition for nurses to begin to integrate plant therapies that are linked to sociocultural traditions into their caring work with patients. That integration can mean providing herb information to patients from a broad knowledge base that includes evidence from both biomedical and traditional paradigms. For some nurses, integration of plant therapies also may mean that they begin to explore the clinical uses of herbs in practice and to design research studies with herbs that will better inform professional nursing care in the future.

An Integrative Paradigm for Plant Use

The concept of using plant therapies as part of nursing practice is certainly not new. As has been discussed, caregivers, including nurses, have used and continue to use plants as part of healing work.

What may be different is the concept of integrating plant with biomedical therapies into current nursing practice in conventional health care settings.

THE VISION OF THE WORLD HEALTH ORGANIZATION:

Integration has been initiated by the World Health Organization's Traditional Medicine Programme. The Alma Ata Declaration of 1978 marked the beginning of a health policy with a goal of health for all in the spirit of social justice. Alma Ata accepted the *primary health care (PHC)* approach defined as "essential health care based on practical, scientifically sound, and socially acceptable methods and technology made universally accessible to individuals and families in the community through their full participation and at a cost that the community and country can afford to maintain at every stage of their development in the spirit of self-reliance and self-determination" (Barnes et al., 1995, p. 8). PHC is not to be confused with the concept of primary care, which is a health care delivery system stressing first contact and maintenance care. PHC has been implemented with the intent of increasing accessibility of affordable health care. Alma Ata also recognized "traditional medical practitioners and birth attendants as important allies in organizing efforts to improve health of the community and recommend that proven traditional remedies should be incorporated in national programmes for the provision of essential drugs for primary health care" (Baba, Akerele, & Kawaguchi, 1992, p. 64). Resolution WHA44.34 of the 44th World Health Assembly urged member states (i.e., countries participating in WHO) to, "identify activities leading to cooperation between those providing traditional medicine and modern health care, respectively, especially in regards to the use of scientifically proven safe and effective traditional remedies to reduce national drug costs" (Baba, Akerele, & Kawaguchi, 1992, p. 65).

For years, WHO and its Traditional Medicine Programme have been pursuing the goal of cooperation between traditional and biomedical practitioners primarily in third world countries. Primary health care is the foundation for this cooperation. Is there a role for nurses in achieving this vision? In 1985, the WHO executive board concluded that the role of nurses "would move from the hospital to everyday life in the community, that nurses would become resources to people, rather than to physicians, and that nurses would become leaders and managers of PHC teams, including supervising nonprofessional community health workers" (Barnes et al., 1995, p. 8). Nurses have an important role to play in the furthering of the plan of primary health care and health for all. Nurses therefore play an important role in cooperating with traditional healers and integrating plant therapies with biomedical services as deemed appropriate for the unique needs of their communities.

A WHO report identifies the advantages of integration of biomedical and traditional healing systems as the following:

- Improving general health care knowledge for the greater welfare of mankind
- Providing wider and more efficient population coverage
- Enhancing the quality and numbers of practitioners
- Promoting dissemination of PHC knowledge
- Providing a means of achieving the goal of health care for all

Some of the obstacles to integration include lack of interest, fear of harmful effects of traditional medicines, doubting the results of integrated trainings, resistance to change by advocates of biomedical or traditional systems, and fear of litigation (WHO, 1978). There have been obstacles to the approach, which ultimately leads to some type of greater recognition of the importance of traditional healing systems, including herbal medicines. In the 1970s, "some medical circles sarcastically denigrated WHO with lead headlines in their journals announcing that the Organization had sold its soul to the 'witch doctors'" (Baba, Akerele, & Kawaguchi, 1992, p. 73). Baba et al. (1992) note that there has been tremendous growth in the acceptance of herbal and other traditional health practices since the early 1970s.

Some nurses are already involved in the integration process in community centers. In the United States, for example, Native American healers in the southwest and indigenous healers in Hawaii participate in the programs of their community health centers led by nurses. In South Africa, new historical research clearly outlines the evolving role of the nurse as a "culture broker . . . whose work was at the intersection of two healthcare worlds . . . they acted as a bridge between the 'modern' western medical model of their training and the African 'traditional' medicine of their patients" (Digby & Sweet, in press).

What actually happens with integration can differ from place to place and nurse to nurse. Bodeker (1995, p. 232) suggests that there are four possible relationships between biomedical and traditional medicine.

1. The health care system can be "monopolistic" where physicians have the sole right to practice medicine.
2. Relationships can be "tolerant" where traditional practitioners freely practice without official recognition and agree not to claim to be medical doctors.
3. There can be a "parallel" relationship, such as exists in India, in which both systems are officially recognized and provide services to patients through equal but separate systems.
4. There can be an "integrated" relationship such as in China where traditional and biomedical systems merge in educational and practice settings.

The question still remains whether or not full integration of traditional and biomedical systems is truly the ultimate answer in health care. For example, one patient who trusts their community elder healer implicitly might not be as comfortable going to that practitioner if the healer had been trained in primary health care (Hoff & WHO, 1995) and had become part of a government-sponsored facility that only allowed the practitioner to use herbs that had been scientifically proven by biomedical standards as set forth in WHO guidelines.

Or vice versa, patients used to being given medications for their asthma might think it odd if their practitioner started recommending acupuncture and herbs. Does the full integration of traditional and biomedical health practices mean that health will become increasingly medicalized? For instance, because the biomedical paradigm is primarily focused on the eradication of disease, will the only herbal applications used in a clinic be those that are approved and proven to treat disease? What would happen to the practice of using herbs for promoting health and longevity? Biomedicine does have a history of "establishing claims to expertise and authority over many areas of life not viewed as medical in other cultures or at other times" (Hufford, 1997, p. 81). The question might be raised about the ability of traditional healers to maintain their individuality within the sphere of conventional medicine if chiropractors and nurses have difficulty maintaining their individuality (Hufford, 1997, p. 82).

Having worked in a clinic with many complementary therapies practitioners, it was my experience that the biomedical practices were often viewed by some team members as superior. The belief was that biomedical practices were to be offered first before traditional practices such as herbal medicine. Some practitioners with a strict biomedical paradigm that focuses on safety and efficacy, may erroneously believe that they must be the gatekeepers to complementary therapies such as herbal medicine. Although they may be well intended, this type of monopolistic approach couched in an expressed desire for integration serves only to alienate patients, traditional practitioners, and biomedical practitioners who are seeking integration without a belief in the superiority of the biomedical health care paradigm.

Biomedical practitioners are starting to understand that they can best serve the consumers of health care when they recognize their own paradigm for what it is—a set of cultural beliefs—and create roundtable discussions about what approaches may be best for an individual patient. The Amish community in the United States, which has chosen what to accept and not accept from the technological world, is an example of an integrative approach. The Amish are able to keep the phone outside the house for emergencies and not have it inside the house where a call might just interrupt their dinner or time with family. This is a healthy expression of a sense of boundaries.

There must be a strong honoring of people's boundaries on the part of both biomedical and traditional practitioners. In an integrated setting, there is no room for ethnocentrism, which only undermines the ultimate goal of health care for all.

INTEGRATIVE INSIGHT:

The understanding of the different plant paradigms and how they interact is operationalized on two occasions: when a nurse enters into a healing relationship with someone using plant therapies and when the nurse learns about an herb from the media, colleagues, educational programs, and books. This text presents information on a number of plants (see chapters 7–18). Both traditional and biomedical sources are used in these chapters to facilitate the development of an integrated knowledge base for the use of plant therapies.

Nurses also experience the interaction of different plant paradigms when they care for patients who have been successfully practicing the integration of herbal and biomedical therapies for many years. Patients are often very adept at integration because often their only goal for health care is to get their needs met. The way that their needs are met may be inconsequential; so they use whatever modality works. Nurses can learn much from their patients about integration.

Regardless of whether nurses have knowledge of herbs or their integration with biomedical therapies, they do have an excellent foundation for the study and practice of herbal medicine. There are some philosophical similarities between herbal and nursing practice. Herbal medicine focuses on concepts of *symptom patterns* and *pattern recognition*. A holistic assessment is completed and the recognition of the symptom pattern is what leads to herb and application choice. Nursing too focuses on the importance of pattern. The writings of Martha Rogers and Margaret Newman provide clear descriptions of the importance of understanding pattern when engaging in a healing relationship with a patient. Pattern is described by Rogers as, "the distinguishing characteristic of an energy field . . . it is an abstraction. . . . Pattern is not directly observable. However, manifestations of field patterning are observable events in the real world. The implications of this for increased individualization of nursing services are explicit" (Rogers, 1992, pp. 30–31).

Margaret Newman (1994) defines pattern as "information that depicts the whole, understanding of the meaning of all the relationships at once. An understanding of pattern is basic to an understanding of health. . . . Pattern recognition comes from within the observer" (pp. 71, 73). Understanding pattern is also the foundation of the herbal assessment of many traditions, to recognize the patterns, relationships and whole picture of health so that a holistic, individualized plan of care can be implemented with a patient.

Other theories, such as the Roy Adaptation Model of nursing (1984), outline symptom-sign assessments that include behaviors assessed by an herbal practitioner such as a TCM practitioner. Both Adaptation Model and TCM practitioners assess health patterns such as energy level, nutritional and fluid intake, elimination, skin, sleep and rest, and emotions to name a few. Practitioners of herbal medicine use a clinically based system of assessment that includes such methods as pulse, tongue, and face diagnosis along with extensive history taking, symptom-sign pattern recognition, and discussion of concerns with patients. The assessment is then matched with the personality of plants. The clinical assessment allows the practitioner to create a unique picture of a patient and then match that picture with the herbs necessary to, in a sense, balance that picture. This type of clinical assessment and pattern recognition represents "biological individuality rather than a standardized nosology. In clinical science, systems of correspondence, that is, whole system models are used as a foundation for practice. Using a whole system model as a foundation for clinical practice makes mastery of botanical medicine, or any therapeutic modality possible" (Kenner, 1998, p. 54). The nursing models mentioned here emphasize wholeness. Nursing process and theories can be used as a foundation for the study of plant therapies. Learning herbal medicine theory such as is part of TCM is often a smooth transition for nurses who have studied nursing theory based on wholeness models.

Reading through this book of plant therapies may induce you to ask how herbs might be integrated into a nursing practice based on biomedicine and technology and caring. In general, the way any caring modality is integrated with biomedical skills is through the creativity of the nurse (Libster, 2001). But before nurses can be creative and integrate all of their skills in a way that uniquely addresses the needs of a patient, they must first have the skills. Before nurses attempt to integrate herbal therapies into practice they must have an understanding of the art and science of the modality. The nurse must have education in herbal therapies.

As with all caring modalities, critical decision making, reflection, and the nurse-patient relationship help determine the appropriateness of the use of herbal therapies with a patient. Nurses educated in both herbal therapies and conventional, biomedically based nursing have a foundation for the successful integration of the two modalities. Nursing's history reveals that using teas and topicals were common among nursing duties. Nurses who are beginning the integration process might consider learning first about the use of herbs in tea form and in topical applications, such as baths and compresses.

Integration is possible. An example of successful integration can be found at hospitals such as the Herdecke Klinic in Germany where nurses provide herbal applications as taught in the Anthroposophical nursing tradition. Anthroposophy is a type of nature-based health care started in Europe in the early 1900s. The nurses who receive their education at the Herdecke Klinic have the option of choosing to take an additional 40 hours of education in herbal compresses and packs and another 80 hours in rhythmical Einreibungen (a type of massage using embrocation). German nurses are not required to study herbs. Nurses who work at Herdecke Klinic are not required to have had the training or be able to provide herbal therapies, but many of the patients who go to the hospital (over 450 beds) may request herbal treatments if their hospital stay permits. Nurses who are knowledgeable of the different herbal applications provide the therapies after consulting with the patient's physician. The nurse makes recommendations to the physician, and the physician must provide the final consent for herbal treatment of the patient under German law (personal communication, Mathias Bertram, May 2000).

Determining how herbal therapies might be integrated into the nursing practice of the twenty-first century is a challenge nurses will face when seeking to provide quality health care that is accessible to all. The pursuit of integration and cooperation between biomedicine and tradition in the use of herbs for patient care necessitates reflection. There is a point during reflection when a certain synergy can occur and a greater understanding of the potential of healing herbs can emerge. It is through this integrative insight that a new spectrum of herbal art and science can manifest, transcending that which has already been viewed through the prism of the current biomedical and traditional paradigms.

CHAPTER 4
Carefulness and Conservation

W HEN NURSES GATHER INFORMATION ABOUT HEALING plants from biomedical and traditional sources, they find that each paradigm has certain recommendations for the wise or safe use of each plant. This includes appropriate choice of plants for an individual, appropriate amount, appropriate form or application, and appropriate time for use. The cautious use of plant therapies is not unlike the nurse's "five rights" of administering pharmaceutical drugs. Biomedical and traditional healers alike give cautionary information related to the use of plants. For example, a botanist might warn that excessive ingestion of comfrey *(Symphytum officinale)* can potentially lead to hepatotoxicity because of the amount of pyrrolizidine alkaloids, and a traditional healer might recommend that a particular plant only be harvested in a special area.

Nurses must be aware not only of the types of plants that grow in the areas where they live but also of the wise and safe use of the plants in their area. Many plant medicines have been used traditionally within the ritual practices of a particular society. It also is possible that the plant medicine is not the same if the plant is used outside of the rituals of that society. The cautions related to the use of the plant may change as the information about the medicinal use of a particular plant is transmitted across cultures. Because plants and their specific cautionary issues vary greatly from place to place, the cautions presented here are general guidelines related to the use of plant therapies. Safety cannot be completely ensured even under the best of circumstances. Children of responsible parents still run out in the road; campfires get out of control; and, despite the safety strategies put in place by communities and the good intentions of well-meaning people, medicines still cause illness, even death, rather than promoting health and life. People who would use herbs responsibly must be careful and not rely solely upon external safety standards and guidelines to direct their health care decisions. Being cautious means using inner wisdom, insight, and common sense in choosing how and when to use an herb. Herbal therapies are best evaluated for an individual person and his or her needs for healing and care. Both biomedicine and tradition support an individualized approach as the foundation for the wise and safe use of herbs.

Biomedicine may have evidence of a particular plant substance being helpful in laboratory studies, but this does not mean that an individual will benefit from the use of that plant. The response of a person to any healing intervention or modality, such as herbs, is unique. Laboratory and clinical studies provide general information, but the practitioner and the patient must always be mindful of the potential for a unique response to an herbal application. In addition, just because a plant is used medicinally by hundreds of people in New Zealand, for example, does not mean that a person in Scandinavia can use the plant without caution. Responses to plant remedies can be as similar or diverse as the people within a particular country. Hypothetically, if a healing plant is a foreigner to a particular country, it is possible that the people of that country will have no biologic history with the plant and its constituents and may have an entirely different response to the plant than those who live where the plant has been grown and used for many years.

Safety Standards and Control

As a healing modality, plant therapies have been shown through scientific study and hundreds of years of traditional use to be quite safe. "Based on published reports, side effects or toxic reactions associated with herbal medicines in any form are rare. . . . Clearly, then, herbal medicines do not present any more of a problem with respect to acting as potential allergenic agents following human ingestion than any other class of widely used foods or drugs" (Farnsworth, 1993, p. 36C-D). Herb safety is related however to the use of the plant and the knowledge base of the user. Potential risks are associated with using plants as ornaments, let alone as foods and medicines. If someone were walking in the woods and thought stinging nettle *(Urtica doica)* leaves were perfect for an arrangement of wild flowers, they would be surprised when they touched the leaf. The plant causes, just as its common name implies, a stinging sensation to the skin when touched. Although traditionally people have not been known to pick nettle for ornamental reasons, there is a possibility it could happen. The concern, and sometimes the conflict, between the scientists and the people is how safe use with nettle or any herb is addressed. How extensive should the controls on a plant be? Should all stinging nettle be exterminated because of its potential to sting a hiker in the woods? How do communities and governments make decisions to protect the public from the potential harm from plants, and how great is the risk from plants, really? It is the responsibility of every individual using a plant as medicine and therapy to exercise prudent care. This includes using a common sense approach to taking herbs and understanding that the complexity of whole plants is a safety feature of herbalism.

COMMON SENSE AND COMPLEXITY:

Having common sense is a very important component of one's ability to be cautious. The wise and safe use of herbs often depends on the user's common sense. Common sense is defined as "sound and prudent but often unsophisticated judgment" (Merriam-Webster, 1999). People do not have to have extensive formal herbal education to be able to reason about how they might use an herb. They can access their common sense. Common sense, if it is not repressed, can be helpful in determining the appropriateness of an herb for the individual and the amount that can be tolerated. Common sense is demonstrated as an intuition or insight related to a particular experience. For example, if someone decided to eat cayenne pepper *(Capsicum frutescens)* to improve circulation, but they took it in capsule form, they could block one way that commonly has been used to measure dose—taste. Taste and other sensory experiences can activate one's common sense. If a person eats whole cayenne peppers and experiences the hot spicy taste of the herb they would, at some point, say, "I think I've had enough." Another example of the importance of using the common sense approach to tasting herbs can be found in the reports of the use of chaparral *(Larrea tridentata)* for cancer. Chaparral has a very unpleasant taste. And yet the three people reported to experience symptoms of liver toxicity related to chaparral ingestion were probably able to take high doses of the herb because they took it in tablet or capsule form (Gordon, Rosenthal, Hart, Sirota, & Baker, 1995; *Morbidity and Mortality Weekly Report [MMWR]*, 1992). Perhaps if they had taken chaparral in tea form, they might not have had the liver toxicity problems because they could have regulated their intake based upon toleration of the taste of the herb. There is one clinical study of patients with terminal cancer who received 16 to 24 ounces of chaparral tea *(Larrea divericata)* per day and the participants who drank the tea did not show any signs of liver toxicity (Smart, Hogle, Vogel, Broom, & Bartholomew, 1970). The difference in responses between the situations may be due to the difference in therapeutic application, species tea versus powdered herb, or the dose; but it is also possible that how an herb is used can potentially have an effect on the ability of the five senses and common sense to provide the necessary safety feedback to the user. Herbs are safer when the user allows them to provide their sensory experience. Common sense works best when the plant is experienced fully by the senses. Taste, smell, vision, and tactile sensation are all important to the proper identification of an herb and its safe use. Common sense can be our own personal, natural regulatory agency!

Complexity is another reason plant therapies are relatively safe. Plants are made up of many different biochemical constituents. Used in whole form, whether decocted as tea or used as an extract or salve, the action of plant therapies is very complex. Most of the chemical constituents occur in very small amounts. When people use herbs, they are taking small doses of particular substances. These substances are in a natural, not synthetic, state and are in formulation as they occur in nature. If people have been shown to take herbs in their natural complex form over a lengthy period of time without toxicity or unhealthy effects, then the herb can be said to be relatively safe. Safe use of a plant does not necessarily mean that it is effective, however. Safety and efficacy are separate issues.

In biomedicine, a single substance remedy is most often used in the treatment of a disease identified through the diagnostic process. Because herbs are complex they can be used in a different way than pharmaceutical drugs in the care of patients. Herbs do not have to be used to target one organ or a specific disease. Herbalism is similar to nursing in that the focus of helping the patient can be to address the patient's *illness* as a whole experience rather than reduce that experience to a disease.

Illness is the total patient response to disease. In the biomedical paradigm, peptic ulcer, for example, is a specific problem related to a specific area of the body. Diseases, such as peptic ulcer, are usually defined or diagnosed by one set of symptoms. All patients with ulcer *disease* are viewed as having the same ulcer *illness*. Herbalism, like nursing, makes a distinction between disease and illness. "Disease refers to a problem that the practitioner views from the biomedical model, in biological terms, as an alteration in structure or function. Illness, on the other hand, is the human experience of symptoms and suffering, and refers to how the disease is perceived, lived with, and responded to by patients and families" (Curtin & Lubkin, 1998, p. 3). The illness addressed by the herbalist is the unique patient's feelings and responses to disharmony of body, mind, and spirit. In herbalism, two people with ulcer disease do not have the same illness.

For instance, in Chinese herbal medicine, an herbal formula for the symptom pattern of illness associated with the biomedical diagnosis of ulcer might warm and dispel "cold" in the organs in the middle of the body (e.g., the stomach). Or a formula for clearing heat from the organs in the middle of the body might be used. The difference in choice of herb formula that will either warm or clear heat from the middle of the body, rests in the determination of a thermal quality of the symptom pattern or illness as the person describes it. Ulcer-type symptoms can, from a holistic herbal perspective, be thermally hot or cold, and the herbs given for treatment would therefore be quite different.

Working with biochemically complex herbs from a holistic perspective allows one to deal with the complexities of an entire illness pattern. To work holistically, the practitioner must customize the remedy for the patient, thereby increasing the safety of the remedy. Clinical herbalists, naturopaths, and traditional Chinese herbalists specialize in the treatment of illness with herbs from this holistic perspective.

SAFETY IN REFERRAL:

Practitioners of herbal medicine, such as doctors of oriental medicine, naturopathic physicians, and clinical herbalists, have extensive education and experience in individualizing herbal therapy for patients. If a person using herbs has a concern about self-medicating with an herb, the most prudent and supportive action for a nurse who does not have education and/or experience in herbal therapies may be to refer the patient to one of these skilled practitioners.

In general, it is wise and safe practice for nurses to consider referring a patient to a herbal practitioner when:

1. The patient is considering taking the herb for the treatment of a health concern or taking any particular herb for more than thirty days (perhaps less, depending upon the individual).
2. The patient taking medicinal amounts of herbs is pregnant, elderly, or is an infant less than fifteen months old.
3. The patient is taking pharmaceutical drugs and herbal remedies simultaneously to treat a specific biomedically diagnosed condition.

Nurses who want to refer to an herbal practitioner can use a strategy similar to that which they would use when referring to any type of specialist. Identifying an appropriate person to refer to can begin by asking questions such as the following (Libster, 1999):

1. What is the herbal practitioner's education and experience? Do they have a specific model for practice that they follow such as traditional Chinese medicine (TCM)?
2. Is the practitioner certified from a formal education program or does the practitioner hold a national certification, if available?

3. Does the herbal practitioner belong to any professional organizations and demonstrate a professional demeanor to which you would expose your patients?
4. Does the practitioner communicate well and is he or she willing to communicate with you?

Nurses who decide to work with patients using herbs and who do not refer to herbal practitioners may take on one or both of the following roles related to herbal therapies. One, the nurse provides information about herbal therapies to patients in the course of discussing health decisions. Two, nurses integrate the use of plant therapies into their own practice and make recommendations for the use of herbs in relation to helping patients adapt to and cope with illness. Regardless of the role the nurse takes in working with patients using herbs, the cautions discussed in this chapter must be considered.

THE MYTH OF "NO RISK":

Some people believe that because a plant remedy is natural that it is safe to use. You may have heard patients actually say that they believe that an herb is safe because it is natural. Nurses often discuss the benefits and risks of a particular intervention with a patient. There are benefits and risks associated with every plant use, especially when one considers that each patient is an individual. Most of the risk of using a plant as medicine or therapy has to do with improper use or amount of herb used. Paracelsus is quoted as having said that "the only difference between medicine and poison is the dose." Dr. Jim Duke, former lead botanist for the U.S. government, writes, "There are probably safe, medicinal, toxic, and lethal doses for all chemicals, natural and synthetic" (Duke, 2000, www.ars-grin.gov/duke/syllabus/module15.htm).

The word "toxic" is taken from the Greek word "toxikon," meaning "poison for arrows" (Mann, 1992). Many cultures have described the use of plants as poison, and not just from the tips of arrows. Socrates (469–399 B.C.E.), after being convicted of corrupting youth and interfering with the religion of the city of Athens, drank poison hemlock *(Conium maculatum),* and died. Although some plants can be deadly, a plant is not labeled toxic or poisonous just because it contains a specific toxic constituent.

> *In order for a plant to be functionally poisonous, however, it must not only contain a toxic secondary compound but also possess effective means of presenting that compound to an animal in sufficient concentration, and the secondary compound must be capable of overcoming whatever physiological or biochemical defenses the animal may possess against it. Thus the presence of a known poison principle, even in toxicologically significant amounts, in a plant does not automatically mean that either man or a given species of animal will ever be effectively poisoned by that plant (Kingsbury, 1979, p. 2).*

Think about tobacco and how deadly it has been shown to be. Alcohol can be deadly also. Even water has been shown to kill people when taken in excess. Yet smoking cigarettes, drinking alcoholic beverages, and consuming water are not known for routinely causing death and therefore are not banned by regulatory agencies.

Establishing toxicity is not a simple matter. "The toxicology of any substance is based on a number of variables: The chemistry of the substance, the dosage, the biochemical individuality of the person ingesting the substance, and any other drugs or foods that might be taken during or near the time of ingestion" (HerbClip, 1994). There are ethical concerns in trying to create data to publish the lethal dose of a substance. Because whole herbs and products are relatively nontoxic, not a lot of data are available regarding toxic amounts of medicinal plants. In 1998 in the United States, "about 100 people died after ingesting common, ordinary nuts. In the same period, fewer than 100 Americans died after consuming an herb in some form, and more than 90% of these people were intentionally abusing certain of the more potent members of our herbal pharmacy" (Duke, 1999, p. 3).

One way to determine the toxicity of a chemical constituent of a plant is by studying the amount (mg/kg) of the substance needed to kill 50% of the mice in a particular population. The result of the study is stated as the median lethal dose (LD_{50}). These numbers are not given to complex substances such as those found in whole plants, so they are often not helpful in herbal medicine. But, to establish perspective about the toxicity of plant substances, it is often helpful to know that the LD_{50} of caffeine, a substance many people take into their bodies everyday, is 192 mg/kg and the LD_{50} of carotatoxin (a substance found in garden carrot *Daucus carota*) is 100 mg/kg (Duke, 2000, www.ars-grin.gov/duke/dosage.html). For a 50 kg person to be poisoned from the caffeine in a cup of coffee containing 48 mg of caffeine, the person would need to drink 200 cups of coffee. The LD_{50} of 192 or 100 is quite low. Many plant constituents found in medicinal plants have significantly higher median lethal doses. To clarify, a higher LD_{50} means that it takes more of the substance to become toxic and a lower LD_{50} means that it takes less of the substance to become toxic. Many people ingest caffeine-containing beverages all the time, and although it may not be the healthiest practice, no deaths have resulted.

Another source of toxicity data is the list that botanists create of those plants that are generally recognized as safe (GRAS), generally recognized as food (GRAF), and generally recognized as poisonous (GRAP). There are limitations to the usefulness of this classification system. A plant may have constituents that are each classified differently. "There are probably carcinogens, mutagens, and poisons, as well as anticarcinogens, antimutagens, and antidotes in all GRAF, GRAP, and GRAS species. . . . Apples are GRAF, and their extracts are GRAS but the cyanide in the seeds are GRAP" (Duke, 1992, intro). Because of the complexity of plants, this system may not really be helpful to people making regulatory decisions based on a specific classification system.

Establishing toxicity of all medicinal plants used by humans is not a simple matter, scientifically speaking. Numerous specialists including botanists and clinical toxicologists would be needed to accomplish the task. Practically speaking, it is debatable whether or not establishing toxicity of plants is very helpful data anyway. A plant may contain a certain toxin that does not cause any problem to a human when ingested. "Toxicity is rarely an all-or-none phenomenon. Species of plants vary in their content of toxic compounds owing to unpredictable extrinsic and genetic factors. Vertebrate species and individual animals vary in susceptibility" (Kingsbury, 1979, p. 5). Toxicity often comes down to a matter of individual dose, right use, and common sense.

So often practitioners write that herbs are horribly understudied, completely unregulated, and have serious potential for toxicity. This is just not the case. The track record of herbal medicines has been evaluated and has been found to "not present a major problem with regard to toxicity. . . . In fact, of all classes of substances reported to cause toxicities of sufficient magnitude to be reported in the United States, plants are the least problematic" (Farnsworth, 1993, p. 36H). There is a huge body of literature on medicinal plants as well as centuries of use in health care systems. Herbs also are regulated in many countries; however, they may not be regulated in the same way as pharmaceutical drugs.

Although many health practitioners in the biomedical paradigm may believe that the system of pharmaceutical drug regulation is the gold standard in ensuring safety with herbal products, the literature does not support this. In the United States, where pharmaceutical drugs are highly regulated, researched, and monitored for safe use, a metanalysis of the incidence of adverse drug reactions in hospitalized patients reported that in 1994, 106,000 patients died from adverse drug reactions and 2,216,000 had serious adverse drug reactions. Adverse drug reactions to *drugs that are properly prescribed and administered* were the fourth to sixth leading cause of death in the country (Lazarou, Pomeranz, & Corey, 1998). The researchers have noted that the adverse drug reaction problem is much the same worldwide and that the incidence has remained stable over the last 30 years. In Hong Kong, for example, where herbal medicines are used quite often, it was reported that 0.2% of general hospital admissions were due to adverse reactions to Chinese herbal medicines as compared with 4.4% of admissions due to adverse reactions to Western drugs (Chan, Chan, & Critchley, 1992).

Rigorous drug standards and controls also have not had much impact on the potential toxic effects of the common, over-the-counter medication, acetaminophen. One study published in the *New England Journal of Medicine* revealed that in one urban hospital alone from 1992 to 1995, 50 patients were reported to have taken acetaminophen during suicide attempts and 21 people accidentally poisoned themselves while attempting to relieve pain (Schiodt, Rochling, Casey, & Lee, 1997, p. 1112). Although some claim that herbs are underregulated in the United States and therefore potentially unsafe, the Food and Drug Administration (FDA) and the herb and supplement industry have been very active in promoting the proper marketing and regulation of herbs. Nurses also might ask what the FDA and biomedicine are doing about the excessive number of deaths related to properly prescribed and administered drugs in hospitals.

One of the roles of the FDA is to evaluate reports of adverse reactions to foods, drugs, and herbs along with other products marketed for human consumption. Some have suggested that adverse reactions to herbs are underreported. Therefore, the FDA has set up a telephone hotline to facilitate reporting. This is a public reporting site, and the detail and accuracy needed to conduct scientific analysis have not been present. The data collected and used by the FDA have been called unreliable and unsubstantiated by the U.S. General Accounting Office (Treasure, 2000, p. 9).

Any nurse who has ever worked on a hotline service, such as at a poison control center, learns that when someone calls in to report an adverse reaction to a substance, a scientific line of inquiry is set in motion as a result of the report. The professional who takes the report does not immediately identify or target the substance suggested by the caller as the cause of the reaction. Linking a reaction to a specific substance is not always as easy as it appears.

In order to establish causality, certain criteria should be met. For example, one source identifies consistency, strength, and specificity of the association as being part of the assessment leading to potential judgment of causality. They identify biologic plausibility and evidence from prior experience and consider confounding or other causal factors (Cantox Health Sciences International, 2000). Most importantly with drugs and herbs, the substance taken by an individual must be clearly identified. For example, if a patient sees a practitioner because of a rash they incurred when playing in the woods, and they say that they started to see the rash after rubbing a plant on their skin, one of the responsibilities of the practitioner is to identify the plant the person rubbed on their skin. If the practitioner does not clearly identify the plant, they might say to the patient that it is possible that the plant caused the rash, but a definitive statement should not be made without proper scientific evaluation.

In one example, there were seven cases of anticholinergic poisoning in New York City in 1994 thought by the patients to be due to drinking Paraguay tea or maté *(Ilex paraguariensis)*. When the emergency room staff obtained samples of the tea and it was analyzed by the police department, it was found that the tea was adulterated with belladonna alkaloids, atropine, scopolamine and hyoscyamine, substances not part of the plant (MMWR, 1995). The maté was not the cause of the poisoning reaction; the adulterants were. Drinking this tea is common and customary in a number of cultures. It is important that nurses wait for a full evaluation before discussing the cause of an adverse reaction with a patient when it may be related to their use of an herb, especially when the herb is a part of a culture's healing traditions.

The purpose of regulation is to promote the safest possible use of the substance. It has been proposed that the safety of a medicinal plant not be judged based on information from one source. "Safety or efficacy of a particular drug can rarely be based upon the results of a single study. In contrast, a combination of information indicating that a specific plant has been used in a local health care system for centuries, together with efficacy and toxicity data can help in deciding whether it should be considered acceptable for medicinal use" (Farnsworth, Akerele, Bingle, Soejarto, & Guo, 1985, p. 965). The World Health Organization (WHO) recommends that member states adopt some form of regulation of herbal medicines to address issues of quality, safety, and efficacy. Regulation does not have to be for purposes of control of behavior of people; it also can be established for education purposes.

Nurses often educate parents about safety issues in the home. Each year, several poisonings in which children have ingested the leaves of a house plant are reported to poison control centers. There are no regulations banning people from acquiring house plants. Pediatric health practitioners inform parents of the potential safety issues with house plants so that they are more aware and can put the plants out of the reach of little explorers.

Some of the guidelines presented by WHO regarding the regulation of herbal medicines have to do with assessment of use of herbs and herbal products, evaluation of manufacturing procedures and product labeling, assessment and evaluation of toxic plant materials, and the establishment of a government agency to keep records on herbal medicines in use (WHO, 1998a). The regulation of herbal medicines varies from country to country. Some countries exempt herbal and traditional medicines from regulatory requirements; some are subject to all requirements. Some countries exempt herbal medicines regarding registration and marketing authorization and some require registration (WHO, 1998b). Canada, for instance, has a system whereby the Health Protection Branch of Health Canada regulates plant medicines under its Food and Drug protectorates. It assigns drug identification numbers (DINs) to an herb based on the therapeutic claims (Awang, 1997). Nurses should contact their regulatory agencies to learn more about their countries' laws regarding the safe use of herbs.

Some areas in nursing—for instance, surgical nursing—have been especially concerned about the safety and control of herbal medicines. Nurses who work in preanesthesia and postanesthesia units are particularly concerned about the interactions of herbal medicines and anesthetic drugs. This is not a new concern. In 1998, a report published in the *British Medical Journal* stated that solanaceous glyco-alkaloids found in potatoes, tomatoes and aubergines [eggplant] may slow the metabolism of muscle relaxants and anesthetic agents such as suxamethonium and cocaine (Tanne, 1998, p. 1102). Thus the patient may take five to ten hours recovering from anesthesia rather than the expected forty to ninety minutes. These are foods, but there is a similar concern with herbal medicines.

While nurses and other perioperative health care team members have begun to ask about the herbs patients may be taking before surgery, what nurses and health care team members should do with the information they gather is not clear. If a patient is taking an herbal formula prescribed by a traditional healer, does the nurse tell the patient to stop taking the herbs, and if so, what effect might that have on the outcome of the surgery? Should patients be told to stop taking their herbal remedies used in self-care two weeks before surgery? Will that take care of the potential problem? These kinds of questions present nurses and perioperative team members with an opportunity to use an integrative approach. From an integrative perspective, the practitioner would not simply tell a patient to stop taking an herb. The herb may have significant meaning to the patient's health and well-being.

The benefits and risks and the timing of all interventions, surgery, and herbs need to be discussed with the individual patient. They must be informed that their caregivers do not have all the answers about potential anesthetic drug and herb or food interactions. In light of the statistics on adverse reactions and deaths related to properly prescribed and administered drugs in hospitals, health team members must address the herb-drug interaction carefully, considerately, and integratively.

Plant Potency: Gentle Greens and Powerful Potions

At times, plant medicines are gentle remedies, such as taking a cup of chamomile *(Matricaria recutita)* tea. At other times, as previously discussed, they can be used as poison. It is often a matter of how the plant is used and how much of the plant is used. Plants and their constituents also have been known throughout history to have a synergistic effect, an ability for the total effect be greater than the sum of the individual effects. In traditional Chinese herbal medicine for instance, certain herbs, such as *Angelica sinensis* and *Peoniae lactiflora,* are almost always used in formulation together because of their synergistic effect. Sections of the Chinese *Materia Medica* explain which herbs can best be used together and which herbs should not be used together. This information from China of herb-herb interactions is the result of hundreds of years of use and scientific observation.

Herb-herb interaction information is often found among traditional herbal healers. Knowing which herbs can and cannot be used together is part of the cautionary information associated with medicinal plant use. There are herbs for which this information may not exist. What can be frustrating to the biomedical practitioner is the paucity of information about the interaction of herbs and pharmaceutical drugs. It is known that grapefruit juice *(Citrus paradisi),* for example, does interact with drugs such as felodipine, nifedipine, verapamil, cyclosporin, and triazolam. Human studies have shown that the psoralens and possibly the flavonoid naringenin in grapefruit diminish the first-pass metabolism of the drugs by suppressing a cytochrome P-450 enzyme in the small intestine and thereby increasing drug concentrations (Fuhr, 1998).

Cytochrome P-450 is the major member of the class of enzymes primarily localized in the liver that is involved in the metabolism of many medications. Certain drugs and substances, such as cigarette smoke and estrogens, can *induce* the P-450 system and therefore detoxify chemical substances. Certain drugs like cimetidine and acute alcohol ingestion *inhibit* cytochrome P-450 and therefore may potentiate other chemical substances, including drugs (Boyd & Nihart, 1998, p. 206; Treasure, 2000). Just as there is a potential for drug-drug interactions every time a patient takes more than one medication, there is a possibility for drug-herb interactions that involve the P-450 system. "The interaction of a given compound with the CYP450 system will determine its fate and possible effects in the body" (Treasure, 2000, p. 3).

The individuality of the patient also exists on the molecular level in the cytochrome P-450 system. The range of responses to drugs and herbs is wide. Factors that influence individual expression of the cytochrome P-450 system include gender, age, race, genetics, and hepatic condition. Just because an herb is shown in in vitro studies to affect P-450 in some way, does not necessarily mean that the herb will affect all people in the same way at all times. It is important for nurses to realize that although plants, such as St. John's wort, may *induce* the P-450 system (inducing CYP3A4 in hepatocyte cells), many plants, including St. John's wort, also contain the bioflavonoid quercetin, which is a 3A4 *inhibitor* (personal communication, Duke, April 2001). What happens in the body when both inhibitors and inducers are present in the same herb? Dosage, environmental, and individual factors must be taken into account. Because of the complexity of plant remedies, it may be possible that there are no clinical sequelae in taking herbs with certain drugs. However, it may be possible that certain herbs and drugs should not be taken simultaneously by the same individual. It may also be possible that the body has the ability to sort out all the chemical interactions and produce the response it needs for greater health.

Nurses are aware of the need to be cognizant of the timing of taking drugs. They know that some drugs are best taken with meals and some are best taken on an empty stomach, for example. Giving foods at certain times in relation to meals is often done to reduce gastric distress (Bates & Florit, 1996). Foods, as in the case of grapefruit, also can potentially alter the metabolism of certain medications, making it more difficult to regulate dosage. It is not possible for a drug in clinical trials to be tested against every food there is, so there are certainly gaps in drug-food interaction information. For similar reasons, there are gaps in the information about drug-herb interactions. For the most part, drug-herb interaction data are speculative because the interactions have not been studied and shown to exist in humans or even animals. Drug-herb interactions are often listed as "potential" interactions based on the biomedical data about certain herb constituents (Newall, Anderson, & Phillipson, 1996, pp. 277-280).

From a traditional Chinese medicine (TCM) perspective, all drugs, herbs, and foods are potentially interactive and/or synergistic. Drugs, herbs, and foods are evaluated from an energetic perspective when helping a patient to heal and find greater balance. For example, patients I have seen over the years who are on thyroid medication have a certain pulse profile, a characteristic about their pulse found on pulse diagnosis, that often indicates excess heat in the body. Because I have found through observation that the thyroid medication may be part of the reason for the excess heat, I consider the energetic qualities of the thyroid medication when formulating the proper tea. It would seem that questioning whether herbs, drugs, and foods interact is not as relevant as asking *how* they interact. And if they interact, the most important clinical question for a practitioner and for a patient is, "What do you do now?" The patient and their caregiver must decide if the herb will be used or not and if so, when.

Some biomedical practitioners would have a patient believe that there is no choice regarding the integrative use of medications and herbs or foods that may interact— the patient must have their medication and therefore should avoid a specific food or herb. Occasionally this works pretty well and patients accept that answer, but more recently, patients are not happy when given no alternatives or choices. They want information and choice. Some patients upon hearing from a biomedical practitioner that they have no choice, such as, "You are on this medication now, so do not take any herbal medicines," opt not to take pharmaceutical drugs at all, which can be life threatening. Some patients choose to take herbs and foods because they have a longer record of safe use. They may think that if combining herbs and foods has not been an issue for all these years, then there probably isn't an issue. We need to know much more about individual responses to drugs and drug-herb interactions before drawing definitive conclusions about how herbs and drugs will or will not be integrated in health care.

The Western world is now catching up, as it were, in the integration of herbs with biomedicine. Schools of nursing may want to follow schools of pharmacy in America where, although not required, 74% of programs offer a course in pharmacognosy with material on herbal therapies (Klepser & Klepser, 1999). In herbal education, nurses would focus on using biomedical and traditional data in herbal, clinical applications, rather than on the biochemistry of plants. This is discussed further in chapter 19.

Integration may not mean that every person takes herbs and drugs for an illness, but it does mean that the health care system acknowledges that people use herbal medicines and sometimes prefer them over pharmaceutical drugs. Ancient health care systems such as the Ayurvedic system in India have had centuries to evaluate what time of day is best to take a particular herb for a particular condition and in a particular form. Ayurvedic medicine is just one example of the extent of the art involved in creating a health care system. The study of drug-herb-food interactions is part of the new frontier of creating an integrative health care system that includes the understanding of science and tradition. Practitioners, both traditional and biomedical, need to be very aware that it is no longer sufficient to tell a patient to only follow their biomedical regimen or only take traditional remedies. People want and use both traditional and biomedical therapies, and they need practitioners who have accepted that both will be considered when health care choices must be made.

STANDARDIZATION:

Plant therapies include teas, liquid extracts, poultices, and other applications. A more modern use of plant medicines is in the form of a standardized extract, the benefits of which are controversial among herbal practitioners. A standardized extract is a plant preparation in which the "active component" has been standardized or made uniform from individual product to individual product. This is seen as beneficial by those practitioners working from a biomedical paradigm because of the belief that the active constituents in a plant can be identified, extracted, purified, and standardized, making the remedy more like a pharmaceutical drug than any other plant preparation. Having the plant remedy standardized means that the practitioner can prescribe a specific dose of a "known" active constituent with the benefit of the constituent being in a "natural" form, as compared to synthetic drugs. Many practitioners and patients prefer drugs that are from a natural source.

The ability to produce a standardized herbal medicine rests upon the ability of researchers to identify the active constituent of a plant. In some plants such as senna *(Cassia senna L.),* a plant that has been traditionally used for constipation, an "active constituent" has been identified. In senna, the active constituent that seems to have a bowel irritant or stimulant effect is identified as "sennasides." Standardization of sennasides means for the consumer that taking a certain amount of herbal product should have a laxative effect. Because the sennasides are identifiable, the sennaside constituents can be researched in much the same way a pharmaceutical drug would be.

The controversy is that sennasides are not the whole plant. The history of relatively safe use of senna has to do with the traditional use of the whole leaf, not sennasides. It is also argued that in many plants, the goal of identifying a single constituent is not possible and that the standardization of a plant medicine to a single constituent is therefore misleading in regard to efficacy and safety. One plant researcher writes, "As there are normally more than one (or one type of) active component in a natural product, standardization based on one particular type of chemical component is not representative of the total activity of the product. Consequently, these arbitrarily selected components can only be useful as a 'marker' of product quality. And these 'markers' are only valid for extracts that are total extractions of the herbs concerned" (Leung & Foster, 1996, p. xv). Standardization is helpful to identify the quality of a particular herb.

Plants grown even in the same field can vary in potency of certain active constituents. Quality markers can help growers identify potential potency of the whole medicinal plant. Whole plants are, in general, less potent than an individual plant constituent. For comparison, take the apple. Most people who have eaten an apple remember the strong outer skin and the crunching sound when biting into the fruit for the first time. There is a lot of pectin and fiber in the apple skin. Now recall eating the fleshy part of the apple. Although some apples are more tart than others, they are basically a sweet fruit. The sugars in fruits are known as fructose. When extracted from fruit and processed, fructose looks much the same as the white crystallized cane sugar you might eat. Think about what it might be like to eat a spoonful of fructose sugar. How might your body respond? Sugars are known to give the body an energy boost. Does your body get the identical energy boost from an apple as it does from a spoonful of fructose? Common sense tells us that extracted (standardized) fructose is not the same as an apple and it does not have the same total effect on the body either.

Standardization is grounded in a reductionist biomedical paradigm that may or may not be helpful for a patient. An example of when standardization may be helpful is in liver damage due to toxic substance exposure from acetaminophen, environmental pollutants, or mushroom poisoning. Milk thistle seed *(Silybum marianum)* has been used traditionally for more than 2000 years for illness related to liver. Milk thistle products are standardized to silymarin, a hepatoprotective and antioxidant constituent. According to research, a therapeutic level of silymarin cannot be achieved by taking teas or simple alcohol extracts of the milk thistle seed because silymarin cannot survive the breakdown by digestive juices and enter the bloodstream via the intestinal wall. Because silymarin is not very soluble in water and is poorly absorbed from the gastrointestinal tract, a concentrated, standardized extract or injectable form of the plant is used to fully provide the desired effects (Blumenthal et al, 2000; Foster & Tyler, 1999). Herbalists and traditional healers may disagree that standardization is necessary for the patient to receive a health benefit from milk thistle. Some herbalists have found that patients with chemical sensitivities even have a negative response to standardized products because of the chemical residue in the product from the standardization process. More research is needed to fully determine the benefits and risks of using standardized herbal products.

Standardization is just one example of manufacturing or processing that goes into the production of plant medicine. Good manufacturing practices have been identified by many, including WHO (1996a), as a target for the improvement of herbal products on the market. Herbalists and traditional healers who use whole herbs have always known the importance of making a proper identification of the plant and finding a pure source of the plant. Plants that have been sprayed with herbicides and pesticides would not be used. For instance, an herbalist would not harvest mullein *(Verbascum officinale)* leaf and flowers from plants growing by the highway. It is important that the plant is grown in a pure environment.

Plants targeted for medicinal use, be they whole dried plant or one of the numerous products on the market, are subject to contamination and deterioration. Just as with buying a vegetable in the supermarket, the medicinal plant must be "ripe" and not decomposing to make a good product. Shelf life is different for different herbs, often based on their constituents. Storage of herbal products is very important. Whole dried herbs, for example, need to be open to the air and therefore are best kept in protective bags that have an opening. Many herbs and herb products lose their potency when exposed to heat, humidity, and/or light and therefore are kept in special areas where the storage climate can be controlled. Herbs are stored separately, sometimes in separate rooms, because of the potency of certain constituents. For example, at the Celestial Seasonings Tea Company in Boulder, Colorado, the peppermint *(Mentha piperita)* is kept in its own special vault. On public tours, the tour guides encourage participants to enter the vault where they receive a literal blast of menthol, the volatile oil that permeates any room it is stored in. For this reason, the peppermint stands alone.

Herb production facilities must be clean, and measures must be taken to prevent cross contamination between products. All products should be labeled and documented with the botanical name of all ingredients; date of harvest and/or date of process; plant source; results of screening for herbicide, pesticide, or other contaminants; the drying system used, if dried; and the results of tests for microbial and aflatoxin contamination. All processing records should be kept up to date (WHO, 1996a). The WHO (1996b) also has guidelines for the assessment of herbal medicines that can be followed for the production of herbal remedies.

Although standardized herbal extracts may be very similar to pharmaceutical drugs, most plant medicines are not. Herbal remedies are not pharmaceuticals. Some practitioners mistakenly tell patients that herbs are "drugs" and should be used cautiously. Although the message about using caution is correct, it is not safe practice to teach the public that herbs are drugs. For years, biomedical practitioners have wrestled with patient noncompliance to pharmaceutical drug regimens. Patients clearly believe that they can and should regulate whether they take a drug or not. They may be quite familiar with self-medication with over-the-counter drugs. By telling people that herbs are drugs, practitioners may be inadvertently telling people that what they know about over-the-counter and prescription drugs can be applied to herbs. This can potentially lead to some serious safety issues, mainly that the patient may not seek understanding about an herb.

Patients should be taught that they can learn more about the herbs that are appearing in exponential numbers on the shelves of their pharmacies and grocery stores. Countries such as Germany, China, and Switzerland have a much more sustained history of people using herbs. In the United States, although self-medication has certainly continued, there has been a significant decrease in people's use of herbal remedies in self-care until recently. This has left more recent generations with a lapse in knowledge of herbal self care.

SELF-CARE WITH HERBS:

"The proper use of medicinal plants in therapy is a necessity and not a luxury. It is one that plays a very important role in self-medication, thereby reducing demands on the precious time of the already overtaxed health professionals" (Akerele, 1993, p. 15). Many health care practitioners have become involved with the promotion of self-care practices in their countries. The WHO recognizes the role of nurses in supporting patients in health care and has written a booklet for pharmacists about their role in supporting self-care and self-medication (WHO, 1998c). From a global health perspective, one way to promote health care for all is for all practitioners, biomedical and traditional, to teach patients what they know. There is an increasing need for self-care related to a number of factors, including socioeconomic factors, lifestyle issues, increased access to drugs, increased recognition of potential to manage illness through self-care, environmental factors, and demographic and epidemiologic factors (WHO, 1998c). Nurses are very aware of the importance of supporting self-care practices of patients. Nurse theorist Dorothea Orem developed a nursing model based on the concept of self-care that has been in use for decades.

There are many reasons for using plant therapies in self-care practices. Herbal therapies work well; they are usually affordable; they have a history of use; and they are, for the most part, very gentle. Describing *whole* herbs as gentle does not mean that they are not potent and active and do not need to be used wisely and safely. Herbs are gentle in how they convey their medicinal properties to humans especially when compared with many pharmaceutical drugs. They may have very toxic constituents in them, but the amounts are often quite small. Even a properly used purgative herb can be experienced without the significant aftereffects felt with many pharmaceutical drugs. People need whole herb medicines and therapies as well as pharmaceutical drugs. Many times when people don't feel well, a cup of the appropriate tea and a nap is just enough to work through the ill feeling. Children are excellent examples of this. As a school nurse, I often found that the five-year-old children who had stomachache often felt better by holding a teddy bear while they had a short rest. Giving a child a cup of tummy tea (I use a spearmint and All-Heal/ *Prunella vulgaris*) when they feel queasy can be medicinal and an opportunity for expression of gentleness and healing. Often pharmaceutical drugs are harsh and very strong. Sensitive people can feel the not-so-subtle differences in their bodies between taking a pharmaceutical drug and an herb. The gentleness of herbal therapies also has to do with the preparation.

When people make their own herbal medicines, there can be a tremendous healing effect. One phenomenologic study by a nurse, called "Understanding Ethnic Women's Experiences with Pharmacopeia," found that the women studied liked to take teas rather than pills (with the exception of aspirin, acetaminophen, and ibuprofen), because, ". . . the substance that makes up the pill is a real unknown and cannot be trusted . . . they feel that the teas are natural and talked about the acts of handling the leaves, boiling the water, and watching the remedy brew as critical to the known therapeutics of the remedy. . . . The role of the folk remedies is important to the continuation of culture and tradition through caregiving activities involving generations of knowledge" (Davis, 1997, p. 433). As reported by the women in this study, there is something inherently special and healing about making one's own medicine. It is a connection with the earth; it is a healing art.

HERBS IN PREGNANCY AND LACTATION:

Women in particular have a history of centuries of use of plants in healing work. Herbs continue to be a routine part of women's health care, especially in relationship to birthing. Historically, women and their caregivers used herbs at risk of peril. In 1590, Agnes Simpson of Keith was burned at the stake, accused of practicing witchcraft for using herbs to alleviate pain during childbirth. She was sentenced to death by ministers who argued that God would not have made illness if people were not meant to suffer (Atkinson, 2000). Women were believed to have been ordained to experience pain in childbirth. Witches were believed to be handmaidens of the devil and their work with healing herbs to be used by those who were "thinking more of their bodily health than of God" (Ehrenreich & English, 1978, p. 36). "Wise wimmin," healers often pegged as witches to be feared by the God-fearing, used herbs that were effective painkillers and digestive aides. "They used ergot for the pain of labor at a time when the Church held that pain in labor was the Lord's punishment for Eve's original sin. . . . Digitalis, still an important drug in treating heart ailments, is said to have been discovered by an English witch" (Ehrenreich & English, 1978, p. 37). Estimates of those executed during the witch hunts from the fifteenth through the sixteenth centuries have numbered in the millions, with women making up 85% of those killed (Ehrenreich & English, 1978).

Much of what American women caregivers and midwives learned about healing with plants, they learned from healers among the Native American Indian tribes and the black slaves from the West Indies (Ehrenreich & English, 1978). As is described in *A Midwife's Tale* and *For Her Own Good*, the American women healers who routinely used herb "potions" in practice were not executed in the 1800s but were effectively stopped from practicing through socioeconomic and political means. In the early 1800s, a movement known as the Thomsonian Medico-botanical movement sprang up in response to the organization of physicians and the thrust to move medicine into the marketplace. Samuel Thomson (1769–1843) began the movement after seeing his wife suffer and his mother die in the hands of doctors. The goal of the movement was to educate patients so that "every man might be his own physician" and to democratize the practice of medicine in the United States. Samuel Thomson was very concerned with the health of women and opposed practices such as tight corseting and the replacement of midwives with physicians, men who had no experience with birthing.

Thomson himself received his education in herbs and healing from an herbal doctor named Mrs. Benton, who had learned from Native Americans (Haller, 1997). Thomson's practice focused on the alleviating of illness by the "assisting and raising of the natural *heat* of the body" (Day, 1833, vii), which he associated with the life force. He used herbs like cayenne and ginger when instructing people how to care for themselves. Thomson wrote of the practice of midwifery,

Thirty years ago the practice of midwifery was principally in the hands of experienced women who had no difficulty; and there was scarce an instance known in those days of a woman dying in childbed, and it was very uncommon for them to lose the child; but at the present time these things are so common that it is hardly talked about. . . . I can account for it in no other way than the unskilful treatment they experience from the doctors, who have now got most of the practice into their own hands. In the country where I was born and where I brought up a family of children, there was no such thing thought of as calling the assistance of a doctor; a midwife was all that was thought necessary, and the instances were very rare that they were not successful, for they used no art, but afforded such assistance as nature requires; gave herb tea to keep them in a per-spiration, and to quiet the nerves; their price was one dollar (as reported in Day, 1833, p. 114).

Today, midwives and pregnant women continue the time-honored tradition of using herbs during pregnancy. Most herbal practitioners are experienced in the use of herbs in pregnancy, yet many herb books recommend that pregnant women abstain from herbs altogether until herbs are sufficiently researched. Herbs may not be researched in pregnancy or in lactation for ethical reasons. Because of ethical issues like potential for harm to the baby in utero, herbs, pharmaceutical drugs, and biomedical therapies may not be tested in pregnant and lactating women. The procedure for clinical use is similar for biomed-icine and herbalism—individualized care and looking at the history of clinical use in pregnant women.

Psychiatric illness during pregnancy is one example of when drugs or herbs may be considered. Practitioners must rely primarily on the history of traditional uses or animal studies of drugs when de-termining the potential risk to the fetus if a mother were to receive an antidepressant medication. "None of the medications used to treat these disorders (anxiety and depression) have been subjected to con-trolled trials in pregnancy, allowing for calculations of the actual risk of teratogenesis. The majority of the data available rely on animal studies, case reports, and retrospective studies" (Diket & Nolan, 1997, p. 551).

The decision to start a pregnant woman on an antidepressant drug is not an easy one. It has been reported that "almost all drugs cross the placenta and reach pharmacologically significant concentra-tions in the fetus after therapeutic treatment of the mother" (Pacifici & Nottoli, 1995, p. 261). The prevalence of depression in pregnancy has been reported to be from 9% to 16% and is the most common psychi-atric illness seen in pregnancy (Diket & Nolan, 1997, p. 554). When practitioners consider the benefits and risks of prescribing an antide-pressant medication, they must consider the prospect of fetal malfor-mation, the possibility of complications during labor and delivery, the effects on the newborn, the long-term sequelae to the child, and then the effects on the breastfeeding infant.

Much of the literature states that the guideline for giving an anti-depressant to a pregnant woman is whether or not the depressive ill-ness poses a threat to her and therefore the fetus. Antidepressant medications are considered when "the mother's depression is severe enough to threaten both herself and her fetus. This includes suicidal intent, vegetative and nutritional disturbances, or severely impaired functioning and judgment not responsive to non-biological interventions including hospitalization" (Kerns, 1986, p. 655).

Pregnant women and developing fetuses are more susceptible to complications of drugs for several reasons.

1. During pregnancy there are changes in drug metabolism relating to the mother's increased absorption of certain nutrients. Total serum protein concentration decreases and total water content and blood volume increases, which therefore influences the distribution of drugs in the body (Robinson, Stewart, & Flak, 1986).
2. The mother's kidney and liver function changes so that excretion of drugs is changed.
3. Fetal cardiac output is greater as compared with adults, and a greater proportion of blood flow goes to the brain. Because a fetus has greater blood-brain permeability, drug exposure to a fetus' brain is more rapid and complete.
4. In the fetus, drugs are primarily metabolized through the liver. A fetus has fewer liver enzymes than an adult. This leads to a delay of excretion and therefore an exaggeration of the effects of the drug. Excretion of the drugs through the placenta and fetal urine also is delayed (Kerns, 1986).

From these reasons, it can be seen that there is tremendous risk to a fetus/infant if it is exposed to any medication including antidepressants in utero. The first line of defense in treatment of a depressed pregnant woman might be nonbiologic methods like psychotherapy, social casework, couples therapy, and hospitalization. Herbs also might be considered, depending on the benefits and risks. Some health practitioners consider herbs a welcome alternative to drugs when making the tough benefit versus risk decisions regarding treatment during pregnancy and lactation.

There is a long history of safe use of herbs in pregnancy. This may be an area where traditional healers can be of help by sharing their wisdom. For example, Hawaiian women have traditionally used several herbs throughout pregnancy and lactation. Women also give their well and sick infants herbal remedies by ingesting them and letting them get the herb's benefits through the breastmilk until they reach a level of maturity at which the baby can take the herbs that the mother has chewed directly (Gutmanis, 1995, p. 41).

Plants used during pregnancy are often used to ripen the cervix and help the woman adapt during the intensity of the birthing process. During lactation, herbs can be used to promote or suppress breast milk production and treat engorgement and sore nipples. I have had patients use herbs such as fenugreek *(Trigonella foenum-graecum)* to successfully increase breast milk supply and chilled green cabbage leaf to successfully relieve engorgement. However, I have had no success so far with my patients in using herbs to suppress lactation. Sage has been used for many years for this purpose, but it has not helped anyone in my practice. I had a referral from a physician who had a mother whose baby weaned himself very early, leaving a grieving mother, who wanted to stop the flow of milk (sage didn't help). We suggested she try topical applications of jasmine *(Jasminum officinale)* flowers because Duke (1997) had reported a study from India in which researchers found the flowers to be as effective as Parlodel in suppressing lactation (p. 92). The jasmine flowers didn't help either in this case, so we continued to help the woman grieve in a healthy way and work on her new relationship with her baby.

The cautions given throughout this book related to pregnancy and lactation are in regard to the medicinal or therapeutic use of herbs. Herbs also are used in beverage teas and foods. Herbs drunk as beverage teas can potentially affect the fetus and pregnant woman. Herbs are best avoided altogether in the first trimester of pregnancy. After that, no herb should be taken on a daily basis, even as a beverage tea, without checking with a knowledgeable herb practitioner. Most practitioners agree that pregnant women can have a number of beverage teas that they rotate drinking throughout the weeks following the first trimester. The teas should be a blend of herbs, not one herb. Herbs that are used in beverage teas include spearmint, lemon balm, and raspberry leaf later in pregnancy. It may be very appropriate for an herb to be offered as a choice for treatment during pregnancy and lactation. It depends on the herb and the patient. When considering using herbs during pregnancy and lactation, it is often best to consult a clinical herbalist and/or a knowledgeable midwife or obstetrician who has used the herbs when caring for pregnant or lactating women.

Conservation: Safe Sampling versus Grazing with Gusto

Medicinal plant populations must be protected and used wisely and safely. Conservation of natural resources consists of any act that follows the belief that the resource is valuable and must be used prudently in the present so that the resource is not depleted for future generations. Plant medicines are valuable and must be conserved, which is why the WHO Traditional Medicine Programme, clinical herbalists, and herb associations focus on the importance of conservation.

To protect medicinal plants, the environment in which they are nourished must be cared for as well. Because plants obviously do not speak out, it is up to humans to understand and provide for their needs. Plants thrive in healthy environments just as people do. The plant itself produces its medicinal constituents in relationship to its environment. For example, Indian studies on the *Ephedra sp.* plant have shown that the amount of rainfall in a particular area has a relationship with the ephedrine content of the plant. The greater the annual rainfall, the smaller the ephedrine content, and occasional heavy showers also lower the ephedrine content (Nadkarni, 1976, p. 501). Altitude affects plants; it also has a great bearing on which plants grow in a particular area. High altitudes have different plant life than those found at sea level. People who live at different altitudes have traditionally learned to use the plants that grow in their areas for healing.

Indigenous peoples use the plants for medicine as directed by what grows in their environment; hence, there has always been a strong connection with the earth and specifically the environment where a specific people live. More recently, increasing agricultural, mining, and lumber industries pose threats to the habitats of medicinal plants. Pollution is also a serious threat to plant life and their environments. In 1950, 30% of the globe was forested, and in 1975 only 12% of the surface of the earth was covered by forest. In 1995, it was reported that the tree populations shrink by 10,000 per minute (Anyinam, 1995). "Transformation of local ecosystems wrought through human economic activities has been exercising severe constraints on the availability and accessibility of specific types of plants and animal species used for medicinal purposes" (Anyinam, 1995, p. 323). Along with the disappearance of the forests is the disappearance of indigenous people, who not only have the expertise in the use of the medicinal plants in a particular location but who also protect and respect the environment. With the numbers of these people who could be considered national treasures dwindling, the habitats of many medicinal plants, the plants themselves, and the knowledge of the use of these plants are at serious risk.

It is up to those who value medicinal plant life to speak up and protect the environments of these plants. People such as Rosita Arvigo, an American herbologist who apprenticed with Don Elijio Panti, one of the last surviving Maya traditional healers in the rainforest in Belize, help preserve the traditional healing methods and the plants of the areas in which they live. Arvigo (1994) has been an advocate for conserving the medicinal plants of the rainforest, and *Sastun,* her story of her relationship with a Mayan healer, can be very inspiring to those who work with the healing power of plants.

WHO has produced numerous documents and guidelines regarding the importance of protecting medicinal plants in their native habitats (WHO, 1991, 1993). In addition, many countries have botanical gardens, even in the inner cities, where plants are preserved for the public so that they can have a place to go to connect with the plants and gain a greater awareness of how the plants grow that are responsible for many of the medications used in healing.

Nurses and nursing organizations also are becoming increasingly aware of the need for greater connection with the environment. Environmental changes and destruction pose significant challenges to human health and well-being. Nursing philosophers such as Jean

Watson have taught extensively on the connection of human beings and their world and that the two cannot be separated. This sense of connection is rooted in what Kleffel (1996), a nurse theorist, calls an "ecocentric" approach. She writes that the ecocentric approach in nursing is "grounded in the cosmos. The whole environment, including inanimate elements such as rocks and minerals, along with animate animals and plants, is assigned intrinsic value" (Kleffel, 1996, p. 4). Kleffel (1996) also describes the egocentric and homocentric approaches of nursing. The egocentric approach assumes that whatever is best for the individual human being is best for society, and the individual is the focus of change. In the egocentric perspective, the environment is defined by its relation to people and not in terms of its own intrinsic value. From the homocentric perspective, humans are considered stewards of the natural world and decisions are made based on common good. The environment is the focus of change in the homocentric perspective and humans manage nature to benefit humans. Kleffel (1996) states that "moving to the ecocentric paradigm will encourage nurses to address worldwide environmental problems that affect the health of everything that exists" (p. 5). Getting closer to the plants that provide medicine or the inspiration for medicine is a perfect way for nurses to move into a more ecocentric paradigm and reconnect with the essence of the earth as "home" and as the source of the natural beauty that surrounds us and provides us with an abundance of unique healing plants.

Safety is a concept that can be oversimplified, leading to gross generalizations. There are risks associated with using plants in healing; that is a given. It is important that nurses and their patients put that risk in context when making health decisions. For example, if a patient just sustained a head injury in a motor vehicle accident, they need a trauma team to administer the best of biomedical interventions. Herbs would not be the best choice in this scenario. However, there are numerous examples of patients with chronic illness, pain, and general discomforts in which herbs are extremely valuable and safe, especially when compared to the risks associated with long-term use of pharmaceutical drugs. Therefore, nurses must exercise caution not only in using herbs or when advising patients who are using herbs; nurses also must be careful not to be overly cautious and fearful when approaching the use of herbs just because they may not have education and experience in herbalism. Nurses are used to working with the strong medicines and therapies of the biomedical world and must be careful not to see herbs through the same lens. Herbs are different. In summary, herbs are gentle healers and have a place in the repertoire of nurses who often care for those who need compassionate, gentle care.

CHAPTER 5
Nursing Care and Plants: Back to the Roots

WHEN PEOPLE CONNECT WITH NATURE THEY CONNECT WITH their roots. The evolution of human beings shows that people were originally hunters and gatherers. For many centuries, humans have been close to the land and have tilled the soil. It is only more recently in human evolution that people have become separated from their agrarian roots as our world has become more industrialized. Being in nature—touching the ground, smelling the trees and flowers, looking up at the sun and the clouds—can be soothing and reassuring. Connecting with the natural world can be a way of reconnecting with one's roots.

Roots anchor a plant deeply in the soil and protect it from being blown about by fierce winds or rain. Roots provide nourishment for the plant and are the point of connection between the soil and the plant. When human beings connect with the natural world, they often find their own roots—a source of security, protection, and nourishment. Direct interaction with the plant world by working with medicinal plants is one way of connecting with nature and one's roots. Not only are medicinal plants potentially healing for the receiver of the remedy, but also those working with the plant remedies can be healed. Making plant medicines is a healing experience.

Growing and harvesting medicinal plants in the wild is a direct experience with nature that can be healing. People who work with plants are exposed to the fragrances, textures, shapes and tastes of the various species of medicinal plants. Gardening, for example, is good exercise with all the bending and stooping. Gardening and interaction with plant life also increases sensory perception. Watching a seed that has been planted grow into a large plant or observing the opening of a new flower bud promotes an interest, even an enthusiasm in the future. People who grow plants receive tremendous satisfaction in being able not only to see the fruit of their labor, but also they get to partake of that fruit as well. They can experience a sense of completion that is often lacking in a fast-paced world. Plants inspire a sense of wonder. They are fascinating to observe through their various life cycles. Plants offer opportunity for experimentation and creativity in addition to providing us with a source of food and medicine.

Making medicine from plants is an art, a science, and a cultural experience. For example, making tea in Japan can be different from making tea in England. Many herbs can be used in various ways to make plant remedies. Nurses can benefit from learning what plant remedies are most prevalent in the local areas where they live. It is also important for nurses to learn how those plants are best used in making remedies. Making plant remedies is an opportunity for nurses to improve their understanding of the plant-human relationship and to develop their skills of exploring nature's way of assisting in the process of human healing. Nurses have historically had a connection with the environment, nature, and plants. Florence Nightingale once said, "Nature alone cures . . . and what nursing has to do is put the patient in the best condition for nature to act upon him" (Nightingale, 1957, p. 75). Learning how to use plants in caring for patients continues a nursing tradition that benefits both patients and nurses alike.

Nature Care

Florence Nightingale, like many caregivers throughout history, emphasized the importance of the relationship between people and their environment in regard to healing. *Nature care* is the inclusion of natural elements in the care of people. Nurses might include water, light, fresh air, and warmth in their intervention strategies. Plant remedies also can be considered because they are inexpensive and effective and can be prepared from local plant populations. Nurses who make their own plant remedies can experience directly from the plant the medicinal properties of the plant. The plant medicine-making information presented here is grounded in the traditional paradigm. Pharmaceutical techniques of extraction of plant constituents is not covered. All of the remedies presented in this chapter are based on the use of whole plants or parts of plants.

Many resources on plant medicine-making are available. Nurses can learn directly from traditional healers and herbalists. They also can learn from their country's formularies, pharmacopoeia, dispensatories, and/or historical texts on medicine making. The following information on the making of herbal remedies includes three areas: oral use, topical applications, and the use of plants in creating a healing environment. The information provided is derived from traditional herbals, my own experience, *The Dispensatory of the United States of America, 1839,* and *A Textbook of Nursing, 1914.*

Plant parts that are used in making remedies are the bulb, bark, twigs, flower, leaf, fruit, skin, juice, pollen, root, rhizome, tuber, seed, and/or whole plant. The quality of a plant medicine is related to the way the plant is grown, harvested, and processed. Plants used for healing should be grown without the aid of synthetic pesticides and herbicides because the chemicals used in these products can be toxic to humans. There is a potential for chemical residues to remain with the plant even after processing and passed on to a patient, so medicinal plants should not be exposed to these strong chemicals. The plants used should be fresh. Dried herbs can maintain a fresh quality for certain periods of time, depending on the plant. Flowers and tiny leaves are more fragile and susceptible to a loss of vitality than whole roots. Using plant materials in pieces that are as whole as possible preserves freshness. Certain plant constituents, such as volatile oils, however, may deteriorate or dissipate quickly. Freshly picked herbs can spoil or lose vitality in a matter of hours or minutes. In general, fresh plants are used immediately, and thoroughly dried plant materials are used as soon as possible but usually have a shelf life of approximately one year, again depending on the plant. Dried herbs for external use may be stored longer, depending on the plant.

Some plant medicine-makers consider how and when the plant or plant part is harvested to be very important. Some plant medicine companies continue the tradition of planting, harvesting, and preparing remedies according to specific lunar, solar, and planetary cycles and configurations. Attention to cosmic forces is known to increase the hardiness of the medicinal plant and the potency and prevalence of medicinal components. Large European pharmaceutical companies, such as Weleeda and WALA, pay close attention to how the medicinal plants used in their remedies are grown in relationship with the whole environment, including the flow of water near the plant, the balance of the soil, and the position of the planets. The plants in one of the medicinal plant garden projects I coordinated had been planted originally by horticulturists who had used traditional astrologic data regarding appropriate timing for planting and the appropriate positioning of plants in a garden. Laboratory testing of herbs grown in that garden revealed exceptional quantity and quality of known active constituents. Perhaps using the astrologic data had been helpful.

The processing of the plant is also important to the quality of the medicinal plant preparation. Traditionally, plants have been said to have healing "properties" and the "medicine" to actually reside in the healer preparing the medicine. Many plant medicine-makers are aware of this and are very careful and meticulous about their preparations. For example, remedies are often thought to be best if hand-harvested. The purity of the menstruum (solvent) used to extract the medicinal constituents of plants, such as water (referred to as the universal solvent), alcohol, glycerine, vinegar, or oil, is very important. Some herbalists recommend using only distilled or soft water in making remedies to facilitate the extraction process because hard, well, or spring waters can foster precipitation.

HEALING FOODS AND ORAL REMEDIES:

The medicinal benefits of plants are most commonly acquired through ingestion in foods and teas. Some medicinal plants, such as saw palmetto *(Serenoa repens)* have a history of also being eaten as staple foods. Herbs are used in many cultures in food preparation. Herbs such as dill *(Anethum graveolens)* and basil *(Ocimum basilicum)* are used in foods because of their supportive effects on digestion. They are used traditionally in small amounts determined by taste.

Oral ingestion of herbal remedies through teas, juices, and foods enables the person to taste the plant. Because many culinary herbs and spices come from plants that also can serve as medicines, they should be used sparingly. As discussed previously, taste is a good way to regulate oral ingestion of herbs because many medicinal plants and many plant constituents are not the most pleasurable to taste. Medicinal plants can be bitter, sour, pungent, astringent, salty, and sweet. Often, tasting a medicinal plant reveals a combination of tastes that is unique to that plant. The understanding of the importance of taste in herbal medicine is highly developed in the Indian system of medicine known as Ayurveda and in the traditional Chinese medicine (TCM) system.

In the Ayurvedic system, bitter taste is said to restore the sense of taste. In many cultures, the use of medicinal plant bitters, a combination of bitter plants, is used in aiding digestion. Typical bitter plants include goldenseal *(Hydrastis canadensis),* yarrow *(Achillea millefolium),* and dandelion *(Taraxicum officinalis).* My mother used to harvest dandelions in the spring to make a vat of dandelion wine that was often drunk with dinner to aid digestion.

Sour taste is helpful in digestion as well. Sour is experienced with lemon *(Citrus limon)* and other citrus fruits as well as rosehips *(Rosa canina)* and hawthorn berries *(Crataegus laevigata).* Pungent taste increases the appetite and promotes digestion and sweating. Examples are black pepper *(Piper nigrum)* and onion *(Allium cepa).* Astringent taste is drying and constricting and is used to promote absorption and restriction of fluid. The astringent taste, associated with the tannin constituents in plants, can be found with raspberry leaf *(Rubus idaeus)* and witch hazel *(Hamamelis virginiana L.).* In addition to its effects on digestion, the salty taste found in plants such as seaweeds also promotes the body's ability to retain fluids. Sweet taste, found in herbs such as licorice *(Glycyrrhiza glabra L.)* and psyllium *(Plantago psyllium L.)* is nutritive and promotes growth of tissues (Lad & Frawley, 1986).

In TCM, practitioners taste teas made from hundreds of medicinal plants as part of their education. Plants are recognized by taste (part of the safe use system). Herbal tea formulations of several carefully selected herbs are prepared for each individual patient. TCM practitioners believe that, despite the strong and often repulsive taste of a formula, a patient will be aware of craving the formula that is designed for their health concern, if that formula is appropriate for them. TCM herbal formulas are designed for the patient with the goal of greater "balance" in mind. The body is said to crave that which assists its natural tendency to seek greater balance and harmony. I have seen this happen time and again in clinical practice.

Teas

Teas, also called "tisanes," are aqueous or water extractions of medicinal plants. Water extractions are often hot but can be cold, especially if the plant has highly volatile active principles. *Infusions* are water extractions of the plant material that is more delicate, such as leaves and flowers. The plant material used is allowed to steep in the water for a period of time. Fresh or dried plant can be infused, but because of the water content in fresh plant, more plant should be used per cup of tea than with dried (approximately 3 teaspoons [9 to 15 g] of fresh herb is equal to 1 teaspoon [3 to 5 g] of dried herb). The *decoction* method of making tea is used when the plant material is hard or woody (i.e., roots or barks) because more heat is needed to release the medicinal constituents in the plant (usually the mineral salts and bitter principles). For decoction, the plant material is simmered and/or boiled for approximately fifteen minutes. In TCM practice, the formulas often contain roots and harder parts of plants, and the usual decoction time generally is $1\frac{1}{2}$ to 2 hours. If the plant material used is dried, the plant material is steeped in warm water for approximately 4 hours before simmering to allow the dried herb to absorb water and expand. Infusions and decoctions can be taken internally and used externally. External uses are discussed in the section "topical applications."

How to Make an Infusion
- *Supplies:*
  - A china or glass teapot (for 2+ cups [500 ml]), a tea ball or net for 1 cup (Note: Do not use aluminum teapots when making herbal teas. Also, tea nets made of cotton do not compact the herb as tightly as the stainless steel tea balls and allow for greater circulation of the water around the plant material during extraction)

- Tea strainer to place in cup to strain tea made from infused loose herb (not teabags or tea net)
- Herb of choice, usually leaf or flower, cut or ground in small but not minute pieces
- Boiling water
- *Method:* Boil the water and select the herb you want to use. When using large dried flowers or leaves, break up the amount of herb needed in the pot or tea net. If using fresh herbs, cut them into pieces and bruise them with a knife so that volatile oils will not be absorbed into the skin of the hands. Measure the herbs for the tea. The rule of thumb for quantities is 1 to 2 rounded teaspoons (about 5 g) per cup of water. Pour the boiling water over the plant material, and cover the cup or teapot to prevent the volatile oils from escaping. These oils will accumulate with water on the underside of the lid. Be sure to shake the condensation on the lid back into the tea. For very thin and tender parts of plants, steep for approximately three to five minutes. For other plant materials, steep for approximately ten minutes. Strain and drink tea hot.

These are general guidelines and following a specific formula may be required, depending on the herb(s) being used. Infusions are made in small quantities on an as-needed basis because they often contain constituents that spoil quite readily after hot water infusion. *Beverage teas* are infusions. They are usually a blend of plant leaves or flowers and are steeped so that a person receives very small amounts of any one plant's medicinal constituents. The concept of a beverage tea can be compared with the use of a blend of herbs in seasoning Italian foods, such as oregano *(Oreganum vulgare L.)*, basil *(Ocimum basilicum)*, and thyme *(Thymus vulgaris L.)*. Instead of making an infusion of thyme and using it medicinally, either drinking it or putting it in a bath, a small amount of thyme is blended with other herbs and put into a sauce for pasta, for example. The intent of the beverage tea infusion is for culinary purposes rather than medicinal use.

How to Make a Decoction

- *Supplies:* The same supplies as for making an infusion are needed, but the plant material used is usually the harder part of a plant such as the root or bark. With roots, the pieces are often much larger than with leaves or flowers.
- *Method:* Use approximately 1 ounce (30 g) of herb per 750 ml (1½ cups) of water. Place dried, hard herbs in a pot and cover completely with cold water. Bring water almost to the boil, cover, and remove from heat. Allow to stand four hours to allow dried herbs to expand. (This step can be skipped when using fresh herbs.) After standing, the herbs are simmered in a pot (not aluminum) for approximately fifteen minutes. Volatile oils will escape during simmering. These instructions are a generalization and specific instructions (as with TCM formulas where the herbs are cooked for 2 hours) should be followed whenever possible. The decoction is strained *after* cooling

slightly and then drunk warm. Decoctions are considered more potent than infusions. Larger quantities of decoction often are made. The rule of thumb is that decoctions can be kept refrigerated for up to 72 hours and portions reheated, without boiling, for use during the day.

Soups and Foods

One very common way of taking small amounts of medicinal plants is to make soups with herbs. For instance, ginger *(Zingiber officinale)* and astragalus *(Astragalus membranicus)* can be added to chicken soup to strengthen the stomach and spleen energy systems and reduce hypertension (Flaws & Wolfe, 1983). As discussed in the herb profile on soy (chapter 8), miso, a fermented soy product, makes a nutritious broth. Is the soup then medicinal instead of strictly nutritional? This is determined by how much herb is used and by the patient and his or her needs.

The question of whether or not foods with added medicinal herbs are actually medicines instead of foods has become a big issue in countries such as the United States where the health food industry has created a new food category called "functional" foods. "Functional foods claim to have added ingredients that provide an extra nutrition boost . . . the classic example: already nutritious orange juice pumped up with bone-strengthening calcium" (Neergaard, 2000, p. 2A). Not only do the claims made by manufacturers suggest a nutritional boost, but they also suggest health benefits related to the medicinal plants used in the food. There are concerns among the biomedical community about deception in advertising such as making false claims about the health benefits of functional foods and that many medicinal plants have not been traditionally or conventionally used as food. One expert pharmacist is quoted as saying that "herbs are drugs . . . and we do not add Viagra to soup" (Neergaard, 2000, p. 2A). Although it is true that drugs (other than vitamin fortification) are not purposefully added to foods, herbs have traditionally been added to soups. Culinary herbs that have medicinal value are added to foods routinely. Defining whether an herb used in food preparation is medicinal or not is a matter of intent and society defining, and perhaps redefining, what it considers medicine. The quantity of an herb that can be taken in foods on any given day is also questionable. Many herbs, such as chamomile, are used traditionally as a decoction or infusion and are not usually ingested as food. This is a concern with herbs that are being sold in capsule and tablet forms as well.

Pills and Capsules

In industrialized countries, herbs are often sold as capsules or pills. Because many people are used to taking pills prescribed from biomedical practitioners, they often prefer taking herbs in these easy-to-use forms as opposed to having to prepare their own medicine. It is actually simple to prepare one's own capsulated herbal medicine. The herb is crushed using a mortar and pestle and the capsules are either filled individually or by using a capsule holder where the herb powder is spread into the open capsules and the excess scraped away. The other half of the capsule is then applied. In terms of safety, capsules that are self-prepared from herbs you have identified may be better quality than those bought in a store. When purchasing herbs in capsule form, the consumer must instead rely on the integrity of the manufacturer and the standards of the governing agency of the country where they live. Because the herb is powdered, it is not easy, if nearly impossible, to identify the herb by visual inspection, smell, and sometimes taste. The risk of adulteration (the wrong plant being added to the product) also can be greater with powdered medicinal plant products.

In addition, the plant in a capsule is not tasted. In traditional medicine systems, such as Ayurveda, taste and sensory experiences of the plant medicine are considered the beginning of the healing process because the nervous system is stimulated by the senses. When viewed from a traditional herbal medicine paradigm, the consumer who ingests the herb in capsule form may not be getting the full benefit of the plant that they would get by tasting the herb in decoction, infusion, or liquid extraction forms. Some traditional herbalists also consider the bulking agents used in making herb capsules and tablets to be unhealthy in daily quantities. In TCM, these filler materials are thought to be stagnating to the liver energy system, an important issue for women, who often have symptoms indicative of liver stagnation even before taking their herbal remedy.

As mentioned previously, not all herbs are meant to be eaten whole. Therefore, they may not be as safe or effective ingested in a supplement or pill form as when used in traditional forms. Many herbs are now sold in pill or capsule form as dietary supplements. Some liken the expansion in the dietary supplements industry in America to the patent medicine era of the 1800s. Traditional herbal *Materia Medica* are specific about which herbs can be eaten after decoction. For example, in the Chinese *Materia Medica, dong quai (Angelica sinensis)* is said to be edible. Many people might find the taste of "dong quai" or any other herb repugnant and therefore may ask to take the herb in capsule or pill form. Some practitioners believe that the benefit of using pills and capsules is that doses of specific plant constituents may be more easily controlled than in tea form. While this may be correct, whole plant dosages can be specifically measured out for teas. Although traditional herbalists create herbal formulas using dosage strategies with precision to $\frac{1}{3}$ of a gram or better that meet the specific needs of a patient, some practitioners and patients are more comfortable with pills. Comfort with one's medicine is an issue nurses know quite well. Nurses who work with herbal medicine programs must address this issue and may be involved in the education of patients regarding the benefits and risks of the use of herbs in various forms.

Tinctures and Liquid Extracts

Tinctures and liquid extracts are preparations in which alcohol is used to extract the medicinal components of a plant. Alcohol is an excellent menstruum (solvent) for most plant constituents, and it also serves as a preservative for the finished product. Because of the alcohol, the shelf life of an herbal tincture or liquid extract is approximately 10 years. According to the 1902 International Protocol (as reported in Green, 1990), tinctures of dried toxic or intense plants should be a 10% or 1:10 plant weight/volume of menstruum. Extracts of dried nontoxic plant should be a 20% or 1:5 solution, and fresh plant extracts are 50% or 1:2 weight/volume solutions. In the marketplace, a tincture is often a 1:10 preparation, meaning one part plant is used to ten parts alcohol. A liquid extract is often a preparation of one part plant to five parts alcohol or less. When buying alcohol preparations, it can be somewhat confusing for the consumer because the words tincture and extract are not always used in a standard fashion by manufacturers. Understanding the preparation is important when buying alcohol products because cost comparisons should include how much plant constituent may actually be extracted.

Making your own alcohol preparations requires some research because some plants are best extracted dry and some fresh. Alcohol preparations are performed by either the percolation method or by maceration. Because percolation involves the use of laboratory equipment that most people do not have in their homes, maceration, a simpler and effective method, is described here.

How to Make an Alcohol Tincture or Extract

- *Supplies:*
  - Fresh or dried herb (see information following method for selecting)
  - Wide-mouthed jar with lid
  - Food grade ethyl alcohol (Pure grain spirits up to 190 proof [e.g., Everclear] are used for maceration.) Amount of alcohol used is discussed after method.

- *Method:* Maceration begins with cutting up fresh herb or powdering (coarse not fine) dried herb and putting the plant material in a wide-mouthed jar. The appropriate amount and type of menstruum is then poured over the plant material and the lid to the jar is placed on tightly. The jar is then put in an accessible but dark corner of the kitchen. Shake the jar at least twice daily so that the menstruum can thoroughly penetrate the plant material. Shake and store the jar for two weeks. Heat is not necessary because of the longer maceration period (Wood & Bache, 1839). At the end of the two weeks, the plant material is strained into a bowl. Use cheesecloth to press out the remaining menstruum from the plant material. Take the alcohol extract, pass it through a coffee filter, and transfer the strained liquid to dark-colored dropper bottles.

Tinctures and liquid extracts lose potency when exposed to light and therefore are prepared and stored away from light. The bottles used to store tinctures and extracts should be dark-colored glass, such as brown, and have glass droppers. Dropper bottles are necessary because the dosages for the concentrated tinctures and liquid extracts are smaller and are given in drops. Be sure to label the bottle with the name of the remedy and the date it was prepared.

The alcohol extraction process entails understanding the water content of the plant material used and then adding the appropriate amount of grain alcohol necessary to extract the medicinal constituents. Different amounts of alcohol are used for fresh and dried plants. Often alcohol is diluted with water for extraction—50% alcohol and 50% water, or 100 proof. "Diluted alcohol or proof spirit is employed, when the substance is soluble both in alcohol and water, or when one or more of the ingredients are soluble in the one fluid, and one or more in the other, as in the case of those vegetables which contain extractive or tannin, or the native salts of the organic alkalies, or gum united with resin or essential oil. As these include the greater number of medicines from which tinctures are prepared, diluted alcohol is most frequently used" (Wood & Bache, 1839, p. 1065).

If dry plant is used, then the amount of menstruum used to extract the plant material to make a 1:5 liquid extract is five times the weight of the plant material. Thus if you have 500 g of dried plant you will need 2500 ml of menstruum for the liquid extraction. If a 1:10 tincture is to be made then ten times the weight of the dried plant, or 5000 ml of menstruum is needed. Generally, the menstruum used for dried plant tinctures is 50% alcohol and 50% water, or 100 proof (vodka). If fresh plant is used, then there is already a significant amount of water present and water is rarely added. A fresh plant can have as much as three times the amount of moisture as a dried plant. The water content can be measured by moisture analysis and then the correct amount of menstruum calculated. In *general*, for fresh plant tinctures, a 1:2 weight-to-volume calculation is made and the plant is extracted in straight 190 proof alcohol (Everclear). For example, if 200 g of fresh plant is collected then 400 ml of alcohol is used for the maceration.

A Note about Homeopathy. Many people ask what the differences are between homeopathic remedies and herbal extracts. A fresh herb tincture made by extracting one part herb in two parts alcohol is often referred to as a "mother tincture." This mother tincture can be shaken and diluted 1:10 to give a "homeopathic" tincture with a potency known as 2X. Then that 2X tincture is shaken and diluted once again 1:10 with alcohol/water and that dilution is known as 3X. This shaking and dilution process is known as "potentization." Samuel Hahnemann, a renowned homeopathic scientist, described his observation of the effect of potentization as, "The more a substance is succussed and diluted, the greater the therapeutic effect while simultaneously nullifying the toxic effect" (Vithoulkas, 1980). The potentization process continues and the potencies are recorded carefully.

Homeopathic medicine includes the use of remedies that have been diluted as many as twenty-four times (Avogadro's number), or the point at which there are no detectable molecules of the original mother (herbal) tincture. Homeopathic remedies are not only derived from plants. Minerals are also used. The remedies are then used based on the "Law of Similars" (like treats like) in which the symptoms of a condition are actually treated with a homeopathic dilution originally made from a substance, such as a plant, known to cause the same symptoms. Thus, homeopathy, although it uses plants as mother tinctures, is not the same science nor the same healing art as herbalism.

Alcohol extracts and tinctures are usually taken in a small amount of warm water, but they can be taken directly in the mouth. Nonsynthetic vegetable glycerin also can be used for maceration of plants. Glycerin is a type of alcohol that also is known as glycerol or glyceric alcohol. Glycerin is not as effective as alcohol in preserving plants, so some plant medicines include a greater volume of glycerin or are a mixture of glycerin and alcohol. Glycerin also is more effective than water but less effective than alcohol in extracting resinous and oily plant constituents. Glycerites are often used with children, who may be repulsed by the smell and taste of alcohol. Some may recommend glycerites for those who are sensitive to alcohol, but I usually recommend teas for these folks and avoid alcohol and glycerin altogether. People who are sensitive to alcohol can be carbohydrate sensitive and do not do well with simple sugars, carbohydrates, or alcohols, which are metabolized quickly.

Another type of maceration is the juice pressed from a plant such as the berries of the elder *(Sambucus nigra)*. The juice, extract, tincture, infusion, or decoction of a plant can be made into a syrup. Syrups are one way to help children get used to the different tastes associated with herbal remedies. Syrups most often are made with sugar or honey and are the boiled and reduced form of the original liquid plant remedy.

Standardized extracts as discussed in chapter 4 are plant preparations in which some plant constituent, an active ingredient, has been adjusted to ensure that the potency of the product is standardized. There is some debate as to whether or not the concept of standardization is misleading to the public because many herbs' healing benefits are not the result of one constituent or active ingredient, but rather the synergy between multiple constituents. Active ingredients have yet to be isolated in many medicinal plants. Standardized extracts are generally more expensive than other extracts and tinctures. Labels on products should disclose the plant constituent and percentage of that constituent to which the product has been standardized.

TOPICAL APPLICATIONS OF PLANTS:

Topical applications are a part of nursing practice. Nurses are already familiar with the use of creams, lotions, water, packs, and other remedies to the exterior of the body. Topical application of herbal remedies is an area of nursing that is ripe for exploration. Although the whole body can be affected by topical applications, the skin and the nervous system are most particularly affected. The skin, as the largest organ of the body, and the peripheral nervous system both have connection with the whole body. Topical remedies are used not only in skin care, such as care of a localized wound (an application called a vulnerary in herbalism), but also are used to address systemic discomfort and imbalances affecting body, mind, and spirit. The importance of skin applications is described by Anthroposophical nurses in Europe. They write, "A 'breathing' can take place between the external curative quality of a substance administered to the body and the body's reaction to it. This 'breathing' process also can be described in terms of question and answer; the questions usually come from the outside, the answer follows from within" (van Bentheim et al., 1980).

Topical application of plant remedies to the skin allows a physical chemical reaction to occur and also creates a healing moment when the patient's attention is focused on that part of the body receiving the external application. The patient can use the moment to tune into the body, even ask the body what it needs for healing, and then perceive or intuit the answer. People often have a very limited awareness of their bodies when they are healthy. When ill or in pain, it is human nature to want the discomfort in a particular area of the body to go away. Applications to the skin provide a comforting way for the patient to stay aware of their body and fully participate in the healing process.

Some nurses, such as enterostomal or wound and skin nurses, specialize in the care of the skin. Historically, all nurses have provided total patient care that has included the hygienic care of the body as well as administering treatments that involve topical applications. For example, nurses have administered hot baths to soothe anxious patients. Nurses also have applied remedies to the skin in the form of poultices, plasters, compresses, salves, ointments, lotions, and more. Herbal medicine also includes the art and science of topical application of remedies. This section discusses the general use of topical remedies in which plants could be considered for use in patient care.

Compresses, Fomentations, and Stupes

A compress, also called a "fomentation" or "stupe," is a folded piece of material, made of a white, natural fiber, that is applied moist to a part of the body so that it presses against that body part. Compresses combine the knowledge of the external use of herbs and the science of hydrotherapy or use of water. Natural fiber cloth such as wool, cotton, silk, and linen is used because they are more absorbent and allow the skin to perspire and breathe during the compress. A compress can be applied hot, warm, or cool and in herbalism is made with an infusion, decoction, tincture, or herbal oil. The cloth is selected so that it can be shaped to fit the area where the compress is to be applied. For example, a compress for the eyes will be smaller than a compress for the kidneys. Some examples of compresses that can be used in patient care are arnica compresses for a sprained ankle, witch hazel compresses for puffy eyes, and mint compresses for fever or heat in the head, back, abdomen, or thighs.

How to Make and Use a Compress

- *Supplies:*
  - Natural fiber cloths cut to size and shape of body part to be covered
  - Cold, warm, or hot herbal infusion, decoction, or tincture to be used
  - Bowl to soak compress
  - Bath and hand towels for warm/hot compress

- *Method:* Cool compresses are made by dipping the cloth into the infusion, decoction, or tincture, wringing out the cloth and applying it to the body part. The compress is not necessarily covered because the compress is changed as soon as the heat from the body warms the compress, as in the case of fever. With warm and hot compresses, the nurse must keep the compress as warm as possible. The cloth is dipped in the hot or warm infusion or decoction and is placed in a wringing towel so that the nurse does not have to touch the steaming compress directly and it can be wrung out thoroughly. Hot compresses are not applied wet and drippy because they cool too quickly. After wringing, the compress temperature is tested against the arm of the nurse and if tolerable to the skin is applied as hot as possible to the patient's skin. After the compress is applied, it is completely covered with another cloth and then a wool cloth or towel to keep the heat in. Each successive cloth covers the previous one by a few centimeters to be sure to seal in the heat. The compress is left in place for about 20 minutes. Some people use a piece of plastic, like a plastic bag, to seal in the heat of a compress but this may not allow the skin to breathe fully. It is best to use other means of keeping the application warm such as changing the compress during the application. If the compress turns cold, the patient will become uncomfortable and it should be removed and replaced with a warm one. If the patient relaxes deeply or falls asleep, the compress is left in place for the 20 minutes. Compresses that are secured and worn for longer periods of time are kept moist by adding a small amount of the infusion, decoction, tincture, or oil at intervals throughout the day. For certain conditions, hot and cold compresses using different herbs may be alternated.

Example of Cold Compress. Use witch hazel *(Hamamelis virginiana)* infusion or tincture. Dip cotton bandaging cut to the size of the eyes in the infusion or tincture and squeeze out the excess. Apply to the outside of the eyes to relieve puffiness.

Example of Hot Compress. Use 4 to 5 oz (120 g) of fresh grated ginger *(Zingiberis officinalis)* root or 1 to 1½ oz (40 g) of ginger powder. Put the ginger into a small cloth bag and add it to 1 gallon (3.8 L) of water that is simmering on the stove. Allow the decoction to gently simmer, not boil, for five minutes. Remove the ginger. Put the compress cloths, the size of the area to be treated, in the ginger decoction. Using a tong, place the compress in the middle of a small towel. Holding both ends of a small towel, wring out the compress over the pot of ginger water. The compress should be steaming and should not be dripping. Apply the compress to the patient. Take care in applying the hot compress to the area of the body to be treated, making sure that the skin does not burn because of the heat. As the compress cools, replace it with another compress by placing the warm cloth on top of the cooled compress and flipping them over. This keeps the skin from cooling off between compresses. Rotate the compresses about every three to four minutes for twenty minutes. The ginger compress creates increased circulation of blood and body fluids to the treated area, thereby turning the skin pink.

The use of compresses is not new to nurses. Compresses have been used historically in nursing care for small areas of the body, and fomentations or stupes have been used for larger areas of the body. "Stupes" is the term used when applying heat to the body. Hot stupes, a hydrotherapy application, have been used to promote circulation and relieve spasm, pain, and edema (see Figure 5-1). Nurses interested in learning the art of hydrotherapies can learn from older nursing *Materia Medica,* such as those by Harmer and Henderson (1955) or Tracy (1938).

To use herbs for wraps, packs, and compresses, the nurse must learn the preparation of the plant infusion, decoction, tincture, or oil and the application aspects. It also is important to think about the timing and rhythm of applying compresses, fomentations, packs, wraps, and stupes. Learning topical applications is similar to learning bed making. A certain "look" must be achieved, so that the patient associates comfort with the application. In bed making, the sheets should not be wrinkled because the bedridden patient's skin is better protected and patients are often more comfortable when their covers are straightened. With compresses and packs, the look of the application should be tight and tucked in. The patient should feel protected by the compress or wrap and not feel as of the pack or compress is going to fall off or move. The compress or wrap should be a comforting temperature, and the patient should be told when it will be applied to their body so that they will not be shocked by a temperature change. Learning topical applications from another nurse or herbalist can convey some of the nuances of using herbs topically. Nurses and herbalists who have used topical applications for years often have their own creative way of doing the application that is best shared through one-to-one interaction.

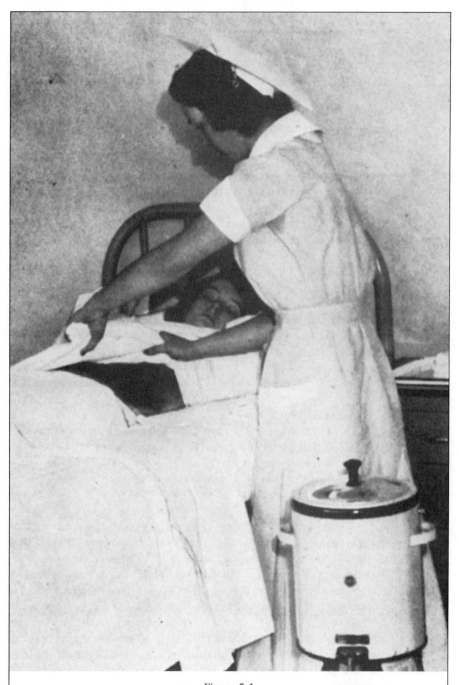

Figure 5-1
Hot stupes, also called hot packs. (From Margaret Tracy, *Nursing: An Art and a Science*. St. Louis, MO: The C.V. Mosby Company, 1938. Used with permission.)

Although each nurse learns basic principles of external applications, individual differences and variations often emerge regarding how compresses and fomentations are actually done in each unique patient situation. One study showed that not only was there great diversity in how nurses performed moist soaks (i.e., regarding temperature, method, duration, frequency, and solution) but also that the nurse has considerable discretion and authority in deciding how the moist soaks are done (Glor & Estes, 1970). Such is the art of nursing. Nurses have tremendous opportunity for growth, theoretically and clinically, in the area of external applications, especially in regard to herbal compresses, fomentations, and stupes.

How to Make and Use an Oil Compress. Herbal oils, such as castor oil *(Racinus communis)* can be used with healing compresses too. I learned the benefits of a warm, soothing castor oil pack or compress from a healer who had been affiliated with the Edgar Cayce Foundation in Virginia Beach, Virginia. Edgar Cayce (1877–1945) was a medical clairvoyant for 43 years whose work included the use of numerous plant remedies. Cayce recommended castor oil packs in cases of impaired lymph flow; inflammation; congestion; constipation; gallbladder, liver, kidney and pelvic disorders; muscle spasms, and back pain (Duggan & Duggan, 1989). Castor oil is very thick compared with other oils and when placed on the skin provides a protective coating that subsequently penetrates the tissues very deeply. With the assistance of heat, the oil is taken up readily by the skin and tissues and provides a deep healing and soothing effect.

- *Supplies:*
  - Cotton flannel cloth (two swatches a size that when doubled will completely cover the body part)
  - Castor oil—warmed
  - One large thin hand towel and one large bath towel for each body part treated
  - Hot water bottle filled and burped
- *Method for Castor Oil Pack to the Feet:* There are two ways of doing a castor oil pack for the feet or any part of the body. The Cayce method is to completely soak the flannel with the warmed castor oil and apply it to the feet or body part. These packs are reusable if refrigerated. In clinical practice, I use another method that is not reusable. I use significantly less oil by applying the oil directly to the feet or body part and then applying the flannel soaked in very hot water. Either way, the pack is applied moist. A piece of thin plastic can be used to protect the heat of the pack. For the feet, large plastic baggies are put easily over the foot after the compress is applied and squeezed next to the foot so that all air escapes. After the plastic is applied, the small hand towel is wrapped around the foot in a way to keep air from entering the pack. After both feet are wrapped and tucked in, they are placed at the center edge of a larger towel, and the

hot water bottle is placed at the bottom of the feet outside the small towels. The edge of the large towel away from the patient is folded up over the bottle and pack. Then the towel ends are wrapped up and around the feet, securing the bottle in place and keeping the warmth in. The patient is covered with warm blankets, and the castor pack is kept in place for up to 1 to 1½ hours. After the castor oil pack is removed be sure to keep warm the body part treated with the pack. People always comment that this herbal application is very comforting.

Poultices and Plasters

Herbal poultices, also known as cataplasms, are similar to compresses, except that instead of putting the cloth in an infusion, decoction, tincture, or oil, the cloth is used to hold a slurry or softened paste of the plant material, which is then applied to the skin. Nurses may be familiar with the historical use of flaxseed, bread, onion, or hops as poultices. In 1924, Bertha Harmer wrote that poultices, "give the patient great relief and a sensation of comfort if properly applied" (p. 208). They can be used as a therapeutic measure for pneumonia; to relieve distention in postoperative patients; and for painful, inflamed, and infected wounds.

According to historian John Haller (1985), poultices were an "essential element in effective therapeutics" throughout history until the later nineteenth century when "germ theory and knowledge of asepsis lead to its gradual extinction" (p. 207), at least in biomedicine. Practitioners varied the temperature of the poultice based on the nature of the disease. They routinely used oats, cornmeal, arrowroot, carrots, chlorinated soda, and charcoal for poultices. With the advent of germ theory, the poultice fell into disuse by many, but not all, physicians because they were "found to be the source of pyogenic bacteria" (1985, p. 208). In some countries, herbalists and nurses, too, continue to successfully use the poultice, prepared fresh, with appropriate attention to hygiene and the possibility of introducing bacteria and infection.

How to Make a Poultice

- *Supplies:*
  - Linen, cheesecloth, or a light natural fiber fabric cut to size
  - Cut or chopped herb chosen for poultice. May be raw and cut or mashed, or may be lightly sautéed
- *Method:* Prepare the herb. Place the slurry of the raw or cooked herb in the center of the cheesecloth or fabric and fold the fabric to enclose the herb. The poultice should be a size that fits the body part to be treated. The poultice is left in place for a certain amount of time determined by the nature of the herb and the tolerance of the patient.

Plasters are a type of poultice in which the plant material is applied directly to the skin or through a thin cloth, but the plaster is often made of a plant powder that has been mixed into a thick paste. The most common plaster used by nurses is the mustard plaster (see chapter 7). More recently, nurses who work with lactating mothers have acknowledged the benefits of green cabbage *(Brassica oleracea L.)* leaf plasters to the breast in cases of engorgement. The cabbage leaf is applied directly to the breast, chilled, without any cloth. (Nikodem, Danziger, Gebka, Gulmezoglu, & Hofmeyr, 1993; Roberts, 1995; Roberts, Reiter, & Schuster, 1995). Another example is the use of aloe vera leaf plasters on first- and second-degree burns (see chapter 10).

Herbal Oils, Liniments, Salves, and Ointments

Herbal oils (also called oil infusions to distinguish them from essential oils) are made by saturating fresh plant material with a fixed oil such as olive, sesame, or canola oil. The oil is massaged into the skin for various reasons, depending on the plant used. For example, the flowers of *Arnica montana* are infused in oil and can be rubbed into sprains and sore muscles.

How to Make an Herbal Infused Oil

- *Supplies:*
  - Use fresh or dried plant material, depending on which plants are best used as oils and whether they must be prepared from fresh or dried herb. You may need to do some research to answer these questions. Some plants such as St. John's wort must be used fresh.
  - Wide mouth glass jar with cheesecloth and rubber band to use as cover
  - Oil
- *Method:* An oil of the flowers and tiny leaves of the St. John's wort *(Hypericum perforatum)* plant is used as an example here. St. John's wort oil is applied to first- and second-degree burns and is used in wound healing and for muscle and trigger point pain. The aerial parts of the *fresh* plant (flowers and small leaves) are collected, chopped, and placed in a wide-mouthed jar. Do not use dried St. John's wort. A little oil (preferably olive) is added to the plant material and then the flowers are crushed again with the back of a spoon. Then more oil is added to cover the plant material completely. The jar is shaken and placed in a warm location for ten days to two weeks.

The oil must be approximately 37.7°C or 100°F during the infusion time. St. John's wort oil turns red. After the oil infusion is completed, the plant material is strained out of the oil. The residual oil is pressed out of the plant material with cheesecloth. Because fresh material is used, some water may still be in the herbal oil even though the cheesecloth covering allows for some evaporation. The water can cause the oil to go rancid over time, so it is best to let the strained oil sit for one to two weeks undisturbed. The oil will rise above any water remaining and can be decanted off into brown glass storage bottles.

If dried plant material is used to make an herbal oil (herbs other than St. John's wort), grind the dried herb to a powder when you are ready to make the oil. Wet the herb thoroughly with oil and stir. Add oil so that the level is a few centimeters above the herb powder. Cap the jar tightly and put in a warm place. The same method is followed except dried herbs absorb the oil. The oil level must be checked after the first twenty-four hours, and more oil is added if needed.

Liniments are lighter topical remedies than oils and are usually alcohol or camphor based for quick absorption by the skin. Liniments have been used traditionally to warm and stimulate muscles and ligaments. They evaporate quickly so that no oil is left on the skin as with herbal oils. Liniments are often used before physical exercise to warm up the body, but they also can be used for local inflammation after exertion. Liniments are used in specific areas of the body, not for full body massage. The herbs traditionally used as liniments are the more warming herbs like cayenne and lobelia. One of my favorite liniments is a camphor-based liniment with lobelia that is applied to the temples for discomfort related to headache, migraine, and eyestrain. The camphor, as with all alcohol-based liniments, is cooling, while the herb is warming. Liniments feel initially cool on the skin and then quickly begin to warm. They cause a beneficial exchange of the blood in a specific area through this cooling and warming action.

Herbal salves and ointments are semisolid plant preparations that are absorbed into the skin. The base for an herbal salve or ointment is the herbal oil (already prepared) and a wax such as beeswax.

How to Make an Herbal Salve
- *Supplies:*
  - Herbal infused oil already prepared or plain oil can be used (Plain vegetable oil is used when drops of essential oils are to be used.)
  - Beeswax (approximately 28 g per 250 ml oil or 1 ounce wax per 1 cup oil)
  - Tincture of benzoin (1 drop per 30 ml or 1 ounce of oil) as a preservative
- *Method:* This is the basic process for making a salve. The ingredients must be adjusted, based on the herbs used and the consistency desired. The oil and shaved beeswax are placed in the top of a double boiler and the wax is melted. Test the consistency by pouring a small amount of the salve into a jar. It should harden quickly and be the consistency that you want. Add more oil if you want the salve to be softer and more wax if you want it harder, depending on the nature of the application. For example, in the care of an open wound, a hard salve would not be used because applying it takes a little more rubbing, which is not helpful when the wound is healing. A softer salve would be needed that smoothes over the wound easily. When the consistency of the salve is right, add the tincture of benzoin as a preservative.

Aromatic essential oils also can be used in making oils, liniments, salves, and ointments for topical application. Essential oils are extracted from aromatic plants. They make up a very small amount of the whole plant. Essential oils evaporate readily and therefore, once extracted, must be kept in sealed bottles. They are sold in small amounts because they are a highly concentrated plant constituent. For medicinal purposes they must be used in pure form. Aromatic oils often are considered precious and valuable and are used in small amounts. Like perfume, essential oils are meant to be used in amounts that do not overpower the sense of smell. Some essential oils are lighter in fragrance than others. For example, lemon verbena is less intense than cinnamon. Herbal oils, often used for massage, are made with drops of essential oils in a light carrier oil such as sweet almond oil, which has no fragrance. Keville and Green (1995) recommend a 2% to 3% dilution (10 to 12 drops per 1 ounce/30 ml of vegetable oil) and a 1% dilution (5 drops per 1 ounce/30 ml oil) for pregnant women, people with illness, and children (p. 23). For a liniment, they recommend the use of essential oils of ginger, eucalyptus, peppermint, and cinnamon (Keville & Green, 1995, p. 75). Patients should always choose their own aromatic massage oil or liniment because fragrance preference is very personal. Essential oils also can be blended for specific medicinal effects related to the absorption of the properties of the oil through the skin and the inhalation of the scent. Through their unique fragrances and their visual beauty, healing plants can contribute to the creation of a healing environment.

PLANTS AND A HEALING ENVIRONMENT:

The creation of a healing environment is very important in the care of patients. Plants as part of the natural environment are an important part of the care of patients. The personality or medicine of a plant is not only ingested or felt through contact with the skin. Plant medicine can be experienced through environmental interaction. It can be inhaled with the air as aromatherapy, steams and inhalations, absorbed with water through herbal baths, "taken in" through vision, and experienced by direct interaction through a garden experience.

Aromatherapy and Inhalations

Aromatherapy, like homeopathy, is related to herbal medicine, but because it is a specific science and art in its own right, it is only mentioned here. The essential oils from aromatic plants can be used to affect the health of body, mind, and spirit. Throughout history, perfumers have known of the medicinal benefits of the aromatic volatile fragrances they used. Religious rituals continue to include the aromatic use of plants as incense, such as frankincense *(Boswellia carterii)*. The olfactory cells are the only place in the human body where the central nervous system comes in direct contact with the external environment (Lawless, 1998). Humans' sense of smell is one direct connection with their environment. Plants often provide that sensory experience. The essential oils from plants used in a practice known as aromatherapy do not just provide a pleasurable or memorable experience. They have been shown through numerous studies to have specific healing properties. Studies have shown the antibacterial, antiviral, and antifungal effects of essential oils in the human body (Buckle, 1997). Studies also have shown other significant effects on mood, alertness, and electroencephalogram patterns (Diego et al., 1998). Scientists such as Dr. Alan Hirsch of the Smell and Taste Treatment and Research Foundation (www.smellandtaste.org) are researching the effects of odor from various plant sources on learning and behavior.

Nurses have become interested in the art and science of aromatherapy. Jane Buckle (1997), a nurse author who has written the book *Clinical Aromatherapy in Nursing,* describes numerous ways that nurses can clinically use and research the healing effects of essential oils. For example, she describes the potential use of aromatherapy in hospitals as "a complete hospital stress management package, producing a happier and more content work force, with more secure and less anxious patients" (p. 23). Buckle (1997) suggests that the integration of clinical aromatherapy into nursing practice may form "a bridge between orthodox and alternative medicine" (p. 266).

In addition to aromatherapy, medicinal herbs also are taken in with the air through the modalities of smoking and steaming. Herbs such as mullein leaf *(Verbascum spp.)* are smoked for their healing effect upon the lungs. The herb is smoked in much the same way a tobacco cigar or cigarette is smoked. Herbal steam inhalations are often used in the healing of the sinuses. Chamomile inhalations are one example.

How to Make an Herbal Steam Inhalation
- *Supplies:*
  - Plant to be infused—usually an aromatic herb such as chamomile or lemon
  - Large bowl
  - 1 large and 1 small towel
  - Hot water bottle
- *Method:* Prepare a warm room and have the patient sit next to a table. The patient should be dressed warmly, with socks on and his feet resting on a hot water bottle. The herb is placed in the bowl and boiling water is poured over the plant material. Cover the patient's head and shoulders with the large towel and place the towel over the bowl so that the vapors do not escape. The patient breathes in the vapors for about fifteen minutes, at which time the patient's head should be dried and covered with a small dry towel to prevent chilling.

Herbal Baths

Some people may consider herbal baths a luxury. They are really a necessity. Hippocrates, the father of modern medicine, stated that the key to good health rested on having a daily aromatic bath and scented massage (Lawless, 1998, p. 13). During herbal baths, the plant medicine surrounds the body, allowing for the intermingling of plant and human in a deeply healing experience. Many herbs are used in baths for their aromatic effects. Plants also can be used to create other effects. Lavender *(Lavendula officinalis),* for example, also can be healing to the skin. Herbal full baths, sitz baths, and foot baths all can be used in the care of patients.

How to Make an Herbal Bath

- *Supplies:*
  - Herbal infusion (i.e., a strong water extraction that can be diluted in the bath)
  - Tub, foot, or sitz basin
  - Towels
- *Method:* To prepare a herbal bath infusion, use one handful of cut herb per liter or quart of water. For a full body tub make 3 quarts/L; use less for smaller basins. Steep the herbs in cold water for a few hours or overnight and then heat almost to boiling, cover and allow the herbs to steep for ten minutes. Strain the infusion and pour into tub or basin filled with warm water. Adjust the temperature and submerge. Baths should last at least twenty minutes because that is the amount of time the pores take to open fully. After the bath, the body should be wrapped warmly in towels and allowed to perspire for a short time. Even the feet will perspire after a foot bath. Dry the body and put on fresh clothing.

Some essential oils such as rose, eucalyptus, and rosemary can be used instead of herbal infusions in a bath. Three to fifteen drops of pure essential oil can be used per large tub, depending on the type of oil. For a foot bath, 5 to 10 drops per liter or quart of water are used (Keville & Green, 1995). Taking an herbal bath and smelling fragrant oils can cause one to remember soothing moments of direct interactions with plants, either during a walk in the woods or through a fragrant garden.

Healing Gardens

Experiences in nature can be very calming to body, mind, and spirit. A stroll through a meadow, a walk in the woods, and gardening too can decrease stress levels and cultivate a positive outlook on life. Landscape architects and artists have created gardens in healing institutions where patients can have the opportunity to interact with nature. Cancer patients can actually see the plants that inspired the drugs they take in botanical gardens housed in the hospitals they go to for treatment. Gardens and gardening provide a connection with the earth, the soil, and the life that springs forth from it. Watching a plant grow gives a sense of the continuation of life. And watching a plant go by or a tree lose its leaves in the winter can give us reassurance that all life, not just human life, is impermanent and has a cycle. When people are sick they can feel isolated and afraid. Being part of nature can reconnect people with the larger processes and cycles present in nature of which they are a part. Reestablishing a connection with nature during illness can be comforting and healing. Even *viewing* pictures of bright, colorful nature scenes has been shown to improve outcome in postoperative cardiac patients undergoing various procedures (Friedrich, 1999).

Horticultural therapy is a specific modality that is described as one of the oldest healing arts. The horticultural therapist is concerned with how people interact in the horticultural environment, how people act working with plants, and how people react to passive involvement with plants. The plant world is often viewed as nonthreatening by patients. They may be given an opportunity to pot plants or seeds either individually to improve hand-eye coordination or attention skills, or with others to improve their socialization skills. "The essence of horticulture is action . . . a person works with plants doing things with them or to them to modify and enhance their growth . . . one explanation for the positive response that man has to working with plants may be because it deals with life cycles and most people make a ready translation between the life cycle of plants and their own human life cycle" (Relf, 2000, p. 4). There are a growing number of horticultural therapy programs in hospitals, community centers, and botanical gardens that offer people an opportunity to dig in the dirt, plant a seed, and be part of the nurturing of life in plants. Master's level educational programs also are available for practitioners who want to use horticulture as their modality for therapy.

Hospitals used to have their own botanical gardens that provided the herbs that practitioners used in remedies for patients. Some facilities continue this tradition for the benefit of staff and patients. Some of the hospitals I have visited have had gardens that were cared for by the nursing students during their education. I worked as a coordinator of an herb program where many of the herbs we raised were used in the remedies provided to patients. I often had patients harvest their own herbs as part of their treatment. They enjoyed this very much.

The staff of botanical gardens are some of those who have taken on the responsibility of educating the public about medicinal plants. Nurses too can benefit greatly from growing their own medicines and tending to plant life. Picking just one plant to study its growth cycle, its personality, and its medicinal properties can be deeply rewarding and healing. A garden can be a small window box on a sunny windowsill or a large community vegetable and herb garden. The size doesn't matter. It's the opportunity to experience the tending of plant life and making your own plant medicine that's important.

Partnering With Plants

In using plant medicines, a person enters into a partnership with a plant. The plant provides the vehicle for healing, but the user must offer an intent. How the plant medicine is used by the nurse and patient is as important to the healing of the patient as the vehicle for healing (the plant). The care expressed in the harvesting and processing of the plant is important to the potency of the resulting medicine. How a nurse or patient applies an herbal oil to the skin, prepares a bath, and serves a tea are important parts of the healing experience using a plant medicine. Nurses can apply the unique ways they demonstrate care to their use of plant therapies.

As nurses around the world grow in their understanding of herbal remedies and medicine making, they can share with others their experiences of how those remedies influence health and illness of patients and their own practice, health, and well-being. This sharing about plant therapies is helpful to the development of herbal remedies as part of nature care and their continued recognition as a part of nursing practice. Nurses who learn the art and science of medicine making can then teach and empower others in their communities to establish plant partnerships that can be instrumental in healing illness, promoting health and long life, and connecting with one's roots.

CHAPTER 6
Plant Profiles

FIFTY-EIGHT PLANTS ARE PROFILED IN DETAIL IN CHAPTERS 7 to 18. These plants were chosen specifically because of their familiarity to nurses and/or potential for use in nursing practice and research. After the herbs were selected for this edition, I asked, "How would *nurses* want to see the herbs presented?" Numerous herb books present herbs in an alphabetized format either by common or botanical name. Books arranged by common name can create a barrier to use because there are numerous common names for a single plant in different parts of the world. Arranging an herb book by botanical name also may be a barrier to use because readers are often not familiar with the botanical name of a medicinal plant. Also, when a health practitioner has no knowledge of botanical or common names for herbs, arranging the book by herb name may not be helpful. When using an herb text, health practitioners often turn to the index to see what herbs may be useful for a particular health concern. Organizing an herb book by health concerns for nurses learning about herbs seemed to be the most practical approach. Having resolved my approach to this text, I then asked, "What health concerns should be used?"

Some herb books are arranged by *disease process* such as "herbs for diabetes or herbs for heart disease." Although this is often helpful for practitioners, including registered and advanced practice nurses, using a disease process or medical diagnosis as the organizational basis for arranging herbs in an herb guide does not directly relate to the paradigm of the practicing nurse whose focus is not medical diagnosis. The focus of nursing is the patient's patterns of response to illness. Although professional nurses use pathophysiologic and psychopathologic concepts in practice, we routinely work with patients who have common health concerns that do not necessarily fall into a category related to disease process or medical diagnosis per se. Patients' health concerns are often related to mild, everyday discomforts or imbalances. It is these concerns that nurses have traditionally included in their care plans, and it is for these types of concerns that nurses have historically used plant remedies. Therefore, the herbs in this book have been arranged by those patterns of response that in this guide are referred to as *health patterns*.

Nurses develop nursing diagnoses after recognition of health patterns rather than disease process. The titles of the health patterns used to organize the herbs in this guide are comfort and pain relief, hormone balance, immune response, skin care, sleep and rest, elimination, digestion, energy, emotions and adaptation, mobility, lifestyle choices, and restoration. Although nurses do not use herbs to treat disease they have and can continue to use herbs in practice to promote patterns of health. Some of the titles of health patterns chosen for this guide may be familiar, while others may be unfamiliar (e.g., restoration). For this reason, chapters 7 through 18 begin with brief introductions to the health pattern and its relationship with plant therapies.

Within each herb profile, the information provided also includes disease-related information. There has been significant research in biomedicine on the effects of herbs on disease processes. Information about traditional or cultural use also is included in the profiles. Traditional information includes data that focus on concerns not necessarily defined as disease. For example, traditional healers may recognize that a person is not sleeping well. The person may be experiencing sleeplessness but not necessarily have a disease such as depression, which often includes symptoms such as insomnia. There is also a recognition in traditional healing that symptoms such as sleeplessness are not the same in all people. Different herbs may be used for different people with sleeplessness. For example, some people may have difficulty falling asleep and some people fall asleep easily but wake frequently during the night. The herb or herbs are adapted for the individual manifestation of the health concern.

The herbs in this guide are assigned to a chapter, based on an outstanding characteristic demonstrating their relationship to the particular health pattern either from a scientific or traditional perspective or both. For example, cinnamon is included in the chapter on mobility because it is traditionally used in herbal formulas for unblocking channels or energy meridians and vessels of the body, allowing warmth, blood, and *qi* to move. Kava-kava is in the chapter on emotions because

Table 6.1

ORGANIZATION OF HERB PROFILES

   I. Latin Name

  II. Family

 III. Common Names

 IV. Health Pattern

  V. Plant Description

 VI. Plant Parts Used

VII. Traditional Evidence
- A. Cultural Use
  1. Asian
  2. North American Indian
  3. Hispanic
  4. Pacific Islander
  5. Australian
  6. African
  7. East Indian
  8. Middle Eastern
  9. Russian/Baltic
  10. European
- B. Culinary Use
- C. Use in Herbalism

VIII. Biomedical Evidence
- A. Studies Related to (Health Pattern)
- B. Studies Related to Other Health Patterns
- C. Mechanism of Action

 IX. Use in Pregnancy or Lactation

  X. Use for Children

 XI. Cautions

XII. Nursing Evidence
- A. Historical Nursing Use
- B. Potential Nursing Applications
- C. Integrative Insight

XIII. Therapeutic Applications
- A. Oral
- B. Topical
- C. Environmental

XIV. Patient Interaction

XV. Nurturing the Nurse-Plant Relationship

research has found it to have an antianxiety effect. In actuality, each plant medicine may have many uses and classifying them by how they may influence one particular health pattern may seem limiting. For this reason, the herb has been included under one primary health pattern to facilitate use of the herb guide, while in addition, there are sections in each profile, such as Use in Herbalism or Studies Related to Other Health Patterns where the herb's other uses are addressed.

The remainder of this chapter details the format used in presenting the information on each of the fifty-eight plants profiled in chapters 7 through 18. Within each herb profile, the data on the plant are organized by headings to facilitate the referencing of the material. The headings are listed in Table 6.1. Each heading, including the cultural uses, is described here.

Introduction to Profiles

The following is an outline and brief summary of the purpose of each section of the herb profiles listed in Table 6.1. Throughout history, books about healing herbs, known as herbals, were written to summarize the information known about an herb. This herbal guide summarizes some of the traditional and biomedical data on the herb profiled and also offers suggestions for the future use of the plant in nursing care.

LATIN NAME AND FAMILY:

Latin is the universal language of plant taxonomy or classification. The Latin name is often descriptive of the plant's features. Latin names have two parts that identify the plant being discussed: (1) the genus name, which is capitalized and (2) the species name, which appears in lower case. Botanical names are italicized. The family name also is given. Throughout the profile chapters, a specific species of plant is identified; however, in some cases more than one species of the genus of the plant profiled is discussed. When using the information from the profiles be sure to clearly identify the genus and species of the medicinal plant you use in all documentation of care and clinical discussion.

COMMON NAMES:

The common names of medicinal plants are, as with all language, culturally defined. They are often too numerous to list. The common names have been presented in the profile to help in communicating with patients who use herbal remedies and often know the remedy by its common name. Common names also have been used in naming the profiles themselves for ease of access; however, there is a cross-reference in the index between common and Latin botanical names in case only one name is known. Some common names in languages other than English are identified in the sections under their respective cultures so that if a nurse were to talk with a patient who only knows the name of the herb in the language of his or her country, the nurse can still find the herb if included in the guide.

HEALTH PATTERN:

This is the main pattern for which the plant is being profiled as previously discussed. Although the focus of the profile is specifically related to the primary health pattern, the herb profiled often has qualities related to other health patterns. Traditional and biomedical data supporting use for other health patterns is presented in the Traditional Evidence section and in Studies Related to Other Health Patterns. Because in tradition, plants grown in a particular area might be used by the people of that area for many different health concerns, the traditional data presented in the herb profile often include a description of multiple uses of the plant other than the specific health pattern under which the herb is arranged here.

PLANT DESCRIPTION:

The plant description identifies specific features of the healing plant such as a leaf or growth pattern. It is important for anyone using plants in healing to be able to accurately identify the plant to be used. One way to learn to identify plants is from a botanist, herbalist, or horticulturist who knows the plant. The descriptions presented here can be used as a general resource for starting to become familiar with the characteristics of plants. It is important to identify such things as the leaf pattern, flower color, growth pattern, smell, and size. Specifics on how to grow and harvest each herb are not included in this herb guide.

PLANT PARTS USED:

This section lists the parts of a plant most commonly used in therapeutic applications, such as the root, flower, seed, or leaf.

TRADITIONAL EVIDENCE:

There are three forms of "evidence" presented in this herb guide that are based in the three paradigms discussed in chapter 3: traditional, biomedical, and nursing evidence. The following sections discuss the subheadings under which traditional evidence has been organized.

Cultural Use

It is fascinating to learn how plants are used as medicine from one country to another. Sometimes the plant is used similarly and sometimes very differently. To speak in general of entire cultures and their use of a plant may seem somewhat limiting because people *within* a specific culture often have diverse and creative ways of using medicinal plants. There are patterns or trends in herb use among cultural groups beginning with whether or not a plant grows in the location where the cultural group is established. Many cultures have shared an understanding of plant medicine as various groups of people have traveled, explored, and even plundered or encroached upon other groups. For example, Europeans moved to North America and learned the traditional plant medicine practices of the North American Indian, who intimately understood the plants of the continent. Yet, from tribe to tribe in North America, there is variation among what herb is used for a particular health pattern as well as what herbs are used at all.

The information in this cultural section was collected from reference texts and reports of ethnobotanical research. Input about herb use among various cultural groups from nurses with personal understanding of those cultures is also included in this section. The intent of this section is to provide a brief accounting of plant use related to cultural groups as a way of shedding some light on the pattern of use from a global perspective.

Asian. Herbs have been used in traditional medicine practices throughout Asia for centuries. There are highly developed systems of medicine, in China, Japan, and Korea, for example, that include the use of plants. Traditional Chinese medicine (TCM) is the system that is the primary focus here. The use of herbs in TCM is based on the principle of balance, a major concept in Taoist philosophy, and on the recognition of patterns of symptoms and signs unique to a given patient. The Chinese system of herbalism recognizes that no two symptoms, such as a headache, are alike when the whole picture, or symptom-sign pattern, is assessed. The Chinese system of herbal medicine has been very successful, not necessarily because of the herbs used, but more so because of the way the herbs are used.

The herbs in a Chinese *Materia Medica* are not herbs that are necessarily native to or cultivated in China. The Chinese actually collected medicinal plants from around the globe to add to their *Materia Medica*. Yet some species of "Chinese" herbs are found primarily, if not exclusively, in Asia. The successful treatment of a patient with Chinese herbs stems from the understanding of the patient's unique *response* to illness, disease, or discomfort. This is similar to the nursing process of understanding and intervening in actual and potential responses to illness.

Response to illness often occurs incrementally. I have noticed this for example when working with patients with back pain. When a thorough history and assessment of the signs and symptoms are taken without discounting any data reported by the patient, a pattern of acute episodes is often easily recognized. Patients might discover that every time they eat a specific food they get slightly constipated and then their back begins to go into spasm, leading to another acute episode. "It is commonly observed by TCM doctors that clearly detectable imbalances in a patient's health and their corresponding symptoms manifest long before they are usually detected as an abnormality in blood chemistry, x-rays, electrical activity, etc. . . . The success of TCM health care is partly due to its ability to detect imbalances in health in their early stages" (Wicke, 1992, p. 14). The assessment process includes history; determination of symptom-sign patterns (a grouping of symptoms), such as whether the person likes cold or hot drinks; the consistency of the patient's stool; the tone of their voice; their skin color; and a diagnosis of the tongue and pulse. Once the pattern or patterns are identified, an herbal tea is formulated specifically for the patient. The formula is designed to promote balance. One example of designing a balancing formula is, if the patient has interior cold, they might receive a formula with herbs that warm the interior.

TCM has its own language related to symptom-sign patterns and classification of herbs that is learned by practitioners and the public. An herb in China might be sold for "yin deficiency" condition. Westerners who use Chinese herbs, those herbs in a Chinese *Materia Medica,* must learn the language and underlying philosophy of the system to be able to effectively apply the principles and methods of the system. Failure to do so can result in ineffective application and treatment. The Asian section includes the language of the TCM system to begin to familiarize the reader with the terminology used in the system. Resources for further learning of the TCM system are included in chapter 19 and in the appendix.

Tea formulation is a major issue in the TCM system of herbal medicine. Herbs are used most commonly in formulation because they are synergistic. Putting two herbs together in the same formula can have a greater effect than giving the herbs separately. It is a phenomenon that may not be able to be fully explained from a conventional pharmaceutical paradigm. The Chinese have had hundreds of years of trial and error and scientific observation that has laid the foundation of a highly effective system of herbal medicine.

The traditional practitioner of Chinese medicine begins treatment with suggesting lifestyle and dietary changes. If the imbalance is not affected by the changes, then herbs and other modalities are introduced. Herbs are used to treat acute and chronic illness in China. For example, since the cultural revolution (until 1975), as many as 20,000 cases of appendicitis have been treated with herbal formulas (different in various hospitals) with a 90% overall cure rate (National Academy of Sciences, 1975). Many herb gardens are situated in traditional medical colleges for students to see as they are studying. Although studies of the herbs are always being done (usually human rather than animal studies), many Chinese oppose the placebo-controlled trial because of ethical issues. They believe that placebo use is deceptive (National Academy of Sciences, 1975, p. 67). Because of the many years of traditional use of herbs in humans, the studies on Chinese herbs are often performed to understand why and how the herbs have worked. Chinese researchers believe that safety is not an issue in human trials because the herbs have already been shown to be safe, and they do not feel that animal trials are necessary.

In China, nurses are educated to work in TCM hospitals. As mentioned in chapter 3, nurses in conventional hospitals also may administer herbal therapies in practice. There are numerous oral, topical, and intravenous applications of herbs. Many of the herbs and prepared herbal products are exported to other countries. Analgesic salves with exotic names like "tiger balm" (does not contain tiger) are becoming more common in Western use. Western practitioners often voice concerns about the quality of some of the Chinese products. Chinese whole dried herbs must be washed thoroughly because of the fertilizers used. When using whole herbs, care must be taken to clearly identify herbs and sources of product. This is a good practice regardless of where the herb comes from. There is also a concern about patent formulations, prepared remedies often in tablet form in which unwanted ingredients might be included. Examples of substances that have been known to be included in patent formulas include steroids and heavy metals such as lead. For this reason, it is recommended that a TCM practitioner be consulted for use of patent formulas.

Kampo medicine, Japanese traditional medicine, is very similar to TCM in philosophy and the herbs used. Kampo is used clinically and also is being researched in hopes of shedding light on the mechanism of action of the successful, time-tested traditional Japanese remedies.

North American Indian. North American Indian traditional medicine is part of the history of nursing in North America. Midwives and caregivers, often the women of the households of the European settlers, learned how to apply plant remedies in caring for themselves and their families from Native American healers. Early North American medical dispensatories included plant medicines commonly used by various Native American groups. Yet the Native American contribution to the medical practices of North Americans is often devalued if not grossly underrecognized.

This section of the herb profile lists some of the traditional uses of the herb by various North American Indian tribes. Often you may notice that it is not uncommon for the same herb to be used for the same action (e.g., as an emetic) but completely different ailments. North American Indian medicine includes the use of plant remedies for wounds, fractures, and numerous illnesses. Some illnesses are not only treated with plant remedies. For example, "persistent internal disease" is thought to be caused by supernatural forces; therefore, other methods of healing besides plant remedies, such as chant, dance, and drumming, also are used in healing.

North American Indian herbalists, called "Mashki-kike-winini," receive a calling to know the various mysterious properties of medicinal plants. "Although these herbalists are aware that certain plants or roots will produce a specified effect upon the human system, they attribute the benefit to the fact that such remedies are distasteful and injurious to the demons who are present in the system and whom the disease is attributed" (Vogel, 1970, p. 23).

The term "medicine" to a North American Indian has meaning that extends well beyond the remedy or treatment. Medicine is equated with the "mysterious, inexplicable, and unaccountable" (Vogel, 1970, p. 25). This section of the herb profile by no means begins to capture the rituals and mystical understanding held by the American Indian traditional healers regarding the individual plant. Much of this plant wisdom and understanding is protected as a valuable treasure and is not shared even by tribal members without the express permission and spiritual guidance of the tribal elders and healers. Ethnobotanical studies have revealed the richness of the healing traditions of various American Indian tribes such as the Zuni and Cheyenne and that knowledge of traditional beliefs and customs in regard to medicinal plant healing is diminishing (Camazine & Bye, 1980; Hart, 1981).

Hispanic. The Hispanic uses of herbal "remedios" or "yerbas" included in this section are from various countries, including Spain, the southwestern United States, and countries in Central and South America. There is a rich history of plant use among Hispanic peoples that, as with the other cultures listed here, greatly exceeds the scope of this guide. It is hoped that this sample of some of the traditional Hispanic uses of plant medicines will give the reader an understanding of some of the ways herbs have been used in the Hispanic culture. The way herbs are used within the Hispanic culture varies greatly from country to country, region to region, and even individual to individual. The remedies used and the value placed on those traditional remedies also depends on the cultural group and the plants that grow in the area where people live.

Among Hispanics, the understanding of the "remedios" is often passed orally from generation to generation. In preparing this book, I met with a Hispanic nurse-herbal healer and her family. The grandchildren of the family use the remedies made by their grandmother from the herbs she grows. As with many cultures, use of traditional remedies can be influenced by the presence of biomedicine, the presence of traditional healers, and the belief system and preferences of the individual.

Women continue the tradition of sharing plant healing knowledge among each other and with their families. Margarita Kay, a nurse-medical anthropologist, has written extensively on medicinal plants of the Mexican and American West. She writes that herb gardens were common among the Aztec people (Kay, 1996, p. 22), and she traces the use of medicinal plants in relationship to the exporting of plants from Spain to the New World. For some Hispanics, use of plant remedies is interwoven with their religious beliefs and practices, especially in the West after the conquests of Holy Roman Emperor Charles V. Charles V studied the indigenous healing and uses of herbs in the West. "He is cited today as the first researcher to use ethnographic techniques in his interviews" (Kay, 1996, p. 23). Under Christian influence, herbs used by Hispanics have been named after saints or religious figures and some rituals around their use have been influenced by religion, such as setting dates for herb harvest on the feast days of certain saints. The first herbal of the Americas is said to have been written in 1552 by Martin de la Cruz, an Aztec, in his native language. The herbal was later translated to Latin (Foster, 1992, p. 12).

The other aspect of Hispanic use of herbs that has drawn much attention is in the area of the rainforests of Central and South America. The indigenous peoples of the Amazonian rainforest have access to an area of the globe that is said to house 80,000 species of higher plants, which is 15% of the world's flora. The Amazon rainforest is a "neglected chemical laboratory" that offers the greatest possibility of new drugs (Schultes, 1994, p. 107). The survival of many regions of the Amazonian rainforest is in jeopardy because of road construction, lumber industry, warfare, tourism, industry encroachment on the land, and governmental attempts to civilize the indigenous peoples. Conservationists continue to call for help for this region of the globe to preserve the rainforest and its wealth of vegetation and medicinal plant knowledge among its indigenous peoples.

Pacific Islander. This section includes information specifically related to the traditional use of herbs among Hawaiian and Polynesian indigenous healers. The essence of Hawaiian herbal healing is spirituality. Plants are an important component of Hawaiian herbal healing but they are only considered the tools of healing. Hawaiian herbal healing includes the belief in God or a Higher Being, belief in prayer, belief in the healer, belief in "mihi" or asking forgiveness, and "kala" or giving forgiveness.

Native Hawaiian herbal healing is called "laau lapaau." In the 1800s under the influence of Western beliefs and power, indigenous Hawaiian healers known as "kahuna" or keepers of the secrets, were driven underground. Today, Hawaiian herbal healers call themselves "kupuna," or "elders," and are once again sharing their plant knowledge and wisdom with others.

Nanette Judd (1997), a Hawaiian nurse, conducted a multi-island study in which she interviewed and extensively studied "kupuna" and their healing practices. Hawaiian herbal healers learn healing "laau" by observing, listening, and doing in apprenticeship with a teacher. Healers learn that they are instruments of God and are not responsible for the healing that takes place. They believe that God channels power through them. Herbalists begin each day with prayer and then pray continuously throughout the day. It is believed that herbal healers must have the following attributes:

- Loving others
- Humility
- Asking for forgiveness
- Forgiving others
- Respecting God
- Having respect and faith in the "laau"
- Respecting others
- Being ready to serve others

Hawaiian herbal healers value living in harmony with nature. Because of this, plants are used for many aspects of daily life. Herbal healers select the strongest "laau" according to smell, taste, color of the leaves, healthy appearance, and place of growth. Access to "kupuna" is through word of mouth, although some clinics in Hawaii now have integrated programs, providing biomedical and traditional healing side by side. The average age of the elders, according to Judd, is 70 years old. The elders are concerned about not finding anyone to pass their knowledge on to and the protection of the environment, the source of "laau."

The foundation of Samoan traditional medicine is also spiritual. Health is believed to be achieved through balance of the three worlds—the natural world, the social world, and the spiritual world— and by avoiding tensions. Samoan healers called "fofo" use plant medicine. The first line of defense for many Samoans is traditional medicine, although biomedicine is very accessible. Samoan medicine is especially important in the treatment of illness in infants. Herbs are used in folk remedies known by the people of Samoa and by the "fofo," whom people go to when their illness is not helped by the folk remedies that are used like first aid. Nurses and physicians are said to be very tolerant of traditional healers and healing practices even if they do not hold the same faith in the healing practices that the people do (Whistler, 1996).

Australian. In Australia, two systems of herbal medicine exist. One is the indigenous herbal practice of the Aborigines and the other is European herbal medicine brought by British settlers. Very little research has been conducted on the plants used by Aboriginals. "Only a handful of people are left who have extensive knowledge of Aboriginal herbal medicine . . . while men know all the plants, the women know the finer details of their respective uses . . . information on medicinal plants is being lost every year as the older generation of Aborigines diminishes in number (Lassak & McCarthy, 1997, p. 14).

The Aborigines have not always readily shared their knowledge of medicinal plants and British settlers have not always shown interest in learning native medicinal practices. The Aboriginal people and the British settlers have interacted at times regarding investigation of native Australian flora. Language barriers regarding the names of medicinal plants have been a challenge to researching and understanding the plants in Australia. "The use of Aboriginal names may confuse matters . . . the white man's rendering of the sound he heard differed from person to person. There are cases where Aborigines have taken English words and changed them so as to be unrecognizable to whites when they boomeranged back under the guise of being genuine Aboriginal names" (Lassak & McCarthy, 1997, p. 18). Some common Australian medicinal flora include various species of *Eucalyptus* and *Melaleuca* trees.

African. African herbal healing can be traced back to approximately 3200 B.C. during the reign of Menes, the first Egyptian pharaoh (Iwu, 1993). The Ebers papyrus, one of the oldest *Materia Medica* in history, lists several medicinal and food plants. "In traditional African medicine, many food plants are used for therapeutic purposes, and medicines are not viewed as 'necessary poisons' as in Western orthodox medicine" (Iwu, 1993, p. 1). Some examples of plants used in African traditional healing are kola, areca nuts, calabar bean *(Physostigma venenosum),* devil's claw *(Harpagophytum procumbens),* and African periwinkle *(Catharanthus roseus).*

African traditional medicine is based on the belief that everything has a life force and that, "Preservation or restoration of health cannot be pursued without involving these life forces all of which have their own personality and cosmic place" (DeSmet, 1999, p. 12). A traditional healer's power manifests in his or her ability to apply understanding of the relationship between all things in nature for the good of the patient and the community. Africans believe that man cannot be separated from nature. Medicine men and women use herbal remedies as part of their holistic service, which includes a consideration of the patient's mind and soul as well as the body. The traditional African system of medicine is "based on persistent faith in the natural order of the world and in healing symbols manifested in cryptic creatures, hidden habits, and artifacts that serve as points of contact between the physical world and the spiritual realm" (Iwu, in DeSmet, 1999, p. 8).

The spiritual significance of the herbal remedy is much more important in the African traditional medicine system than the biochemical properties of the plant used in healing. Patients take herbal remedies for the healing benefit of the life force in the plant. The remedies also are taken because they are endowed with powers by the healer, such as the power of ancestors or other spirits that have been asked to overshadow the remedy. "The African healer therefore questions strongly any form of treatment that focuses only on the organic diseased state and ignores the spiritual side of the illness" (Iwu, 1993, p. 310). African traditional healers continue in the lineage of some of the most outstanding healers in the history of man, the Egyptians. Although some think that African healers are simply, "witch doctors" who may have only a knowledge of magic and charms, African healers often have an understanding of the medical sciences. "Ancient Egyptian medicine, like all African medicine, has baffled scholars because of the complete interpenetration of 'magicospiritual' and 'rational' elements" (Iwu, 1993, p. 313).

Plant remedies are common in Africa. For instance, in South Africa, between 12 and 15 million people use traditional remedies from as many as 700 species of plants. Ethnographic studies in one province alone have shown that thirty-eight plant species are used externally as washings or poultices in the treatment of wounds (Grierson & Afolayan, 1999). In addition to skin applications, herbal remedies are applied to the body by enema, inhalation, oral forms, drops for the ears and nose, and lotions. "The cures dispensed by the medicine man are not all products of chance, but results of years of careful experimentation and painstaking observations. The pharmacopoeia of the medicine man is rich with cures . . . for many intractable human diseases, such as cancer and various immune deficiency disorders" (Iwu, 1993, p. 5). Africans today continue to seek a better understanding of the integration of traditional and biomedical healing knowledge and practice.

East Indian. The two primary traditional medicine systems in India are known as Ayurveda and Unani. The focus here is Ayurveda or the "science of life." The *Caraka Samhita,* "Collection of Caraka," is the oldest known Sanskrit text on the practice of traditional medicine in India. The date of its exact composition and its exact author are unknown. Some historians conclude from the actual writing, that *Caraka* was written between 300 B.C. and 600 B.C. *Caraka Samhita* is said to have been the result of a meeting of sages somewhere in the Himalayas. The major portion of the work is written in the form of questions and answers between a teacher and disciple. According to *Caraka*, life is everlasting and without beginning and therefore Ayurveda, the science of life, has always been in existence (Ray & Gupta, 1980).

The philosophy of the *Caraka* is related to the Hindi doctrines "Samkhya" and "Vedanta." *Caraka* philosophy holds that each person is a replica of the universal; man is an epitome of the macrocosm. Spirit and matter are an integrated whole. It is also written in *Caraka Samhita* that the aim of the study of medical science is the pursuit of the sound mind and body as prerequisites for the beatific experience of "Brahman," or the "divine." The sound mind and body are pursued as an aid to fulfillment of the four purposes of life: "dharma," or duty; "artha," or acquisition of wealth; "kama," or satisfaction of desire; and "moksa," or self-realization. The nurse or "attendant" is clearly defined in the *Caraka* as one of four basic factors of treatment of patients. "The physician, the drugs, the attendant, and the patient constitute the four basic factors of treatment" (Ghai & Ghai, 1997, p. 131).

The foundation of Ayurvedic medical theory is "tridosha," similar to humoral theory. In Ayurveda, three "dosha" exist in the body: "vayu" or "vata," "pitta," and "kapha." Different parts of the body are associated with each of the "dosha." Health is defined as the balance of the three "dosha"; however, every individual is believed to be born with a predominant "dosha," which has the tendency to create imbalances or disease. For example if a person is "vata" predominant and eats foods that aggravate "vata," they can become ill with a "vata" type illness. Understanding "tridosha" theory takes years of study and is well beyond the scope of this book. *Caraka Samhita's* vast scope includes such topics as "sarira" (anatomy), "vyadhi" (pathology), "karma" (treatment), and "karana" (medicines and appliances). Diet is an integral part of *Caraka Samhita.*

In Ayurveda, no distinction is made between herbs, medicines, and foods. All foods and medicines are believed to have both a nutritive and a therapeutic action in the body. The actions of various herbal remedies are understood and applied in terms of their effect on the "doshas." Indian remedies, also called "bazaar" medicines, are used extensively throughout India. Pure vegetable drugs are considered more "powerful" in their efficacy than those drugs that have undergone processing in a laboratory (Nadkarni, 1976).

Middle Eastern. This section contains information from countries such as what are now known as Israel and Saudi Arabia. The Bible records a number of herbs used for centuries in this part of the world. Herbs such as lemon, onion, myrrh, willow bark, cinnamon, greater celandine, wormwood, and aloe are mentioned (De Waal, 1980). Israel has been involved in the research of herbal medicines for a number of years. Israeli researchers have published their reports on chamomile and elderberry to name a few.

Historically, Arabian medicine has had a tremendous influence on herbal medicine and modern biomedicine. Arabian medicine, that "body of medical doctrine which is enshrined in books written in the Arabic language, is for the most part Greek in origin" (Browne, 1921, p. 2). In addition to its connection with the Greeks, Arabian medicine is connected with the history of Islam. Muslim physicians view themselves as practitioners of the art of healing and of maintaining health. Two of the most noted Muslim physicians of all time are Abu Bakr Muhammad Ibn Zakariyya Ar-Razi, known as "Rhazes" (864–930 C.E., uncertain), and Abu Ali Husayn Ibn Abdullah Ibn Sina, known as "Avicenna" (981–1036 C.E.). Both physicians were prolific writers on medicine and were highly recognized for their research and understanding of disease. Rhazes wrote a 20-volume medical encyclopedia called *al-Hawi,* the "Comprehensive book," which includes the medical knowledge of Greeks, Syrians, and the early Arabs. Avicenna wrote the *Qanum fi al-Tibb,* "The Canons of Medicine," an encyclopedia of medicine of over one million words. This canon, which included a description of over 760 medicinal plants and the drugs that could be derived from them, was used as a reference and teaching guide in medicine well into the nineteenth century. Avicenna, physician, healer, philosopher, scientist, poet, and musician, has been called the "prince of physicians." His work has greatly influenced European herbal and biomedicine. A renowned botanist, Ibn El Beithar, born at the end of the twelfth century, wrote *Le Traite des Simples* (in French), a complete work on medicinal plant drugs used by the Arabs to that date (Fleurentin, Mazars, & Pelt, 1983).

The Muslim people also developed the science of pharmacy. They believe that "God has provided a remedy for every illness and that Muslims should search for those remedies and use them with skill and compassion" (Tschanz, 1997). Arab pharmacopoeia are highly developed and extensive, including the geographical origin, properties, and application and methods of medicinal substances used in the cure of disease. "Saydalani," Arab pharmacists, are credited with the introduction of the use of the following plants in health practice: senna, sandalwood, myrrh, tamarind, nutmeg, and cloves, to name a few. They also are credited with the extensive use of aromatic oils and the development of syrups and juleps and orange-blossom and rose water as a means of administering medicines (Browne, 1921).

Russian/Baltic. Russian herbal medicine of today was originally based in the medicine of the people, the folk medicine of the Skif and Clavac tribes, and was largely influenced by the Greek tradition of Galen and Dioscorides. Russian herbal medicine also has also drawn from the knowledge of Arab, Scandinavian, Tartar, Mongolian, and Turkish cultures (Zevin, 1997). Russian physicians are unique in that they are taught both their traditional and folk medicines as well as conventional biomedicine. Russia has long-established, state-sponsored facilities for herbal medicine research. The All-Union Institute of Herbs and Aromatherapy is said to be one of the largest herbal research centers in the world (Zevin, 1997). In Russian herbal medicine, special techniques, including the infusion and decoction of herbs by water bath or "banya," which uses an apparatus similar to a double-boiler, have been perfected and are thought to increase the medicinal value of the herbal remedies.

European. The Greeks and Arabs also have significantly influenced European and Western herbalism. The philosophies and writings of Hippocrates and Avicenna as great men of medicine were very influential. However, two other major influences on herbalism in Europe are Saint Hildegard of Bingen, Germany, and the philosopher Goethe, with his influence on Rudolf Steiner and what has come to be known as Anthroposophical medicine.

Anthroposophical medicine is part of the culture of Germany and Switzerland. Rudolf Steiner (1861–1925), philosopher, writer, and scientist, emphasized that every person has the potential to know the spiritual world. He opened a college in Switzerland specifically for the study of the "sciences of the spirit." He used his research with the assistance of a Dutch physician named Ita Wegman to develop a spiritual medical doctrine that was connected to nature. Plants and plant therapies are a very important part of Anthroposophical healing practices.

Anthroposophical practitioners, including nurses, not only use plants in their interventions with patients, they also value interaction with and observation of the live plants they use in practice. The nursing students who receive their education at Anthroposophical hospitals (I have visited hospitals with as many as 450 beds) in Germany and Switzerland tend the plants in the medicinal herb gardens. Pharmacists at these hospitals prepare herbal remedies for patient care on site. Nurses' clean utility and medication rooms are stocked with herbal oils and other plant-based remedies. Nurses can receive instruction on Anthroposophical herbal applications, such as rhythmical embrocation with herbal oils, in addition to conventional nursing curriculum. Anthroposophical nurses have a system of practice and education that has integrated the use of herbs, primarily topicals, into patient care. Nurses who work in Anthroposophical hospitals do not have to be formal students of the Steiner teachings to learn and apply the wisdom and techniques of plant use that have been developed in Anthroposophical healing practices.

Hildegard von Bingen (1098–1179) of Germany was a mystic, prophet, poet, musician, physician, and political moralist. Her principal writing, *Scivias* (meaning Know the Ways), contains accounts of the numerous visions she received beginning at the age of six. These visions included discourse on the universe, the structure of man, birth, death, and the nature of the soul. *Scivias* also includes an explanation of the concept of "viriditas" or greenness—the life principle. "According to Hildegard, and other thinkers of her time, life from God was transmitted into the plants, animals, and precious gems. People, in turn, ate the plants and animals and acquired some of the gems, thereby obtaining 'viriditas.' People then gave out 'viriditas' through virtues" (Hozeski, 1986).

Hildegard von Bingen wrote extensively about the use of plants and their utility to humans either as food or medicine. Her book entitled *Natural History* covers more than 200 plants. She writes about plants such as yarrow, hemp, aloe, and fennel and describes their healing actions relative to her version of humoral medicine such as whether the plant is hot, cold, wet, or dry (Flanagan, 1996). Both Hildegard of Bingen and Anthroposophical plant remedies continue to be used not only in Germany and Switzerland but also throughout the world.

Culinary Use

This section includes descriptions of the plant's use in food preparation.

Use in Herbalism

This section includes historical and present day uses of the herb in healing and care outside the conventional biomedical arena. The uses of the plant described in Use in Herbalism have been gathered from sources on Western herbalism, associated with herb applications developed in Europe and North America. Herb uses that are specific to a particular cultural group or planetary location such as Africa or Asia are included in their respective Cultural Use sections. The cosmetic uses of an herb are included at the end of this section on herbalism.

BIOMEDICAL EVIDENCE:

The information included in the Biomedical Evidence sections focuses on human clinical trials whenever possible, although some in vitro and animal data have been included. The profile does not present an exhaustive search of the literature, outlining every study ever done on the plant. The studies presented here have been selected for their potential relevance to nurses and the science of nursing as a human science. In a number of the profiles, plants or a phytochemical constituent are often shown in animal or in vitro studies to have a certain action that is the exact opposite of the action in humans as demonstrated in the clinical trial. Although this kind of scientific evidence and conflicting data may be helpful overall in leading to greater understanding of a particular plant's personality, the focus here is the research on humans.

Studies Related to this Health Pattern

In this section, studies related to the primary health pattern, such as sleep and rest or skin care, are summarized and may be analyzed here or in the sections on Nursing Evidence.

Studies Related to Other Health Patterns

This section is organized by health patterns other than the health pattern the chapter is devoted to. The studies are summarized and are analyzed in this section or in the Nursing Evidence section.

Mechanism of Action

The mechanism of action is a pharmacologic concept that is applied here to summarize the research data about how a particular phytochemical, or plant constituent, works. Often this type of data comes from in vitro or animal studies. Human data have been presented here whenever possible. This section should be read carefully for two reasons. One, the type of study is important. How a plant works in an animal may be completely different than in humans. Secondly, the information provided often refers to plant constituents rather than the whole plants that patients and nurses may be using. For example, hypericin, a plant constituent of St. John's wort, may have a relationship to the overall action of the plant in raising a person's spirit when they feel depressed. Hypericin is not the same thing as *Hypericum perforatum*, or whole plant St. John's wort, and does not necessarily have the same action. Be sure to read carefully because the plant or constituent will be identified in this section.

USE IN PREGNANCY OR LACTATION:

In general, herbs should not be used by anyone during pregnancy or lactation unless they have specifically learned how to use the plant during this sensitive time. All plant medicine experts are educated about any herbs recommended during pregnancy. Some herbs have been used for centuries during pregnancy and lactation and are safe when used appropriately such as during the last trimester or at the time of delivery. Conversely, some herbs should be avoided during pregnancy altogether because they are known to stimulate the uterus thereby potentially causing miscarriage.

The information presented here includes the traditional uses of an herb in pregnancy and cautionary data based on that same use. Some cautions about use in pregnant and lactating women are presented based on what is known from a biomedical perspective about the use of the plant as a whole or the plant constituents. The reader is encouraged to be clear about what plant, plant constituent, or plant product is being discussed and then weigh all sources of information carefully when making clinical decisions regarding the use of a particular medicinal plant during pregnancy or lactation. Chapter 4 has additional information about the importance of weighing the benefits and risks to the use of herbs in pregnancy and lactation. Often herbs have fewer potential side effects than pharmaceutical drugs and therefore need to be included in the list of remedies being considered for use in women who become ill during pregnancy.

USE FOR CHILDREN:

The ethical issues regarding health care treatment and research that exist for pregnant and lactating women exist also for infants and children. Like pharmaceuticals, clinical trials of herbal remedies used in children have rarely been done, although this is changing. In general, herbal remedies are not used in infants because the liver of a newborn is very immature and plants are often metabolized through the liver. There are some herbal remedies that are commonly used in infants and children, such as mild chamomile tea for colic or chamomile or calendula salve for diaper rash. In these cases, small amounts of herb teas or topical applications are used. In some cultures such as in Hawaii, herbs are given to lactating women to benefit the breastfeeding baby (Gutmanis, 1995).

Homeopathic remedies are often used instead of herbs. They are more often recommended for the infant because babies often respond very well to the most subtle and gentlest of medicine. For example, I have observed a midwife trained in Britain giving a homeopathic remedy to a newborn with hyperbilirubinemia. The baby's bilirubin level went from 17 to 12 overnight and the baby never stopped nursing. The key in medicating infants, as well as children and adults, is to give the gentlest remedy possible first. As for dosing, there is usually a range for an effective dose in herbal medicine and the smallest amounts should be tried first and more given if necessary. The philosophy here is exemplified in the caregiver who sponges a child with a mild fever and brings the child's fever down 2° F to a more comfortable level for the child, before considering having to use herbs or acetaminophen.

Children over one year of age are given herbal medicines in many cultures. Children who learn about plant therapies develop a repertoire of ideas for self-care for minor illnesses and discomfort. For example, if a child is only given acetaminophen every time they have a fever, they will never think to ask for an alternative or complementary solution such as sponging or an herb to cool them down. Children often respond very well to an herbal tea or bath. "It is very often the case that gentle ('mite') or weak medicinal actions are perfectly adequate in the treatment of childhood diseases" (Schilcher, 1992, p. 16). Herbs have fewer side effects and therefore parents are not as hesitant to use them. They also are usually less expensive than pharmaceutical drugs. Children also benefit greatly from the attention given them by a caregiver who makes their medicine for them such as making a *special* tea or ointment that is used when the child is not feeling well.

A major consideration when using herbs in children is the dosage primarily related to oral use. In general, when using We'stern herbal medicine in children, the quantity of herbal remedy given is calculated using Cowling's, Clark's, or Young's rule. Cowling's and Young's rules are calculated based on age, so I prefer to calculate dosage for children based on weight or Clark's rule: Divide the weight (in pounds) of the child by 150 to give the approximate fraction of the adult dose. So if an adult is to take 6 ml of a liquid herbal extract, a 50-pound child would take one-third or 2 ml of the extract.

CAUTIONS:

The cautions section contains information alerts to specific actual or potential concerns of using a particular herb and potential risks to either humans or plant populations. Herbs have been shown to be very safe over hundreds of years of use. They are a much milder form of treatment as compared with pharmaceuticals. Both pharmaceuticals and herbs have their place in health care, and the health practitioner recommending herbs has the responsibility of first observing the patient and assessing the appropriateness of herbs for the individual patient and any potential safety issues. For example, I once had a patient come in to the clinic I worked in with a huge finger laceration. She had cut her finger with a knife at work and had wrapped the wound in a piece of a sheet of *nori* (a seaweed) to stop the bleeding. Traditionally, *nori* has been known to help blood to clot. She had never taken a first-aid class and didn't know about direct pressure. Direct pressure would have been very effective and the herb unnecessary. It is the responsibility of the user and practitioner of herbal remedies to understand their options for care as well as the herbal remedy and to choose the most appropriate for the individual situation. Appropriate use and thorough understanding passed through oral tradition is one reason why herbs have had such a strong record of safe use.

NURSING EVIDENCE:

Historical Nursing Use

This section includes any use of the herb known to date by nurses or midwives. The information included here may be taken from historical sources that predate the formalization of nursing and therefore may refer to caregivers.

Potential Nursing Applications

This section describes the ways, based on traditional evidence, biomedical evidence, and historical nursing use, that nurses might consider using the herb in clinical practice or researching it for further understanding.

Integrative Insight

This section is a summary, integration, and/or synergy of the biomedical, traditional, and nursing evidence about the herb. This section is included to inspire reflective herbal practice.

THERAPEUTIC APPLICATIONS:

The following three sections describe the potential uses of the profiled herb. Although nurses might wish to be told the preferred application for a particular plant, this information is not provided because the preferred application is not determined by the information about the plant. It is determined through interaction with the individual patient and gaining an understanding of the relationship between plant and patient.

To determine the best application for a given patient, it is recommended that the nurse evaluate the biomedical, traditional, and nursing evidence given and then, after reading the integrative insight, talk with the patient again using the guideline in chapter 20, "Talking with Patients About Herbs—Nine Questions and Interventions." After talking with the patient, the nurse can reflect on the interaction, at which time she or he may have a better idea of which application is best for the patient.

Oral

This section describes the oral uses of the plant being profiled and can include actual recipes for making the remedy. Oral forms of herbal remedies are described in detail in chapter 5 and therefore this section is not used to provide instruction on how to make an infusion, decoction, or syrup for example. The information is general, stating that the herb is commonly used in a particular form. All dosages reported are meant to be a guideline for understanding and are not meant to be viewed as a recommendation for the uneducated practitioner to then make recommendations for patients. For example, if a patient talks about taking a whole bottle of goldenseal capsules to "cleanse the liver" before urine drug screening at his place of employment, the guideline dosages given in the profile and the cautionary information will provide the nurse with adequate information to formulate an understanding of the benefits and risks with the patient. Although herbs are often taken for self-care in uniformly established amounts such as 1 spoonful of dried herb per cup of water for tea, when used clinically, amounts must be individualized for each patient and the patient observed closely, just as with any nursing intervention or recommendation.

Topical

This section includes a description of the topical applications for the herb profiled, such as ointments, liniments, and poultices. Again, the standard methods for preparing each topical application can be found in chapter 5 and may not be described in detail in this section unless there is additional information about the application that is specific to the herb profiled.

Environmental

This section of the profile describes any "environmental" uses of the plant such as inhalation or aromatherapy and herbal baths.

PATIENT INTERACTION:

This section of the profile is a brief summary of the highlights of the information about the herb that could be discussed with a patient who is considering using the herb for self-care. This section is written for the herb consumer. It can be copied and used as a patient handout.

NURTURING THE NURSE-PLANT RELATIONSHIP:

This section of the profile contains suggestions and recipes to be used by the reader as a way of getting to know the plant more intimately through personal use. Suggestions include tea tastings and herbal stress-reducing techniques with topical applications. Enjoy the personal experience of learning about herbs!

CHAPTER 7
Comfort and Pain Relief

INTRODUCTION

P AIN IS WHAT A PERSON SAYS IT IS. IT IS SUBJEC-
tive and personal. Pain, as opposed to an infectious rash or a broken
bone, is often not apparent to the observer. People with chronic back pain
or migraine, for example, may go to work, eat their meals, take care of their
families, and spend the rest of their time trying to adapt to or manage their
pain. No one may ever know that these people are in pain unless they reveal their agony through verbal cues or body language such as a wince or a
moment of weeping.

Many nurses work with people in pain on a daily basis. Nurses observe the numerous manifestations of pain as being as unique as each individual patient. Pain can be acute or chronic. Acute pain is a signal via
the nervous system that something in the body needs attention. Acute
pain can be a call to action and, if ignored, has the uncanny ability of becoming louder and louder until recognized and attended to. There are
many triggers for acute pain, including injury, allergic reaction, and
stress.

Chronic pain is a major cause of debility. People with chronic pain
suffer from the "terrible triad of suffering, sleeplessness, and sadness, a
calamity that is as hard on the family as it is on the victim" (National Institutes of Health, 1998, http://www.ninds.nih.gov/health_and_medical/

pubs/chronic_pain_htr.htm#Pain). Chronic pain, as opposed to acute pain, is persistent and does not really get "better" or heal. Pain signals can keep firing long after the person has become aware of the body part needing attention and long after the person has attempted to address the pain. Chronic pain sufferers often find that few if any conventional remedies such as drug therapies help over time.

The theories about how pain occurs in the body can be simplified by saying pain is a sensory experience involving the nervous system and a person's perception of that sensory experience. What is painful for one person may not be painful for another, and what is painful for one person at a particular moment may not be painful for them at another time. For example, women who go through childbirth the first time often have a different perception of the pain involved with the experience than they do with subsequent deliveries. Pain threshold, sensitivity, and tolerance are determining factors in the experience of pain. These factors can change over time. People learn what acute pain is and how to deal with it. They also learn to live with chronic pain and carry on with their lives despite the challenge of daily discomfort.

What brings comfort and pain relief is as subjective and personal as the pain and discomfort a person feels to begin with. What comforts one person may exacerbate pain in another, and therefore people must often explore many options before finding and creating comfort and pain relief if at all. Herbs are one option that can be explored for comforting those with acute and chronic pain. The herbs in this chapter—feverfew, lavender, evening primrose, and mustard—have different ways of addressing pain and discomfort. For example, they may primarily address a certain type of pain such as migraine or provide comfort through a soothing aroma. For centuries, herbs have been used traditionally and successfully to comfort and soothe peoples' aches and pains, whether minor, acute, or chronic.

"Pain is regularly undertreated by health care professionals . . . health professionals focus more on identifying and treating the underlying condition that is causing the pain" (Lubkin, 1998, p. 151). Often while diagnostic tests are being done, people continue to suffer. Nurses, concerned about causing secondary problems such as opiate addiction or because of the somewhat obscure nature of patients' pain, often do not provide the necessary care that addresses the unique pain experience of the patient. Herbs offer an opportunity for providing alternative and complementary care to patients with pain and discomfort.

Some people do not have the type of discomfort or the perception of discomfort that warrants taking a drug, but they would take a comforting tea or have a massage with a pain-relieving herbal oil. Herbs can add breadth to the list of noninvasive modalities that patients and their caregivers need in order to address the full range of discomfort and pain responses.

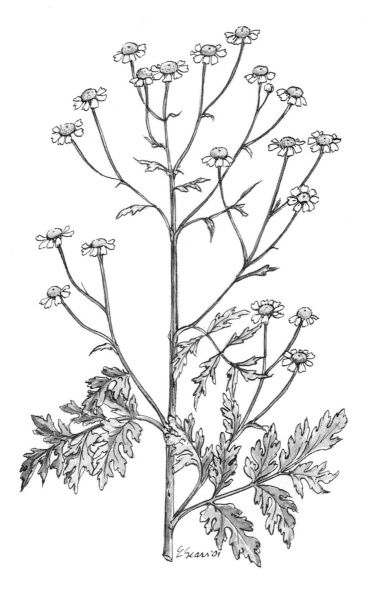

Tanacetum parthenium

Feverfew

- **LATIN NAME:** *Tanacetum parthenium*

- **FAMILY:** Asteraceae

- **COMMON NAMES:** Feverfew, featherfew, febrifuge plant, featherfoil, midsummer daisy, flirtwort, bachelor's buttons, Mutterkraut (mother herb), medieval aspirin.

- **HEALTH PATTERN:** Comfort and pain relief

- **PLANT DESCRIPTION:**

The name "feverfew" is related to its Latin name *febrifugia,* meaning "fever reducer" (Foster & Tyler, 1999). Feverfew is an abundantly growing perennial about 2 feet (½ meter) high. The stems are finely furrowed and downy, with leaves that are alternating on the stem. The leaves are either downy or nearly smooth, and up to 4½ inches (about 11 cm) long and 2 inches (5 cm) wide, with toothed edges. The numerous flowers are small and daisylike with white outer petals and flat yellow centers. To the untrained eye, feverfew and chamomile plants might be confused, but feverfew's leaves are wider and not as bushy or feathery as chamomile leaves. The entire feverfew plant also has a strong, aromatic smell and a very bitter taste, which is not present with chamomile. The cultivated feverfew's leaves are slightly more yellow than the wild variety. According to one source, many of the biologic and chemical investigations of feverfew have been carried out on the wild variety (Groenewegen, Knight, & Heptinstall, 1992).

- **PLANT PART USED:** Leaf

- **TRADITIONAL EVIDENCE:**

Cultural Use

North American Indian. The Cherokee use an infusion of feverfew to bathe swollen feet. Other tribes use it internally to treat rheumatism (Moerman, 1998). Feverfew has been used to relieve hyperemic conditions of the mucous membranes in instances of colic; for flatulence, indigestion, decreased urine output, and colds; to help expel worms; and in some febrile diseases. It also has been used for scanty or delayed menses (Hutchens, 1992).

Hispanic. In Latin America, feverfew is used to promote digestion and alleviate colic and for earache, stomachache, morning sickness, and kidney pains (Leung & Foster, 1996). In Mexico, feverfew is used as an insecticide. Mexicans also use it as an antispasmodic, emmenagogue, tonic, and in sitz baths to stop menstruation (Duke, 1985).

Costa Ricans use feverfew for conditions associated with digestion and the heart and to promote menstruation. It is used in Guatemala for diarrhea. In Venezuela, a decoction of feverfew is used for earache (Duke, 1985).

European. Feverfew has been used in the United Kingdom for relieving rheumatic and arthritic joint inflammation and to prevent migraines (Johnson, Kadam, Anderson, Jenkinson, Dewdney, & Blowers, 1987; Anderson, Jenkinson, Dewdney, Blowers, Johnson, & Kadam, 1988; Murphy, Heptinstall, & Mitchell, 1988).

Culinary Use

Feverfew is generally not used in foods.

Use in Herbalism

It is believed that the first written record of feverfew occurred in the *Materia Medica* by Diocorides. Since at least 78 A.D., feverfew has been used to treat headache, stomach pain, menstrual irregularities, and fever. Early Europeans believed that the herb was ruled by the planet Venus and therefore was a good herb for women. Feverfew is used in a bath or drunk as a wine for women's conditions. It is used to strengthen the womb, help expel afterbirth, and promote menstruation. Some women use feverfew tincture to promote delayed menstruation by taking 40 drops every three hours for four days (Weed, 1986). Feverfew is used for pains in the head, dizziness, shortness of breath, and depression. A syrup can be made of the plant during the summer months to be stored and used during the winter when the fresh plant is not available. Feverfew also has been used historically as a remedy "against opium taken too liberally" (Culpeper, 1990, p. 73).

Feverfew traditionally has been used in herbalism to relieve intestinal gas and dental pain; promote the onset of menstruation; as a mild laxative; and as a "bitter," an agent that promotes digestion. It has been used for nervous complaints, depression, and as a general tonic. At one time, feverfew was mixed with sugar or honey and used to treat coughs, wheezing, and difficult breathing. An oil made from feverfew was applied externally to relieve gas and colic. A tincture of feverfew applied topically was used traditionally for insect bites and stings (Grieve, 1971). More recently, feverfew is used especially for the painful symptoms of migraine and arthritis. Fresh leaves picked before flowering are thought to be most medicinal.

BIOMEDICAL EVIDENCE:

There are at least two varieties of feverfew, cultivated *Tanacetum parthenium aureus* and a wild variety. Many of the biologic and chemical investigations of feverfew have been carried out on the wild variety (Groenewegen et al., 1992).

Studies Related to Comfort and Pain Relief

Pain and symptoms commonly associated with migraine (e.g., nausea, vomiting, and sensitivity to light) all were reduced significantly in 57 patients (age 9 to 65 years) who received daily doses of feverfew, 100 mg capsulized powdered leaf with a demonstrated parthenolide content of 0.2%, during a double-blind, placebo-controlled, crossover study, conducted at an outpatient pain clinic over the course of four months. Symptoms not only improved when the participant was given the feverfew capsule but also worsened when given the parsley placebo capsule (Palevitch, Earon, & Carasso, 1997).

In a randomized, double-blind, placebo-controlled study of 60 patients with migraine, those given one capsule of dried powdered feverfew leaf per day (82 mg per day containing about 2.19 μmol parthenolide per capsule) experienced a 24% reduction in the number of attacks and a significant reduction in nausea and vomiting associated with their migraines. There was also a trend, although statistically insignificant, of a reduction in severity of migraine with feverfew (Murphy et al., 1988).

In a double-blind, placebo-controlled trial of 17 patients with migraine who took capsules of freeze-dried feverfew powder (50 mg per day) prophylactically to prevent migraine, the treatment group showed no change in the frequency or severity of symptoms of migraine, whereas the placebo group had a significant increase in severity and frequency of migraine (Johnson et al., 1985).

There were no significant differences in the pain, stiffness, laboratory values or grip strength of 41 female patients with diagnosed rheumatoid arthritis who received 70 to 86 mg of dried chopped feverfew in capsules once daily for six weeks; however, the investigators acknowledge that they chose their dose based on folkloric treatment for migraine, not arthritis, and that the participants were taking nonsteroidal, anti-inflammatory drugs concomitantly with the feverfew capsules, a practice thought to reduce the efficacy of feverfew (Pattrick, Heptinstall, & Doherty, 1989).

Studies Related to Other Health Patterns

No data are available at this time.

Mechanism of Action

Feverfew contains compounds that act to prevent spasms of the smooth muscles in the walls of the cerebral blood vessels. It is believed that these compounds may produce the antimigraine effect similar to methysergide, a serotonin antagonist (Foster & Tyler, 1999).

Constituents in feverfew have been found to inhibit prostaglandin production and arachidonic acid release in vitro and in animal studies. This may account for its antiplatelet and antifebrile actions. Changes in the chemistry of platelets in human patients taking feverfew have not been detected (Groenewegen et al., 1992). Extracts also inhibit secretion of serotonin from platelets and proteins from polymorphonuclear leukocytes (PMNs). "The pattern of the effects of the feverfew extracts on platelets is different from that obtained with other inhibitors of platelet aggregation and the effect of PMNs is more pronounced than with high concentrations of non-streroidal anti-inflammatory agents" (Heptinstall, White, Williamson, & Mitchell, 1985, p. 1071). Because serotonin is implicated in the cause of migraines, and PMNs are increased in rheumatoid arthritis, feverfew may be of use in relieving the pain and discomfort associated with these conditions. Because feverfew inhibits the release of damaging chemicals from white cells in inflamed joints, it has been used in the treatment of arthritis (Bradley, 1992).

A sesquiterpene lactone constituent called "parthenolide" has been shown to reduce calcium secretion in animals. It has been suggested that feverfew may be useful in treating hypercalciuria and related conditions in humans (Wren, 1988). The exact mechanism of action is unknown. Regional variations of parthenolide, in Mexico for example, have been found to occur. One of the active constituents found in feverfew in Mexico is santamarine, a constituent closely related to parthenolide (Groenewegen et al., 1992). Parthenolide inhibits the growth of gram-positive bacteria, yeast, and some fungi and is thought to act as a protector of the plant against pathogens.

USE IN PREGNANCY OR LACTATION:

Feverfew has been demonstrated to cause abortion in cows. It has not been documented to cause the same effect in humans. Feverfew has the ability to promote the onset of menstruation. One source suggests that this herb not be used during pregnancy because of the possibility of disrupting gestation (Brinker, 1998). No effect of feverfew on lactation has been noted (DeSmet, 1992).

Herbal Caveat—Pregnancy or Lactation

Some herbs are contraindicated in pregnancy because of a risk of the herb or one of its constituents stimulating the uterus and therefore possibly promoting fetal loss. Many herbal practitioners do not recommend herbal remedies, in particular oral doses of herbs, during the first trimester of pregnancy and seek an alternative. However, herbs are successfully used during pregnancy, especially to prepare the body for the birth. Herbs are relatively unstudied in pregnancy and lactation, so patients need to be made aware through education of the potential benefits and risks of using herbs for health conditions that arise during pregnancy or lactation. The use of herbal remedies during pregnancy often warrants a referral to a knowledgeable herbal practitioner.

✅ USE FOR CHILDREN:

Although feverfew has not been studied in children, it may be suitable for helping children with pain related to headaches (Schilcher, 1992). For headache in children, my usual preference is to try a chamomile compress to the back and neck (see chamomile profile in chapter 11), followed by a gentle massage with an herbal oil such as St. John's wort or arnica before giving oral remedies such as bitter-tasting feverfew.

Herbal Caveat—Children

Children have special needs in regard to herbal therapies. They require lesser amounts of herbs and often respond well to mild teas and topical applications such as compresses and baths. The lowest dose of oral preparations should be tried first before increasing the amount given children. Caregivers should observe children closely for responses to herbal remedies. Younger children, particularly infants, have traditionally been given herbs either through their mother's breast milk or in the form of a homeopathic remedy because of their sensitivity to medicines and treatments and the immaturity of their liver. It is recommended that a person knowledgeable in the herbal treatment of children be consulted before the offering of any herb to a child for the first time.

✅ CAUTIONS:

In the studies by Johnson et al. (1985) and Murphy et al. (1988), it is noted that no serious side effects have been reported in those patients taking feverfew for years. Side effects such as mouth ulceration and gastric disturbance have been noted in 6% to 15% of users, usually within the first week of use (McGuffin, Hobbs, Upton, & Goldberg, 1997).

It is suggested that those who experience allergic reactions to plants in the Asteraceae family should exercise caution when using feverfew. Plants in the Asteraceae family contain chemicals known as "sesquiterpene lactones" that are known to cause contact dermatitis and other allergic effects. Allergic reactions to one of the plants in the Asteraceae family could possibly mean an allergic reaction to all such plants. Those who are sensitive to chamomile, yarrow, and ragweed, for example, can have reactions to the fresh, dried, or extracted forms of feverfew. One study has shown that there can be a high degree of cross-reactivity between feverfew and ragweed, in particular (Sriramarao & Rao, 1993). Skin contact with feverfew may cause topical irritation (Duke, 1985), although contact dermatitis may not manifest for several hours or days after contact with the plant (Brinker, 1998). Even though a patient may have had an allergic reaction to a plant in the Asteraceae family or a chemical constituent of the plant, such as a lactone, the clinical relevance is determined by the clinical history. It is possible for patients to react to plants or plant constituents to which they have never been exposed (Rodriguez, Epstein, & Mitchell, 1977).

Some sources cite the findings of in vitro studies of feverfew that the plant exhibits an ability to inhibit platelet activity as reason to avoid the use of feverfew in patients taking anticoagulant pharmaceutical drugs (Miller, 1998); however, changes in the chemistry of platelets in human patients taking feverfew have not been detected (Groenewegen et al, 1992).

Human studies have shown that both prophylactic use and daily consumption of feverfew have not resulted in an increase in chromosomal aberrations or sister chromatid exchanges in peripheral lymphocytes (Anderson et al., 1988; Johnson et al., 1987).

NURSING EVIDENCE:

Historical Nursing Use

No data are available at this time.

Potential Nursing Applications

Feverfew has potential for use in pain management, especially in those patients who have been treated medically and continue to experience chronic pain symptoms. Nurses may want to consider using feverfew for those with migraines, tension headaches, and arthritis. Nurses may want to consider researching the effects of feverfew leaf in either fresh, encapsulated, or liquid extract form, in patients being treated for chronic pain symptoms.

Integrative Insight

Pain, such as occurs with headache, migraine, or arthritis, can be excruciating and debilitating. The biomedical approach to care is to suppress the pain. Biomedical and traditional evidence both show that feverfew can be a very effective way of addressing the patient's need for comfort and pain relief. Integrative care also includes recognition that pain is often a symptom of an underlying and perhaps unrecognized concern. For example, a patient's pain may occur as a result of a reaction to something in their environment. While feverfew may be helpful in suppressing pain and promoting comfort, it is also important for nurses to provide patients with information regarding potential underlying patterns that create and re-create pain, the body's signal of need for attention. It is also important to take time to help the patient begin to identify personal and environmental triggers for their pain. Holistic evaluation of those patients with chronic pain or chronic use of plant therapies for pain reduction must be done.

THERAPEUTIC APPLICATIONS:

Oral

Dried Leaves. The suggested dosage of feverfew needed to prevent migraine headaches is 25 mg of the dried powdered leaves taken twice daily or 82 mg of dried powdered leaves taken once daily. A higher dose (up to 2 g) may be necessary to reduce inflammation in rheumatoid arthritis (Werbach & Murray, 1994).

Capsules or Tablets. Dried herb tablets or capsules (50 to 200 mg) may be taken daily (Bradley, 1992). Feverfew is standardized to 0.2% parthenolide (Leung & Foster, 1996).

Fresh Leaves. As a preventative for migraines, fresh leaves can be eaten daily (Wren, 1988). One to two leaves per day are used for prevention.

Tincture. (1:5 g/ml, 25% ethanol) 5 to 20 drops daily (Bradley, 1992)

Leaf Tea. Pour 1 cup (240 ml) of boiled water over 1 teaspoon (3 to 5 g) of the herb. Allow this to steep for three to five minutes, then strain. Drink 2 cups daily in small mouthful doses (Hutchens, 1992).

Topical

The boiled leaves of feverfew can be used to make hot compresses for pain due to congestion and inflammation of the lungs, stomach, and abdomen (Hutchens, 1992).

Environmental

An old folk belief is that feverfew, planted around dwellings, will purify the air and ward off disease (Grieve, 1971). It is said that bees dislike feverfew so much that placing the herb around the vicinity causes them to keep their distance (Hutchens, 1992). Many insects tend to avoid landing on feverfew, thereby making it an excellent natural insect repellent.

Herbal Caveat—Therapeutic Applications

In traditional and conventional herbal medicine, amounts of herbs given to patients are based on individual needs. The amounts or "doses" recorded here are provided so that the health practitioner has a general idea of the amounts recommended for an adult patient. Dosing in herbalism not only refers to amount of plant used but also includes when, where, and how to take a plant medicine. These dosages should not be used as guidelines for indiscriminate intervention without proper assessment, critical thinking, and patient education on the part of the practitioner.

Note: Please see chapter 5 for detailed descriptions of how to prepare various applications.

PATIENT INTERACTION:

Although herbs, including feverfew, are often helpful in providing pain relief and comfort for those with headache, identifying those substances and activities that precipitate a migraine is helpful in prevention as well. Some common precipitating factors in migraine headaches include excessive and/or unmanaged stress; alcohol, especially red wines; weather changes; constipation; hormonal changes;

poor vision or eye strain; too little or too much sleep; extreme emotions such as anger; nitrates such as those found in meats; monosodium glutamate; cheeses; chocolate; onions; avocado; caffeine; withdrawal from caffeine or other vasopressors; and allergic reactions to foods, herbs, drugs (including pain medications), vitamins, or environmental stimuli. Feverfew has been shown to decrease the frequency and/or intensity of migraine headaches and may be helpful in relieving the pain associated with arthritis as well. People with allergies to plants in the Asteraceae or daisy family, such as ragweed, may want to consider feverfew carefully before using it because it has been known to cause allergies among those who are allergic to ragweed.

Herbal Caveat—Patient Interaction

Patients considering the use of an herb or formula of herbs in self-care benefit from education about the plant itself and the use of the plant in healing. This education can come through many sources, including local herbalists; plant specialists such as botanists; health practitioners such as nurses, nutritionists, naturopaths, and other physicians; and various written references including the scientific literature. Patients need to remember that their unique health care needs are not necessarily represented in any literature they may encounter. Therefore, it is recommended that a knowledgeable mentor be consulted before initiating self-care with any herb being used for the first time.

NURTURING THE NURSE-PLANT RELATIONSHIP:

Note: You may want to keep a journal of your experiences with the herb.

To get to know feverfew's pain relieving action, consider putting some drops of feverfew liquid extract in a half cup of warm water and sipping it down the next time head pain, especially of the throbbing type, starts. Don't forget to close your eyes and rest as you take note of the effects of feverfew.

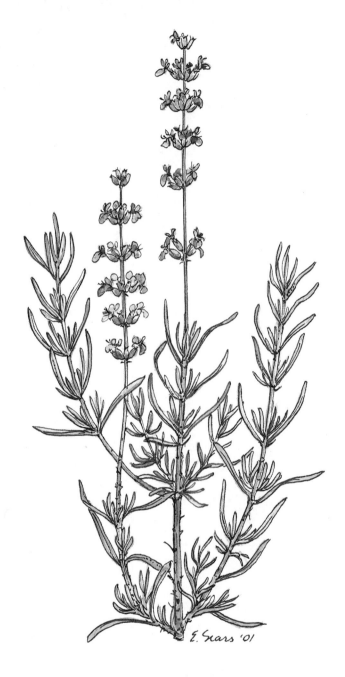

Lavandula angustifolia

Lavender

🌿 **LATIN NAMES:** *Lavandula angustifolia, Lavandula officinalis, Lavandula vera*

🌿 **FAMILY:** Lamiaceae

🌿 **COMMON NAMES:** Lavender, English lavender, garden lavender, true lavender

🌿 **HEALTH PATTERN:** Comfort and pain relief

🌿 **PLANT DESCRIPTION:**

Lavender's botanical name comes from the Latin *lavare,* meaning "to wash." Lavender is a bushy plant that grows from 1 to 3 feet (up to 1 meter) tall. It has short, crooked stems with many branches that are covered with a shaggy yellowish-gray bark. The leaves are opposite each other on the stems, and are narrow, slightly white, and downy. Extending vertically from the main body of the plant are numerous straight branches that bear the flower spikes. The spikes are comprised of from six to ten blue-violet colored flowers. The flowers are described as having a sweet odor that is both floral and herbal, with balsamic undertones (Keville & Green, 1995).

Lavender is indigenous to the mountains of the western Mediterranean and is cultivated extensively in France, Italy, England, Norway, and Australia. The flowers are best harvested in July and August.

🌿 **PLANT PART USED:** Flowers

🌿 **TRADITIONAL EVIDENCE:**

Cultural Use

Asian. Lavender is still used today in the form of an edible medicinal butter by Tibetan Buddhist medical practitioners for treating insanity and psychoses (Blumenthal, Goldberg, & Brinckman, 2000).

East Indian. As early as the eighth century B.C., lavender was described in an ancient Indian medical text as useful for psychiatric disorders. Lavender is used specifically for depressive states associated with chronic digestive disturbances. It is used to expel intestinal gas and as an antispasmodic, sedative, antidepressant, and antirheumatic. Lavender oil is used topically to increase circulation to the skin (Blumenthal et al., 2000).

In India, lavender roots are made into a paste with water and applied topically to stings of "wild animals." As a supposed antidote for snake poisoning, the powdered leaves are inhaled to prevent sleep. In Ayurvedic medicine, lavender is called the "broom of the brain" because its use is said to sweep away sluggishness of thought, strengthen brain power, and clarify the intellect. It also is used as a stimulant, carminative, diaphoretic, expectorant, antispasmodic, and emmena-gogue. The essential oil is used for colic and chest congestion and to relieve biliary complaints and headaches. Warm, moist applications of the flower help relieve pain associated with rheumatism and neural-gia (Nadkarni, 1976).

Middle Eastern. Arabs have used lavender as an expectorant and antispasmodic (Grieve, 1971).

European. Lavender is licensed in Germany as a medicinal tea for sleep problems and for nervous stomach. It also is used in various sedative preparations and for promoting the flow of bile from the biliary tract. It is used for restlessness, lack of appetite, and intestinal gas. In European lore, lavender was one of the herbs dedicated to the goddess Hecate, who was sacred to witches and sorcerers. It was thought that a sprig of lavender could avert the "evil eye" and was placed in churches and homes to ward off the plague. Elizabethan ladies sewed sachets of lavender into their dresses to create a pleas-ant scent and to deter clothing moths (Lawless, 1998). Lavender also was woven into nosegays to help ward off the plague.

Culinary Use

All species of lavender are very attractive to bees and make a tasty honey. Extracts from lavender are used to flavor alcoholic and non-alcoholic beverages, frozen dairy desserts, candy, baked goods, gelatins, puddings, and aromatic vinegars. The flowers and oil are used to flavor various teas.

Use in Herbalism

Lavender flowers to be used medicinally should be collected right before they have fully opened. In ancient Greece, Arabia, and Rome, lavender was used as an antiseptic, a bactericide, and to disinfect hospitals and sick rooms. Lavender was used to dispel gas and for its sedative properties. It has been used to mask disagreeable odors in ointments and other preparations. A tea brewed from lavender flowers was useful to relieve headaches caused by fatigue and ex-haustion. Topically, a few drops of essence of lavender were used in footbaths to alleviate fatigue. External applications were used for toothache, neuralgia, sprains, and rheumatism and to cleanse wounds, varicose ulcers, burns, and scalds. Lavender was used as a stimulant in hysteria, palsy, and other nervous conditions. At one time, it was common for the French to keep a bottle of lavender essence in the home to be used for bruises, bites, aches, and pains—both internal and external.

Lavender is used for restlessness, insomnia, nervous stomach ir-ritations, and nervous intestinal discomfort. It is used in baths to treat functional circulatory disorders. Lavender is reported to be effective for intestinal gas and as an antispasmodic, sedative, tonic, and stimulant. It is used for various spasms, colic, nervous headache, migraine, toothache, sprains, neuralgia, rheumatism, nausea, vomiting, acne, pimples, and sores (Leung & Foster, 1996).

Lavender essential oil is considered one of the safest and most widely used oils in aromatherapy (Keville & Green, 1995). It is one of the few essential oils that can be used on the skin neat (no dilution), without irritating the skin. The essential oil is used to scent medicinal skin preparations. Although most essential oils have pain-relieving qualities, lavender oil is considered to be especially analgesic (Buckle, 1997). The essential oil is used to treat infections, including *Candida*. It is also used for laryngitis, asthma, muscle pain, insect bites, cystitis, digestive problems, colic, inflammation, and to help boost immunity. Lavender essential oil is considered to be safe for all skin types and is believed to regenerate skin cells. It acts to prevent the formation of scars and stretch marks and slows the formation of wrinkles. It can be used on burns, sun-damaged skin, rashes, wounds, and skin infections. The essential oil of lavender is used as a restorative during fainting and to treat nervous palpitations, spasms, and colic. It stimulates the appetite and helps to relieve depression. In addition to depression, Lavender essential oil is used in aromatherapy for the treatment of emotional disorders, such as nervousness, irritability, insomnia, and manic depression. Old medical books document its use in "raising the spirits" and "comforting the brain." Lavender essential oil has the ability to bring balance to body and spirit because it both relaxes and stimulates.

Cosmetic Use. Lavender flowers and essential oil are used as fragrance ingredients in cosmetics, soaps, detergents, creams, lotions, perfumes, and colognes (Leung & Foster, 1996). The ancient Greeks who called the plant "nardus" and the Romans who called it "asarum" used lavender extensively as a perfume for the bath. Lavender essential oil applied to the skin also is used as an insect repellent. Lavender has been used in sachets to scent linens and clothing. Moths and other insects are repelled by its scent, so they tend to stay away from fabrics that have been stored with lavender. Lavender oil also has been used in the embalming process.

BIOMEDICAL EVIDENCE:

Studies Related to Comfort and Pain Relief

One blinded, randomized clinical trial of 635 postpartum women by two midwifery sisters in England, demonstrated that adding 6 drops of pure lavender oil to the bath for ten days postpartum was not statistically significant in reducing perineal discomfort as compared with synthetic lavender oil or an inert aromatic placebo; however, clinical significance may have been achieved between days three and five when the mothers did record lower discomfort scores and found the lavender bath to be a "pleasant experience." This study does not fully support the traditional use of lavender bath for perineal discomfort and further study is required; however, the investigators did not report whether the six drops were added to a sitz bath or a full body bath (Dale & Cornwell, 1994). This is significant because the six drops used for a full body bath would be considered very dilute by herbal standards. To treat perineal pain with lavender oil, given the low toxicity of the topical use of the pure oil, up to 10 drops usually would be recommended in a sitz bath, not a full body bath.

Studies Related to Other Health Patterns

Sleep and Rest. In a small, uncontrolled study, 9 elderly patients had one drop of lavender essential oil placed on their pillow at night for one week, and then one week followed without lavender. Eight of the participants demonstrated improved alertness and awakeness as well as less confusion when receiving lavender (Hudson, 1995). With a more stringent design (e.g., increasing the sample size, adding a control group, and using a standardized evaluation instrument), this study is repeated easily and the results are potentially more significant.

Skin Care. In a randomized, controlled, double-blind trial of 86 patients with alopecia areata, a combination of essential oils of lavender, rosemary, thyme, and cedarwood in a carrier oil was found to improve hair regrowth in 44% of the test group. In their discussion of the limitations of the study, the investigators note they were unable to control for fragrance between the active and control groups and only one of the essential oils may have been responsible for the outstanding results, as compared with a 38% result with a leading pharmaceutical therapy (Hay, Jamieson, & Ormerod, 1998).

Restoration. Perillyl alcohol, a constituent found in lavender, has been found to prevent and completely regress advanced mammary tumors in rats and is being studied as a potential alternative to tamoxifen (Ziegler, 1996).

Emotions and Adaptation. A controlled study of the effect of lavender aromatherapy on the anxiety levels of 134 women undergoing mammography screening demonstrated a significant decrease in state trait anxiety as measured by Spielberger's inventory in those women having their mammogram in a treatment room where *Lavender officinalis* essential oil was being atomized for four minutes every twenty-five minutes by a diffuser with a 115 volt, 60 Hz, 4.0 watt capacity (Blake, 1998).

A pilot study of the effect of lavender oil as aromatherapy on cardiovascular measures after exercise showed positive effects in the general descriptive statistics obtained in 20 men, but the effects were found not to be statistically significant. The investigators plan further study with a larger sample to clarify the effects noted in the pilot study (Romine, Bush, & Geist, 1999).

Mechanism of Action

In vitro studies of guinea pig ileum smooth muscle preparation have indicated that lavender oil and one of its constituents, linalool, create a spasmolytic action through a rise in intracellular cAMP (Lis-Balchin & Hart, 1999). Linalool and linalyl aldehyde seem to reduce the flow of nerve impulses such as those that transmit pain (Duke, 1997). Lavender has been shown to be most effective in vitro against *Clostridium sporogenes, Moraxella* spp., *Staphylococcus aureus,* and *Brevibacterium* linens (Buckle, 1997).

🍃 USE IN PREGNANCY OR LACTATION:

Traditional use has shown that lavender has the ability to promote the onset of menstruation. For this reason, it is speculated that excessive internal use should be avoided in early pregnancy (Brinker, 1998).

Herbal Caveat—Pregnancy or Lactation
Some herbs are contraindicated in pregnancy because of a risk of the herb or one of its constituents stimulating the uterus and therefore possibly promoting fetal loss. Many herbal practitioners do not recommend herbal remedies, in particular oral doses of herbs, during the first trimester of pregnancy and seek an alternative. However, herbs are successfully used during pregnancy, especially to prepare the body for the birth. Herbs are relatively unstudied in pregnancy and lactation, so patients need to be made aware through education of the potential benefits and risks of using herbs for health conditions that arise during pregnancy or lactation. The use of herbal remedies during pregnancy often warrants a referral to a knowledgeable herbal practitioner.

🍃 USE FOR CHILDREN:

Bundles or bags of lavender flowers are hung beside children's beds in France to promote relaxation and sleep. Lavender baths are given to children for its sedative effects (Schilcher, 1992).

Herbal Caveat—Children
Children have special needs in regard to herbal therapies. They require lesser amounts of herbs and often respond well to mild teas and topical applications such as compresses and baths. The lowest dose of oral preparations should be tried first before increasing the amount given children. Caregivers should observe children closely for responses to herbal remedies. Younger children, particularly infants, have traditionally been given herbs either through their mother's breast milk or in the form of a homeopathic remedy because of their sensitivity to medicines and treatments and the immaturity of their liver. It is recommended that a person knowledgeable in the herbal treatment of children be consulted before the offering of any herb to a child for the first time.

🍃 CAUTIONS:

Lavender has long been used to help promote sleep through relaxation. It may, therefore, potentiate the effects of pharmaceutical sedatives, antihistamines, and tranquilizers and lead to reduced alertness. Some suggest that lavender not be used in combination with alcohol or other sedatives (Brinker, 1998). There have been few reports of contact dermatitis in those exposed to lavender. A strong positive reaction to lavender oil during patch testing was reported in a hairdresser in Portugal who was exposed to lavender shampoo several times over the course of a day (Brandao, 1986).

NURSING EVIDENCE:

Historical Nursing Use

Nurses have used lavender baths postnatally to reduce perineal discomfort and to reduce discomfort associated with mammography.

Potential Nursing Applications

Lavender has tremendous potential in nursing practice because of its versatility. Lavender can be considered for the elderly and for those undergoing rehabilitation. These patients often have chronic aches, pains, and discomfort that are easily relieved by nursing care rather than pharmaceuticals. Nurses may want to consider using hot lavender fomentations or lavender massage oil for patients with localized aches and pains. Oleum Spicae, lavender mixed with three quarters turpentine or wine spirit, is a formula renowned for healing sprains, relieving stiffness in joints, and stimulating paralyzed extremities (Grieve, 1971).

Lavender can be considered for use in burn unit patients who have a need for its wound healing capabilities and calming and pain relief effects. Specific uses for lavender include comfort measures. Some nurses have found that giving their intubated patients a gentle hand massage with dilute lavender essential oil twenty minutes before extubation allowed the patient to relax and not struggle against the tube. The patients were able to relax in preparation for extubation, but not so deeply that they weren't able to breathe on their own (Buckle, 1997). "The Dales Occupational Therapy service in Derbyshire, England uses aromatherapy to improve quality of life of patients with Alzheimer's disease" (Buckle, 1997, p. 195). Lavender essential oil also can be considered for numerous applications in which its antibacterial effects and ability to speed wound healing might be appreciated. Lavender oil could be used as a disinfectant for the sick room if patients or their caregivers are chemically sensitive to synthetically fragranced or disinfectant products.

Integrative Insight

Lavender, especially the essential oil, has extensive traditional evidence supporting its use in the care of those with pain related to various health concerns. Lavender eases pain by promoting physical and emotional relaxation and by soothing irritation and inflammation in or on the body. It promotes comfort and rest with its balanced aroma. Lavender has so much potential to help patients: It helps relieve daily aches and pains and heal burns and wounds. It calms the nerves and promotes sleep and rest. It helps restore a patient's appetite and raises the spirit. It also can disinfect a sick room! Lavender and its essential oil just might prove to be nursing "care alls."

THERAPEUTIC APPLICATIONS:

Oral

Tea. Use 1 to 2 teaspoons (5 to 10 g) of the herb in 5 ounces (150 ml) of water.

Essential Oil Internal Use. Use 1 to 4 drops of the essential oil on a sugar cube (Blumenthal et al., 2000) to relieve pain.

Topical

Massage. Add 2 drops of lavender essential oil to 1 tablespoon (15 ml) of sweet almond oil to be used for a massage to relieve symptoms of premenstrual tension, grief, mood swings, menopausal problems, and depression. A few drops of lavender essential oil can be gently massaged on the temples to relieve headache or can be dabbed directly on affected areas to ease the pain associated with burns (Lawless, 1998).

Environmental

Bath. Add 5 to 10 drops of lavender essential oil to a full bath to relieve insomnia, restlessness, anxiety, nervousness, fears, sunburn, sunstroke, and other stress-related problems (Lawless, 1998).

Inhalation. Lavender essential oil can be used in a diffuser or vaporizer in the home to purify the air and create a relaxed atmosphere. A few drops can be put on pillows or pajamas so that the inhaled scent produces relaxation and restful sleep. A few drops can be put on a handkerchief or tissue and inhaled to relieve nausea, travel sickness, faintness, and migraine (Lawless, 1998).

The healing benefits of lavender flowers also can be enjoyed in potpourris and dried arrangements.

Herbal Caveat—Therapeutic Applications

In traditional and conventional herbal medicine, amounts of herbs given to patients are based on individual needs. The amounts or "doses" recorded here are provided so that the health practitioner has a general idea of the amounts recommended for an adult patient. Dosing in herbalism not only refers to amount of plant used but also includes when, where, and how to take a plant medicine. These dosages should not be used as guidelines for indiscriminate intervention without proper assessment, critical thinking, and patient education on the part of the practitioner.

Note: Please see chapter 5 for detailed descriptions of how to prepare various applications.

PATIENT INTERACTION:

Lavender and pure lavender essential oil can be added to any first-aid kit. The oil can be safely applied on burns and wounds to help heal the skin. Lavender oil can be applied to the temples for easing pain associated with headache. It can be applied to the skin in a bath or as a massage oil to ease the aches and pains of daily life. The scent can be very relaxing to the spirit and calming to the emotions.

Herbal Caveat—Patient Interaction

Patients considering the use of an herb or formula of herbs in self-care benefit from education about the plant itself and the use of the plant in healing. This education can come through many sources, including local herbalists; plant specialists such as botanists; health practitioners such as nurses, nutritionists, naturopaths, and other physicians; and various written references including the scientific literature. Patients need to remember that their unique health care needs are not necessarily represented in any literature they may encounter. Therefore, it is recommended that a knowledgeable mentor be consulted before initiating self-care with any herb being used for the first time.

NURTURING THE NURSE-PLANT RELATIONSHIP:

Note: You may want to keep a journal of your experiences with the herb.

Lavender and lavender essential oil are good additions to every nurse's home remedy kit. As long as the scent of lavender is perceived as pleasing, it can be used for the common aches, pains, and stresses on body and spirit associated with hard work. Lavender baths are especially soothing after a physically and emotionally taxing day. To get to know the soothing benefits of lavender, try a lavender bath as soon as you get home from work. Use either a whole herb bath infusion or some drops of essential oil and see if you don't have some energy left for fun times with your family!

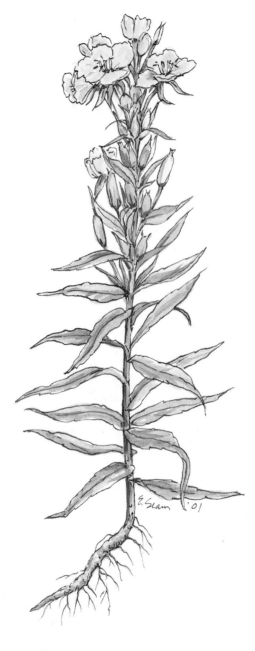

Oenothera biennis

Evening Primrose

- **LATIN NAME:** *Oenothera biennis*

- **FAMILY:** Onagraceae

- **COMMON NAMES:** Evening primrose, tree primrose, sun drop, king's cure-all, night willow herb

- **HEALTH PATTERN:** Comfort and pain relief

- **PLANT DESCRIPTION:**

  Evening primrose is a biennial, a plant that lives for two years. Its stem grows erect, reaches 2 to 5 feet (1 to 2 meters) in height, and is downy with many branches. The downy leaves are opposite each other on the stem and are 3 to 6 inches (1 to 2.5 cm) long and oval shaped with pointed ends. The pale yellow flowers appear in July and August. They are nocturnal, that is, they open in the evening and at night. The seed capsule is oblong and contains numerous seeds. It has been said that on dark nights when no objects are visible, the flowers of evening primrose can be seen from a distance. Some speculate that this is due to some phosphoric property in the flowers (Felter & Lloyd, 1983).

  Evening primrose is a hardy plant that thrives in almost any soil condition, but it seems to prefer good sandy soil that is in a sunny location. It is found growing wild throughout North America in pastures, old fields, and roadsides and is cultivated in Europe, North America, and elsewhere for its seed oil.

- **PLANT PARTS USED:** Leaves, bark, twigs, seeds, roots, and oil extracted from the seeds

- **TRADITIONAL EVIDENCE:**

  Cultural Use

  North American Indian. The Cherokee use evening primrose as an infusion to help weight loss, a condition they refer to as "overfatness." They use a hot root poultice topically for hemorrhoids. As a food source, the Cherokee cook the leaves and eat them as greens and boil the root as a potato. The Iroquois use the plant for boils, internally and externally for hemorrhoids, and believe that the chewed roots rubbed on the body promote strength. The Lakota use evening primrose seeds as an aromatic incense (Moerman, 1998).

  Hispanic. Some Hispanics chop the root of the evening primrose, boil it, and make it into a cough syrup. The root and the flower are boiled and strained and then the infusion is used in the bath to relax smooth muscles and relieve skin inflammation.

European. Evening primrose oil is used clinically in Britain to treat eczema, premenstrual syndrome (PMS), and breast pain.

Culinary Use

In some European countries, the roots of evening primrose are used for garnishing salads (Grieve, 1971).

Use in Herbalism

Historically, evening primrose twigs, leaves, and bark were boiled in lard or tallow to make an ointment to apply to cutaneous inflammations in infants. The fresh bruised leaves were applied to skin ulcers. The plant was used internally in cases of gastrointestinal disorders, specifically in patients who had sallow skin and a gloomy, despondent nature. In these conditions, it was used for dyspepsia, liver disorders, enlargement of the spleen, and for female reproductive disorders in which the woman had a sensation of pelvic fullness and was lethargic. Evening primrose leaves, bark, and twigs were used for dyspepsia associated with vomiting, nausea, restlessness, and urinary urgency. It was used in infantile cholera, watery diarrhea, and dysentery with tenesmus and bloody stools. Evening primrose also was used to relieve difficult respirations and chronic asthma with gastric complications (Felter & Lloyd, 1983). It also has been used in the treatment of whooping cough (Grieve, 1971).

The fatty oil derived from the small, reddish-brown seeds of the evening primrose has caused a resurgence of interest in the plant in recent years. The oil of evening primrose seeds contains gamma-linolenic acid (GLA), which is the precursor of linoleic acid and prostaglandin E_1. This natural polyunsaturated fatty acid is used for the pain and discomfort associated with diabetic neuropathy and mastalgia. It is used for dry skin conditions that accompany viral infections, alcoholism, smoking, and chronic diseases. Additionally, it is used in the treatment of many inflammatory diseases, such as rheumatoid arthritis and eczema. Evening primrose oil is used for weight loss, to lower blood cholesterol, decrease blood pressure, alleviate premenstrual pain, slow the progress of multiple sclerosis, and provide relief from hangovers (Foster & Tyler, 1999). Oil of evening primrose may be applied to the edges of wounds to facilitate the healing process (Buckle, 1997).

Evening primrose oil currently is sold in some countries as a dietary supplement in capsule form. The oil is expensive. Other less expensive oils are currently on the market that contain from 6% to 9% GLA (evening primrose contains 2%). These oils are derived from the seeds of two other plants, black currant and borage. However, evening primrose is considered safer than borage for long-term use because borage seed oil may contain enough toxic pyrrolizidine alkaloids, as does the whole plant, that it may make long-term therapeutic use unsafe (Duke, 1999).

Cosmetic Use. The oil also is used in cosmetic products such as soaps, hand lotions, and shampoos.

BIOMEDICAL EVIDENCE:

Evening primrose oil has been the subject of several studies. Because the human body needs a balance of omega-6 and omega-3 essential fatty acids (EFAs), evening primrose oil has often been studied with fish oil, a rich source of omega-3 EFAs. Although studying a supplement containing more than one substance is not ideal, given the knowledge of the importance of a balance of EFAs, investigators should consider the ethical issue regarding the potential harm of providing high doses of omega-6 EFA without omega-3. Although the studies included in this section were selected for their specificity to evening primrose, I have chosen to acknowledge the many other studies that use a more balanced and perhaps healthier approach to investigating the effects of evening primrose in combination with omega-3 EFAs.

Studies Related to Comfort and Pain Relief

In a multicenter, double-blind, randomized parallel trial of 111 patients with diabetic neuropathy conducted over the course of one year, those patients receiving 12 capsules daily of evening primrose (EF4 brand with a known GLA content of 40 mg per capsule, totaling 480 mg of GLA daily) showed significant reverses of symptoms of polyneuropathy or deterioration of symptoms as compared with patients receiving the placebo, especially if the patient's baseline Hb A_1 was lower. Sex, age, and type of diabetes are reported not to have influenced the results. No adverse events occurred in this trial. Although diabetic control levels, as measured by Hb A_1, deteriorated during the study, it occurred in both treatment and control groups (Keen et al., 1993).

In a double-blind placebo-controlled study of 22 patients with diabetic neuropathy, patients exhibited significant improvement when receiving 2000 mg of evening primrose oil twice a day (total 360 mg GLA) as compared with patients receiving the placebo (Jamal & Carmichael, 1990).

In a randomized, double-blind, placebo-controlled crossover study of 73 patients, those receiving evening primrose oil daily for three months (dose not published) demonstrated significant improvement in cyclical mastalgia (i.e., breast pain) (Pashby, Mansel, Hughes, Hanslip, & Preece, 1981). When used as a first-line treatment, evening primrose oil significantly reduced pain and discomfort in 58% of those patients with cyclical mastalgia and 38% of those with noncyclical mastalgia. Evening primrose oil was less effective than danazol

(Danol) and equally effective as bromocriptine (Parlodel) but had fewer adverse events than either drug (Gateley, Miers, Mansel, & Hughes, 1992).

Evening primrose oil given orally, 6 capsules per day for three to six months (dosage not reported), significantly reduced severe and persistent mastalgia (breast pain) in 45% of participants with cyclical mastalgia and in 27% of patients with noncyclical mastalgia. Ninety-five percent of those who responded to evening primrose oil did so within three months and 2% of the patients in both groups complained of a bloated feeling with nausea after taking the evening primrose oil (Pye, Mansel, & Hughes, 1985).

Although one survey of 310 women showed that the women rated evening primrose oil as one of the effective interventions for reducing premenstrual symptoms (Campbell, Peterkin, O'Grady, & Sanson-Fisher, 1997), according to a metanalysis of the literature on the subject, the two most well-controlled trials failed to show any beneficial effects from evening primrose oil. However, the samples in these studies were small (Budeiri, Li Wan Po, & Dorman, 1996).

Studies Related to Other Health Patterns

Elimination. One preliminary British study of 43 patients with stable ulcerative colitis, using sigmoidoscopy, histology, and diary cards for clinical evaluation, demonstrated that 19 patients in the group given a combination of evening primrose and borage oil in a 250 mg capsule (15.5% GLA) had a slight improvement in stool consistency. The patients were given 12 capsules daily for one month and 6 capsules daily for five months. There was no effect on stool frequency or rectal bleeding in the test group (Greenfield, Green, Teare, Jenkins, Punchard, Ainley, & Thompson, 1993).

Immune Response. After three months of daily treatment with 4000 mg evening primrose oil (Epogam) and fish oil, 85% of patients in the treatment group diagnosed with postviral fatigue syndrome demonstrated significant improvement as compared with the placebo group in a double-blind, placebo-controlled trial of 63 adults (Behan, Behan, & Horrobin, 1990).

Skin Care. Although evening primrose oil is licensed for the treatment of atopic dermatitis in some European countries, evidence of its efficacy is conflicting. Several studies have found that there is no significant improvement in symptoms related to atopic dermatitis, eczema, chronic hand dermatitis, or psoriasis (Berth-Jones & Graham-Brown, 1994; Hederos & Berg, 1996; Oliwiecki & Burton, 1994; Whitaker, Cilliers, & de Beer, 1996).

In a double-blind study, significant improvement in skin redness and surface damage occurred in those eczema patients ($N = 52$) who received 6000 mg of evening primrose oil daily as compared with the placebo group. Women who reported a premenstrual flare of their eczema showed an even greater improvement than the other participants (Humphreys, Symons, Brown, Duff, & Hunter, 1994).

Mechanism of Action

Evening primrose oil, extracted from the seed of the plant, is a rich source of EFAs. EFAs are unsaturated long carbon chain molecules that contain their first double bond at either the n-3 or n-6 position. The parents of EFAs are linoleic acid and alpha-linolenic acid, which are found in significant concentrations in plants. Evening primrose oil, an omega-6 EFA, contains high amounts of GLA. The GLA content of evening primrose oil is of interest because it is a precursor of prostaglandins, especially PGE_1. Prostaglandins help regulate many metabolic functions. PGE_1 is important in nerve cell transmission and is both anti-inflammatory and immunostimulating. Affecting the PGE_1 pathway has been shown to improve conditions such as depression and schizophrenia, multiple sclerosis, PMS, and attention deficit hyperactivity disorder (Schmidt, 1997). GLA has the ability to inhibit platelet aggregation, reduce blood pressure, and restore motility of red blood cells in multiple sclerosis (Leung & Foster, 1996). Normal synthesis of GLA from linoleic acid in the body may be blocked or reduced by aging, diabetes, fasting, or excessive carbohydrate intake (Leung & Foster, 1996). It is thought that people with these (and other) conditions lack an enzyme (delta-6 desaturase) necessary for the conversion of linoleic acid to GLA and then to PGE_1. This is why evening primrose oil may be helpful in alleviating the symptoms of many chronic diseases.

Evening primrose is also a source of tryptophan, an amino acid that may help reduce sensitivity to pain. Sensitivity to pain is partly affected by the serotonin levels in the brain, and tryptophan is a precursor for serotonin. Duke (1997) suggests taking the powdered seed instead of the oil because much of the tryptophan is lost in the oil extraction process.

USE IN PREGNANCY OR LACTATION:

Animal studies suggest that evening primrose oil does not cause abnormalities in fetal development. Data on the safety of evening primrose oil during human pregnancy are not available. Midwives often recommend 3 capsules of evening primrose oil daily to ripen the cervix and shorten labor. In cases of a rigid os or firm unripe cervix that is impeding dilation and slowing labor, midwives will rub evening primrose oil directly on the cervix to encourage softening and opening (Weed, 1986). In a survey of 169 certified nurse midwives in the United States, evening primrose oil was reported to be the most efficacious herbal preparation for cervical ripening and had no reported complications (McFarlin, Gibson, O'Rear, & Harman, 1999). One source reports that the topical application of evening primrose oil to the cervix has not been investigated (Dove & Johnson, 1999).

"Small adjustments to the proportions of dietary fatty acids in the mother in late pregnancy or in the postnatal period, or in the newborn infant, can have significant effects on the levels of long-chain polyunsaturated fatty acids in the mother and docosahexaenoic acid and arachidonic acid in her infant.... The full effects of fatty acid supplementation in women and their babies is unknown" (Sattar, Berry, & Greer, 1998, p. 1253). Oral administration of evening primrose oil from the thirty-seventh week of gestation, 500 mg three times a day for one week and then 500 mg per day until the onset of labor, was not shown to shorten gestation or labor in a two-group, retrospective quasi-experimental study of 108 women. This study had some limitations, however, such as its limited generalizability because the sample was comprised of a unique population of low-risk, nulliparous women and the lack of control of variables that might influence cervical ripening such as sexual intercourse and use of other remedies (Dove & Johnson, 1999).

Often, women make drastic cuts to the fat in their diets and end up decreasing their intake of EFAs. Although general guidelines regarding healthy fat intake can be helpful, they are often inadequate in addressing the special needs of the individual, especially if the individual is a woman. For example, in pregnancy, a developing fetus must have adequate fat from the mother to promote healthy growth of the brain. Infants must get 50% of their calories from fat and nursing mothers must have sufficient fat in their diets to meet this need. It is, however, the omega-3 EFAs, such as those found in fish oils, that have often been found to be deficient in the pregnant woman, not the omega-6, as is found in evening primrose oil. Omega-6 linoleic acid levels are often found to be too high (Schmidt, 1997). Because GLA is normally present in breast milk, evening primrose oil may be safe to take orally during lactation. Again, the importance of having a balanced intake of omega-6 and omega-3 EFAs at all times, but especially during pregnancy and lactation, cannot be stressed enough.

Herbal Caveat—Pregnancy or Lactation

Some herbs are contraindicated in pregnancy because of a risk of the herb or one of its constituents stimulating the uterus and therefore possibly promoting fetal loss. Many herbal practitioners do not recommend herbal remedies, in particular oral doses of herbs, during the first trimester of pregnancy and seek an alternative. However, herbs are successfully used during pregnancy, especially to prepare the body for the birth. Herbs are relatively unstudied in pregnancy and lactation, so patients need to be made aware through education of the potential benefits and risks of using herbs for health conditions that arise during pregnancy or lactation. The use of herbal remedies during pregnancy often warrants a referral to a knowledgeable herbal practitioner.

USE FOR CHILDREN:

 In Germany, infants with seborrheic dermatitis (e.g., milk crust, cradle cap) and chronic eczema are given oral doses of evening primrose oil. It is believed that the GLA content of the oil helps correct the inflammatory condition of the skin (Schilcher, 1992). Long-chain polyunsaturated fatty acids, such as are found in evening primrose oil, are critical to the healthy neurologic development of the fetus and infant. The major transfer of EFAs to a fetus occurs in the third trimester. Premature infants often have a significant deficiency of EFAs. Supplementation with n-3 and n-6 long-chain polyunsaturated fatty acids in premature infants is recommended. Supplementation in formula of term infants is controversial (Sattar, Berry, & Greer, 1998).

Herbal Caveat—Children

Children have special needs in regard to herbal therapies. They require lesser amounts of herbs and often respond well to mild teas and topical applications such as compresses and baths. The lowest dose of oral preparations should be tried first before increasing the amount given children. Caregivers should observe children closely for responses to herbal remedies. Younger children, particularly infants, have traditionally been given herbs either through their mother's breast milk or in the form of a homeopathic remedy because of their sensitivity to medicines and treatments and the immaturity of their liver. It is recommended that a person knowledgeable in the herbal treatment of children be consulted before the offering of any herb to a child for the first time.

CAUTIONS:

Evening primrose oil may have to be taken daily for three months before a clinical response is noticed (Newall, Anderson, & Phillipson, 1996). Evening primrose oil seems to be well tolerated orally with very few side effects noted. Occasional side effects that have been reported are mild gastrointestinal effects such as indigestion, nausea, and softening of stools. Headaches also have been reported.

Evening primrose oil may bring out undiagnosed temporal lobe epilepsy in patients, such as those with schizophrenia and/or those taking epileptogenic drugs such as phenothiazines (Newall et al., 1996). Overdosage of evening primrose oil has resulted in loose stools and abdominal pain (Newall et al., 1996).

NURSING EVIDENCE:

Historical Nursing Use

Oral evening primrose oil is widely used by midwives to promote cervical ripening (Dove & Johnson, 1999).

Potential Nursing Applications

Evening primrose, in particular the oil from the seed, has potential for use in nursing. Numerous chronic conditions are either caused or exacerbated by an imbalance or deficiency in EFAs. Nurses might consider evening primrose for its applications in pain management, in particular in patients with mastalgia and neuropathy, and in the promotion of healthy skin. Nurses also might consider being part of an interdisciplinary team to study the effects of oral and topical applications of evening primrose. Nurses performing manual lymph drainage might consider using evening primrose oil topically. This is a specific touch therapy in which light pressure strokes are applied to an engorged limb to facilitate movement of the lymphatic fluid and reduce swelling, such as with lymphedema. The strokes are directed toward the main lymph ducts, away from the periphery, and toward the thoracic duct. Daily sessions may dramatically reduce engorgement. Evening primrose oil applied to the skin during the sessions may help the skin maintain elasticity when lymphedema is present (Buckle, 1997).

Integrative Insight

Biomedical and traditional evidence support the use of evening primrose for several health patterns including comfort and pain relief. The ability of evening primrose to relieve pain is thought to be related to its fatty acid and tryptophan content. Its constituents and its name indicate that evening primrose's beneficial effects may have something to do with nighttime and sleep. I have often recommended that patients take evening primrose before bed. Pain is a complex process that often is relieved by a good night's sleep. The unfortunate thing for pain sufferers is that the pain they feel often precludes sound sleep. Evening primrose may reduce sensitivity to pain. Part of the understanding that can be gained from working with evening primrose is the importance of a holistic approach to finding pain relief measures that include promoting sound and refreshing sleep. Also, evening primrose is a good example of how plants and plant therapies can help lead to greater understanding of the body, mind, and emotions.

Consideration of nutritional imbalances is important to all specialties of nursing practice. Because nurses assess and intervene from a holistic perspective, diet has always been important in helping a patient create and maintain their unique picture of health. There is extensive support for the importance of a diet that is balanced in omega-3 and omega-6 EFAs. Evening primrose oil is a ready source of omega-6 and can be considered as a supplement in the diets of those patients, especially women, who have discomfort related to chronic skin conditions, mastalgia, fibrocystic breasts, and diabetes. Many nurses are looking closely at the effects of low-fat diets, especially on women's health. Often when women drastically reduce their fat intake, they often decrease their intake of

EFAs, which can become a health risk. Understanding EFA balance is important to providing integrative nutritional care. EFA balance is not achieved by taking one substance such as the GLA found in evening primrose oil; taking evening primrose affects the total EFA system.

THERAPEUTIC APPLICATIONS:

Oral

Oil extracted from seed. Daily doses used in the treatment of atopic dermatitis of evening primrose oil standardized to 8% are 6 to 8 g for adults and 2 to 4 g for children. For cyclical mastalgia, it is recommended to take 3 to 4 g daily. The oil may be taken plain or mixed with food or liquid.

Topical

Although evening primrose oil has been recommended for internal use, nurses have begun to use the oil for skin care as well (Buckle, 1997).

Environmental

No data are available at this time.

Herbal Caveat—Therapeutic Applications

In traditional and conventional herbal medicine, amounts of herbs given to patients are based on individual needs. The amounts or "doses" recorded here are provided so that the health practitioner has a general idea of the amounts recommended for an adult patient. Dosing in herbalism not only refers to amount of plant used but also includes when, where, and how to take a plant medicine. These dosages should not be used as guidelines for indiscriminate intervention without proper assessment, critical thinking, and patient education on the part of the practitioner.

Note: Please see chapter 5 for detailed descriptions of how to prepare various applications.

PATIENT INTERACTION:

Evening primrose oil is a plant source of omega-6 EFAs, a substance that is important for the healthy functioning of many of the organ systems in the body. Although evening primrose root has been used traditionally for several purposes, the primary plant part used today is the seed from which the oil is pressed. Evening primrose has been shown to be helpful in patients with discomfort related to breast pain, diabetic neuropathy, and chronic skin conditions. It is important when taking evening primrose oil as a supplement, that omega-3 EFAs be taken as well. In many industrialized countries, it is quite easy to have a diet rich in omega-6 EFAs but not omega-3. A good source of omega-3 EFAs is fish and fish oil.

Herbal Caveat—Patient Interaction

Patients considering the use of an herb or formula of herbs in self-care benefit from education about the plant itself and the use of the plant in healing. This education can come through many sources, including local herbalists; plant specialists such as botanists; health practitioners such as nurses, nutritionists, naturopaths, and other physicians; and various written references including the scientific literature. Patients need to remember that their unique health care needs are not necessarily represented in any literature they may encounter. Therefore, it is recommended that a knowledgeable mentor be consulted before initiating self-care with any herb being used for the first time.

NURTURING THE NURSE-PLANT RELATIONSHIP:

Note: You may want to keep a journal of your experiences with the herb.

One way to get to know a medicinal plant is to first get to know its seed. Evening primrose oil is produced from pressed small seeds. Each seed is said to contain about 14% fixed oil. If at all possible, try to plant this herb and watch its growth cycle. When it goes to seed think about how many seeds would be needed to press enough oil to fill a supplement capsule. The work it takes for an evening primrose plant to produce enough oil to fulfill the need for a supplement is often underestimated and perhaps even undervalued. Growing the plant is the best way to be able to appreciate the work it takes for the grower and the plant to produce the oil.

In addition, if you would like to know your fatty acid status, contact your health care practitioner and ask to have the blood work done. The following is one laboratory that will perform this test:

Great Smokies Diagnostic Laboratory
63 Zillicoa Street
Asheville, NC 28801
1-800-522-4762
cs@gsdl.com

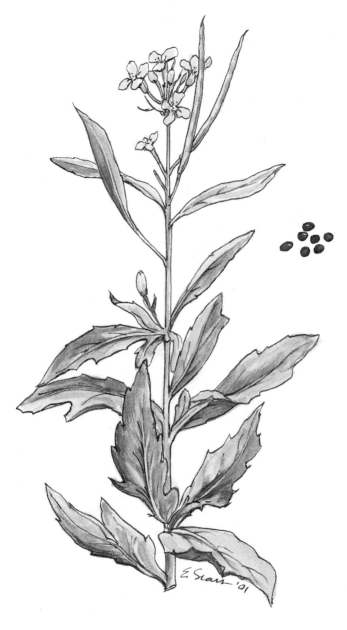

Brassica nigra

Mustard

- **LATIN NAMES:** *Brassica nigra, Brassica alba, Brassica juncea*

- **FAMILY:** Brassicaceae

- **COMMON NAMES:** Mustard; *Brassica nigra*: black mustard; *Brassica alba*: white mustard, yellow mustard; *Brassica juncea*: Chinese mustard, Indian mustard, brown mustard

- **HEALTH PATTERN:** Comfort and pain relief

- **PLANT DESCRIPTION:**
White mustard plant is native to Europe and is commonly found along roadsides and in fields. It is also widely cultivated. It is an annual, growing 12 or more inches (30 cm) tall with large yellow flowers that have four petals. It is very similar to the black mustard plant, except that it is smaller. The seed pods of the white mustard plant grow horizontally and appear hairy, while those of black mustard are more erect and smooth. The white mustard pods are round, ribbed, and have a spike at the end. Each pod contains four to six globular seeds. The seeds are tiny (1 to 2.5 mm in diameter), with a pungent taste and odor when ground.

- **PLANT PARTS USED:** Dried, ripe seeds; leaves; and the oil of the seed

- **TRADITIONAL EVIDENCE:**
Cultural Use

Asian. Traditional Chinese medicine (TCM) recognizes white mustard seed as warming to the lung energy system and having the ability to help expel cold phlegm. It is known as "bai jie zi" in China, "hakugaishi" in Japanese, and "paekkaecha" in Korean and is used for chest congestion, chronic pain, and conditions involving the coughing up of excessive thin sputum. Mustard has been used in TCM to reduce swellings and nodules and for symptoms of joint pain, body aches, boils, bedsores, and oozing wounds. It is contraindicated in cases of cough due to lung deficiency, and in yin deficiency with heat signs. It is not used topically on those patients with skin sensitivities (Bensky & Gamble, 1993).

Japanese herbal medicine uses white mustard seed to dry fluids in the body, calm wheezing, and transform phlegm. The seed is used for rheumatic conditions, flu, inflammation of the nerves, lung conditions, and urinary tract infections. Mustard seed plasters and teas are used topically for many kinds of skin fungi. Some clinicians have been known to inject specific mustard preparations into acupuncture points on the body. This procedure has been used to treat chronic bronchitis, colds, wheezing, and difficulty expectorating phlegm. Mustard seed plasters also are used for the same purposes. White and black mustard seeds are considered equally effective plasters (Rister, 1999).

North American Indian. The Cherokee use black mustard as a dietary aid to increase the appetite and as a fever reducer. They use it as a poultice for croup. Other North American Indian tribes use the ground seeds for head colds and make topical applications of the seeds or leaves for body pains, toothaches, and headaches. Various tribes boil the young spring leaves and eat them as a green vegetable. The leaves are cooked with salt, pepper, and butter. Some tribes even cook mustard greens with other wild plants such as the leaves of nettle, dock, and plantain. Some tribes use mustard seeds as a spice (Moerman, 1998).

Hispanic. Known as "mostaza," mustard leaf, either fresh or dried, is boiled, steeped, and strained, and the infusion is added to the bath water of patients suffering from pain related to rheumatic disease. Mostaza footbaths are given to those with severe colds. Mustard plasters, made with flour and water, are used for backache and chest congestion and are placed on the skin after a protecting salve has been applied. Mustard seed also is used in cooking and canning.

East Indian. In India, white mustard is known as "svetasarisha" and black mustard, "sarshapah." Several varieties of mustard are cultivated in India for food and medicinal uses of the seeds, oil, and leaves. The oil extracted from the seeds is used as an external application to the chest for children's respiratory problems. Mustard oil with camphor topical ointment is used for muscular rheumatism and neck stiffness. A poultice of the powdered seeds is applied to the skin in cases of certain inflammations, abdominal colic, gout, low back pain, and vomiting. External applications also are used for sore throat, fevers, inflammatory swellings, and internal congestion. In India, an external mustard application is never in contact with the skin for longer than ten minutes because of the risk of blistering. Mustard also is used for snakebites (Nadkarni, 1976).

Russian/Baltic. Russians continue to use mustard plasters extensively for pain, congestion, pneumonia, tuberculosis, hypertension, cardiac ischemia, arthritis, and headache (Kunovski, 1982).

European. In Europe, mustard is generally recognized as safe (GRAS). In Germany, white mustard seed has been officially declared an effective external poultice for upper respiratory congestion and for the supportive treatment of joint and soft tissue diseases (Leung & Foster, 1996).

Practitioners of Anthroposophical nursing and medicine regard mustard as a highly stimulating substance because of its sulfur content. It is stimulating to the head region, the nervous and sensory systems, and metabolism. Black mustard seed is applied as a poultice (Husemann & Wolff, 1982).

Culinary Use

Romans used the leaves of black mustard as a vegetable (Grieve, 1971). Mustard greens can be purchased today and, although somewhat bitter, are quite palatable and offer a good alternative to other green leafy vegetables. Currently, mustard seeds are widely used in prepared condiments in which they are ground and mixed with vinegar and other spices, such as turmeric. Mustard seeds also are used commercially in baked goods, meats, vegetables, fats and oils, gravies, snack foods, and nut products. Mustard oil is used as a flavoring in nonalcoholic beverages, frozen dairy desserts, gelatins, puddings, condiments and relishes, candy, and other foods. The Italians mix black mustard seeds with orange and lemon peel to make a condiment. Dijon mustard is prepared with black mustard seeds, anchovies, capers, tarragon, and various spices (Grieve, 1971). In India, oil of mustard is used to flavor curries and vegetables and the whole seeds are used in relishes. The leaves and green seed pods are eaten as vegetables (Nadkarni, 1976).

Use in Herbalism

Mustard is best known for its ability to increase the sensation of heat in the body and to relieve pain and congestion. Historically, topical applications of mustard have been used for sciatica, gout, and other joint pains. It was believed that the blistering of the skin caused by the mustard drew the "disease" to the outside of the body. Now it is believed that mustard works by increasing circulation at the surface of the body, thereby relieving congestion in the organs below (Grieve, 1971). This process of stimulating the skin with mustard is known as counterirritation. Oil of mustard is a very strong irritant and rubefacient. If it is applied to the skin in its pure state, it will cause immediate blistering. But if, like mustard, it is properly prepared and diluted, it is an effective treatment for colic and mild frostbite and pain that is associated with chronic rheumatism and arthritis.

Hot water poured over black mustard seeds can be used as a stimulating footbath to help with pain and discomfort related to colds and headaches (Grieve, 1971). The rationale for the mustard footbath is that the mustard and the footbath are both stimulating to the circulation. Stimulating the feet relieves congestion and pain in the head and upper body. The mustard contains antibiotic principles that are absorbed through the sensitive skin of the feet (Griggs, 1991). Mustard plasters, poultices, and footbaths were commonly used until the mid-1900s.

The crushed seeds can be mixed with honey and applied to bruises, rough and scabby skin, leprosy, and lice infestations (Culpeper, 1990). The dried, ripe seeds of black and white mustard are powdered to create a mustard flour that is used as poultices for inflammation, pneumonia, bronchitis, and other conditions of the respiratory tract. Mustard seed also can be mixed with Indian meal and vinegar after bruising the seed and made into a paste or plaster (Beach, 1843). Mustard poultices also have been used historically for "comatose affections, prevention of return of convulsions, gout, cholera and low typhus fever" (Beach, 1843, p. 674).

Mustard seed is an appetite stimulant. Historical references state that mustard seed was ground with cinnamon, prepared into tablets, and taken an hour before meals. This preparation was used by those who had difficulty digesting meats (Culpeper, 1990). Mustard was sometimes chewed to relieve toothache pain and gargled for sore throats. A sauce can be made of mustard and taken for the treatment of "weak stomach," by those who are aged and troubled by "cold diseases."

Mustard is known to promote menstruation, to increase mental alertness, and to assist in the treatment of colds and coughs. Herbalists also use mustard internally to treat mushroom poisoning, stings from scorpions and other venomous creatures, and to decrease chills and fever. Mustard flour added to a glass of tepid water and taken internally induces vomiting.

Mustard oil is sometimes added to ointments and liniments and used for the relief of cold symptoms. When applied topically, the properly prepared oil is taken up by the skin and directed to the lungs for excretion through exhalation. For this reason, mustard liniments can relieve lung congestion (Leung & Foster, 1996).

BIOMEDICAL EVIDENCE:

The studies on the therapeutic use of mustard are primarily in Russian. Very few studies have been done on mustard, and it has not been used in some countries for several years.

Studies Related to Comfort and Pain Relief

One uncontrolled Russian study of the use of mustard plaster for pain and breathing difficulty associated with pneumonia, chronic bronchitis, or asthma showed that the majority of the sample of 150 patients who received mustard plasters experienced a decrease in pleural pain, an improvement in volume and speed of respiration, and an increase in expectoration (Kirsanov, 1982).

Studies Related to Other Health Patterns

No data are available at this time.

Mechanism of Action

Allyl isothiocyanate is the plant constituent thought to be responsible for the counterirritant action as well as the contact dermatitis and hyperpigmentation some patients experience as the result of mustard external applications (Linder, Mele, & Harries, 1996).

USE IN PREGNANCY OR LACTATION:

Empirical evidence suggests that pregnant women should avoid using mustard therapeutically because it has emmenagogic and abortifacient effects when taken in large amounts (Brinker, 1998).

Herbal Caveat—Pregnancy or Lactation

Some herbs are contraindicated in pregnancy because of a risk of the herb or one of its constituents stimulating the uterus and therefore possibly promoting fetal loss. Many herbal practitioners do not recommend herbal remedies, in particular oral doses of herbs, during the first trimester of pregnancy and seek an alternative. However, herbs are successfully used during pregnancy, especially to prepare the body for the birth. Herbs are relatively unstudied in pregnancy and lactation, so patients need to be made aware through education of the potential benefits and risks of using herbs for health conditions that arise during pregnancy or lactation. The use of herbal remedies during pregnancy often warrants a referral to a knowledgeable herbal practitioner.

USE FOR CHILDREN:

According to one source, mustard should not be used on children under six years of age (McGuffin et al., 1997), yet some countries routinely use mustard plasters on children and modify the plaster application. The application time is shorter; the plaster is moved more frequently on the body; and in Russia, the plaster is put in a plastic bag so that the child does not have to tolerate the smell. Children should always be closely attended during the application of a mustard plaster to make sure they do not get the mustard on their hands and spread it to their eyes or other sensitive areas.

Herbal Caveat—Children

Children have special needs in regard to herbal therapies. They require lesser amounts of herbs and often respond well to mild teas and topical applications such as compresses and baths. The lowest dose of oral preparations should be tried first before increasing the amount given children. Caregivers should observe children closely for responses to herbal remedies. Younger children, particularly infants, have traditionally been given herbs either through their mother's breast milk or in the form of a homeopathic remedy because of their sensitivity to medicines and treatments and the immaturity of their liver. It is recommended that a person knowledgeable in the herbal treatment of children be consulted before the offering of any herb to a child for the first time.

CAUTIONS:

Internal use of mustard is contraindicated in those who have preexisting inflammation in the gastrointestinal tract due to the irritant effect of the constituent allyl isothiocyanate. Mustard should not be used to induce vomiting in cases of corrosive poisonings because of the danger of reexposure of the esophagus to both the irritative effects of the mustard and the corrosive agent. Pure mustard powder should not be used on unprotected skin for more than fifteen to twenty minutes because severe burns could occur (Brinker, 1998; McGuffin et al., 1997). Russian sources recommend using the plaster for five minutes for the first application, ten minutes for the second, and fifteen minutes for the third in adults (Kunovskii, 1982). It is suggested that mustard not be used topically for more than two weeks because of the possibility of blistering and ulceration of the skin (Brinker, 1998; McGuffin et al., 1997). The internal and external use of white mustard is contraindicated in those who have a kidney disorder because of the possibility of irritant poisoning (Brinker, 1998).

One case of acute respiratory distress in a 15-month-old boy has been reported as the result of his ingestion and inhalation of ground black mustard seed purchased in El Salvador (Gulbransen & Esernio-Jenssen, 1998). Another case of a 34-year-old woman was reported in 1990. The woman had used a mustard compress for ten minutes when she felt a burning sensation. She left the compress on for another ten minutes and then removed the compress to find that her skin was erythematous. She then applied an "anti-inflammatory lotion" and the skin healed, but five days later, after eating a German sausage with mustard, she developed a severe exacerbation of the skin condition. Allergy tests were normal one month later, and after four months, she was able to eat mustard again without event (Kohl & Frosch, 1990). This demonstrates the importance of observing conservative guidelines in the topical application of mustard. Twenty minutes was too long, especially for the first application and because the person was feeling burning and did not heed her body's warning.

One case of chronic hyperpigmentation related to a heated mustard compress burn was reported (Linder et al., 1996). This type of side effect did not occur simply as a result of the potency of the mustard. It occurred as a result of a lack of knowledge on the part of the patient. The patient used a heating pad with the mustard compress. Heat potentiated the herb that was, energetically, already very "hot." Mustard is an example of a plant remedy that is "extreme" by energetic and thermal standards. Herbalists exercise caution when using "extreme" applications and either supervise the remedy closely or recommend a different application for patient self-care. Extreme plant remedies should be recommended and used with caution and common sense. Patients should not use heat in addition to a mustard compress, especially the heat of a heating pad that is difficult to regulate. There is an art and a science to the use of the mustard plaster that must be learned before use.

While mustard greens are one of the best food sources of tyrosine, a compound that can contribute to the production of the hormone thyroxine (Duke, 1997), constituents found in the mustard and cabbage families have been implicated in hypothyroidism with thyroid enlargement (goiter) (Leung & Foster, 1996).

The volatile oil of mustard is prepared by steam distillation of seeds. It contains a powerful irritant, allyl isothiocyanate, one of the most toxic essential oil constituents. It should not be inhaled or used in any way (Keville & Green, 1995).

The disciplines of medicine and pharmacy have worked together to develop a medicine known as nitrogen mustard that has been used in the treatment of cancers such as Hodgkin's disease, lymphosarcoma, and chronic lymphoid myeloid leukemia as well as rheumatoid arthritis and nephritis. Nitrogen mustard is not derived from the mustard plant. It is a synthetic product, the oldest chemotherapy drug in existence, and has been in use since World War I. It is a white powder that, when prepared for use, becomes a clear, colorless liquid that is given by intravenous route only.

Nitrogen mustard was derived from and is a less toxic form of the mustard gas originally used in World War I. Mustard gas is a poison that results in a painful and often slow death. Soldiers who are exposed to the chemical warfare agent, sulfur mustard, or mustard gas, potentially suffer from reduced numbers of white blood cells, especially lymphocytes; severe skin blistering; lung damage, if the gas is inhaled; and blindness. Mustard gas is not very soluble in water and therefore is difficult to wash off. It also doesn't disappear readily.

Mustard agent is very simple to manufacture and is often a "first choice" when a country decides to build up a capacity for chemical warfare. During the Iran–Iraq war of 1979 to 1988, many Iranians died as a result of mustard gas and many were severely injured. Although the mustard plant has not been directly involved in the development of mustard gas or nitrogen mustard and there is no link between the plant and these chemical products (personal communication Professor Andrew Ternay, December 13, 2000), there is a clear similarity between the caustic nature of the chemical products and the potential effects of overuse or misuse of the mustard plant applications. By example, the mustard plant teaches the power of the interaction between its chemical substances and the human body. When using the mustard plant, people must be acutely aware of the potential strength of the medicine and the potential for *creating* pain and discomfort rather than relieving it.

NURSING EVIDENCE:

Historical Nursing Use

Nurses have historically used mustard plasters for the relief of pain and/or congestion, particularly lung congestion. Mustard footbaths also have been used for relief from colds and headache.

Potential Nursing Applications

Nurses in some areas of the world continue to use mustard in external applications for pain and discomfort related to several health concerns. Nurses may want to consider learning the art and science of mustard applications and documenting the observations they make of the clinical results of their use. Nurses may want to consider performing more in-depth studies of the effects of the external application of mustard, using the significant visible interaction of mustard with the skin as a marker for therapeutic activity.

Integrative Insight

Pain is often a call to action. It gets a person's attention and potentially can have a powerful influence. Mustard is a complement to pain. It too is powerful and gets people's attention when they come in contact with it, especially if they try to ignore that contact and the plant starts to create a burning sensation. To use mustard therapeutically, one must be attentive and observant of its power. Its healing power is felt in its ability to stimulate and warm. The power of a compress or plaster may even have the ability to distract a patient from the initial sense of pain they were experiencing before the introduction of mustard. When the compress or plaster is removed, the distraction has caused a change, a lessening of the original pain response. Using mustard effectively entails being able to recognize just how much distraction the painful body needs. It also entails knowing the limits to the interaction between people and plant.

Biomedical and traditional evidence demonstrate that mustard must be used judiciously. It also must be used by people who are able to exercise their common sense. Biomedical evidence of how to use a mustard application, regardless of sample size, can never replace common sense responses to the observation of the body's reaction to the plant in the moment. To use mustard, the person using the plant must be in the moment, and if they cannot be because of the pain or discomfort they are feeling, then the message from mustard is that the application must be done by a friend, a spouse, or a nurse who can monitor, observe closely, and ensure that the experience with mustard is as therapeutic as it can be and has been during hundreds of years of use.

THERAPEUTIC APPLICATIONS:
Oral

Mustard can be ingested in small amounts in foods.

Topical

Mustard Seed Plaster. Mix two handfuls of ground mustard seed with enough water to make a thick cream. Heat it in a pan to no more than 140°F (60°C) because temperatures greater than 140°F deactivate a necessary enzyme (Kunovskii, 1982; Rister, 1999). After heating, remove it from the stove and allow it to cool until just warm. Spread it on a piece of paper towel or wax paper twice the size of the area to be treated. Fold the paper in half. Spread the mustard paste on one half of the paper. Fold the other half over on top of the paste to cover it. Place a very thin cotton towel over the area of the body to be treated. Place the mustard plaster on top of the towel and cover it all with a warm second towel. After about ten to twenty minutes, a sensation of heat should be noticed. At this time, the plaster should be removed. The skin beneath will normally appear reddened. The plaster *must not* be allowed to directly contact the skin because of the blistering that may occur. Mustard seed plasters should not be used on any part of the body that has compromised circulation or on varicose veins or areas of decreased sensation. If blisters should occur due to inaccurate application, gently rinse the area in warm water without applying friction to the skin.

In the 1980s, Russian health practitioners began recommending putting the mustard plaster in a plastic bag and applying it to the skin in the bag. According to one article, this method was started by Solovev and found to produce similar responses without the risks associated with putting mustard directly on the skin. Solovev also promoted the plastic bag technique because the static electricity of the plastic bag enables the plaster to stay in place on the body and not slip. This technique is used with tuberculosis patients and others who are very ill or have sensitive skin. After a ten- to twenty-minute application with the plaster, a counterirritant effect can be noticed for up to two days (Kunovskii, 1982).

Environmental

Mustard must not be inhaled.

Herbal Caveat—Therapeutic Applications

In traditional and conventional herbal medicine, amounts of herbs given to patients are based on individual needs. The amounts or "doses" recorded here are provided so that the health practitioner has a general idea of the amounts recommended for an adult patient. Dosing in herbalism not only refers to amount of plant used but also includes when, where, and how to take a plant medicine. These dosages should not be used as guidelines for indiscriminate intervention without proper assessment, critical thinking, and patient education on the part of the practitioner.

Note: Please see chapter 5 for detailed descriptions of how to prepare various applications.

PATIENT INTERACTION:

Mustard is a powerful and warming herb. When using mustard for medicinal purposes, as opposed to using it in culinary endeavors, extra care should be taken. A long history of external use has shown that mustard poultices, footbaths, and plasters can be helpful in relieving pain and discomfort associated with conditions such as rheumatism, back pain, headache, and lung congestion. It is highly recommended to learn how to use mustard from someone experienced in the use of the plant.

Herbal Caveat—Patient Interaction

Patients considering the use of an herb or formula of herbs in self-care benefit from education about the plant itself and the use of the plant in healing. This education can come through many sources, including local herbalists; plant specialists such as botanists; health practitioners such as nurses, nutritionists, naturopaths, and other physicians; and various written references including the scientific literature. Patients need to remember that their unique health care needs are not necessarily represented in any literature they may encounter. Therefore, it is recommended that a knowledgeable mentor be consulted before initiating self-care with any herb being used for the first time.

NURTURING THE NURSE-PLANT RELATIONSHIP:

Note: You may want to keep a journal of your experiences with the herb.

If you'd like to get to know this plant, it is best to be "introduced." Find an herbalist, Anthroposophical nurse, or older nurse experienced in the topical use of mustard, and experience the soothing heat of mustard when useds as a poultice or plaster on an aching joint. Senior nurses who were taught to use mustard as part of their practice often have fascinating stories to tell about nursing care during their active days of practice. As you relax while the mustard performs its action, ask if there are any mustard plaster stories they might like to tell. Record your experience.

CHAPTER 8

Hormone Balance

INTRODUCTION

THIS CHAPTER DISCUSSES SIX HERBS—WILD YAM, fenugreek, soy, black cohosh, angelica, and kelp—and their influence on hormone balance in the body. Hormones, although not completely understood from a biomedical perspective, seem to enable connection and communication within the body, either through the connection of one organ to another or through communication and connection between body systems. The concept of *balancing* hormones in the body has to do with "bringing into harmony or proportion" (Merriam-Webster, 1999) and the process of finding a centered place of strength and health where hormonal activity occurs smoothly and effortlessly. Think of the trays of a scale as representing hormone balance. The trays hang on either side of a central point. As things are added to one of the scale's trays a shift occurs, and the other tray is affected by the activity on the first tray. For centering to occur and the scale to be balanced, something has to happen to the other tray or perhaps to both trays.

What occurs in terms of hormone balance in the human body is similar to the trays of a scale. The human body is subject to numerous stimuli throughout any given day. It must adapt, center, and rebalance often. Because they are involved in connection and communication within the body, hormones also are subject to daily changes and the call for constant

179

adaptation. Consider changes in blood sugar levels, for example. When people are well they may never notice the "balancing act" that their body goes through when they eat. But the diabetic patient knows very well how delicate the balance of sugar and insulin can be.

Biomedicine has had many successes in helping patients with hormonal imbalances such as diabetes. Nurses work with the diabetic patient in learning such things as foot care, monitoring exercise tolerance, and giving themselves insulin injections to replace their missing hormone. The hormone replacement concept is familiar to nurses. It is one of the biomedical solutions offered people with hormone imbalances.

Hormone replacement alone, however, does not necessarily create hormone balance. Hormone balance is unique to each patient. Nurses are familiar with having to titrate insulin doses in diabetic patients because not every diabetic patient is alike. Nor is every patient's need for hormone balance the same at all times. Internal and external influences can change the insulin needs of a patient. Nurses who work with the diabetic patient who takes a unit too much or too little insulin observe that the patient's physical, mental, and emotional well-being are affected. Because nurses have witnessed this, they are extremely precise in administering insulin to the patient. When dealing with the little insulin syringes and the almost minute doses of insulin, nurses glimpse the delicate nature of hormonal balance and the power of these tiny substances called hormones. With all the hormones scientists have identified in the body and all the processes regulated by them, reflecting on the complexity of the body and its inner workings can be both fascinating and mind-boggling. The concern in hormone-related disorders goes far beyond the question of how much hormone to replace. The challenge is supporting and maintaining the balance of hormones in the body.

Many women and their practitioners are now questioning the practice of hormone replacement therapy during menopause and perimenopause. Replacing estrogen and progesterone and finding the balance of what, when, and how much to give the woman continues to be a tremendous challenge. The practice of estrogen and progesterone replacement therapy has not been the same as insulin replacement therapy. Finding the proper balance for the individual is not usually addressed. Women often receive the same, not unique, doses of the hormone.

There is also concern that what may correct the woman's current hormonal imbalance may affect the total balance of the body in a different, perhaps less desirable way, in the future. For example, long-term biomedical studies have shown an increased risk of breast cancer in those women who use hormone replacement therapy, even when progestins are added to estrogen therapy, compared with those who do not use hormone therapy at all (Colditz et al., 1995).

For centuries, traditional herbal therapies have been used to help bring greater balance to the body, mind, and spirit; however, the concept of using herbs to affect *hormone* balance is much newer. Herbs such as black cohosh have been used traditionally for women's complaints but only more recently are being investigated and used in the biomedical treatment of hormone replacement. Herbs do not contain human hormones, however. They also are very different from single-substance pharmaceuticals such as insulin or estrogen. Herbal remedies contain numerous substances that may or may not have hormonal activity in the strictest scientific meaning of the word. However, herbs do affect hormone balance and conditions such as menopause that biomedical practitioners associate with hormone balance.

Nurses must understand that the way herbs affect hormone balance is different from the hormone replacement model with which they are familiar. The actions of herbs are better compared with the body's stress response. For example, women under extreme stress often stop menstruating, a bodily process related to hormonal activity. Although stress and plant remedies are not human hormones, they both have the potential to affect hormone balance. The ability of plants to affect human hormone balance is being studied. Much of the research is devoted to answering the question of whether or not the plant has hormonal activity, that is, plant hormonal activity that affects human hormone activity such as through occupying hormone receptor sites. Some of this preliminary science is included in these profiles.

Herbs do not contain human hormones—they contain plant hormones or "phytosterols," sometimes referred to in the literature as "phytoestrogens." Phytosterols are substances in the plant that are necessary for the growth and sexual development of the plant itself. Unlike the hormones used in hormone replacement therapy, phytosterols do not have just one action in the human body. They often have potential for more than one effect and perhaps even opposite effects. Science has found through in vitro studies that phytosterols such as lignans and isoflavones can have both estrogen-like and antiestrogen effects (Beckham, 1995). Interaction with estrogen receptors is one way scientists define phytosterol activity. Studies show that phytosterols can compete with estrogen receptor cells (Martin, Horwitz, Ryan, & McGuire, 1978).

The action of phytosterols is thought to be determined by the unique needs of the individual patient. When endogenous estrogens are low, phytosterols can add to the estrogen bank. When there is no need for estrogen, "weaker phytoestrogens can compete with more potent endogenous oestrogens, thereby reducing the overall oestrogen load" (Beckham, 1995, p. 14). Thus the hormonal balancing action occurs. The body, with its innate intelligence and wisdom, communicates its need hormonally and is somehow able to select those plant substances that it needs for greater balance and block those substances it does not need.

There is much to be learned from the hormone-balancing, adaptogen action of herbs. A new paradigm of study may be needed to further understand substances such as phytosterols that seem to have the potential to perform multiple and divergent roles to bring a greater balance determined by the need of the whole.

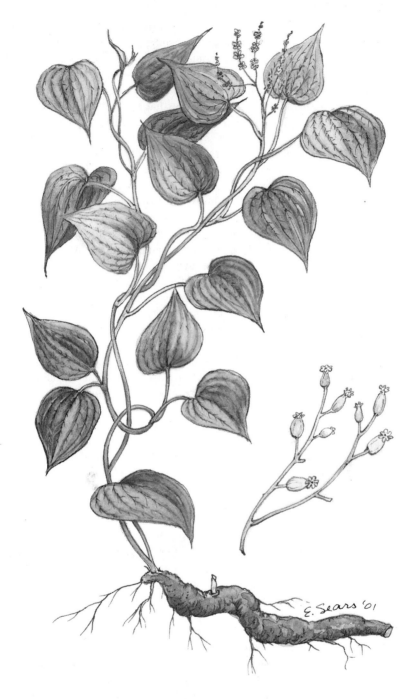

Dioscorea villosa

Wild Yam

🍃 **LATIN NAMES:** *Dioscorea villosa, Dioscorea barbasco, Dioscorea floribunda, Dioscorea opposita*
Note: There are over 850 species of *Dioscorea* (Foster & Tyler, 1999), and few can distinguish them all (Duke, 1985). Species names are included throughout the profile for clarification.

🍃 **FAMILY NAME:** Dioscoreaceae

🍃 **COMMON NAMES:** Wild yam, true wild yam, colic root, rheumatism root

🍃 **HEALTH PATTERN:** Hormone balance

🍃 **PLANT DESCRIPTION:**
Wild yam is a slender vine that grows in warm, temperate, and tropical climates where the vines can climb to impressive heights, sometimes as much as 20 feet (over 6 meters). The smooth green stem twines over fences and bushes. The leaves are heart-shaped with smooth edges and prominent veins. The underside of the leaves is downy. The greenish-yellow flowers are very small and appear in June and July. The plant bears separate male and female flowers. The female flowers are succeeded by a dry, brown fruit that remains hanging on the vine throughout the winter. The rhizome, the root found just below the surface of the soil, is from ¼ to ½ inch (6 to 12.5 mm) in diameter and may be as long as 2 feet (about 1.5 meters). The outside is brown and scaly with a lighter interior. It is one of the hardest of rhizomes and is difficult to powder or crush. It tends to be odorless and has a slightly acrid taste (Felter & Lloyd, 1983).

🍃 **PLANT PART USED:** Rhizome

🍃 **TRADITIONAL EVIDENCE:**
Cultural Use
Asian. "Shan yao" or *D. opposita*, one species of wild yam, is used in traditional Chinese medicine (TCM), for tonifying the energy systems of the spleen and stomach. It is used in cases of diarrhea, fatigue, spontaneous sweating, lack of appetite, and to tonify the energy system of the lung in cases of chronic cough and wheezing. TCM practitioners use wild yam to tonify the kidney energy system when symptoms of excessive undesired weight loss and thirst are present. In these instances it also is used for frequent urination and vaginal discharge. Wild yam is contraindicated in conditions of "excess" (a specific TCM symptom pattern) accompanied by symptoms of dampness, stagnation of qi and/or blood, or accumulation, because the tonifying (building up) quality of the herb would then increase the "excess"

dampness and stagnation already present in the body (Bensky & Gamble, 1993).

Traditional Japanese medicine uses wild yam as a laxative and digestive tonic. It is used to treat symptoms such as coughing, diabetes, frequent urination, involuntary flow of semen, night sweats, and general weakness (Rister, 1999).

North American Indian. Some North American Indian women have used the root of wild yam *(D. villosa)* to ease the pain of childbirth (Moerman, 1998).

Pacific Islander. Several species of wild yam have been used as a food in the Hawaiian Islands. The bitter fruit of *D. bulbifera,* called "air yam," is cooked, grated, and washed several times, then strained and eaten. Other species of *Dioscorea* yield tubers that are baked and eaten or made into a drink for the sick. Native Hawaiians may scrape the bulbs and mix the shavings with water to be given for fevers and excessive sweating (Moerman, 1998).

Australian. The wild yam that is found growing in Australia has been prepared as a decoction to be applied topically for the treatment of skin cancer (Lassak & McCarthy, 1983).

East Indian. Many varieties of wild yam are found in India. The plant has been used as food and medicine since ancient times. Some varieties have a small, potato-like tuber that is powdered and used as a topical application to skin sores. The tubers are used to make plasters to reduce swelling and for scorpion stings and snakebites. The powder is also mixed with cumin, milk, and sugar and given internally as a remedy for syphilis, hemorrhoids, and dysentery. The powder also may be mixed with butter and given rectally to relieve diarrhea (Nadkarni, 1976).

A wild yam *(D. triphylla)* found in Burma causes inflammation of the mouth and throat, vomiting of blood, drowsiness, exhaustion, and a sense of suffocation. A piece of this tuber the size of an apple has been known to cause death if eaten. However, the Burmese are said to know how to prepare the tuber so that it can be eaten safely (Nadkarni, 1976).

Culinary Use

There are over 150 varieties of wild yam and many of these are edible (Grieve, 1971). The sweet potato *(Ipomoea batatas L.)* known as yam (i.e., candied yams), eaten in countries such as the United States, are not the same plants as the yams (*Dioscorea* spp.) being discussed in this profile. Powdered wild yam rhizome is used as a thickening agent in foods (Rister, 1999). Some species of *Dioscorea* are used as coffee substitutes (Duke, 1985).

Use in Herbalism

In the late 1800s, wild yam was primarily used as an antispasmodic for biliary colic. It was given as a decoction, $\frac{1}{2}$ pint every thirty to sixty minutes. It was found to give prompt and permanent relief, even in cases of severe pain. Wild yam also was used successfully in other cases of colic, abdominal pain, and gastrointestinal irritation. It was given with gelsemium *(Gelsemium sempervirens)* to treat pain associated with the passage of gallstones. Wild yam also was given for spasmodic hiccoughs, nervous conditions with spasms, obstinate vomiting, and spasmodic asthma. It was used for nausea, bowel spasms, menstrual cramps, and combined with swamp dogwood *(Cornus sericea)* for the nausea and vomiting of pregnancy. Wild yam's effectiveness was attributed to its action upon irritable tissues that become painful because of underlying muscle fiber spasms. Wild yam also is used for indigestion with hepatic involvement, gastritis associated with alcoholism, and easing uterine pains after childbirth. The tincture of wild yam has been used as an expectorant and diaphoretic and in large doses to produce emesis (Felter & Lloyd, 1983).

In current times, wild yam rhizome has been found to contain steroid glycosides such as diosgenin, plant-steroid compounds that can be processed into pharmaceutical steroids. Diosgenin was first converted to progesterone in the early 1900s and continues to be used directly or indirectly for the production of steroid drugs such as oral contraceptives. Wild yam is an inexpensive source of building blocks for cortisones, androgens, estrogens, progestogens, and topical hormones (Duke, 1985; Foster & Tyler, 1999). These drugs are used to treat menopause, dysmenorrhea, premenstrual tension, testicular deficiency, Addison's disease, allergies, dermatitis, psoriasis, impotency, prostatic hypertrophy, and many others (Duke, 1985). In addition to providing the blueprint for the development of these drugs, wild yam also serves as a source of diosgenin for "natural" hormone pharmaceutical products such as natural progesterone creams. Natural progesterone can be made from animals or plants.

Some bio-identical or natural progesterone products on the market contain only wild yam. Some contain wild yam and progesterone that has been converted in a laboratory from the diosgenin extracted from the wild yam rhizome. This converted progesterone resembles human progesterone and is the most effective product. The herb, in any form other than the laboratory converted product, is poorly absorbed by the body. At this point, scientists believe that humans lack the enzyme necessary to convert diosgenin to human progesterone. Many practitioners I have worked with prescribe the cream for women with perimenopausal and menopausal symptoms. The cream is applied to the chest, inner thighs, or inner arms usually twice a day and may be absorbed at different rates, depending on the woman. While the cream can be very effective in relieving menopausal symptoms, exact dosage of progesterone received by the patient is not as easily calculated as with oral pharmaceutical preparations of synthetic progesterone (progestins) and/or estrogen.

Women have used wild yam rhizome, believing that it prevents fertility and, thereby, conception. It is thought that the steroidal effects may cause sterility when used in appropriate dosages. The inner part of the root is made into a salve and applied topically for vaginal dryness related to menopause (Weed, 1986). In North and Central America, wild yam is used as a relaxing treatment for menstrual cramps and ovarian pain. It also is used in the treatment of asthma, coughing, and to help expectorate phlegm. Wild yam also is used in formulation with other antispasmodic and anti-inflammatory herbs, such as peppermint, to relieve the symptoms associated with diverticulitis.

BIOMEDICAL EVIDENCE:

No published studies were found that support the traditional uses of whole plant infusions and extracts of wild yam; however, some research has been devoted to the wild yam plant constituent, diosgenin, from which steroid medications have been developed. Diosgenin can be converted into steroid hormones by chemists, but the same chemical synthesis does not occur when diosgenin is taken internally or applied externally to the human body. Because of the focus on wild yam as a plant that directly and indirectly affects hormone balance, the studies on diosgenin, in particular the studies on progesterone creams, have been included here. Although clinical reports from physicians such as John Lee (1990a; 1990b; 1991) have shown that wild yam cream as a part of a health care regimen that includes dietary changes, exercise, and vitamin supplements can benefit women with osteoporosis, no published clinical trials with conclusive biomedical evidence were found.

Studies Related to Hormone Balance

According to one small study with 6 women of the use of transdermal estrogen plus Pro-gest cream, a progesterone cream derived from wild yam, 30 mg per day for two weeks and then 60 mg per day for two weeks, there was a significant absorption of progesterone from the cream. The investigators report that the optimum dose required to protect a woman against endometrial cancer has still not been defined (Burry, Patton, & Hermsmeyer, 1999).

In 1998, Cooper et al. reported that the absorption of progesterone from Pro-gest cream was not therapeutic in their study of 20 women using Pro-gest cream. This conclusion was based on testing urinary pregnanediol-3α-glucuronide and plasma progesterone levels. The manufacturer of Pro-gest cream disputed the results of the Cooper study writing, "Since the measurement of progesterone in Pro-gest cream was inaccurate and unsupported by regular laboratory testing in the UK as well as the USA, the results of all the tests reported by Cooper and co-workers are questionable" (MacFarland, 1998, p. 905). Lee (1998) writes that saliva values are far more accurate than plasma or serum concentrations for measurement of the true bioavailable fraction of progesterone when it is delivered transdermally, ". . . progesterone is lipophilic and non-polar and therefore enters the bloodstream by seeking out a similar or non-polar environment such as the fatty membrane of the red blood cells, and not by absorption into plasma" (p. 905). Some practitioners also question the use of progesterone alone, as opposed to progestogens, because of the lack of evidence of the beneficial effect to the human skeleton (Stevenson & Purdie, 1998).

A German study showed that progesterone ointment is better absorbed when applied to the breast than when applied to the abdomen or thigh (Krause et al. as reported in Burry et al., 1999).

A methanol extract of the root of wild yam *(D. dumetorum)* significantly lowered blood sugar in diabetic and normoglycemic rabbits when administered intraperitoneally (Iwu et al., 1990).

Studies Related to Other Health Patterns
No data are available at this time.

Mechanism of Action
Diosgenin, a glycoside derived from wild yam, can be converted into steroid hormones by chemists in the laboratory, but the same chemical synthesis does not occur in the human body (Foster & Tyler, 1999). Diosgenin does have medicinal properties. It is a phytosterol or plant hormone and may produce hormonal effects in humans in addition to reducing inflammation, fatigue, and stress (Dentali, 1994). It is believed that ingesting wild yam rhizome may provide the building blocks for various hormones. The richest source of steroidal precursors is found in *D. floribunda* and *D. composita*, both native to Mexico (Foster & Tyler, 1999); however, diosgenin is poorly absorbed when taken orally or topically by animals and humans and one study using saliva testing demonstrated that diosgenin is not converted to progesterone in the human body (Zava, Dollbaum, & Blen, 1998).

USE IN PREGNANCY OR LACTATION:
Midwives have safely used wild yam rhizome *(D. villosa)* infusion to treat the nausea of pregnancy. The woman takes sips of the infusion throughout the day or teaspoons of the decoction several times daily. A dropper full of the tincture in a glass of water also has been effective (Weed, 1986).

Midwives use an infusion of wild yam rhizome *(D. villosa)* to prevent threatened miscarriage. Two to four ounces (60 to 120 ml) of the infusion are given orally every thirty minutes. Results should be apparent by the second dose. The tincture has proved to be less effective than the infusion, and large doses of the tincture may provoke nausea and vomiting. In addition, wild yam is said to be antispasmodic to uterine muscles (Weed, 1986).

Herbal Caveat—Pregnancy or Lactation

Some herbs are contraindicated in pregnancy because of a risk of the herb or one of its constituents stimulating the uterus and therefore possibly promoting fetal loss. Many herbal practitioners do not recommend herbal remedies, in particular oral doses of herbs, during the first trimester of pregnancy and seek an alternative. However, herbs are successfully used during pregnancy, especially to prepare the body for the birth. Herbs are relatively unstudied in pregnancy and lactation, so patients need to be made aware through education of the potential benefits and risks of using herbs for health conditions that arise during pregnancy or lactation. The use of herbal remedies during pregnancy often warrants a referral to a knowledgeable herbal practitioner.

USE FOR CHILDREN:

There are no specific usages or contraindications for wild yam in children. Some species of wild yam are edible and therefore might be considered safe for medicinal use in some cultures for such things as the discomfort associated with intestinal colic.

Herbal Caveat—Children

Children have special needs in regard to herbal therapies. They require lesser amounts of herbs and often respond well to mild teas and topical applications such as compresses and baths. The lowest dose of oral preparations should be tried first before increasing the amount given children. Caregivers should observe children closely for responses to herbal remedies. Younger children, particularly infants, have traditionally been given herbs either through their mother's breast milk or in the form of a homeopathic remedy because of their sensitivity to medicines and treatments and the immaturity of their liver. It is recommended that a person knowledgeable in the herbal treatment of children be consulted before the offering of any herb to a child for the first time.

CAUTIONS:

Large doses of the tincture of wild yam *(D. villosa* not *D. opposita)* cause vomiting (McGuffin, Hobbs, Upton, & Goldberg, 1997). Let the buyer beware! The buyer must understand that wild yam in cream or any other form is not assimilated by the human body and converted into human progesterone. Nor does the body directly create dehydroepiandrosterone (DHEA) from wild yam. Some manufacturers of natural wild yam creams and their consultant scientists continue to miseducate the public regarding the health benefits of the products they sell. One example of specious advertising is discussed in an editorial in the newsletter of the American Herb Association, which corrects the misleading marketing information provided by one company, stating that wild yam extracts provide the body with what it needs to produce its own DHEA. The marketing information also incorrectly stated that Mexican wild yam *(D. villosa)* was first mentioned by the Chinese in 25 B.C. (Moore as reported in Keville, 1996).

How could the Chinese have known about a Mexican plant in 25 B.C. that does not even grow in China?

Although transdermal creams have benefits such as allowing the use of lower dosages over a period of time, overdose may still be a risk. The pharmacokinetics of transdermal steroid delivery are not well known and there have been two reports of abnormally elevated hormone levels in women taking progesterone cream (not reported as wild yam derived) who experienced gradual water retention and weight gain, breast engorgement, and mild depression (Ilyia, McClure, & Farhat, 1998).

NURSING EVIDENCE:

Historical Nursing Use

No data are available at this time.

Potential Nursing Applications

Nurses observe the benefits of wild yam each time a steroid medication is given. How a steroid medication affects the overall hormone balance of the body is not necessarily known. Greater understanding of the body's delicate hormonal balance and the interaction of hormones are needed. It is known that wild yam does contain phytosterols and diosgenin, a substance that can, with the help of science, affect hormonal balance, especially in women. Nurses might consider following and/or participating in the ongoing research in the development of natural hormone therapies. In the search for greater hormonal balance, it may be found that seeking to replace the body's lack of hormones with synthetic or natural hormones is just a Band-Aid approach. Medicinal benefits of whole plants, including wild yam, hold potential for the understanding of achieving a greater balance of body, mind, and spirit (including hormonal balance) that may not be gleaned from the dissection of the single constituent. Nurses may want to become familiar with wild yam and consider researching the traditional uses of wild yam for easing the pain associated with childbirth and decreasing the threat of miscarriage during pregnancy.

Integrative Insight

The question about how women can achieve hormone balance has not been fully answered. Many physicians now recommend that women themselves make the decision as to whether or not they will begin hormone replacement therapy to prevent osteoporosis or relieve discomfort related to menopause. Many women prefer to take a hormone product that is similar to their own body's hormones. Natural progesterone creams containing whole plant wild yam are not effective for balancing hormones. Progesterone that has been converted from diosgenin in a laboratory is more efficacious.

In her book *Women's Encyclopedia of Natural Medicine,* Tori Hudson (1999), a naturopathic physician, recommends the dosage schedule for natural progesterone cream listed under Therapeutic Applications. The following company is a resource for natural progesterone cream:

Women's International Pharmacy
5708 Monona Drive
Madison, WI 53719-3152
800-279-5708
608-221-7800
Fax 608-221-7819
www.wipws.com

Biomedicine has constructed the concept of hormone "replacement" as one option for women with menopausal discomfort. The Nurse's Health Study (Grodstein et al., 1997) revealed that mortality was initially lower in women who used hormone replacement therapy, but the risk of breast cancer in those taking the hormones for more than ten years was increased. This kind of long-term data concerns patients and practitioners alike. Perhaps it is time to consider changing the treatment approach. Perhaps the answer to whether or not herbal products can help balance hormones eludes women because the question needs revision. The question is not whether a natural hormone replacement may be safer for long-term use than a synthetic hormone replacement. The use of the replacement option or model, whether applied to synthetic or natural hormone products, may be what needs to be questioned. Perhaps the answer lies in adaptation, helping the body adapt to new hormone levels. The body is highly adaptive, so nurses might ask why there are so many concerns regarding hormonal discomfort in industrialized countries. Discomfort associated with menopause in some cultures, such as the traditional Navajo, is virtually unknown (Northrup, 1994).

Although herbal substitutions may be a "next step" in moving away from the risks associated with long-term synthetic hormone replacement therapy, it is certainly not the final word. Hormone balance in the human body is an area that needs further research. The pattern of symptoms related to hormone balance must be studied. Perhaps epidemiologic studies might demonstrate whether or not women living in areas of the world where wild yam is eaten as food or medicine have fewer symptoms identified as being related to hormone balance in biomedicine.

THERAPEUTIC APPLICATIONS:

Oral

Liquid Extract. About ½ teaspoon (2 to 4 ml) (Wren, 1988)

Topical

Natural Progesterone Cream. Postmenopausal women should use ¼ teaspoon cream one to two times per day on days 8 to 30 or 31 of the menstrual cycle and no cream on days 1 to 7. Perimenopausal women should not use the cream during menstruation. Use $\frac{1}{4}$ tea-spoon two times a day on days 8 to 21 and $\frac{1}{4}$ to $\frac{1}{2}$ teaspoon two times a day on days 22 to 28. The dosage range of natural progesterone creams derived from diosgenin is less than 2 mg per ounce (28 g) and up to 400 mg per ounce (28 g) (Hudson, 1999).

Environmental
No data are available at this time.

Herbal Caveat—Therapeutic Applications

In traditional and conventional herbal medicine, amounts of herbs given to patients are based on individual needs. The amounts or "doses" recorded here are provided so that the health practitioner has a general idea of the amounts recommended for an adult patient. Dosing in herbalism not only refers to amount of plant used but also includes when, where, and how to take a plant medicine. These dosages should not be used as guidelines for indiscriminate intervention without proper assessment, critical thinking, and patient education on the part of the practitioner.

Note: Please see chapter 5 for detailed descriptions of how to prepare various applications.

PATIENT INTERACTION:
Wild yam has been used in the pharmaceutical industry for several years in the production of steroid medications. Risks and benefits are associated with most, if not all, medications, and the decision to use natural progesterone cream derived from wild yam must be an informed one. The products made from wild yam rhizome cannot be converted by the human body into progesterone and therefore are considered ineffective for the biomedical treatment known as "hormone replacement." Natural progesterone creams containing progesterone derived from diosgenin, a plant constituent in wild yam, are assimilated by the human body, but the dosages can potentially vary from product to product. If using progesterone cream for hormone replacement, a biomedical treatment, it is best to be under the care of a knowledgeable biomedical health practitioner. The scientific community continues to examine the results of using wild yam–based progesterone creams for the prevention of osteoporosis as a substitute for hormone replacement therapy.

Herbal Caveat—Patient Interaction

Patients considering the use of an herb or formula of herbs in self-care benefit from education about the plant itself and the use of the plant in healing. This education can come through many sources, including local herbalists; plant specialists such as botanists; health practitioners such as nurses, nutritionists, naturopaths, and other physicians; and various written references including the scientific literature. Patients need to remember that their unique health care needs are not necessarily represented in any literature they may encounter. Therefore, it is recommended that a knowledgeable mentor be consulted before initiating self-care with any herb being used for the first time.

Note: You may want to keep a journal of your experiences with the herb.

For this experience, *D. opposita*, the species used to tonify "qi" in TCM, is used to make a decoction. Find a reputable Chinese herb pharmacy near your home or contact one of the herb stores listed below and purchase a small amount of "shan yao." The root is white and looks like a few other herbs, so be sure to read the label in Latin and Chinese. Put approximately ⅓ ounce (9 g) of whole root into a small saucepan and rinse the herb thoroughly with cool water. Cover the herb with water and bring it almost to a boil. Take the pot off the stove, cover the pan with a lid, and let it sit for four hours. After presoaking, the roots will have expanded. Add enough water to cover the herb with water by at least 1 inch (2.5 cm). Put the pot back on the stove and gently simmer the herb (steam rising from the water but not boiling) for about two hours. The decoction from the herb can be drunk and a small amount of the herb can be tasted. This decoction can be quite viscous and often is prepared and drunk separately from the rest of an herbal formula.

Prepare for your herb tasting the way students of Chinese herbal medicine do by centering and meditating before the tasting. During the tasting, sit quietly and observe your body's response to the herb. Where do you feel the effects of the herb in your body? Is the herb energetically cold, hot, or somewhere in between? How does the herb taste—sweet, sour, pungent, salty, astringent, or a combination? How do you feel after the tasting?

You may contact the following company to order this herb:
Nuherbs
3820 Penniman Avenue
Oakland, CA 94619
800-233-4307
Fax: 800-550-1928
www.nuherbs.com

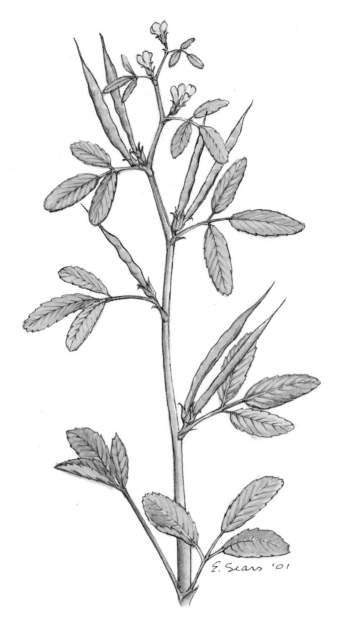

Trigonella foenum-graecum

Fenugreek

🌿 **LATIN NAME:** *Trigonella foenum-graecum*

🌿 **FAMILY NAME:** Fabaceae

🌿 **COMMON NAMES:** Fenugreek, fenugreek seed, Greek hay, trigonella, bird's foot, Greek clover

🌿 **HEALTH PATTERN:** Hormone balance

🌿 **PLANT DESCRIPTION:**

Fenugreek is an annual plant that is native to the Mediterranean area, India, China, and the Ukraine. It is cultivated in these areas for commercial use. The plant grows either erect or horizontally and produces pale yellow flowers that bloom in the summer. The seeds take four months to mature and have a distinctive, somewhat caramel-like scent. Some liken the scent to celery. I find that both descriptions are correct. The pale brownish-yellow seeds are small and approximately $\frac{1}{8}$ inch (approximately 4 mm) long and $\frac{1}{8}$ inch (approximately 4 mm) wide and $\frac{1}{12}$ inch (approximately 2 mm) thick and very hard (Felter & Lloyd, 1983).

🌿 **PLANT PARTS USED:** Ripe, dried seed, seed pods, and leaves

🌿 **TRADITIONAL EVIDENCE:**

Cultural Use

Asian. Fenugreek was introduced into Chinese medicine in the eleventh century where it continues to be used for pain and coldness in the lower abdomen, hernias, and weakness and edema of the legs. In TCM, fenugreek seed, "hu lu ba," is used to tonify yang, warm the kidney energy system, disperse dampness, and alleviate cold damp pain of the lower body. These conditions are recognized by abdominal or flank distention, pain, or hernia. It is contraindicated in persons with a condition known in TCM as yin deficiency with heat. Fenugreek seeds have been used to increase milk production in lactating mothers. It also has been used in the treatment and prevention of mountain sickness (Bensky & Gamble, 1993).

Pacific Islander. Fenugreek seeds reportedly have been used in Java in hair tonics to cure baldness (Leung & Foster, 1996).

African. The use of fenugreek dates back to ancient Egypt where it was used in the embalming process (Buckle, 1997) and as a medicine to induce labor and childbirth (Blumenthal, Goldberg, & Brinckman, 2000). The Egyptians also used fenugreek by soaking the seeds in water until they swelled into a thick paste known as "helba" that currently is said to be as effective as quinine in reducing fevers, is comforting to the stomach, and is helpful for diabetics (Grieve, 1971).

The seeds are used as an oral antidiabetic agent and to increase milk production in lactating mothers. They also are used in the treatment of rheumatism, cough, and as a general tonic. The leaves are used for the relief of indigestion and other stomach disorders (Iwu, 1993).

East Indian. Fenugreek "medhika" is found growing wild in India where the seeds, pods, and leaves are used as food and traditional medicine. The young plants and aromatic leaves are eaten as a vegetable (called "alu methi"). The seeds are used as a condiment and an ingredient of curry powders. The leaves may be boiled and then fried in butter and given for digestive complaints. The green plants are used as food for cattle and horses (Nadkarni, 1976).

Fenugreek seeds are widely used by the people of India for colic, intestinal gas, dysentery, diarrhea, loss of appetite, cough, edema in the lower extremities, and enlargement of the liver and spleen. The seeds may be used to make a cooling drink or a coffee substitute. Fenugreek is used as a substitute for cod liver oil for conditions such as rickets, anemia, recovering after infectious diseases, gout, and diabetes. Topical applications are used for hair loss, skin inflammations, swellings, burns, and as a cosmetic (Nadkarni, 1976). For diarrhea and dysentery, the seeds are fried in ghee (clarified butter) and mixed with anise seed and salt and made into a paste that is eaten. Fenugreek seed gruel is given to nursing mothers to increase lactation. Fenugreek leaf is used as a poultice for burns and swelling.

Arabic. Fenugreek is known in Iraq as "helba." It is used to relieve intestinal and menstrual pain and to increase milk secretion during lactation (Abdo & Al-Kafawi, 1969).

European. Fenugreek seed is used in Germany to prepare a water-based poultice that is used topically to reduce inflammation. It also is used as an internal preparation that has cholagogic actions and as a remedy for gastrointestinal complaints (Blumenthal et al., 2000) and poor appetite (Leung & Foster, 1996).

Culinary Use

Fenugreek seeds are used as a flavoring ingredient in the manufacture of imitation maple syrup. The seeds also can be soaked in water and allowed to sprout. When the sprouts are approximately 2 or 3 inches (5 to 7.5 cm) long, they can be eaten raw with the seeds (Grieve, 1971). The powdered seeds are used as an ingredient in curry powder and other spice blends. An extract from the seeds is used to flavor many food items, including alcoholic and nonalcoholic beverages, frozen dairy desserts, candies, baked goods, meats, gelatins, and many others (Leung & Foster, 1996).

Fenugreek seeds are very nutritious and rich in vitamin A, choline, iron, thiamine, phosphorus, fats, and protein. Fenugreek has been compared to cod liver oil because of its choline and vitamin A content. The protein in fenugreek is rich in lysine and tryptophan and low in sulphur-containing amino acids (Pedersen, 1998).

Use in Herbalism

In the nineteenth century in the United States, fenugreek was one of the main ingredients in Lydia Pinkham's famous "Vegetable Compound" for menstrual pain and postmenopausal vaginal dryness (Blumenthal et al., 2000). In the late 1800s, fenugreek seeds were powdered and made into a poultice, plaster, or decoction and applied topically to inflammations. The decoction has been used as a wash for inflamed rectal or vaginal tissues, and as a gargle for sore throats. It also is used to relieve irritation of the bronchial tubes. An oil prepared with fenugreek seed is used topically for burns. The tincture improves digestion, relieves uterine irritation, and is an emmenagogue (Felter & Lloyd, 1983).

Fenugreek seeds are used in herbalism for the treatment of mouth ulcers, chronic cough, fevers, swollen glands, and digestive problems. A decoction of fenugreek seeds is used internally for inflamed conditions of the stomach and intestines. Externally it is used as a poultice for boils and abscesses (Grieve, 1971), leg ulcers, gout, and wounds (Newall, Anderson, & Phillipson, 1996).

Cosmetic Use. Fenugreek extracts are used to scent perfumes, soaps, detergents, creams, and lotions (Leung & Foster, 1996).

BIOMEDICAL EVIDENCE:

Studies of the hormone-related effects of fenugreek presented here include its ability to lower blood sugar. No studies were found supporting the traditional use of fenugreek to increase milk production in lactating women.

Studies Related to Hormone Balance

In a study of 10 insulin-dependent diabetic patients, fenugreek seed (50 g given twice a day prepared in chapattis, a type of unleavened bread) reduced twenty-four-hour urinary glucose excretion by 54%, significantly reduced fasting blood sugar, improved glucose tolerance, and significantly improved serum lipid profiles (Sharma, Raghuram, & Rao, 1990).

Twenty-one patients with noninsulin-dependent diabetes who received 15 g of fenugreek seed with each meal had lower postprandial blood sugar levels but no change in insulin levels (Madar, Abel, Samish, & Arad, 1988).

Fenugreek seed has been shown to potentiate the secretion of insulin in animal and human in vitro studies (Sauvaire et al., 1998).

Studies Related to Other Health Patterns

No data are available at this time.

Mechanism of Action

Fenugreek seeds contain diosgenin, the same steroidal glycoside found in wild yam. Diosgenin is a building block for hormones and related drugs. It cannot be converted by the human body into human hormones such as progesterone, but can be converted in a laboratory (Foster & Tyler, 1999). Fenugreek seed may be more advantageous to the pharmaceutical industry than wild yam because its seed production cycle is much shorter than the rhizome production cycle for wild yam.

Human and animal in vitro studies suggest that 4-hydroxyisoleucine, an amino acid found only in plants, in particular fenugreek seed, is a potentiator of insulin secretion through a direct action on pancreatic beta-cells (Sauvaire et al., 1998). Fenugreek lowers blood glucose levels by improving the body's sensitivity to insulin (Sharma et al., 1990) and may be able to lower blood sugar because of its high fiber content of 60% (Madar et al., 1988).

Fenugreek's ability to increase milk production in lactating women may be related to its ability to increase sweat production. The breasts are modified sweat glands, and therefore the fenugreek may act similarly on them (Jensen, 1992).

USE IN PREGNANCY OR LACTATION:

Fenugreek is not recommended for use during pregnancy (Blumenthal et al., 2000; Brinker, 1998; McGuffin et al., 1997). Water and alcohol extracts of fenugreek have been found to stimulate the uteruses of guinea pigs and have been considered as oxytocin replacements for use during labor (Abdo & Al-Kafawi, 1969).

Fenugreek has been used in many countries throughout the world in lactating women for increasing milk production. Although anecdotal reports indicate that fenugreek tea made from the seed is effective in increasing milk supply, practitioners in some countries such as the United States, recommend that the woman take up to 15 capsules per day of powdered fenugreek. Fenugreek is said not only to increase milk supply but also the flow of milk, which is very helpful for some babies (Jensen, 1992). Several mothers in my practice have used fenugreek seed successfully for increasing milk production and flow.

Herbal Caveat—Pregnangy or Lactation

Some herbs are contraindicated in pregnancy because of a risk of the herb or one of its constituents stimulating the uterus and therefore possibly promoting fetal loss. Many herbal practitioners do not recommend herbal remedies, in particular oral doses of herbs, during the first trimester of pregnancy and seek an alternative. However, herbs are successfully used during pregnancy, especially to prepare the body for the birth. Herbs are relatively unstudied in pregnancy and lactation, so patients need to be made aware through education of the potential benefits and risks of using herbs for health conditions that arise during pregnancy or lactation. The use of herbal remedies during pregnancy often warrants a referral to a knowledgeable herbal practitioner.

USE FOR CHILDREN:

Fenugreek tea is traditionally given to infants and children to reduce flatulence. However, it is given in small amounts. German physicians report having treated a 5-week-old Egyptian infant for a brief period of unconsciousness that occurred after drinking a bottle of fenugreek tea (preparation not described). The baby's urine smelled like "maggi" (a flavoring the smell of which is often associated with maple sugar disease) and his urine contained sotolone, a compound found in fenugreek tea and also found to be responsible for the smell in patients with maple syrup disease (Sewell, Mosandl, & Bohles, 1999).

Herbal Caveat—Children

Children have special needs in regard to herbal therapies. They require lesser amounts of herbs and often respond well to mild teas and topical applications such as compresses and baths. The lowest dose of oral preparations should be tried first before increasing the amount given children. Caregivers should observe children closely for responses to herbal remedies. Younger children, particularly infants, have traditionally been given herbs either through their mother's breast milk or in the form of a homeopathic remedy because of their sensitivity to medicines and treatments and the immaturity of their liver. It is recommended that a person knowledgeable in the herbal treatment of children be consulted before the offering of any herb to a child for the first time.

CAUTIONS:

Repeated topical applications can cause uncomfortable skin reactions (Blumenthal et al., 2000). Fenugreek seeds are rich in a compound called mucilage that may have the ability to bind to oral drugs in the gastrointestinal tract and prevent or delay their absorption, but this is speculative. It may be wise to avoid taking fenugreek at the same time as pharmaceutical drugs (Brinker, 1998; Madar et al., 1988). Because the mucilage absorbs fluids, it is always advisable to drink plenty of water to keep the fenugreek seed moving through the gastrointestinal tract.

Human clinical studies have demonstrated the blood sugar lowering activity of a component in fenugreek known as trigonelline. People who are taking insulin may need to have their dosages adjusted if also taking fenugreek (Brinker, 1998). Some diabetic research subjects, when taking fenugreek in their diets, experienced diarrhea and excess flatulence for three to four days, after which the symptoms subsided (Sharma et al., 1990).

There have been a few reports of the regular home use of fenugreek causing allergic reactions (Patil, Niphadkar, & Bapat, 1997).

NURSING EVIDENCE:

Historical Nursing Use

Some lactation consultants suggest fenugreek to lactating women to increase milk production and secretion.

Potential Nursing Applications

Nurses might want to consider the clinical use of fenugreek seed for hormone balance in diabetic patients and for increasing milk production and secretion in lactating women as necessary. As a tea, fenugreek may be helpful in the care of patients who are anorexic or recuperating from illness or have indigestion, fever, or extensive wounds or ulcers on the lower extremities. A tea also could be gargled and swished in the mouth in patients with ulcers of the mouth. Fenugreek seed poultices might be considered for the care of patients who have inflammation of the skin such as boils, swelling, and abscesses.

Integrative Insight

There is extensive traditional evidence of the successful use of fenugreek in the care of lactating women and diabetics and in the care of wounds and ulcers. Biomedical evidence is lacking. Many of the conditions fenugreek has been used for, nurses encounter quite often. Some nurses are already recommending fenugreek to help lactating women (especially first-time mothers who may be anxious about breastfeeding). Nurses may want to consider further the potential benefits of researching and developing the use of fenugreek in patient care and how the plant affects hormonal balance and other health patterns such as the skin.

Botanically, fenugreek seed contains mucilage, a substance that combined with water expands into a gel. Plant mucilage has traditionally been helpful for the relief of inflammation of the mucous membranes such as those in the gastrointestinal tract. When used for soothing the inside of the body, fenugreek is a demulcent. When used for soothing the outside of the body, fenugreek is an emollient. Mucilage, such as is found in fenugreek, is hydrating and anti-inflammatory. Fenugreek affects the balance of fluids in the body. Research has shown that hormones are part of the regulatory process in the body having to do with fluid balance. The signature of fluid balance can be seen in fenugreek's ability to be helpful in the care of diabetics who waste and thirst, to help heal wounds and burns when healing of the skin can be impaired because of fluid loss, and in lactation when women need help generating and secreting fluid. Fenugreek may have a broader effect on the processes in the body responsible for fluid-related adaptogen action.

THERAPEUTIC APPLICATIONS:

Oral

Infusion. Macerate 0.5 g of cut seed in 5 ounces (150 ml) of cold water for three hours. Strain and drink several cups daily.

Fluid Extract. 1:1 (g/ml): A little more than 1 teaspoon (6 ml) daily (Blumenthal et al., 2000)

Tincture. 1:5 (g/ml): 1 ounce (30 ml) daily (Blumenthal et al., 2000)

Decoction. Use 1 ounce (28 g) of seeds to 1 pint (470 ml) of water (Grieve, 1971).

Topical

Liniment. Apply topically a liquid preparation containing the infusion or tincture mixed with vegetable oil or alcohol.

Poultice. Prepare a semisolid paste prepared from about 2 ounces (50 g) of powdered seed and 1 quart (1 L) water. (Blumenthal et al., 2000).

Environmental

Bath. Mix about 2 ounces (50 g) of the powdered seed with 1 cup (240 ml) of water. Add this to a hot bath.

Inhalant. The steam vapor of the hot water infusion can be inhaled to help break up mucous congestion.

Herbal Caveat—Therapeutic Applications

In traditional and conventional herbal medicine, amounts of herbs given to patients are based on individual needs. The amounts or "doses" recorded here are provided so that the health practitioner has a general idea of the amounts recommended for an adult patient. Dosing in herbalism not only refers to amount of plant used but also includes when, where, and how to take a plant medicine. These dosages should not be used as guidelines for indiscriminate intervention without proper assessment, critical thinking, and patient education on the part of the practitioner.

Note: Please see chapter 5 for detailed descriptions of how to prepare various applications.

PATIENT INTERACTION:

Fenugreek seed has been used as a spice and as a medicinal plant remedy for centuries. Fenugreek tea can be taken internally for stomach and intestinal complaints such as lack of appetite and diarrhea. Fenugreek seeds make excellent poultices for wounds that do not heal and local inflammations on the skin. Fenugreek seeds are excellent home remedies but should not be taken in medicinal amounts during pregnancy because they may cause miscarriage. Fenugreek seed, in medicinal amounts, can significantly lower blood sugar and should be used by diabetics under the guidance of a health practitioner. The high amount of fiber in fenugreek may slow down the emptying of the stomach when taken internally and therefore may interfere with the body's ability to utilize certain drugs. It is best to discuss this issue with a health practitioner if you are taking medications routinely before taking medicinal amounts of fenugreek so that timing of medications can be adjusted if necessary.

Herbal Caveat—Patient Interaction

Patients considering the use of an herb or formula of herbs in self-care benefit from education about the plant itself and the use of the plant in healing. This education can come through many sources, including local herbalists; plant specialists such as botanists; health practitioners such as nurses, nutritionists, naturopaths, and other physicians; and various written references including the scientific literature. Patients need to remember that their unique health care needs are not necessarily represented in any literature they may encounter. Therefore, it is recommended that a knowledgeable mentor be consulted before initiating self-care with any herb being used for the first time.

NURTURING THE NURSE-PLANT RELATIONSHIP:

Note: You may want to keep a journal of your experiences with the herb.

There are two ways to get to know fenugreek. First, try the leaves and seeds in the foods of the Indian people who have used this herb in cooking and healing for centuries. Try the leaves in a dish known as "alu methi" and the seeds in a curry dish.

The second way to learn about the healing properties of fenugreek is to make a poultice by preparing "helba," the Egyptian preparation. Watch as the seeds soaking in water release their mucilage into the water, forming a wonderful, gooey paste that can be applied to skin inflammations. Smell the odor of the fenugreek, similar to the smell of caramel or celery.

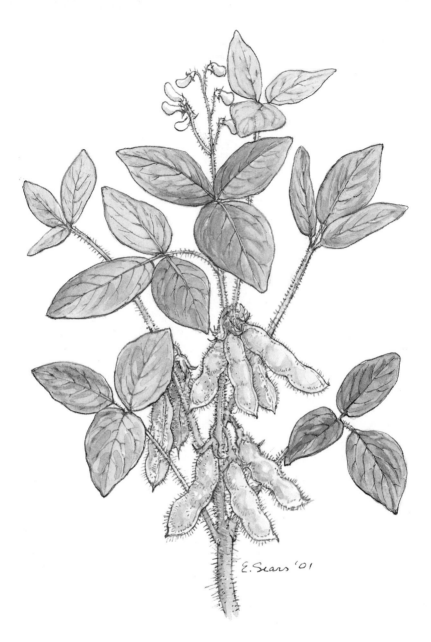

Glycine max

Soy

- **LATIN NAME:** *Glycine max*

- **FAMILY NAME:** Fabaceae

- **COMMON NAMES:** Soy, soybean

- **HEALTH PATTERN:** Hormone balance

- **PLANT DESCRIPTION:**

Soy is an annual plant that grows from 1 to 5 feet (0.3 to 1.5 meters) tall. The entire plant, including the bean pods, is covered with short, fine hairs. The clusters of pods contain from two to four beans per pod. Soy prefers to grow in a subtropical environment that is moist and shady, but it has been successfully cultivated in more temperate regions. It is planted in the spring and the beans are harvested in October and November. Currently, farmers cultivate more than 2500 different varieties, with 49% of the world's soybeans being grown in the United States. Soy yields 25% more protein per acre than beef, so it has the reputation of being a much more cost-effective food source. In addition, soy requires less water per acre than beef so its cultivation as a protein source helps save valuable water resources (McCaleb, Leigh, & Morien, 2000).

- **PLANT PART USED:** Seed, also known as the soybean

- **TRADITIONAL EVIDENCE:**

Cultural Use

Asian. Soybean cultivation is thought to have begun in China sometime between 2967 B.C.E. and 2597 B.C.E. Soy was called one of the five sacred crops. Soybeans were used for symptoms relating to kidney disease, poisoning, and edema (Blumenthal et al., 2000). The fresh crushed leaves of the soybean plant have been applied topically to relieve discomfort from bee and wasp stings (Kushi, 1993).

Currently, TCM uses soybean preparations for patterns of yin deficiency, irritability, restlessness, insomnia following fevers, and for tightness in the chest. TCM practitioners believe that soy should not be given to nursing mothers because it inhibits lactation. Soybeans are prepared with other herbs and given for many different symptoms. The beans are prepared by steaming and then fermenting the mixture (Bensky & Gamble, 1993).

The Chinese classify soy/tofu in general as cooling, slightly sweet and somewhat damp. If someone were to have a condition that has qualities of cold and damp, soy or tofu would be contraindicated. An extreme dampness condition in TCM is known as "phlegm." The phlegm condition can be hot or cold and is aggravated by poor digestion. The condition of phlegm can manifest in what is called in the West, a tumor. Health care providers who are not aware of the energetics of foods, as are TCM practitioners, often recommend soy, based on its plant constituents, in extreme amounts to people with tumors in particular. I have heard well-meaning practitioners say, "Eat as much soy as you can!" From a TCM standpoint, if the cancer patient has a cold phlegm condition or spleen qi deficiency, soy and tofu would not be recommended. Soy also should not be eaten when coming down with a cold when there is excess mucous with a wet, productive cough.

After the bombing of Nagasaki, Japan, in 1945, Tatsuichiro Akizuki, the medical director of internal medicine at St. Francis Hospital (located 1 mile from ground zero), fed all patients and staff who survived (most survived the initial blast) a strict macrobiotic diet of brown rice, miso (fermented soybean paste) and tamari (soy sauce) soup, wakame and other sea vegetables, Hokkaido pumpkin, and sea salt. Although many people died from radiation sickness in Nagasaki, Dr. Akizuki saved everyone in his hospital. Japanese medical researchers continue to study the effects of miso and sea vegetables in particular for protection against radiation sickness, as well as cancer and heart disease (Kushi & Kushi, 1985, p. 249).

East Indian. In India, soy *(Glycine max)* is known by the Hindi name "bhat" and is used as a food for animals and as a source of soybean oil. Another species of *Glycine (labialis, Linn.)* is used for consumption, fever, and certain blood disorders (Nadkarni, 1976).

European. The German Commission E has approved soy *lecithin* for treating disturbances of fat metabolism, such as hypercholesterolemia in cases in which dietary management is not effective (Blumenthal et al., 2000).

Culinary Use

Tofu, a protein-rich curd made from soybeans, was developed in China around 2800 B.C. It was introduced into Japan and Korea by Buddhist missionaries between the second and seventh centuries. Historically, tofu has been a highly esteemed food of the royal courts of China. Asian people continue to use tofu as a dietary staple. Soybeans were introduced into the United States in the late nineteenth century by Chinese immigrants. Currently, soybeans are converted into a variety of food products such as soy milk, soy sauce, tofu, miso (fermented soybean paste), tempeh (fermented soybean), soy flour, and soy oil. Soybean is often fermented, as in the case of miso and tempeh. The fermentation process increases the digestibility of the protein in the soy. Soy milk is used as a substitute by those who have digestive problems associated with ingesting cow's milk products. It is also the base of an alternative infant formula.

Recent technologic improvements have allowed soy protein to be isolated from the soybean and used to make high protein soy burgers

(Barnes, 1998). Soybeans can be cooked with carrots, onions, and tamari soy sauce or sea salt for a delicious dish that traditional Oriental herbalists believe is good for excessive thinness, fatigue, and decreased sexual vitality (Kushi, 1993). Soybeans are low in saturated fat, cholesterol-free, and a good source of protein and omega-3 fatty acids (Messina, 1995).

Because soy is classified energetically as cooling, it can impede digestive fire in healthy people. It can be prepared with spices such as ginger to provide a more energetically balanced meal. Although Asians have eaten soy products for many centuries, people of other races often find soy to be indigestible. This may be due to the difference in digestive enzymes between races, and therefore, people who have not grown up in a culture where soy products are eaten as part of a staple diet may want to ingest soy sparingly, or perhaps not at all (Wicke, 1992).

Use in Herbalism

Soy is used today for skin diseases, leg ulcers, vitamin deficiency, toxemia of pregnancy, and gastrointestinal disorders (Blumenthal et al., 2000). Phospholipids derived from soybeans are useful for treating elevated cholesterol that is not aided by dietary changes, exercise, or weight loss alone (Schulz, Hansel, & Tyler, 1998). Soy has been used for symptoms of menopause such as hot flashes, vaginal dryness, decreased bone density and osteoporosis, fuzzy thinking, heart disease, high cholesterol, and for the prevention of breast and uterine cancer (Hudson, 1999).

Those who subscribe to the macrobiotic lifestyle and diet, and the healing principles associated with it, use soy extensively. Miso, a salty, fermented soybean paste, is used in preparing soups and sauces. It contains enzymes that aid digestion and minerals that aid metabolism. Miso also is used for preventing allergies and tuberculosis (Kushi, 1993).

Tofu, prepared from soybeans, is applied topically to cool burns. Tofu plasters (the water of the tofu is squeezed out thoroughly and grated ginger and flour are added to make a sticky paste that is spread on a piece of gauze and applied to the body) are used to "absorb fever, extinguish inflammatory processes and prevent or decrease swelling" (Kushi, 1993, p. 131). Black soybeans are eaten to relieve cough and asthma and improving reproductive organ function. The beans are only eaten if cooked thoroughly by soaking for ten hours, cooking for two hours, washing with cold water, and then cooking again for two to four hours more (Kushi, 1993).

BIOMEDICAL EVIDENCE:

Although there have been some inconsistencies in the data, there appears to be an effect of the phytosterols in the form of isoflavones in soy on hormone balance in humans and on the incidence of some diseases such as breast cancer and heart disease. Animal and in vitro studies suggest that the protective effects of soy may be equally applicable to both hormone and nonhormone-related cancers (Persky & Van Horn, 1995). One limitation often found in the biomedical literature is that investigators do not clarify the individual soy product used in their studies.

Studies Related to Hormone Balance

The administration of soy protein powder, 60 g, containing 76 mg isoflavones, given daily to postmenopausal women in a double-blind, placebo-controlled study with 104 subjects, led to a 45% reduction of hot flushes over a twelve-week period as compared with the placebo group, which experienced a 30% reduction (Albertazzi et al., 1998).

Soy protein, 40 g per day containing either 1.39 mg or 2.25 mg of isoflavones per gram protein, was found to significantly lower risk factors associated with cardiovascular disease for both levels of isoflavone, and the 2.25 mg level significantly lowered the risk of spinal bone loss in those of 66 hypercholesterolemic, postmenopausal women who received the soy protein. All participants were on a United States National cholesterol education Step I diet (Potter et al., 1998).

Daily intake of 60 g (45 mg isoflavones) of soy protein (Protoveg) for one month in 6 premenopausal women with regular ovulatory cycles significantly increased follicular phase length and delayed menstruation one to five days (Cassidy, Bingham, & Setchell, 1994). In another study of 6 women, decreased estradiol levels and increased menstrual cycle length were observed after one month of feeding the women 12 ounces of soy milk three times a day. (Daily isoflavone intakes were 100 mg each of genistein and daidzein.) Decreases in estradiol levels persisted for two to three cycles after stopping the soy milk feedings (Lu, Anderson, Grady, & Nagamani, 1996).

In a comparison of Adventist vegetarian and nonvegetarian adolescent girls, vegetarian girls who ingested high amounts of soy products in their diet as compared with nonvegetarians had higher levels of follicular and luteal dehydroepiandrosterone sulfate (DHS); however, no significant differences were found related to testosterone, estradiol, or percent free estradiol levels (Persky & Van Horn, 1995).

Soy product intake was not positively related to menstrual cycle length in a study of 50 healthy premenopausal Japanese women (Nagata, Kabuto, Kurisu, Shimizu, 1997). In the same study individual soy foods were assessed. Tofu and miso were found to be inversely correlated with estradiol concentration on days 11 and 22 of the menstrual cycle. An inverse correlation between soy intake and estradiol concentration was demonstrated in one study of 50 premenopausal Japanese women.

Studies Related to Other Health Patterns

Restoration. Four healthy humans receiving soy beverage (42 mg genistein and 27 mg daidzein per day) demonstrated that genistein is absorbed and is present in peripheral blood at concentrations of 0.5 to 1.0 μM, which is not high enough, based on other in vitro studies, to inhibit the growth of most cultured cancer cells but may still have a chemopreventive effect (Barnes, Sfakianos, Coward, & Kirk, 1996).

In a case-controlled study, a significant reduction in breast cancer risk among women with a high dietary intake of phytosterols as measured by excretion was demonstrated in 144 women newly diagnosed with breast cancer (Ingram, Sanders, Kolybaba, & Lopez, 1997).

Hormone Balance. Soy protein powder 60 g per day for twenty-eight days, when administered as a supplement to 20 male subjects in a randomized controlled trial increased plasma concentrations of isoflavones, but did not demonstrate a significant effect on total or high-density lipoprotein (HDL) plasma cholesterol levels or platelet aggregation. Investigators identify a limitation of the study as being that the soy powder was given only as a supplement to, not a replacement for, the high-fat, low-fiber diets that many of the subjects were eating (Gooderham, Aldercreutz, Ojala, Wahala, & Holub, 1996).

Mechanism of Action

Soy contains four main isoflavones (i.e., genistein, daidzein, genistin, and daidzin) that have phytosterol activity and are thought to act as estrogen antagonists. Genistein, the most active phytosterol, has the highest affinity for estrogen receptors (Brandi, 1997). It is absorbed in the gut (Barnes et al., 1996). In vitro studies of human breast cancer cell lines found that genistein effectively inhibits cell growth whether or not the cells express an estrogen receptor, "suggesting that the mechanism of action of the isoflavones in preventing appearance of mammary tumors may not be a direct antiestrogenic effect . . . the target of isoflavones may be signal transduction pathways induced by interaction of growth factors with their receptors on tumors" (Barnes, Peterson, Grubbs, & Setchell, 1994, p. 144). Although the isoflavones are one of the most promising of these agents (anticancer), the role of interactions between the components of the soybean are largely unexplored (Barnes, 1998).

Human estrogens have a dual, dose-dependent effect on breast tumor growth. Large doses have been found to inhibit tumor growth and lower injected doses have been found to promote growth (Horwitz & McGuire, 1977). Scientists speculate that "phytoestrogens may have similar dual potentials" (Martin et al., 1978, p. 1866).

The influence of soy-protein-containing dietary estrogens on the menstrual cycle may explain the reduced rate for breast cancer in premenopausal women consuming soy-protein products. Isoflavones and their metabolites may alter intestinal steroid hormone metabolism, which effects estradiol concentration (Nagata et al., 1997). Studies have determined that fermented soy products such as miso and natto contain much higher levels of the isoflavone genistein than those that are not fermented (Fukutake et al., 1996), and that fermentation of soy increases the availability of isoflavones to the body (Slavin, Karr, Hutchins, & Lampe, 1998). Some soy products have been processed in such a manner that the isoflavones have been removed. Soy protein isolates are one example. When purchasing soy products, it is important to look at the label to check the isoflavone content. Foods known to contain isoflavones are soy protein granules, roasted soy nuts, tofu, tempeh, soy beverages, soy butter, and cooked soybeans (Hudson, 1999).

USE IN PREGNANCY OR LACTATION:

Vegetarian women in particular often eat soy products as part of their regular diet. *Sojae Praeparatum*, or prepared soybean, also known as "dou chi" in Chinese and "tantoshi" in Japanese, is contraindicated in lactating mothers (Bensky & Gamble, 1993). There are no contraindications reported for regular soy.

Herbal Caveat—Pregnancy or Lactation

Some herbs are contraindicated in pregnancy because of a risk of the herb or one of its constituents stimulating the uterus and therefore possibly promoting fetal loss. Many herbal practitioners do not recommend herbal remedies, in particular oral doses of herbs, during the first trimester of pregnancy and seek an alternative. However, herbs are successfully used during pregnancy, especially to prepare the body for the birth. Herbs are relatively unstudied in pregnancy and lactation, so patients need to be made aware through education of the potential benefits and risks of using herbs for health conditions that arise during pregnancy or lactation. The use of herbal remedies during pregnancy often warrants a referral to a knowledgeable herbal practitioner.

USE FOR CHILDREN:

Children can consume soy products in small amounts as part of a well-balanced diet, but they may find them hard to digest. Some parents choose soy infant formulas as an alternative to cow's milk formula. Soy formula is hard for some babies to digest and can cause excessive gas. Baby's digestive systems are immature, and they must be observed closely when given soy formula to be sure that they tolerate it well.

Herbal Caveat—Children

Children have special needs in regard to herbal therapies. They require lesser amounts of herbs and often respond well to mild teas and topical applications such as compresses and baths. The lowest dose of oral preparations should be tried first before increasing the amount given children. Caregivers should observe children closely for responses to herbal reme-

---

dies. Younger children, particularly infants, have traditionally been given herbs either through their mother's breast milk or in the form of a homeopathic remedy because of their sensitivity to medicines and treatments and the immaturity of their liver. It is recommended that a person knowledgeable in the herbal treatment of children be consulted before the offering of any herb to a child for the first time.

CAUTIONS:

Soy is used as a food and is generally recognized as safe (GRAS) by the United States Food and Drug Administration. The digestion and assimilation of soy can be variable among individuals. Some people have a very poor tolerance to soy foods and experience indigestion, bloating, constipation, and irregular bowel habits when they consume soy products.

Raw soybeans contain trypsin inhibitors that interfere with protein metabolism by the pancreatic enzyme trypsin. This process may damage the pancreas. One study demonstrated that eating raw soy products over a long period of time resulted in the development of hyperplastic and neoplastic nodules of the pancreas of rats (Liener, 1995). Soybeans contain phytates, chemicals that bind with iron and zinc to prevent their absorption in the intestinal tract. However, cooking and fermentation destroy most of the phytates (as reported in McCaleb et al., 2000). Soybeans contain substances that can reduce the absorption of iodine by the thyroid gland. It is recommended that those with diminished thyroid function avoid eating soy to prevent further aggravation of this condition (Brinker, 1998).

Soy may not be easily digested by those who have not grown up in cultures where it is eaten traditionally as part of the diet. "We should only adopt traditions from other cultures carefully and gradually. It is now known that people of East Asia are genetically endowed with a greater ability to digest soy products, but even these people carefully process the soybeans according to traditional methods. To suddenly introduce for mass consumption a food product from another culture, and moreover, commercially processed in ways not even used in that culture, may be a recipe for disaster" (Wicke, 2000).

NURSING EVIDENCE:

Historical Nursing Use

Pediatric nurses have historically worked with pediatricians in determining the effectiveness and tolerance of soy infant formulas in the feeding of infants who do not tolerate cow's milk protein.

Potential Nursing Applications

For years, nurses have served beef or chicken bouillon as part of a clear liquid diet for postoperative patients and those who are on restricted diets. Although bouillon may be naturally derived from animal stocks, one of its primary ingredients is the flavor enhancer monosodium glutamate (MSG). MSG has significant physiologic effects on the body. It is used in the treatment of mental retardation and hepatic coma that is due to high blood ammonia levels and has been demonstrated to cause brain damage in infant animals and to cause what is often called "Chinese restaurant syndrome" (i.e., chest pain, facial pressure, and burning sensation) in humans (Leung & Foster, 1996). MSG also can cause increased heart rate and palpitations in some people. A substitute is needed, especially for those who are ill.

Nurses and dieticians might want to consider the substitution of a (soy) miso broth for the bouillon. See the recipe in the Nurturing the Nurse-Plant Relationship section. It is salty just like bouillon and is full of vitamins and minerals rather than a stimulating flavor enhancer.

Many nurses, including those in radiology and those serving in the military may be concerned about the risks to their patients and themselves from exposure to radiation. Nurses may want to consider developing clinical guidelines for dietary recommendations for those exposed to radiation to help support the body's adaptive processes. Japanese nurses with access to the data from Hiroshima and Nagasaki survivors may wish to analyze the data and begin creating guidelines for the use of miso, salt, rice, and sea and land vegetables in the promotion of health following radiation exposure.

Integrative Insight

From a biomedical perspective, there may be significant reasons why women would want to eat high amounts of soy in their diet. Constituents in soy have been shown to be protective against cancer, heart disease, and radiation sickness, to name a few. But traditionally, soy may not be appropriate for everyone, especially in medicinal amounts. Although grown extensively in the United States, soy has been eaten as a large part of the Asian diet, not the American diet. Soy is part of the Asian culture and was lifesaving for some after the bombing of Japan. Now, many women of many countries wonder about adding soy to their diet.

It is not clear that there ever will be a definitive answer regarding if or how much soy should be part of a healthy diet. Nurses need to evaluate each patient as an individual in their practice. From a Chinese perspective, recommending that a patient eat excessive amounts of soy products may actually increase excess phlegm (which can potentially lead to tumor growth). From a biomedical perspective, the woman eating large amounts of soy at the right time in her life just might protect her from breast tumor growth. How does a nurse know what to recommend? Soy shows us the necessity of the integrative approach, in which the answer to the question emerges as the nurse gets to know the patient and the herb, soy, and individualizes care based upon knowledge of the two. Soy has the potential to be effective in preventing death and disease. The questions are in whom, when, and how much?

THERAPEUTIC APPLICATIONS:

Oral

Soy isoflavones are found in products such as roasted soybeans, miso, tofu, and tempeh.

For Regulating Cholesterol. About 1 ounce (25 g) or more of soy protein daily

For Menopause. 50 to 75 mg of isoflavones daily

For Osteoporosis Prevention. 55 to 90 mg of isoflavones daily (McCaleb et al., 2000)

Topical

Tofu, a food prepared from soybeans, can be applied topically for burns. To make a tofu plaster, put the tofu into a cheesecloth or towel and squeeze it to remove excess water. Then mash the tofu in a bowl. Add approximately 5% grated ginger and about 10% to 15% white flour. Mix it well to form a sticky paste. Spread this on a cotton towel or piece of wax paper or a paper towel. Apply the plaster so that the paste directly contacts the skin. Cover over with another towel. Replace the plaster after approximately one or two hours, or sooner if it dries out. It has been reported that the tofu helps reduce pain, promote skin regeneration, and prevent the formation of scars and keloids (Kushi, 1993). Note: Although I have known of this remedy for years I have never recommended it for second- or third-degree burns because of the concern about infection of the wound and the possible need for debridement. There are some herbs that when applied to wounds (as salves for instance) seem to deter infection; so there may be a possibility that tofu could be useful for burns. Study of those who have used tofu for burns would be helpful in this case.

Environmental

No data are available at this time.

Herbal Caveat—Therapeutic Applications

In traditional and conventional herbal medicine, amounts of herbs given to patients are based on individual needs. The amounts or "doses" recorded here are provided so that the health practitioner has a general idea of the amounts recommended for an adult patient. Dosing in herbalism not only refers to amount of plant used but also includes when, where, and how to take a plant medicine. These dosages should not be used as guidelines for indiscriminate intervention without proper assessment, critical thinking, and patient education on the part of the practitioner.

Note: Please see chapter 5 for detailed descriptions of how to prepare various applications.

PATIENT INTERACTION:

Soy is a source of vegetable protein and plant constituents known as isoflavones that may help promote healthy hormone balance in men and women. Soy products include tempeh, tofu, miso, soy powder, soy milk, soy cheese, and roasted soy nuts. Regularly including soy products as part of a healthy diet may lower cholesterol levels and prevent cancer and osteoporosis; however, eating soy is not recommended for all people. Some people, Caucasians in particular, may experience bloating, indigestion, constipation, and irregularity of bowel habits as a result of ingesting soy products. Some infants who ingest soy formula have similar discomfort. Allergies to soy products are possible. It is best to eat soybeans cooked and fermented. Do not eat raw soybeans. One source recommends that people with low thyroid function not eat soy products. Do not eat soy when you are coming down with a cold and are producing a lot of mucus. Exercise caution when considering taking excessive amounts of any food, including soy.

Herbal Caveat—Patient Interaction

Patients considering the use of an herb or formula of herbs in self-care benefit from education about the plant itself and the use of the plant in healing. This education can come through many sources, including local herbalists; plant specialists such as botanists; health practitioners such as nurses, nutritionists, naturopaths, and other physicians; and various written references including the scientific literature. Patients need to remember that their unique health care needs are not necessarily represented in any literature they may encounter. Therefore, it is recommended that a knowledgeable mentor be consulted before initiating self-care with any herb being used for the first time.

NURTURING THE NURSE-PLANT RELATIONSHIP:

Note: You may want to keep a journal of your experiences with the herb.

To learn about soybeans, try replacing the peanuts on your coffee table with roasted soy nuts. They're chock full of isoflavones and make a great crunchy snack.

Recipe for Miso Soup:

Miso is a dark paste made from soybeans, sea salt, and fermented rice or barley that are aged together. Miso contains enzymes that are thought to facilitate digestion and strengthen the quality of the blood and alkalize the body (Kushi & Kushi, 1985). To make miso soup, purchase some dark brown miso paste. Boil 1 cup of water. Add a small amount of the boiled water to approximately 1 tablespoon (14 g) of miso. The strength of the miso broth can be adjusted to taste. After the paste is thinned with a little water, add it to the rest of the boiled water. Do not boil the miso soup. The soup can be drunk plain or a small amount of green onion can be added for flavor and color along with a few drops of brown sesame oil. This is a great home remedy when you are feeling out of balance. I like to have miso soup when traveling, especially on long, international flights. For travel purposes, dried, powdered miso is available.

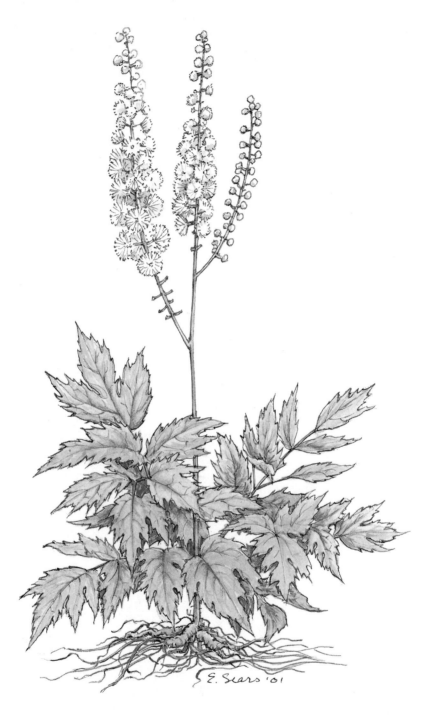

Cimicifuga racemosa

Black Cohosh

🌿 **LATIN NAMES:** *Cimicifuga racemosa, Actaea racemosa*

🌿 **FAMILY NAME:** Ranunculaceae

🌿 **COMMON NAMES:** Black cohosh, black snakeroot, macrotys, bugbane, bugwort, rattleroot, rattlewort, rattleweed, richweed, squawroot

>   NOTE: Do not confuse black cohosh with blue cohosh *(Caulophyllum thalictroides).*

🌿 **HEALTH PATTERN:** Hormone balance

🌿 **PLANT DESCRIPTION:**

The name *Cimicifuga* means "repel bugs" and this is one of black cohosh's uses. Black cohosh is native to North America, especially in the woodlands of the southeastern United States. It is a tall, leafy perennial that grows from 3 to 9 feet (1 to 3 meters) tall. Its root is knotty with many long, slender fibers branching from it. The flowers are small, white, and appear feathery on the ends of the stalks. It blooms from June through August in rich woodlands, on the sides of hills, and in shady fields. It has been determined that the plant produces more of its medically active constituents when it is under stress "such as that caused by insect injury, bright summer light, and fungal infection" (Bruneton, 1995, p. 296). Black cohosh can be cultivated as an attractive ornamental in the yard. It will grow rather easily in many environments, prefers shady areas with some sun, and moist soil. Its roots are harvested after two to four years (McCaleb et al., 2000).

🌿 **PLANT PARTS USED:** Dried roots and rhizome

🌿 **TRADITIONAL EVIDENCE:**

Cultural Use

   Asian. Black cohosh rhizome, called "sheng ma," is classified in TCM as an herb that relieves wind heat. The species is *Cimicifuga foetida.* Chinese black cohosh is used for headaches and releases the exterior of the body so that rashes, such as measles, can erupt. Black cohosh is not used after measles have already erupted. It is commonly used for toothaches, swollen gums, mouth ulcers, canker sores, sore throat, and skin conditions caused by fevers. If too much *C. foetida* is taken, symptoms such as headaches, dizziness, vomiting, gastroenteritis, pathogenic erections, and tremors can occur (Bensky & Gamble, 1993).

   Traditional Japanese medicine uses black cohosh, called "shoma" to relieve symptoms of heat that occur on the surface of the body such as the eruptions of measles and chicken pox. The plant also is used for bad breath, acne associated with the menstrual cycle, mastitis, sore throat, and inflammation of the mouth and breasts (Rister, 1999).

North American Indian. The Cherokee use black cohosh to promote menstruation; as a pain reliever; and for rheumatism, colds, and coughs. It also is used internally for hives, as a diuretic, for constipation, and as a stimulant for fatigue. It was sometimes given to infants to help them sleep. The Iroquois use a decoction of the roots or whole plants as a soak or steam bath for rheumatism. They also use it internally as a "blood purifier" and to increase breast milk in nursing mothers. Other North American Indian tribes used black cohosh for kidney trouble (Moerman, 1998). In some tribes, the women used the root extensively during childbirth and for relieving pain during the menstrual period. The pounded root was both applied topically and taken internally as an antidote for snakebites (Hutchens, 1992). Some tribes call black cohosh "black snakeroot" and use it as a treatment for yellow fever and as a diuretic (Vogel, 1970).

Hispanic. Although not native to the southwestern United States, some Hispanics use black cohosh as a compress for boils, a tea for relaxation purposes, and for discomfort related to rheumatism and neuralgia.

East Indian. Ayurvedic physicians have used their indigenous species of *C. foetida* as a nerve depressant (Nadkarni, 1976).

European. Although not native to Europe, black cohosh is cultivated there (Grieve, 1971). It is used currently in Europe for its estrogen-like action and to suppress luteinizing hormone in menstrual disorders such as premenstrual syndrome, dysmenorrhea, and uterine spasms and in the treatment of symptoms related to menopause (Foster & Tyler, 1999; Leung & Foster, 1996).

Culinary Use

There are no culinary uses for black cohosh.

Use in Herbalism

As early as 1785, black cohosh was used by American Eclectic botanical practitioners. In 1801, records state that the North American Indians also held the plant in high esteem. During this time, it was used for sore throats, itchy skin, and for conditions related to women's reproductive symptoms. In 1832, black cohosh was introduced to the medical profession and became a valuable and commonly used remedy of physicians (Felter & Lloyd, 1983).

In the mid-1800s, physicians in the United States used the resin extracted from the roots of black cohosh for a variety of symptoms. It was used internally for intermittent fevers, leukorrhea, amenorrhea, painful menses, threatened miscarriage, sterility, joint pain, and prolapsed uterus. It also was used for dyspepsia, chronic gonorrhea, and smallpox. The tincture was used as a local application in conjunctivitis. Black cohosh was combined with wild yam for intestinal colic and flatulence. It was combined with other herbs for the relief of painful menses, cramps in pregnant women, and other muscle spasms (Felter & Lloyd, 1983). Black cohosh also was used for chorea but was given with iron. It was used in the treatment of neuralgia, chronic bronchitis, frontal headache, tenderness of the womb, "fatty and irritable heart," and during labor to produce normal contractions (Hare, 1892).

The effect black cohosh exerted over the nervous system was well-known. It was believed to improve digestion and the appetite in small doses and improve excretion via the skin and kidneys. It also was used to support the secretions from the bronchial mucous surfaces and to gently tone the heart and circulatory system. It was used to decrease a fast heartbeat and to increase the power of each beat, which, although compared to the action of digitalis, was much less pronounced. In large doses, however, black cohosh was found to produce vertigo, impaired vision, nausea, dilation of the pupils, and a reduction in circulation. However, it was used in appropriate doses to promote menstrual bleeding and childbirth because of its action on the muscle fibers of the uterus (Felter & Lloyd, 1983).

In the early 1840s, black cohosh was a popular remedy for rheumatism and neuralgia. It was used for all kinds of muscular pain and tension, especially abdominal muscle soreness, tension in the neck and back, and internal abdominal pain. Black cohosh tincture was used as a topical application for inflammation of the nerves, spine, ovaries, and the eyes or old skin ulcers; tic-douloureux; rheumatism; and stiffness in the neck, back, or side (Felter & Lloyd, 1983). It also was used for diseases of the ear and for eyestrain with headaches. Black cohosh was believed to tone the tissues of the female reproductive tract. This was perhaps why it was able to relieve pelvic pain associated with menstruation and restore delayed menses. It was used for sterility and ovarian pain in women, and aching sensations of the prostate gland in men (Felter & Lloyd, 1983). Black cohosh has been used during labor to produce natural intermittent uterine contractions, rather than the constant contractions produced by ergot. It stimulated and toned the uterus to produce the normal contractions necessary for childbirth. After birth, it was given to decrease the after-pains and to relax the nervous system taxed by the exertions of labor. It was thought that a strong decoction of the recently dug roots in tablespoon doses was most effective for these conditions (Felter & Lloyd, 1983).

Black cohosh has been used as a remedy for poisoning and snakebite. It also is given for cough that accompanies tuberculosis and whooping-cough (Grieve, 1971). Other uses identified for black cohosh are for high blood pressure and migraine and as a tonic and sedative (Hutchens, 1992).

In more current times, black cohosh is recommended for use in relieving some symptoms of premenstrual discomfort, painful menses, and menopause. Acteina, a constituent of black cohosh, has been studied for use in the treatment of peripheral arterial disease (Blumenthal et al., 2000). Black cohosh is used to prevent hot flashes, nervousness, and depression associated with menopause. Black cohosh is helpful in treating blurred vision and migraines associated with premenstrual syndrome (Rister, 1999). Black cohosh has been found to be able to increase male fertility and when combined with goldenseal is helpful with the symptom of ringing in the ears (Rister, 1999). Black cohosh also is given in homeopathic form for stimulating and balancing the female reproductive system, for symptoms of menstrual irregularities, menopausal difficulties, arthritis, rheumatism, and in childbirth (Duke, 1985).

BIOMEDICAL EVIDENCE:

Many of the studies that have evaluated the effects of black cohosh on symptoms related to hormone balance (e.g., menopause) have used a standardized ethanol extract of black cohosh called Remifemin. Several of the studies involving Remifemin have been conducted by the manufacturer of the product.

Studies Related to Hormone Balance

In a six- to eight-week multicenter trial, 80% of 629 women, mean age 51 years, demonstrated significant improvement in neurovegetative symptoms (i.e., hot flushes, headache, vertigo, tinnitus, heart palpitations) when taking black cohosh ethanol extract 80 drops per day after the first four weeks of the study, and many had no symptoms by the end of the trial (study by Stolze, 1982 in German as reported by Liske, 1998).

Using the Kupperman index for evaluation (measuring menopausal symptoms such as sweating, hot flushes, irritability, insomnia, depression, vertigo, concentration, and heart palpitations), a randomized, controlled study of 60 women demonstrated that black cohosh ethanol extract, 80 drops per day for three months, was equal to conjugated estrogens (0.625 mg/day) and diazepam (2 mg/day) in significantly decreasing neurovegetative and psychiatric symptoms in women (study by Warnecke, 1985 in German as reported by Liske, 1998).

Luteinizing hormone levels dropped significantly in menopausal women who were given 8 mg per day of Remifemin orally in a study of 110 women, pointing to an "estrogenic effect" of black cohosh preparations (Duker, Kopanski, Jarry, & Wuttke, 1991).

Studies Related to Other Health Patterns

No data are available at this time.

Mechanism of Action

The biologic activity of black cohosh is thought to be related to the triterpene glycoside constituents—actein, cimicifugocide, deoxyacetylacteol, and 27-deoxyactein (Pepping, 1999). Each 20-mg tablet of the standardized product called Remifemin contains 1 mg of deoxyactein.

Although isoflavones are usually found in plants in the Fabaceae family, such as red clover and soy, some have suggested that black cohosh contains isoflavones. However, evidence regarding whether or not black cohosh contains isoflavones (formononetin) or any other substance classified as estrogenic is conflicting (Wade, Kronenberg, Kelly, & Murphy, 1999). Duke lists formononetin as a constituent of the root (Duke, 2000).

The rise in luteinizing hormone (LH) that often occurs during menopause as estrogen levels drop has been linked to the increase in hot flushes. Black cohosh has been shown to lower LH in menopausal women. "Probably several compounds contribute to the LH suppressive effect of *Cimicifuga racemosa* preparations, i.e., those compounds structurally related to estrogen (fractions IV to VI) and those which do not bind to the estrogen receptor (fraction I). . . . This activity of fraction I may be explained by the possibility that it contains pro-estrogenic substances." (Duker et al., 1991, p. 424).

USE IN PREGNANCY OR LACTATION:

Black cohosh is used during pregnancy, but the timing must be right. Black cohosh is usually given to help regulate contractions. It is contraindicated during the first trimester of pregnancy because of reports of its ability to promote uterine bleeding (Brinker, 1998). Black cohosh tincture used in doses of 10 drops under the tongue every hour is given by midwives to facilitate the softening of the cervix. It is especially helpful if labor is to be induced before the cervix has had time to ripen naturally (Weed, 1986).

Black cohosh is combined with blue cohosh and given by midwives when labor needs to be encouraged. It has been used to strengthen or restart contractions. Fetal monitoring has shown that the blue cohosh may increase the heart rate of the baby. It may also decrease blood pressure in the mother (Weed, 1986).

Herbal Caveat—Pregnancy or Lactation
Some herbs are contraindicated in pregnancy because of a risk of the herb or one of its constituents stimulating the uterus and therefore possibly promoting fetal loss. Many herbal practitioners do not recommend herbal remedies, in particular oral doses of herbs, during the first trimester of pregnancy and seek an alternative. However, herbs are successfully used during pregnancy, especially to prepare the body for the birth. Herbs are relatively unstudied in pregnancy and lactation, so patients need to be made aware through education of the potential benefits and risks of using herbs for health conditions that arise during pregnancy or lactation. The use of herbal remedies during pregnancy often warrants a referral to a knowledgeable herbal practitioner.

USE FOR CHILDREN:

Black cohosh has been given to children in syrup form for diarrhea and nervous conditions such as chorea (Grieve, 1971).

CAUTIONS:

Note: A number of these cautions do not specify whether the substance causing the discomfort was the herb black cohosh or the standardized extract product.

The German Commission E recommends that the use of black cohosh be limited to six months (McGuffin et al., 1997). Others recommend that it should be used only for three months (Schulz et al., 1998). Although no long-term studies clarify the safety in long-term use, black cohosh has been traditionally used for much longer than six months.

Experimental studies have shown no toxic, mutagenic, carcinogenic, or teratogenic properties of black cohosh standardized extracts (Liske, 1998). Gastric distress occasionally has been reported from the oral intake of black cohosh. There are no known interactions of black cohosh with other drugs (Blumenthal et al., 2000). In large doses, black cohosh may cause vertigo, nausea, vomiting, headache, impaired vision, impaired circulation (McGuffin et al., 1997), and reduced pulse rate and increased perspiration (Newall et al., 1996). Black cohosh may lower blood pressure (McGuffin et al., 1997).

Black cohosh is considered an at-risk plant by the United Plant Savers because of high demand and overharvesting in the wild. It is recommended that black cohosh be purchased from cultivated sources. No data are available on how much black cohosh exists in the wild. Plant populations are monitored in some parts of the United States. Attempts are now being made to cultivate it in order to preserve the remaining native plants. For more information about the at-risk status of black cohosh and how to grow it, contact United Plant Savers at their website www.plantsavers.org.

NURSING EVIDENCE:

Historical Nursing Use

Some nurse midwives use black cohosh in promoting cervical ripening.

Potential Nursing Applications

Nurses such as women's health practitioners might want to consider recommending black cohosh for women with discomfort related to their menstrual cycle. Midwives may want to research the use of decoction or alcohol extract to promote regular labor, ease after pain, and promote lactation.

In a national survey of 500 members of the American College of Nurse Midwives (ACNM), 90 members said that they use herbs in practice to stimulate labor and of those 90 members, 45% use black cohosh. Of those responders that use herbs in practice, 69% learned to use the plants from other nurse-midwives and none learned about the plants in their formal education (McFarlin, Gibson, O'Rear, & Harman, 1999). This survey is a good source of descriptive data regarding the demographics of the midwives and their use or lack of use of herbs in practice. It also demonstrates the extensive interest in the use of herbs during labor among certified nurse midwives and raises the question of how education programs might be improved in regard to provision of education about plant therapies.

One extensive source of information on the use of herbs in pregnancy, including the use of black cohosh during labor, is the writings of the Thomsonian and Eclectic physicians of the 1800s in America. Much of this literature is housed at the Lloyd Library in Cincinnati, Ohio. The Lloyd Library material is indexed online through the University of Cincinnati at www.libraries.uc.edu.

Integrative Insight

Black cohosh has been used for decades in the health care of women. There is strong traditional evidence on the use of black cohosh for a number of women's health issues, including discomfort related to menopause and menstruation and to help ripen the cervix and regulate contractions during labor. Black cohosh seems to have a hormonal effect, but the mechanism of action is not exactly clear. Rather than in the laboratory, it may be in close clinical observation of the action of the herb in women that we learn the most about the mechanism of action. For example, black cohosh affects physical symptoms related to hormone imbalance such as hot flushes, and it also has been used to treat cardiac conditions. Scientific evidence has shown that there is a relationship between increased risk of cardiac disease and lower estrogen levels in postmenopausal women (Northrup, 1994). Traditional data about black cohosh seems to support the connection between cardiac risk and hormonal changes in women in that the plant is used in both conditions. But traditional data do not necessarily support the concept of the whole of the plant's action being specific to estrogen. While some may identify low estrogen as the "cause" and estrogen replacement therapy as the "cure," black cohosh's action suggests that more than one pathway is affected during the hormonal changes in menopause and therefore another remedy might be needed. Not just one substance affects a positive change in symptoms. This is what is not completely understood. And black cohosh affects not only the physical symptoms women experience but also the psychologic symptoms such as depression, suggesting involvement of other hormonal pathways in the plant's effect.

Herbs such as black cohosh have numerous constituents that are presented to the body in one "package." The body may use what it needs. Black cohosh may block estrogen receptors, and it may have a number of other actions as well. Because women who use black cohosh as a remedy for discomfort are using a substance that has a number of chemical and energetic qualities, using the scientific approach to focus on one action, such as the estrogenic quality, may lead to oversight. In addition to quantitative studies, qualitative studies of those who use black cohosh might be helpful in exploring the full extent of black cohosh's holistic healing action.

THERAPEUTIC APPLICATIONS:

Oral

Dried Rhizome and Root. 40 mg daily in divided doses

Capsules/Tablets. One 500-mg capsule three times per day (McCaleb et al., 2000)

Decoction. 1.5 to 9 g (Bensky & Gamble, 1993).

Note: Tea may not be as effective as other forms (McCaleb et al., 2000). Boiling the root in water releases only a portion of the constituents. Proper immersion in food-grade alcohol fully dissolves the constituents (Hutchens, 1992).

Fluid Extract. 1:1 (g/ml), 40% to 60% alcohol: 0.04 ml daily (Blumenthal et al, 2000)

Tincture. 1:10 (g/ml), 40% to 60% alcohol: 0.4 ml daily (Blumenthal et al, 2000)

Standardized Extract. (1:1[g/ml], standardized to 1% 27-deoxyactein): 4 to 8 mg of 27-deoxyactein daily (Blumenthal et al., 2000; Pepping, 1999)

Topical

No data are available at this time.

Environmental

No data are available at this time.

Herbal Caveat—Therapeutic Applications

In traditional and conventional herbal medicine, amounts of herbs given to patients are based on individual needs. The amounts or "doses" recorded here are provided so that the health practitioner has a general idea of the amounts recommended for an adult patient. Dosing in herbalism not only refers to amount of plant used but also includes when, where, and how to take a plant medicine. These dosages should not be used as guidelines for indiscriminate intervention without proper assessment, critical thinking, and patient education on the part of the practitioner.

Note: Please see chapter 5 for detailed descriptions of how to prepare various applications.

PATIENT INTERACTION:

Historically, black cohosh has been used for numerous discomforts, particularly rheumatic and women's discomforts. Black cohosh has been getting a lot of exposure in some countries like Germany and the United States because of the studies that have been done, primarily on a standardized black cohosh extract called Remifemin. Although the research and results in many women are promising, consumers must still educate themselves about their choices when it comes to dealing with health issues regarding hormone balance. Some women experience little or no discomfort related to menstruation or menopause and therefore need little or no intervention, either medical or herbal. Black cohosh is a plant remedy that has years of safe and effective use and can be considered as one of many options in assisting hormone balance. Science has not clearly shown how black cohosh affects hormone balance in humans; however, it does seem to relieve symptoms related to conditions, such as menopause, that are associated with hormone balance. This herb is best used at first under the guidance of a knowledgeable practitioner.

Herbal Caveat—Patient Interaction

Patients considering the use of an herb or formula of herbs in self-care benefit from education about the plant itself and the use of the plant in healing. This education can come through many sources, including local herbalists; plant specialists such as botanists; health practitioners such as nurses, nutritionists, naturopaths, and other physicians; and various written references including the scientific literature. Patients need to remember that their unique health care needs are not necessarily represented in any literature they may encounter. Therefore, it is recommended that a knowledgeable mentor be consulted before initiating self-care with any herb being used for the first time.

NURTURING THE NURSE-PLANT RELATIONSHIP:

Note: You may want to keep a journal of your experiences with the herb.

Black cohosh, in addition to its renowned status as an herb for women's discomforts, also has been used extensively for muscular and rheumatic pain, headache, and eyestrain. Because black cohosh may be extracted best in alcohol, to get to know this plant's personality and action, try a small amount of tincture (15 to 30 drops) in a small amount of warm water for rheumatic aches and pains. Record your experience.

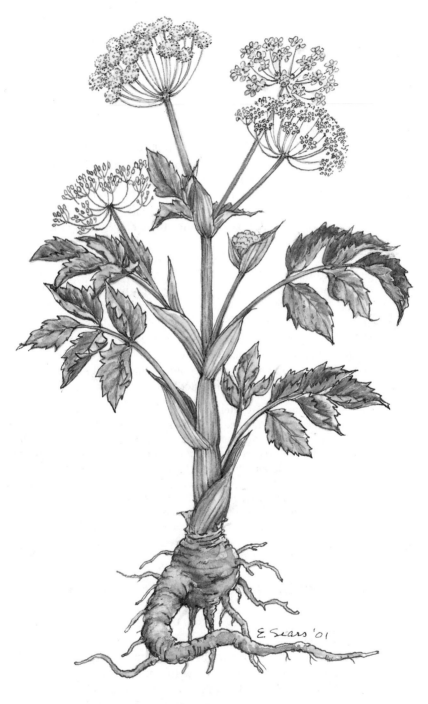

Angelica sinensis

CHAPTER 8

Angelica

🌿 **LATIN NAMES:** *Angelica sinensis, Angelica archangelica*
Note: This section profiles both species.

🌿 **FAMILY NAME:** Apiaceae

🌿 **COMMON NAMES:** *Angelica sinensis*: dong quai, tang kuei, Chinese angelica;
Angelica archangelica: angelica, garden angelica, angelica officinalis, European angelica

🌿 **HEALTH PATTERN:** Hormone balance

🌿 **PLANT DESCRIPTION:**
Angelica has a bold appearance with its large, bright green leaves with toothed edges. The plant grows from 4 to 6 feet (1 to 2 meters) tall and has sturdy but hollow stems. The flower heads have small stems of equal length that form rounded clusters called umbels and are shaped like very small umbrellas. The greenish yellow umbels bloom in July and are succeeded by pale yellow oblong fruits (Grieve, 1971). The seeds have an aromatic fragrance and a pungent, sweet, and bitter taste (Felter & Lloyd, 1983). The fragrant and aromatic roots of angelica are long, thick, and fleshy, sometimes weighing as much as 3 pounds (1360 g). The fresh roots, when cut, yield a golden liquid that has all the aromatic properties of the plant. Angelica likes to grow in rich, moist soil in shady areas, especially near running water (Grieve, 1971).

A. sinensis comes mainly from three western provinces in China. It grows best in higher altitudes (up to 8000 feet [2667 meters]) and in cold, shaded, moist conditions (Foster & Chongxi, 1992). The plant is a perennial that can grow to 3 to 4 feet (over 1 meter) tall with oval, toothed leaves divided into three parts. The flower heads, as with other plants in the same family, have many small flowers. The root is quite large, up to 10 inches (25 cm) long, and is yellow-brown with a very strong aromatic fragrance that some think resembles celery. Its taste is sweet, warm, and aromatic.

🌿 **PLANT PARTS USED:** *A. archangelica:* roots, stalks, leaves, seeds;
A. sinensis: root

🌿 **TRADITIONAL EVIDENCE:**
Cultural Use

Asian. In Chinese medicine, 10 or more species of angelica are used. The most popular one, *A. sinensis*, also known as "dong quai," is a well-known remedy for female disorders. It has been used in China for several thousand years. Asian women take *A. sinensis* as a tea or in soup as a health promotion measure for maintaining a healthy reproductive system. Angelica is used for the treatment of menstrual disorders, hemorrhage, colds, gastrointestinal complaints, and many other conditions. It is believed that the plant has the ability to increase blood flow to the female reproductive organs and therefore creates balanced menstruation and acts as an aphrodisiac and a post-partum healing agent. It is used for its beneficial effects on the energetic systems of the liver, uterus, heart, and nervous system. A specific therapy is used in which carefully prepared extracts of dong quai are injected into acupuncture points to relieve pain and spasms associated with rheumatism, sciatica, and pinched nerves. Chinese physicians also use intravenous *A. sinensis* as an antithrombotic agent to treat stroke (Qi-bing, Jing-yi, & Bo, 1991).

TCM classifies angelica as an herb that tonifies and moves blood. It is often included in formulas used for symptoms related to menstrual irregularities, amenorrhea and dysmenorrhea, tinnitus, blurred vision, heart palpitations, and pallid complexion. Angelica also is used for symptoms such as abdominal pain and trauma and to reduce swelling, promote healing of tissues, and alleviate pain (Bensky & Gamble, 1993).

In China, *A. sinensis* is most often used in formulation, not as a single herb. Chinese herbalists know that angelica, like many herbs, works synergistically in combination with certain other herbs. For example, in formulas taken by women, *A. sinensis* is often used in combination with *Paeonia lactiflora*, *Ligusticum sinensis,* and *Rehmannia glutinosa*. Angelica has been used as a single herb in clinical situations in the treatment of thromboangiitis, ischemic apoplexy, chronic cor pulmonale, headache, and neuralgia (Qi-bing et al., 1991).

Angelica root has three sections, the head, the body, and the tail. Sometimes only a particular section of the root is included in a formula because the different sections have different actions. The head is the uppermost part of the root and is thought to be the most tonifying, but the least effective part for moving blood. The tail, the lowest part of the root, is said to be the least tonifying but the most effective in moving blood. The body of the herb is thought to be more tonifying.

In TCM, medicinal teas, including those with angelica, are not usually taken during menstruation. Chinese herbalists do not recommend angelica root for use in diarrhea or abdominal distention caused by "damp obstruction." It is contraindicated for symptoms associated with a condition known as yin deficiency with accompanying heat signs (Bensky & Gamble, 1993).

Japanese herbalists use angelica to stimulate blood circulation to traumatized tissues to promote healing and expulsion of toxins. The plant is used for constipation and to relieve swelling, alleviate pain, assist in the recovery from wounds, and regulate the menses. Dong quai is used by the Japanese much the same as it is used in China. It is also used to increase male fertility, increase coronary blood flow, prevent the formation of blood clots, and treat pernicious anemia. The plant is a traditional remedy for eczema, psoriasis, arthritis, chronic kidney inflammation, and pain along the course of nerves (Rister, 1999).

North American Indian. North American Indian tribes throughout the United States use several angelica species. The root of *A. atropurpurea* is used by Cherokee women to promote menstrual flow. It is taken for flatulence and abdominal colic, headache, and as a gargle for sore throats and gums. The Delaware tribe uses the roots for stomach disorders. The Iroquois make an infusion of angelica that is used in steam baths to "sweat out" headaches. An infusion of the roots is used as an antidote for poison and for pneumonia. The Blackfoot use the root of *A. dawsonii* medicinally and as a religious medicine. The plant is considered a good luck charm in many tribes (Moerman, 1998). North American Indians on the East coast rub a specific angelica on their hands to attract fish and game. They called it "hunting and fishing root" (Lawless, 1998). Tribes in Virginia mix angelica with bear's oil and other herbs to rub on the skin to repel lice, fleas, and other biting insects (Vogel, 1970).

East Indian. In India, *A. archangelica* is used to treat symptoms of anorexia nervosa and flatulent dyspepsia (Karnick as reported in Blumenthal et al., 2000).

Russian/Baltic. Russian folk tradition uses the roots, seeds, and leaves of *A. archangelica* for various disorders. It is used to relax smooth muscle spasms and to increase the natural secretions from the stomach and bronchial areas. It is thought that angelica contains a bactericidal substance that suppresses gastric fermentation. The plant is used for its tonic effect on the cardiovascular and nervous systems. It is used to promote the flow of bile into the intestines and the secretion of pancreatic juices. It is also used as a diuretic. Russian folk healers use angelica to treat hysteria, epilepsy, insomnia, and lung conditions. It is used to treat rheumatism and low back pain. The leaves are made into a decoction to help expel intestinal worms (Zevin, 1997).

European. Early Europeans held *A. archangelica* in high esteem and used the plant in pagan festivals. In European traditional herbal medicine, *A. archangelica* has been used to treat symptoms of plague and other diseases. In Germany, *A. archangelica* is listed as an official remedy. It is mainly used as an aromatic and bitter preparation for digestion, to stimulate the appetite, and for symptoms of digestive disturbance. It is used for symptoms related to dysfunctions of the liver, gallbladder, and gastrointestinal tract. Germany has licensed angelica for the treatment of symptoms such as bloating, flatulence, mild gastrointestinal cramps, and insufficient gastric juice (Blumenthal et al., 2000).

Culinary Use

The root of *A. sinensis* is edible. Chinese traditional folk healers believe that the warming, tonifying properties of angelica are accentuated when the root is cooked in soup and other dishes. It has traditionally been added to chicken soup to which other tonic herbs are added and eaten while recovering from illnesses or to improve circulation. Whole roots are also steamed and sliced, then dried. One to two pieces can be eaten daily (McCaleb et al., 2000).

A popular historical recipe calls for using the stems of *A. archangelica* that are cut up and candied with sugar. This sweet is considered a delicacy (Grieve, 1971). Angelica also is used as a flavoring in alcoholic and nonalcoholic beverages, frozen dairy desserts, candy, baked goods, puddings, and gelatins. The dried seeds and powdered roots are used as flavorings for teas (Leung & Foster, 1996).

Cosmetic Use. Extracts of *A. archangelica* are used as a fragrance in soaps, detergents, creams, lotions, and perfumes.

Use in Herbalism

A. archangelica has an interesting history. After the introduction of Christianity, the plant became associated with angels and the springtime celebration of the Annunciation. It was considered to be protective against witchcraft and evil spirits, spells, and enchantments. Angelica has been called "the root of the Holy Ghost" (Grieve, 1971).

It is used to comfort a cold stomach by steeping the root in vinegar and taking it before meals. The root and stalks are used for lung problems such as coughs, shortness of breath, and tuberculosis. It also was used for urinary tract pain, to promote menstrual bleeding, to help expel afterbirth, and for problems with the liver and spleen. The juice or tea is dropped into the eyes to help poor vision and into the ears for deafness. The juice of the plant can be dropped into dental cavities to help relieve toothache. The juice or tea from the plant, or powder of the root is applied to ulcers to promote new skin growth. Preparations of the plant have been used topically for sciatica, gout (Culpeper, 1990), and swelling (Felter & Lloyd, 1983).

The plant has been used for colds, rheumatism, and problems with the kidneys and bladder. Traditionally it has not been given to diabetics because it is believed that it can cause an increase of sugar in the urine. It has been used as a stimulating expectorant, for fevers, and as a diaphoretic. A specific preparation of the roots has been used to treat typhoid fever. The stems were chewed for digestive weakness and flatulence. It was said to help heal bites from mad dogs (Grieve, 1971).

Currently, a common use of *A. archangelica* is as an antispasmodic and cholagogue. It stimulates the secretion of gastric juices and is helpful in loss of appetite, mild spasms of the gastrointestinal tract, flatulence, and bloating. Some herbalists recommend the use of *A. archangelica* root tincture or infusion to promote menstruation if the flow is no more than two weeks overdue. *A. sinensis,* in combination with other herbs, is used for normalizing menstrual periods, especially in young girls. A tea of the root is taken during the days between ovulation and menstruation, and then discontinued from the beginning of the menstrual flow to ovulation (Weed, 1986).

The essential oil of angelica is used for symptoms of all types of nervous debility; as a general restorative; and for those who are timid, weak, and have trouble making decisions. It is said to help those with an unbalanced nervous system (Lawless, 1998). Buckle (1997) reports "tremendous effects" using angelica essential oil topically in the treatment of shock patients in a critical unit where they are protected from exposure to ultraviolet light (p. 199).

BIOMEDICAL EVIDENCE:

No human clinical trials were found on the traditional use of *A. archangelica*. There are some human studies on *A. sinensis*. Although it may be preferable to have clinical studies that investigate a single plant, this profile includes research in which *A. sinensis* is studied in formulation. *A. sinensis* is often used and researched in formulation in the traditional Chinese medical system. In reviewing plant medicine research of formulas rather than single herbs or constituents, the reader must consider the formula as a whole unit of measurement.

Studies Related to Hormone Balance

In a study of 31 females, ages 20 to 34, given *A. sinensis* (30 g) in formulation with *Astragalus membranaceus* (30 g), *Zingiberis officinalis* (3 slices fresh), *Ziziphus jujuba* (10 fruits), *Epimedium sagittatum* (15 g), and *Cuscuta chinensis* (30 g) for thirty days, 9 of 15 women with deficiency type amenorrhea (includes dizziness, weakness, poor appetite, constipation, feeling cold, paleness, and sore lower back), and 10 of 16 with asymptomatic amenorrhea demonstrated marked improvement in symptoms as measured by return of menstruation, recurrence of ovulation, increased hemoglobin level, and increased eosinocyte index of vaginal epithelial cells (indicated increased level of estrogen). Investigators suggest that amenorrhea symptoms improve in women who drink this (tea) formula that tonifies both qi and blood because amenorrhea, especially in women with deficiency symptoms, is related to blood and qi deficiency, not just blood deficiency (Zhiping, Dazeng, Lingyi, & Zuqian, 1986).

Studies Related to Other Health Patterns

No data are available at this time.

Mechanism of Action

Although the study by Zhiping et al. (1986) demonstrated an estrogen effect of angelica in formulation on vaginal cells, *A. sinensis*, used alone, does not seem to affect estrogen levels in humans (Hirata, Swiersz, Zell, Small, & Ettinger, 1997). The Chinese have known for years that angelica's effect in women is not related to any plant hormone activity. *A. sinensis* does have an effect on the uterus, however.

It both stimulates and relaxes the uterus. The volatile oil component of the plant is believed to be responsible for the relaxing effect on the uterus and a nonvolatile component seems to stimulate the uterus (Zhu, 1987). Ligustilide may be the active constituent in the essential oil, which is able to inhibit the smooth muscle of the uterus (Qi-bing et al., 1991).

A. sinensis' vitamin B_{12} and folic acid content, although less than daily requirements, could explain its use in Chinese medicine as a blood tonic. *A. sinensis* also contains ferulic acid, which is thought to account for the herb's antithrombotic activity (Qi-bing et al., 1991). Ferulic acid, one of the chemicals in angelica, is thought to increase sperm motility and viability (Rister, 1999). *A. archangelica* contains fifteen compounds that act like calcium channel blockers, which may account for angelica's ability to relieve pain associated with angina (Duke, 1997).

USE IN PREGNANCY OR LACTATION:

The use of *A. sinensis* and *A. archangelica* is contraindicated during pregnancy. They are known to stimulate and relax the uterus, thereby possibly interfering with pregnancy or diminishing effective labor (Brinker, 1998; McGuffin et al., 1997). Traditionally, midwives use angelica to facilitate the birth of an adhered placenta by using a single dose of 30 to 50 drops of the root tincture under the tongue. It is reported that uterine contractions should resume within fifteen minutes and the placenta should be delivered promptly. If contractions do not resume after the initial dose, the dose is repeated (Weed, 1986).

There are no known restrictions for using *A. archangelica* during lactation (Blumenthal et al., 2000).

Herbal Caveat—Pregnancy or Lactation

Some herbs are contraindicated in pregnancy because of a risk of the herb or one of its constituents stimulating the uterus and therefore possibly promoting fetal loss. Many herbal practitioners do not recommend herbal remedies, in particular oral doses of herbs, during the first trimester of pregnancy and seek an alternative. However, herbs are successfully used during pregnancy, especially to prepare the body for the birth. Herbs are relatively unstudied in pregnancy and lactation, so patients need to be made aware through education of the potential benefits and risks of using herbs for health conditions that arise during pregnancy or lactation. The use of herbal remedies during pregnancy often warrants a referral to a knowledgeable herbal practitioner.

USE FOR CHILDREN:

The fluid extract (1.5 to 3 g of 1:1 g/ml) or tincture (1.5 g of 1:5 g/ml) of the root of *A. archangelica* is given to children for discomfort related to gastrointestinal problems and loss of appetite. No contraindications have been reported in children (Schilcher, 1992).

CAUTIONS:

Certain substances known as furanocoumarins that are present in *A. archangelica* may sensitize the skin to sunlight and cause inflammation with sun exposure. Although these substances (also known as "psoralens") may help the person with psoriasis if they sit in the sun for a short period of time, it is generally recommended to avoid prolonged sun bathing and exposure to intense ultraviolet radiation while using *A. archangelica* topically (Blumenthal et al., 2000; Duke, 1997). Photosensitivity with angelica essential oil only occurs with topical applications—not when inhaling (Buckle, 1997).

From animal studies, scientists conclude that *A. sinensis*, when taken with warfarin at steady state, exhibits a pharmacodynamic but not a pharmacokinetic interaction (Page & Lawrence, 1999). Excessive doses of *A. archangelica* may interfere with anticoagulant therapy because of the coumarin content; however, the mechanism of interaction between warfarin and angelica is unknown (Newall et al., 1996; Page & Lawrence, 1999).

Do not use *A. sinensis* tincture for insufficient menstrual flow because it may act to further decrease the flow (Rister, 1999).

A. archangelica can lose its volatile oil if the root is not used within eighteen months of being cut (as reported in Blumenthal et al., 2000).

NURSING EVIDENCE:

Historical Nursing Use
No data are available at this time.

Potential Nursing Applications
Young women with serious menstrual and premenstrual discomfort often go without help. They are expected to learn to cope with the pain associated with menstruation. Angelica root tea can often help relieve these young women's monthly discomfort. School and pediatric nurses may want to consider developing a referral base with local Chinese or western herbalists who can create a tea to help these

young women. Getting young women to cook their own medicinal tea under the guidance of their mothers not only leads to pain relief, but also can help to reestablish a highly successful, centuries-old healing tradition practiced by women of caring for themselves, other women, and their daughters.

Nurses also might consider the use of the essential oil in caring for postoperative patients. Some patients who have elective open-heart surgery can experience postoperative psychosis characterized by tachycardia, hyperventilation, disorientation, paranoid delusions, and auditory hallucinations. Presurgery discussion between the patient and nurse about what to expect after surgery may help the patient cope better postoperatively. This discussion could include allowing the patient to choose an essential oil they find pleasant and relaxing that would be used as aromatherapy after surgery. The essential oil of *A. archangelica* root may be inhaled to reduce the symptoms of postpump depression and promote sleep and has been used by nurses to ease the transitions occurring during the postoperative period (Buckle, 1997).

Integrative Insight

Little evidence supports the traditional use of angelica for conditions that biomedically relate to hormone balance. Some scientific studies have shown that angelica, at least by itself, does not have any estrogen-like effects, yet it does seem to affect processes in the body related to hormone balance. It is important that nurses continue to explore the use of angelica and its lengthy tradition of use in women.

Understanding how to help women maintain balance in their lives is very difficult in a fast-paced modern world. The Chinese understand the concept of balance from a tradition founded in the principles of Taoism—the balance of yin and yang, masculine and feminine. While the yang or masculine principle is associated with heat, light, and moving outward, the yin or feminine principle is associated with cold, dark, and a spiraling inward. Womanhood traditionally has been associated with "keeping the hearth" at home, a yin activity. Women who constantly go outward (e.g., work, exercise classes, and social activities) need to remember to have time to go inward and rekindle their inner (yin) nature. This does not mean that women must stay in the home. It just means that women must have periods for inward reflection.

Traditional Chinese herbalists are taught that the first step in healing is to look at the patient's lifestyle and consider with the patient what changes might effect a change in overall health. After consideration of lifestyle, then diet is considered. After dietary changes are made, if there is still a need, then the practitioner recommends herbs to the patient. The successful traditional use of *A. sinensis* must be understood not only from a scientific standpoint—hormone balance—but also from the cultural perspective of the balance of yin and yang.

Many nurses realize the importance of understanding the cycles of each female patient from a broader perspective and are helping their patients be more attuned to their lifestyle practices and their own cycles and rhythms, such as occur with the menstrual cycle. The menstrual cycle does not just represent a time for the flow of blood, but it also represents a time to "come forth." The cycle before the menses represents a time of accumulation of essence (blood) and a preparation for going forth. It is a time for inward focus and contemplation.

For years, in suggesting the use of a formula including *A. sinensis* for various female patients, I have found that the healing experienced by the patient is quite profound when I adhere to the principle of lifestyle first, then diet and herbs and remember to discuss the concept of the patient attending to her life cycles and how she guards her time for inward reflection. With this focus, the patients experience angelica decoction working at mental, emotional, and spiritual levels, as well as at the physical level.

THERAPEUTIC APPLICATIONS:

Oral

A. archangelica. Unless otherwise prescribed, it is recommended to take about 1 teaspoon (3 to 5 g) daily of the cut dried root or other preparations of *A. archangelica.*

Dried Root. ¼ to ½ teaspoon (1 to 2 g) three times daily

Decoction. Place ¼ teaspoon (1.5 g) of the finely cut root into 5 to 6 ounces (150 to 250 ml) of cold water.

Infusion. Steep ½ to ¾ teaspoons (2 to 4 g) of the root in 5 ounces (150 ml) of boiled water for approximately ten minutes.

Tincture. 1:5 (g/ml): Take up to about ½ teaspoon (0.5 to 2.0 ml) three times daily (Blumenthal et al., 2000).

A. sinensis. Doses vary when formulated by TCM herbalists. The suggested dosages in the following sections are for use as single herb.

Dried Root (or as a Tea). ¼ to ½ teaspoon (1 to 2 g) three times daily

Tincture. 1:5: ½ to 1 teaspoon (3 to 5 ml) three times daily

Solid Extract. 4:1: 125 to 500 mg three times daily (Werbach & Murray, 1994)

Topical

Essential Oil of Angelica. Six drops can be added to 1 tablespoon (15 ml) of almond oil and used during massage to stimulate circulation and nerves (Lawless, 1998).

Environmental

Five to 10 drops added to the bath is said to help mental fatigue, migraine, headaches, nervous depression, and debility. Drops of the essential oil can be added to a vaporizer to create an uplifting, purifying incense for meditation, to promote respiration, and to prevent the spread of infection (Lawless, 1998).

Herbal Caveat—Therapeutic Applications

In traditional and conventional herbal medicine, amounts of herbs given to patients are based on individual needs. The amounts or "doses" recorded here are provided so that the health practitioner has a general idea of the amounts recommended for an adult patient. Dosing in herbalism not only refers to amount of plant used but also includes when, where, and how to take a plant medicine. These dosages should not be used as guidelines for indiscriminate intervention without proper assessment, critical thinking, and patient education on the part of the practitioner.

Note: Please see chapter 5 for detailed descriptions of how to prepare various applications.

PATIENT INTERACTION:

There are numerous species of angelica, so be sure to learn about the plant you are considering for use. If you are thinking about using angelica for menstrual complaints or other disorders related to a woman's reproductive system, and you are planning to use angelica for more than two weeks, it is best to seek the assistance of a Chinese or western herbalist. Over the course of centuries in China, angelica has been found to best be used in formulations (tea) with other herbs in which the medicinal benefits of each of the individual herbs is multiplied (synergy) because they are combined. Traditional Chinese herbalists specialize in formulating teas specifically for each patient.

Herbal Caveat—Patient Interaction

Patients considering the use of an herb or formula of herbs in self-care benefit from education about the plant itself and the use of the plant in healing. This education can come through many sources, including local herbalists; plant specialists such as botanists; health practitioners such as nurses, nutritionists, naturopaths, and other physicians; and various written references including the scientific literature. Patients need to remember that their unique health care needs are not necessarily represented in any literature they may encounter. Therefore, it is recommended that a knowledgeable mentor be consulted before initiating self-care with any herb being used for the first time.

NURTURING THE NURSE-PLANT RELATIONSHIP:

Note: You may want to keep a journal of your experiences with the herb.

(Caution: It is best not to try this when you have diarrhea.) For this experience, *A. sinensis*, the species used to tonify and move blood in TCM, is used. Find a Chinese herb pharmacy near your home or contact an herb store, such as the one below, and purchase a small amount of the dried root. The dried sliced root is a golden color. Be sure to clearly identify the herb you purchase by reading the label in Latin and Chinese. Reflect for a moment on how much time and energy it took for this root to form. Put approximately ¼ ounce (9 g) of whole, dried root into a small saucepan and rinse the herb thoroughly with cool water. Cover the herb with water and bring it almost to a boil. Take the pot off the stove, cover the pan with a lid, and let it sit for two hours. After presoaking, the root will have expanded. Add enough water to cover the herb with water by at least 1 inch (2.5 cm). Put the pot back on the stove and gently simmer the herb (steam rising from the water but not boiling) for about two hours. The decoction or tea from the herb can be drunk and the herb can be eaten in small amounts.

The decoction of *A. sinensis* is bitter, sweet, and spicy. Prepare for your herb tasting the way students of Chinese herbal medicine do by centering and meditating before the tasting. During the tasting, sit quietly and observe your body's response to the herb. Where do you feel the herb going in your body? Is the herb energetically cold, hot, or somewhere in between? How does the herb taste—sweet, sour, pungent, salty, astringent, or a combination? How do you feel after the tasting? Record your experience.

You also can add a few drops of *A. archangelica* essential oil to your bath. Breathe deeply as you relax in the tub. Reflect on the experience of tasting angelica and how the experience of feeling and smelling angelica differs from the tasting experience.

A. sinensis can be ordered from the following company:
Nuherbs
3820 Penniman Avenue
Oakland, CA 94619
800-233-4307
Fax: 800-550-1928
www.nuherbs.com

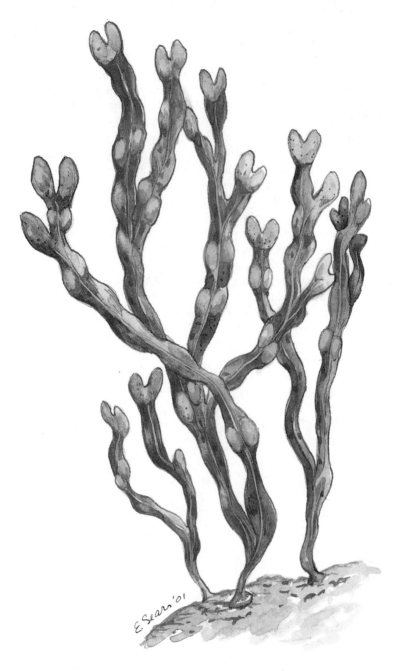

Fucus vesiculosus

Kelp

- **LATIN NAMES:** *Nereocystis luetkeana, Laminaria japonica, Macro-cystic pyrifera*

  Class: Phaeophyceae (Brown Algae); Orders: Fucoles (Fucus, Sargassum) and Laminariales (Laminaria, Nereocystis, Macrocystis)

- **FAMILY NAMES:** Sargassaceae (Sargassum), Lessoniaceae (Macrocystis)

- **COMMON NAMES:** Kelp, bladderwrack (Fucus), sea-wrack (Fucus)

- **HEALTH PATTERN:** Hormone balance

- **PLANT DESCRIPTION:**

Carrageenan, algin, and sodium/calcium alginate are often recognized as substances used either in commercial or medical arenas. Kelp is the common name often given to a group of perennial seaweeds with large, flat, leaflike fronds that are usually found attached to rocks in the ocean. Kelp often refers to *Nereocystis luetkeana* and also has been used in reference to other genera of plants, including Macrocystis, Fucus, and Laminaria, and Sargassum. The kelp plant is one of the fastest growing large plants in the world. The long strips of kelp are like leaves and are called lamina. There are bulbs on the lamina that are full of carbon monoxide as are the hollow stalks that are like stems. The carbon monoxide gas in the bulbs serves the purpose of allowing the lamina to float to the surface of the ocean where the plant can photosynthesize and then reproduce. The stocks can grow up to 90 feet (30 meters) long and the lamina another 60 feet (20 meters). The root is a flat disk.

Because of its incredible metabolism, kelp can become quite hot, but does not self-decompose because of its cooling environment, the ocean water. If you ever try putting some kelp inside your boots while walking the beach, steam may start to come out of your boots! The heat generated by the plant makes it an excellent compost activator, too. The cells that produce the slimy mucopolysaccharide substance in the plant are like the goblet cells in the human throat. These brown algae have the pigments fucoxanthin, chlorophyll *a* and *c,* and carotenes. They use laminarin as a storage product and contain the gels algin and fucoidan. Seaweeds are highly clathritic, meaning that they absorb the nutrients they need from the seawater.

- **PLANT PART USED:** The characteristic plant body of the seaweed, known as the thallus, that lacks distinct leaves and stems like land plants

TRADITIONAL EVIDENCE:

Cultural Use

Asian. The seaweed Sargassum, or "hai zao," is classified as salty, cold, and bitter in TCM and is used to clear heat and phlegm conditions. It is used for the treatment of symptoms often related to diagnoses of both hypothyroidism and hyperthyroidism. Sargassum also is used to reduce neck nodules, to promote urination, reduce edema, and to help pain associated with hernia disorders (Bensky & Gamble, 1993).

In Japanese herbal medicine, kelp is taken internally to reduce sticky phlegm that interferes with normal breathing. It also is used to reduce lymph accumulation in the neck that causes swellings. Kelp is thought to gently enhance urination and relieve swellings throughout the body. It is used as a gentle laxative because up to 45% of its weight consists of a complex carbohydrate that swells in the presence of water.

North American Indian. Common kelp *(Nereocystis)* was used as a topical dressing for burns by some North American Indian tribes. It also was used topically for wounds and for nonpigmented spots on the skin. Kelp has been dried, powdered, and rubbed into children's heads to encourage hair growth. It has been used to make a skin cream for protection from the sun, wind, and cold. Some tribes have used the dried, salty strips as an expectorant by sucking on the stalks when they have colds and sore throats. This method also is used to clear mucus. Kelp also has been used as a food source by eating it with herring roe. The enlarged upper portion of the plant is large enough to be used as a container for oil and other liquids. It was used as a mold into which melted fat-based medicinal ointments were poured. After the fat hardened, the mold was cut open and the ball of ointment removed for use (Moerman, 1998).

Eskimos traditionally eat large amounts of *Laminaria* and other seaweeds and are known to have a low breast cancer rate (Teas, 1983).

Australian. Off the coast of Tasmania and Victoria live huge kelp forests that have been called the rainforests of the sea. No data are available at this time on the medicinal use of kelp in this region.

European. German health authorities do not recommend kelp for any therapeutic purpose (Foster & Tyler, 1999).

Culinary Use

A gel-forming agent known as algin is obtained from brown algaes such as *Laminaria* and *Macrocystis*. It is used in the dairy and baking industries to improve food texture, body, and smoothness of their products (Newall et al., 1996). Algin is used in almost every category of food product and therefore may be eaten as much as once a day by some people. In Asia, kelp is used to flavor soups. Asian cooks toast seaweeds until crisp, then grind them into a powder to sprinkle over foods as a condiment. Toasted sesame seeds are sometimes added before grinding (Kushi, 1993).

The seaweed nori is perhaps the best known by people who do not routinely ingest sea vegetables. It is used to wrap sushi (rice formed into little rolls often with fish or vegetables inside and then sliced horizontally). Nori is a Porphyra, different from the kelp discussed here. The vitamin C content of nori is greater than that of raw oranges. Ireland and Wales have traditionally eaten nori, as have the Asian cultures.

Use in Herbalism

Kelp contains an essential trace element, iodine, that is required for normal functioning of the thyroid gland. It has been determined that the total amount of iodine present in the human body ranges from 20 to 50 mg, of which 60% to 80% is present in the thyroid gland. Iodine is recommended by health care practitioners for symptoms associated with iodine deficiency disorders such as goiter and hypothyroidism. Iodine also is given to prevent goiter disease in areas of the world where the diet or soil is deficient in iodine. The only abundant, naturally occurring sources of iodine are in seaweeds and sea vegetables. Vegetables grown on land have very minute amounts of iodine compared to those found in the ocean (McGuffin et al., 1997). Kelp, depending upon when it is harvested, can have 100 to 500 times more iodine than shellfish. Kelp and other sea vegetables are food sources with a rich mineral content. For example, sea vegetables such as hijiki and wakame contain more than 10 times the calcium in milk, and wakame and kelp contain four times the iron in beef (Pitchford, 1993).

Kelp is used medicinally for its ability to balance hormonal activity of the thyroid. It is often used in herbalism for the treatment of symptoms related to hypothyroidism and obesity. It also has been used as a blood purifier and for atherosclerosis, rheumatism, and benign and malignant tumors (Felter & Lloyd, 1983). It is believed to help these conditions because its mucilage content is very absorptive of toxins in the bowel. The algin from the plant also is used in making the material used to make dental impressions.

BIOMEDICAL EVIDENCE:

There are two major uses for kelp in relation to hormone balance. One is the centuries-old use of kelp as a mechanical way of dilating the cervix in women during labor or for purposes of abortion. The other use of kelp is in relation to improving the hormone balance of the thyroid. Studies regarding these two effects are presented here. Identifying information regarding the plants used in these studies is often lacking in the reporting of the data.

Studies Related to Hormone Balance

Several recent studies have compared various methods for cervical ripening, a process associated with hormonal action. One randomized controlled study comparing *Laminaria* tent, prostaglandin E_2 gel, and extra-amniotic saline for labor induction found no differences in cesarean section rate among all three. Saline infusion was found to result in significantly shorter labor. This study showed that prostaglandin gel was not as successful as *Laminaria* or saline infusion. Identified advantages of *Laminaria* include low cost, ease of placement, and the ability to remove the substance quickly. As a result of the study, saline infusion was accepted as the primary method of cervical ripening (Guinn, Goepfert, Christine, Owen, & Hauth, 2000).

Another randomized trial found that *Laminaria* was comparable to saline infusion in terms of fetal and maternal morbidity but that saline infusion was preferable to *Laminaria* tent because it works more quickly (Lin, Kupferminc, & Dooley, 1995). *Laminaria* tents also have been used successfully in the cervical dilation of female oncology patients undergoing radiation treatments when general anesthesia is contraindicated because of high risk of complication. Complication rates are extremely low with the use of *Laminaria* (Peeples, Given, & Bakri, 1983).

In a study of two women with a history of cervical stenosis undergoing embryo transfer (ET), *Laminaria* tent placement was shown to be a safe and effective option for dilating the cervix. The *Laminaria* can be placed easily without significant discomfort, factors that are very important to the success of the ET procedure (Glatstein, Pang, & McShane, 1997).

Studies in coastal areas such as Japan where kelp proliferates have shown that the prevalence of hypothyroidism in iodine sufficient areas may be associated with the amount of iodine ingested (Konno, Makita, Yuri, Iizuka, & Kawasaki, 1994). Case studies also have reported that when excessive intake of seaweed (genus and species not reported) is stopped, goiter and hyperthyroidism, and/or weight loss resolve (Liewendahl & Gordin, 1974; Shilo & Hirsch, 1986; Tajiri, Higashi, Morita, Umeda, & Sato, 1986).

One animal study showed that kelp, *Laminaria japonica,* when ingested may have a protective effect on the thyroid and prevent internal radiation injury and carcinogenesis in the thyroid (Maruyama & Yamamoto, 1992).

Studies Related to Other Health Patterns

Restoration. Kelp and its constituent sodium alginate have been shown to effectively reduce the absorption of heavy metals and radiation, such as strontium 90 and cesium, in humans. The kelp absorbs the radioactive substance or heavy metal and carries it out in the stool.

In a human trial of 40 people in which 10 ingested stable strontium, sodium alginate from *Sargassum siliquastrum* (12 to 15 g of 2% solution in orange syrup or 6% in bread) was found to significantly reduce absorption of radiostrontium, a hazardous nuclide that has a half-life of twenty-nine years (Yifeng et al., 1991).

A review of animal in vivo studies have shown that hot water extracts of *Laminaria* and *Sargassum* demonstrate significant tumor inhibition effects, in particular with Ehrlich ascites carcinoma and Sarcoma 180 tumors (as reported in Teas, 1983).

As seaweeds have been shown to have the ability to scavenge hydroxyl radicals, *Sargassum* has demonstrated high antioxidative activity in vitro (Yan, Nagata, & Fan, 1998).

Skin. Calcium alginate dressings have been used extensively in the treatment of exuding pressure and leg ulcers. Eleven patients in one study of calcium alginate dressing use for exuding wounds reported significantly less discomfort with dressing changes, especially in those patients with lower extremity ulcerations. In addition to the increased comfort to the patient, calcium alginate dressings were found to be easy to use, conforming to the wound surface, and absorptive without macerating healthy surrounding tissue (McMullen, 1991).

Mechanism of Action

The mechanism of action of kelp relates directly to the personality or qualities of the plant itself. The seaweed receives its own nourishment from the seawater by being able to absorb nutrients from the passing water. Kelp also swells considerably when in the presence of water. In the body, one of kelp's therapeutic actions is related to the algin, a viscous fiber found in the plant, and its ability to absorb water and remove toxins (and possibly minerals too) from the digestive tract.

Kelp, specifically *Laminaria japonica,* has been used for more than a century for cervical ripening. The *Laminaria* tent, when placed in the cervix, extracts water from the cervical tissue and swells to three to four times its original diameter causing the cervix to expand as well. Maximal dilation usually occurs within six to twelve hours. "Mechanical stimulation or irritation of the cervix has been shown to trigger endogenous prostaglandin synthesis and release, which reduces cervical stiffness and thus helps cervical ripening and labor induction" (Summers, 1997, p. 78). Kelp contains significant quantities of iodine, calcium, and potassium. Kelp also is known to contain heavy metals such as arsenic, lead, and mercury. The heavy metals are in biologically unavailable forms and are fully excreted from the body in sixty hours (Fukui, Hirayama, Nohara, & Sakagami, 1981). Potassium alginate, the potassium salt of algin, acts as a scavenger in the digestive tract, a demulcent, and a hypotensive agent.

The iodine content in kelp is believed to be responsible for correcting the function of hypothyroid disorders and also to temporarily improve the symptoms of hyperthyroidism (Bensky & Gamble, 1993). Kelp's algin content forms a gel in the intestines that soothes the lining of the intestines and acts to soften the stool. It is believed that the algin's bulk-producing effect decreases bowel transit time, which decreases the time that harmful estrogens are present in the intestines. Decreased bowel transit can result in less estrogen being absorbed back into the bloodstream and thereby potentially decreasing the risk of breast cancer (Teas, 1983).

USE IN PREGNANCY OR LACTATION:

It is recommended to avoid excessive consumption of iodine (kelp is rich in iodine) during pregnancy because infantile goiter has been observed (McGuffin et al., 1997). Some midwives advocate the moderate use of kelp as a food source of iron and calcium during pregnancy (Weed, 1986). Kelp also is used in cervical dilation.

Herbal Caveat—Pregnancy or Lactation

Some herbs are contraindicated in pregnancy because of a risk of the herb or one of its constituents stimulating the uterus and therefore possibly promoting fetal loss. Many herbal practitioners do not recommend herbal remedies, in particular oral doses of herbs, during the first trimester of pregnancy and seek an alternative. However, herbs are successfully used during pregnancy, especially to prepare the body for the birth. Herbs are relatively unstudied in pregnancy and lactation, so patients need to be made aware through education of the potential benefits and risks of using herbs for health conditions that arise during pregnancy or lactation. The use of herbal remedies during pregnancy often warrants a referral to a knowledgeable herbal practitioner.

USE FOR CHILDREN:

Excessive ingestion of seaweeds by children is not advised because of the possibility of causing hyperthyroidism or hypothyroidism (Newall et al., 1996); however, children can eat kelp in small amounts, in soups or as a condiment with rice, for instance.

Herbal Caveat—Children

Children have special needs in regard to herbal therapies. They require lesser amounts of herbs and often respond well to mild teas and topical applications such as compresses and baths. The lowest dose of oral preparations should be tried first before increasing the amount given children. Caregivers should observe children closely for responses to herbal remedies. Younger children, particularly infants, have traditionally been given herbs either through their mother's breast milk or in the form of a homeopathic remedy because of their sensitivity to medicines and treatments and the immaturity of their liver. It is recommended that a person knowledgeable in the herbal treatment of children be consulted before the offering of any herb to a child for the first time.

Both a deficiency and an excess of iodine in the diet can cause a variety of health concerns associated with the thyroid gland. Some of these symptoms include goiter; irritation of the eyes; severe skin eruptions; inflammation of the mouth, throat, and gastrointestinal tract; diarrhea; and increased salivation (McGuffin et al., 1997). The use of kelp is contraindicated in those with excess thyroid activity because of the high iodine content that could further stimulate the thyroid (Brinker, 1998). Too much iodine can inhibit thyroid activity. It seems that constant consumption of kelp will first stimulate, then deplete, thyroid function. Therefore, to avoid consuming too much iodine, it is suggested that kelp not be eaten every day. Iodine also has been associated with acnelike skin eruptions and the aggravation of preexisting acne (Newall et al., 1996). Eat kelp in moderation, such as using it for the stock for miso soup or as a condiment.

The iodine content in seaweeds may interfere with existing treatment for hypothyroid or hyperthyroid conditions. For example, Japanese physicians instruct their patients not to eat seaweeds one to two weeks before radioactive iodine uptake tests because kelp can prevent radiation uptake by the thyroid (Maruyama & Yamamoto, 1992).

Kelp supplements have been sold for many years. The kelp used in these tablets and powders is harvested en masse by large barges that go through the ocean water cutting the kelp much the way a lawnmower cuts grass. Because the kelp is put into the barge and it has such a high metabolic rate, formalin is used to keep the kelp from decomposing. Those who are chemically sensitive may want to be careful to purchase kelp in as whole a form as possible for which preservatives have not been necessary. Fresh kelp powder should be greenish in color, not brown. Because of the clathritic nature of kelp and its ability to easily absorb chemicals from its environment, it is best to purchase plant product that has been harvested as far away as possible from sewer outfalls, industrial sites, and mining operations. Also, kelp in tablet form contains varying amounts of iodine because the iodine evaporates during storage (Liewendahl & Gordin, 1974). People should drink plenty of water when adding sea vegetables to their diet. In TCM, kelp (Sargassum) is contraindicated when using licorice root (Bensky & Gamble, 1993).

NURSING EVIDENCE:

Historical Nursing Use

Nurses have used algin dressings in the care of wounds and midwives have historically used *Laminaria* tents for cervical dilation.

Potential Nursing Applications

In addition to the use of calcium alginate dressings for exuding wounds and the use of *Laminaria* for cervical dilation, nurses may want to consider researching the protective effects of kelp against radioactive substances such as strontium and cesium. Nurses are involved in interdisciplinary work related to preventing disasters associated with biologic and chemical warfare and can consider creating protocols for evaluating radioactivity levels and exposure in patients. Because they are not easily perceived with the five senses, radioactive substances are rarely thought of as a possible cause of illness. Although Chernobyl disasters do not happen everyday, because of technologic advances, radioactive fallout poses a clear and present danger to human health. Nurses not only need to know about the dangers but also the potential antidotes. Kelp has been shown to successfully remove toxic substances, such as strontium and cesium, from the body.

Integrative Insight

Kelp is a clear example of the importance of knowing the nature or personality of a plant to understanding its medicinal benefit. Kelp's clathritic nature, its ability to absorb fluid and nutrients from its environment, provides a signature for its action in the body. Kelp has demonstrated health benefits to humans, most importantly the ability to remove heavy metals and radioactive toxins from the body without harming the body in the process. Its ability to absorb fluid from its environment has made it effective in cervical dilation and wound care. Biomedical evidence shows that the rich iodine content in kelp does affect thyroid function and therefore weight. Weight loss and weight gain also fit with the signature of kelp's ability to expand (absorb and swell) and contract (pull out). Kelp demonstrates how the plant's nature alone can help define its safe and responsible use. Biomedical evidence shows that excessive use of kelp can upset hormone balance, in particular within the thyroid. Therefore it is important for patients and practitioners to work together to decide on the appropriate use of this plant for the individual.

THERAPEUTIC APPLICATIONS:

Oral

Whether you use whole or powdered kelp, take it with lots of water and start with the smallest amounts. A water extraction of Kelp, in particular *Laminaria,* can be used as the stock for making miso soup rather than using plain water.

Fresh Plant. ¼ to ½ cup daily

Dried Plant. Dried kelp powder should be green in color, which denotes freshness. Take up to 2 to 4 teaspoons daily (Pedersen, 1998).

Infusion. 5 to 20 drops every three hours for bladder irritation (Felter & Lloyd, 1983)

Topical

Algin from seaweeds is used in facial masks, creams, and lotions. Facial masks can be used to revitalize and soften the skin.

Environmental

Seaweed baths are very revitalizing to the skin. Kelp is also used for its ability to remove harmful environmental toxins such as radioactive strontium and cesium from the human body without harming the body.

Herbal Caveat—Therapeutic Applications

In traditional and conventional herbal medicine, amounts of herbs given to patients are based on individual needs. The amounts or "doses" recorded here are provided so that the health practitioner has a general idea of the amounts recommended for an adult patient. Dosing in herbalism not only refers to amount of plant used but also includes when, where, and how to take a plant medicine. These dosages should not be used as guidelines for indiscriminate intervention without proper assessment, critical thinking, and patient education on the part of the practitioner.

Note: Please see chapter 5 for detailed descriptions of how to prepare various applications.

PATIENT INTERACTION:

Kelp can be a healthy addition to a rotation diet. It has lots of minerals and is able to remove toxic substances such as radioactive strontium and cesium from the human body. It is best to begin eating sea vegetables in small amounts, such as a crushed whole herb condiment, with lots of water so that the body can get used to metabolizing them. Do not eat excessive amounts of kelp. Macrobiotic cookbooks have excellent condiment recipes. It takes up to four months for the body to adjust to digesting sea vegetables, so be sure to chew them thoroughly. Stop eating kelp if excessive weight loss; goiter; irritation of the eyes; severe skin eruptions; inflammation of the mouth, throat, and gastrointestinal tract; diarrhea; or increased salivation occur. Do not eat kelp if you have a known hyperthyroid condition (goiter). It is best to eat kelp from a known source because kelp readily absorbs pollutants from its environment.

Herbal Caveat—Patient Interaction

Patients considering the use of an herb or formula of herbs in self-care benefit from education about the plant itself and the use of the plant in healing. This education can come through many sources, including local herbalists; plant specialists such as botanists; health practitioners such as nurses, nutritionists, naturopaths, and other physicians; and various written references including the scientific literature. Patients need to remember that their unique health care needs are not necessarily represented in any literature they may encounter. Therefore, it is recommended that a knowledgeable mentor be consulted before initiating self-care with any herb being used for the first time.

NURTURING THE NURSE-PLANT RELATIONSHIP:

Note: You may want to keep a journal of your experiences with the herb.

There are many ways to get to know kelp. It is always best to learn about the plant in its natural state, so if you live near an ocean, try finding a piece of kelp that may have just washed ashore. It is often easiest to find some after a storm. Open one of the bubbles on the frond and hear and smell the carbon monoxide as it escapes. Feel the sliminess of the plant. Try putting some in your shoes and feel the heat of the plant grow as you walk the beach.

If you have never eaten kelp or any sea vegetables and you'd like to try some, start off slowly as it takes the body up to three to four months to adjust to the addition of marine plant polysaccharides in the digestive tract. Get some dried brown algae such as kombu *(Laminaria)* or wakame *(Undaria),* preferably whole pieces rather than powder, and soak the seaweed for a few minutes. You can add the kombu to a pot of rice you are cooking and taste it afterward. After soaking, wakame is bright green in color and can be thinly sliced and added to miso soup (see recipe in soy profile). You must chew the sea vegetables thoroughly or they will expand exponentially and be excreted pretty much in the same form in which they are ingested. It is important to drink plenty of plain water when eating kelp or sea vegetables in any form.

Nori, although not a kelp, is a fun sea vegetable to taste. It can be purchased in flat sheets that can be lightly cooked over the flame on a gas stove. This crisps the nori and then it can be eaten as a crunchy snack or crumbled and used as a condiment for rice and land vegetables. Nori is the sea vegetable that is used to wrap sushi. Don't forget to read the labels on the foods you buy. If the food has carrageenan, agar, or algin in it, you are eating seaweed!

CHAPTER 9
Immune Response

INTRODUCTION

NURSES, DATING BACK TO THE TIME OF FLORENCE Nightingale and earlier, in their careful observation of health patterns, have recognized that not all people exposed to an identical illness become sick. This same phenomenon occurs when people are exposed to a microorganism that is said to be the cause of a particular infectious disease. Even though people are exposed and perhaps even interact immunologically with a particular pathogen, there is no assurance that the person will contract a disease. What makes one person contract an infectious disease and another not? The answer has to do with a person's immune response.

The leading theory regarding infectious disease dates back to the late 1800s and Louis Pasteur and holds the view that disease is caused by a microbe or invader from outside the body. It also includes that the microbe only ever had one form, a theory known as "monomorphism" (Enby, Gosch, & Sheehan, 1990). This view has been supported, for example, by the evidence that practitioners' washing their hands in between patients results in fewer deaths related to care. This was important during the time of Ignaz Semmelweis who suggested that residents disinfect their hands with chlorinated water after examining cadavers and before examining pregnant women.

Scientists such as Antoine Bechamp (a contemporary of Pasteur), Max Gruber, and Guenther Enderlein challenged the concept of monomorphism and believed that microorganisms actually evolve and go through different stages of development, a theory known as "pleomorphism" (Enby et al., 1990). Enderlein's theory states that in early development, the body's immune response to microorganisms is harmonious and even health promoting. It is only later, when and if the body's internal environment changes, that the microbes are "forced to advance to later stages of growth in order to survive and can become pathogenic and lead to disease" (Enby et al., 1990, p. 13). This concept of changing microbes originating inside the body is contrary to the monomorphous theory of Pasteur and others who believed that disease is caused by bacteria already in existence that invade from outside the body. Florence Nightingale (1980) herself in *Notes on Nursing* seemed to take a position on infectious disease closer to the pleomorphic position. She wrote, "Is it not living in a continual mistake to look upon diseases, as we do now, as separate entities, which must exist like cats and dogs instead of looking upon them as conditions like a dirty and a clean condition, and just as much under our own control; or rather as the reactions of kindly nature, against the conditions in which we have placed ourselves" (p. 23).

Disease is a condition that is not fully understood. Immune response, the reaction of the body to such things as viruses and microbes either inside or outside the body, also is not fully understood. Nurses often observe that there are more variables influencing the development of disease and when and how the immune system responds, than the type and presence of a particular microbe. For instance, the research of psychoneuroimmunologists such as Dr. Candace Pert (1997) shows that viruses use the same receptors as neuropeptides to enter a cell. A virus that fits that receptor will have an easier or harder time getting into the cell, depending on how much of the peptide for a particular receptor is around. In her research, Pert has linked neuropeptides to emotions. Pert (1997) writes, "Immune cells are making the same chemicals that we conceive of as controlling mood in the brain. . . . Because the molecules of emotion are involved in the process of a virus entering a cell, it seems logical to assume that the state of our emotions will affect whether or not we succumb to viral infection" (pp. 183, 190). Emotions and neuropeptides' receptors are just two of the other variables potentially involved in immune response.

Physicians, nurses, and researchers wonder about the immune response of the body, how people develop disease, and how they stay healthy despite the presence of microbes thought to cause disease. Herbalists too have made observations of people's differences and similarities in immune response, especially in regard to the use of herbs. Herbs have been known throughout history to somehow protect individuals from disease. For example, it is said that many perfumers, such as those in Bucklersbury, England, escaped the plague. In Bucklersbury, this phenomenon was said to be due to the town's position as the center of the lavender trade (Keville & Green, 1995). The herbs included in this chapter—goldenseal, echinacea, elder, garlic, sage, thyme, and onion—all have demonstrated a prominent influence on the health pattern, immune response.

Nurses entering the world of healing plants must remember that herbs are not exactly like the pharmaceutical antibiotics with which they are familiar. Although herbs do not necessarily kill, attack, or destroy microbes, this does not mean that herbs cannot or do not somehow affect the cell structure of microbes in some way. However, they may influence the immune response in a manner similar to that of the pleomorphic perspective. Herbs may alter the "terrain" or inner environment of the body in such a way that disease just does not occur, a concept similar to the idea that emotions affect neuropeptide receptors and therefore viruses just may not find a cell with which to merge. It is important to explore medicinal plants with the possibility that their effect on immune response may not fit with conventional biomedical understanding. There may be several ways in which herbs, such as those discussed here, support the health of immune response, the health pattern that symbolizes each person's unique adaptation to and connection with their environment, both inside and out.

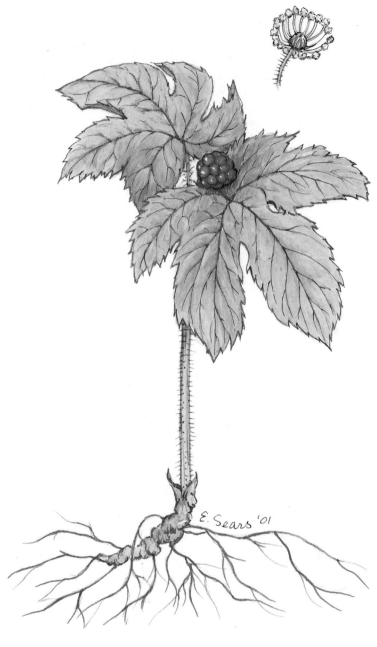

Hydrastis canadensis

Goldenseal

- **LATIN NAME:** *Hydrastis canadensis*

- **FAMILY:** Ranunculaceae

- **COMMON NAMES:** Goldenseal, jaundice root, eye balm, eye root, yellow puccoon, tumeric root, yellowroot, orangeroot, Indian plant, ground raspberry, Indian turmeric

- **HEALTH PATTERN:** Immune response

- **PLANT DESCRIPTION:**

Goldenseal is native to North America and is found growing in shady woods, rich soil, and damp meadows. It is found growing from Vermont to Minnesota and south to Georgia and Arkansas. It is a perennial with an erect stem from 6 to 12 inches (15 to 30 cm) tall. It can have as few as two or three leaves. They grow opposite each other and have three to five lobes with toothed edges. The flowers appear at the end of the erect stem around May and are small and green-white or rosy. The plant produces a fruit that resembles a red raspberry and has many little two-seeded compartments. The root appears knotty with many long fibers protruding from it and is bright yellow internally (Felter & Lloyd, 1983).

- **PLANT PARTS USED:** Roots and rhizome

- **TRADITIONAL EVIDENCE:**

Cultural Use

North American Indian. Goldenseal is commonly used by the Indian tribes that live in the areas where it grows. The Cherokee have a history of using the plant as a treatment for cancer, but it is not known exactly how it was used. They also used goldenseal as a skin wash for local inflammations. They take it internally to improve the appetite, for general debility, and for dyspepsia (Moerman, 1998). Goldenseal also has been mixed with bear's grease and used as an insect repellant (Vogel, 1970). The Iroquois have used goldenseal internally for diarrhea, whooping cough, flatulence, bloating, fever, liver and gallbladder problems, sour stomach, pneumonia, and tuberculosis. The roots are infused with whisky and taken for heart problems. In addition to its topical use for skin inflammations, it is also used topically as eyedrops and eardrops. The Micmac tribe uses the root to make a preparation for chapped or cut lips (Moerman, 1998).

European. In Great Britain, goldenseal is approved for use related to menorrhagia, atonic dyspepsia, gastritis, and as an eyewash (McCaleb, Leigh, & Morien, 2000).

Culinary Use

Goldenseal is not usually used in cooking.

Use in Herbalism

It is said that the early settlers in the United States learned of goldenseal from the Native Americans who used it as a medicine. Goldenseal became popular in the United States around the mid-1800s (Grieve, 1971) and was declared an official drug in the U.S. Pharmacopoeia in 1830 (Leung & Foster, 1996). It was considered a specific remedy for inflammation of the mucous membranes, especially if chronic. One exception to this was in cases of acute otitis media, in which goldenseal was said to work better than in chronic cases. It has been used for gastric inflammation, poor circulation, bleeding from the uterus and other pelvic tissues, and for skin diseases associated with gastric problems. It also has been used in cases of muscular tenderness that was worse with pressure or motion (Felter & Lloyd, 1983).

Goldenseal appears to stimulate the respiratory and circulatory systems, bring tone to the arteries, increase blood pressure in the capillaries, and result in decreased blood stasis. It is thought that this action brings more nutrition to the muscles and helps in various cases of muscular debility. Early physicians discovered that goldenseal stimulates the salivary glands and the appetite, and it was thought that it also stimulated the liver, stomach, and intestinal mucosa. It is used for inflammation and sores in the mouth and in chronic conditions of the gastric mucosa such as gastritis and ulcers. It is not used in cases of acute inflammation. Goldenseal is used in cases of inflammation of the gallbladder ducts, hepatic congestion, severe diarrhea, and dysentery. It is taken internally and applied topically to hemorrhoids, anal fissures, rectal ulcers and eczema, and prolapsed rectum (Felter & Lloyd, 1983).

Goldenseal is applied topically to conditions of the nose and throat. It is used for sore throat, rhinitis, inflammations of the tonsils, and in diphtheria (Felter & Lloyd, 1983). Powdered goldenseal used to be snuffed into the nostrils for nasal inflammation (Grieve, 1971), and today some sinus sprays have goldenseal in them. It has been applied in weak dilutions to eye conditions such as conjunctivitis and corneal ulcerations. The journals of nineteenth century American explorers Lewis and Clark describe Native American tribes using goldenseal for eye inflammations (McGuffin, Hobbs, Upton, & Goldberg, 1997). A preparation also is dropped into the ear for various symptoms, although this procedure is controversial because of the possibility of dropping it into an already ruptured eardrum. Goldenseal also has been used for disorders of the uterus and prostate, for gonorrhea, bladder inflammation and cystitis, eczema, acne, boils, skin ulcers, and in the treatment of cancer (Felter & Lloyd, 1983).

Goldenseal is often used in combination with echinacea today or as a single preparation in capsules, tablets, tinctures, and teas. It is used as an antiseptic, diuretic, laxative, tonic, and anti-inflammatory for the mucous membranes (Leung & Foster, 1996).

Some people mistakenly believe that goldenseal can mask the presence of illicit drugs in urine tests. When I was the director for the Herb Research Foundation Natural Healthcare Hotline, this was definitely the rumor. There were a number of calls everyday asking about goldenseal and how to use it to "clean out the body" before a drug test. Some people who called said that their urine drug tests had been positive for marijuana in the past even though they had not smoked it in ten years, so they wanted to take an herb that would "detoxify their liver." No data support the use of goldenseal in this manner. The rumor probably started in the early days of urine testing in methadone maintenance programs where thin layer chromatography was used to test for morphine glucuronide. Because of the way those tests were done a few years ago, some compounds in goldenseal possibly could have interfered with the test, giving it the reputation for being able to "mask" drugs in urine tests (Morgan, 1994). Some trace the rumor back to a novel written by pharmacist John Uri Lloyd (Foster & Tyler, 1999). The tests commonly used today for drug testing such as immunoassays are not affected in any way by goldenseal, and the large doses people take in some cases to "clean out" before drug testing could be harmful and therefore should be discouraged.

BIOMEDICAL EVIDENCE:

No published human studies were found on the traditional uses of goldenseal root for any infectious diseases such as dysentery, sore throat, cystitis, or otitis. Several studies have been conducted on berberine, one of the active constituents in goldenseal, and its effect on infection in the human body. Goldenseal contains active principles isoquinoline alkaloids, consisting mainly of hydrastine and berberine (0.5% to 6%) (Leung & Foster, 1996). Some of the studies on berberine are included here because their results may suggest that goldenseal, with its berberine content, may be effective against certain types of microorganisms. One animal study of goldenseal extract is included.

Studies Related to Immune Response

One animal study demonstrated that rats given 6.6 g of goldenseal root liquid extract per liter of drinking water had higher levels of immunoglobulin (Ig) M following initial exposure to the antigen used in the study. Goldenseal appears to enhance or accelerate antibody production in rats during the first two weeks of treatment. There was no IgG response with goldenseal (Rehman et al., 1999).

Preliminary studies of berberine, from a plant called *Berberis aristata,* 10 mg/kg per day, has been found to be effective in producing negative stool samples and decreased symptoms related to giardiasis in children 5 months to 14 years (Gupte, 1975).

In one double-blind, placebo-controlled trial, men from Bangladesh with diagnosed *Escherichia coli* diarrhea infection, given berberine sulfate 400 mg orally as a single dose, experienced a 48% reduction in stool volume and 42% had stopped having watery stools within twenty-four hours as compared with 20% in the control group ($p < .05$) (Rabbani, Butler, Knight, Sanyal, & Alam, 1987).

Studies Related to Other Health Patterns

No data are available at this time.

Mechanism of Action

The medicinal action of goldenseal is thought to be due to its isoquinolines, hydrastine and berberine, constituents that have been determined to have broad-spectrum antibiotic action. Berberine is bacteriostatic at low doses and bactericidal at high doses, is fungicidal, and toxic to protozoans such as *Leishmania* and *Plasmodium*. Berberine also decreases intestinal peristalsis (Bruneton, 1999). Berberine and hydrastine are not absorbed following oral ingestion so no systemic effects have been shown. When given by injection, berberine has been shown to stimulate digestion and bile secretion, lower blood pressure, and inhibit the action of adrenaline (Foster & Tyler, 1999).

Goldenseal and berberine do not have a systemic antibiotic-like effect unless coming in direct contact with some infected tissue such as in wound care. According to Bergner (1996–1997), goldenseal, while stimulating the mucous membranes to secrete, increases the IgA that naturally flows at the beginning of a cold or flu as the body attempts to shed the virus on its own. Therefore goldenseal is not needed when the body is producing enough mucous and antibodies. Goldenseal does not act like an antibiotic in that it does not work systemically to scavenge and kill harmful or healthy bacteria. "We have no evidence either from traditional use or from scientific experiments that either berberine or goldenseal cause this problem [disrupt the balance of normal bacteria in the intestine] (Bergner, 1996–1997, p. 6). Berberine does have an antisecretory effect in the case of patients with *E. coli* diarrhea and a mild antisecretory effect in those with *Vibrio cholerae*. Berberine was not as effective as tetracycline or tetracycline in combination with berberine in reducing symptoms associated with cholera (Khin-Maung-U, Myo-Khin, Nyunt-Nyunt-Wai, Aye-Kyaw, Tin-U, 1985). Goldenseal has been reported to increase the blood supply to the spleen, and berberine is said to activate macrophages in the body (Duke, 1997).

USE IN PREGNANCY OR LACTATION:

The oral use of goldenseal is contraindicated in pregnancy because of the uterine stimulant effect of its alkaloids berberine, hydrastine, canadine, and hydrastinine (Brinker, 1998; McGuffin et al., 1997).

Midwives often recommend herbal sitz baths to aid in the healing of perineal tears or sutures after the birth. Goldenseal is frequently one of the ingredients included in the sitz (Weed, 1986).

Herbal Caveat—Pregnancy or Lactation

Some herbs are contraindicated in pregnancy because of a risk of the herb or one of its constituents stimulating the uterus and therefore possibly promoting fetal loss. Many herbal practitioners do not recommend herbal remedies, in particular oral doses of herbs, during the first trimester of pregnancy and seek an alternative. However, herbs are successfully used during pregnancy, especially to prepare the body for the birth. Herbs are relatively unstudied in pregnancy and lactation, so patients need to be made aware through education of the potential benefits and risks of using herbs for health conditions that arise during pregnancy or lactation. The use of herbal remedies during pregnancy often warrants a referral to a knowledgeable herbal practitioner.

USE FOR CHILDREN:

Some midwives recommend the use of goldenseal eye drops for newborns rather than the silver nitrate eye drops commonly used to prevent gonorrheal eye infections that the infant may have acquired from the mother during the birth. Some think that the silver nitrate drops are very irritating to the baby's eyes and may cause long-term ill effects not to mention disruption of bonding the first days of life. An eyewash of goldenseal and eyebright is considered an effective and less irritating eyewash. One half ounce of eyebright is steeped with two whole goldenseal roots for eight hours. The decoction is strained thoroughly through a coffee filter or cotton cloth. Goldenseal whole root, not powder, is used because it is very difficult to strain out the particles of the powder that could be irritating to the eye. Mothers have used this preparation for a variety of other minor childhood eye problems (Weed, 1986).

Thrush is an overgrowth of *Candida albicans* on moist mucous membranes in the body. It can be seen as white patches in the affected baby's mouth. Goldenseal has been used to relieve the discomfort associated with this condition, although, it tastes very bitter and children often do not like it (Weed, 1986).

Herbal Caveat—Children

Children have special needs in regard to herbal therapies. They require lesser amounts of herbs and often respond well to mild teas and topical applications such as compresses and baths. The lowest dose of oral preparations should be tried first before increasing the amount given children. Caregivers should observe children closely for responses to herbal remedies. Younger children, particularly infants, have traditionally been given herbs either through their mother's breast milk or in the form of a homeopathic remedy because of their sensitivity to medicines and treatments and the immaturity of their liver. It is recommended that a person knowledgeable in the herbal treatment of children be consulted before the offering of any herb to a child for the first time.

Goldenseal is contraindicated in individuals with elevated blood pressure. Prolonged use of the root may decrease vitamin B absorption. It is speculated that because berberine has been shown to have coagulant activity, it may oppose the action of heparin (Newall, Anderson, & Phillipson, 1996). An external overdose of goldenseal may produce skin ulceration (Duke, 1985). Canadian regulation does not allow goldenseal to be used as a nonmedicinal ingredient for oral products (Michols, 1995 as reported in McGuffin et al., 1997). Goldenseal is not recommended to be applied topically to diaper rash because it can further irritate sensitive genital skin (Weed, 1986). Some do not recommend using goldenseal in the ear canal during ear infections because of the possibility of the presence of a ruptured ear drum (Brinker, 1998).

Western herbalists warn that taking goldenseal for *viral* illness such as colds and flu, as seems to have become popular in the United States, is not recommended. They also warn against taking excessive doses of goldenseal because it can overstimulate the mucous membranes and cause a reflexive drying and weaken the immune response.

Traditional Chinese medicine (TCM) also suggests caution in the use of any cold bitter herb, such as goldenseal, because it can damage the spleen energy system resulting in symptoms such as diarrhea, loss of appetite, and poor digestion. A healthy digestive tract is helpful when fighting infection, and weakening the digestive tract with excessive doses of cold bitter herbs is contraindicated.

In 1997, Foster reported that 250,000 pounds of goldenseal is sold every year. Because goldenseal has become a very popular herb and is often misused because of misinformation, plant populations are at risk. The Convention on International Trade in Endangered Species (CITES), lists goldenseal as an Appendix II plant (www.wcmc.org.uk/CITES/index.shtml). This means that although it may not be currently threatened with extinction, it may become so if the trade of the plant is not strictly regulated. Whenever a root of a plant is used medicinally, the risk of depleting plant populations is greater. It takes years to grow a root sufficient for harvest. Herb growers are being encouraged to cultivate goldenseal, and in the meantime, health practitioners and the public can help prevent the loss of goldenseal by becoming educated regarding the proper use of the plant.

⚜ NURSING EVIDENCE:

Historical Nursing Use

Mary Ann Bickerdyke, an American nurse-herbalist who is highly regarded for her service during the Civil War, was known to dose the soldiers/patients suffering from infection with smallpox with "black root and goldenseal, sassafras tea and beet juice, and all the milk and fresh vegetables they would take" (Baker, 1952, p. 142), after which a large number recovered.

Potential Nursing Applications

Nurses might want to consider researching the effects of goldenseal whole root decoction or extract in patients with discomfort related to gastrointestinal infection, in particular, cholera. Goldenseal also has been shown to be effective topically and nurses may want to explore the clinical use of goldenseal as an antiseptic for use in eye, skin, and wound care and as a gargle for sore throat.

Integrative Insight

Although berberine, a constituent in goldenseal, has demonstrated both in vitro and in vivo activity against a broad spectrum of microbes including *Candida, E. coli,* and *Shigella*, it is not meant to be used like a pharmaceutical antibiotic. Oral ingestion of neither goldenseal nor berberine produces a systemic pharmaceutical-like antibiotic effect; however, research has supported the traditional use of goldenseal as an immune stimulant, in animals, and as an antiseptic. Goldenseal affects microorganisms in the intestines in particular.

Noted British infectious disease physician, Edward Bach, who performed original research in bacteriology and homeopathy eventually creating the Bach flower remedies, found that gram-negative bacilli, in particular those found in the intestines that are often regarded as having no significance in relationship to disease processes, are actually associated with chronic disease (Howard & Ramsell, 1990). Perhaps goldenseal's effective antiseptic action on the intestines and its immune stimulating effect should be studied further in relation to its potential to be preventive and/or healing for some chronic illnesses.

Goldenseal serves as a good reminder that herbs need to be used for the right situation, at the right time, and in the right amount. Goldenseal must be used for the right condition and in the right amount because it has been overharvested, and its existence may be endangered if its populations are not conserved. Goldenseal also must be used at the right time. For example, in the case of intestinal infection, it is best used for chronic conditions. "As a remedy for various *gastric disorders* it will take a leading place, especially if it be born in mind that it is never beneficial, but on the contrary, does harm, in acute inflammatory conditions" (Felter & Lloyd, 1983, p. 1026).

THERAPEUTIC APPLICATIONS:

Oral

Dried Root. Up to four 500 mg capsules daily (McCaleb et al, 2000)

Tincture. (1:10 [g/ml], 60% alcohol): ½ to ¾ teaspoon (2 to 4 ml) three times daily

Liquid Extract. (1:1 [g/ml], 60% alcohol): 0.3 to 1.0 ml three times daily (McGuffin et al., 1997)

Topical

Compress. For antiseptic purposes, make a decoction and apply it to the skin with a flannel or cotton ball.

Mouth Rinse for Thrush. One half teaspoon of goldenseal powder is stirred into a cup (240 ml) of boiled water. One dose of the room temperature tea is ½ teaspoon (2.5 ml) per 10 pounds (4.5 kg) of body weight taken by mouth; swish and swallow, two to three times daily (Weed, 1986).

Environmental

As previously mentioned, goldenseal must be used judiciously because it may be nearing endangerment.

Sitz Bath (Used for Perineal Tears). Pour ½ gallon (about 2 liters) of boiling water over 4 ounces (112 g) of herb. Steep for eight hours. Strain and pour the "tea" into a shallow basin or pan. Sit in this liquid for fifteen minutes once or twice daily (Weed, 1986).

Herbal Caveat—Therapeutic Applications

In traditional and conventional herbal medicine, amounts of herbs given to patients are based on individual needs. The amounts or "doses" recorded here are provided so that the health practitioner has a general idea of the amounts recommended for an adult patient. Dosing in herbalism not only refers to amount of plant used but also includes when, where, and how to take a plant medicine. These dosages should not be used as guidelines for indiscriminate intervention without proper assessment, critical thinking, and patient education on the part of the practitioner.

Note: Please see chapter 5 for detailed descriptions of how to prepare various applications.

PATIENT INTERACTION:

Goldenseal and one of its major healing constituents, berberine, have demonstrated strong antibacterial and antifungal activity. However, there is no published scientific support for the use of goldenseal as a "replacement" for pharmaceutical antibiotics. It has been shown in animal studies to stimulate the immune system, and it does have many years of effective use in the treatment of symptoms related to infectious diseases, especially those of a chronic nature and those involving the intestines. Goldenseal should not be used to cleanse or detoxify the body before urine drug testing because the laboratory tests used today are not affected by goldenseal. Goldenseal must be used at the right time in the right amount. Plant populations of goldenseal are at risk because of high volume of use. It should be used judiciously.

Herbal Caveat—Patient Interaction

Patients considering the use of an herb or formula of herbs in self-care benefit from education about the plant itself and the use of the plant in healing. This education can come through many sources, including local herbalists; plant specialists such as botanists; health practitioners such as nurses, nutritionists, naturopaths, and other physicians; and various written references including the scientific literature. Patients need to remember that their unique health care needs are not necessarily represented in any literature they may encounter. Therefore, it is recommended that a knowledgeable mentor be consulted before initiating self-care with any herb being used for the first time.

☙ NURTURING THE NURSE-PLANT RELATIONSHIP:

Note: You may want to keep a journal of your experiences with the herb.

Goldenseal has a very distinctive bitter taste. Make a strong tea using goldenseal powder. The powder can be steeped in boiled water for twenty minutes. Then strain it through cheesecloth and allow it to cool. When tasting the tea, allow it to stay in your mouth for one minute. Notice how the tea affects the mucous membrane of your mouth. Swish and swallow. If your gums are sore, try brushing your teeth with a little goldenseal tea. Record your experience.

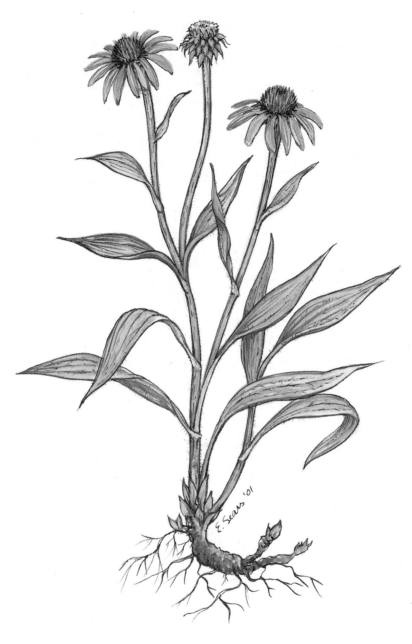

Echinacea purpurea

Echinacea

🍃 **LATIN NAME:** *Echinacea angustifolia, Echinacea pallida, Echinacea purpurea*

🍃 **FAMILY:** Asteraceae

🍃 **COMMON NAMES:** *Echinacea angustifolia* and *Echinacea pallida*: echinacea, Kansas snake root, narrow-leaved echinacea, narrow-leaved purple coneflower, pale-flowered echinacea, pale purple coneflower, black sampson, scurvy root, Indian head, comb flower, black Susans, hedge hog; *Echinacea purpurea*: echinacea, coneflower, purple coneflower, purple echinacea, black sampson

🍃 **HEALTH PATTERN:** Immune response

🍃 **PLANT DESCRIPTION:**

The name "echinacea" is derived from the Greek word "echinos," meaning "hedge-hog," and referring to the many spines on the cone. The genus Echinacea includes nine indigenous species in North America. In general, echinacea has a thick, black, pungent root that sends up a stout stem that reaches 24 to 48 inches (60 to 120 cm) high (Leung & Foster, 1996). The leaves, opposite each other on the stem, can be rather narrow with fine bristly hairs, and reach 4 to 8 inches (10 to 20 cm) in length. The flower has a central brownish-red cone, with numerous stiff projections. The cone is surrounded by 15 to 20 narrow petals that are purple-violet (Felter & Lloyd, 1983). *E. purpurea* root is fibrous and *E. angustifolia* and *E. pallida* have tap roots. The roots have a slightly sweet taste that quickly becomes bitter on the tongue and leaves a tingling sensation (World Health Organization [WHO], 1999). Echinacea is commonly cultivated in home and public gardens for its beauty and durability.

🍃 **PLANT PARTS USED:** Roots, aerial parts, and seed

🍃 **TRADITIONAL EVIDENCE:**

Cultural Use

North American Indian. Many Native American tribes have used *E. purpurea, E. pallida*, and *E. angustifolia* to treat a variety of symptoms. The roots are chewed to cause numbing of the pain associated with toothaches. Infusions of the roots are taken internally for sore mouth, gums, and throat. The juice from the plant is applied topically for burns, and poultices of the chewed roots are applied to swollen areas. The plant also is used for various venomous bites and stings, especially those from snakes. In some cases, a poultice of the roots is applied directly to the snakebite. The plant has been used in a smoke treatment for headache. Some tribes make a decoction of the roots for smallpox, mumps, measles, and sore eyes (Moerman, 1998). It has been reported that the plant so numbs the mouth that one man was able to put a hot coal in his mouth just to show off (Vogel, 1970). The cone, "mika-hi," was used by the Omaha and Poncas tribes as a comb for the hair, and the root was chewed to stimulate the flow of saliva, especially during the sun dance to prevent thirst. In addition to these uses, the Dakotas use echinacea to "cure" hydrophobia (Kindscher, 1992).

African. Echinacea has been introduced as a cultivated plant from North America and is grown in parts of north and eastern Africa (Iwu, 1993).

Russian/Baltic. Although not native to Russia, echinacea is used in Russia. The Russians use it as an antiseptic both internally and externally. It is used to reduce pain and improve blood quality to strengthen the constitution of the patient so that they can resist infection better. Echinacea is used in caring for the skin, wounds, ulcers, burns, and decubiti (Hutchens, 1992).

European. Topical, oral, and parenteral preparations of echinacea are used in Germany to treat a wide variety of conditions. External applications are used for hard-to-heal wounds, eczema, burns, psoriasis, and herpes simplex. Internal preparations are used to stimulate the immune system at the onset of colds and flu symptoms and for treatment of *C. albicans* infections, chronic respiratory infections, prostatitis, and rheumatoid arthritis. More than 280 pharmaceutical echinacea products are currently available in Europe (Leung & Foster, 1996).

The German Commission E no longer approves the use of parenteral preparations of echinacea because of the risks associated with parenteral application. As of 1992, the German Commission E listed the following uses of echinacea but stated that there was not enough scientific data for a recommendation for therapeutic use: promoting natural powers of resistance, infectious conditions in the nose and throat, influenza, inflammatory and purulent wounds, abscesses, headaches, metabolic disturbances, and as a diaphoretic and antiseptic (Blumenthal, Goldberg, & Brinckman, 2000).

Culinary Use

No data are available at this time.

Use in Herbalism

The North American Indians were very familiar with the medicinal use of echinacea and shared their knowledge with white settlers. Among the first uses of echinacea by U.S. physicians was for septicemia in 1888. It gained popularity and came to be used for infected injuries and cases of venomous bites from snakes, spiders, scorpions, and wasps. It was used with other preparations for the treatment of meningitis. Echinacea also was used for diphtheria, tonsillitis, sinus inflammation, and other respiratory tract problems. It has been specifically indicated for ulcerated or infected mucous membranes with general debility. It has been used effectively for bronchitis, pneumonia, and other lung infections.

Echinacea is used to stimulate the appetite, improve digestion, and treat fevers, including those of malaria, typhoid, and puerperal fever. The recovery time from influenza has been observed to be shortened by the use of echinacea. Echinacea is also effective in wound care (Awang & Kindack, 1991). It has been used topically for cleansing and deodorizing cancerous growths, for cleansing infected wounds, and to wash surgical sites postoperatively. Preparations of echinacea have been applied to eczema and psoriasis with good results (Felter & Lloyd, 1983).

Echinacea is thought to increase one's resistance to infection and has been used for boils, septicemia, cancer, syphilis, hemorrhoids, and as an antiseptic. It is believed to be useful as an aphrodisiac as well (Grieve, 1971). Echinacea is currently used in many popular cold and flu remedies. Some current herbalists believe that different species of echinacea have to be prepared in different ways to maximize their effects on the immune system. It is thought that the active constituents can vary greatly among the different species. Some herbalists recommended using *E. angustifolia* for bacterial infections, *E. pallida* for infections of unknown cause, and *E. purpurea* for viral infections (but only if it is in an alcohol-based tincture). *E. angustifolia* is thought to be most effective if taken in the form of a water-based infusion, with *E. pallida* effective as either tincture or infusion (Rister, 1999). Regardless of the differences between species, one species of echinacea has not been found to be more *medicinal* than another. *E. purpurea* may be easier to grow and is found in common use (Foster & Tyler, 1999).

Cosmetic Use. Extracts are being commonly used in cosmetics, lip balms, shampoos, toothpaste, and other product categories (Leung & Foster, 1996).

BIOMEDICAL EVIDENCE:

Many of the studies conducted on echinacea have been done in Germany on the injectable form of the aerial part of the plant. (Parenteral use of echinacea is no longer approved by German Commission E.) I worked in a clinic where patients were given injections of echinacea as an immune system stimulant often with excellent results. The majority of people, however, do not have access nor would they necessarily choose to take echinacea in injectable form. The studies presented here have been conducted with oral echinacea.

One review of 26 controlled clinical trials investigating the immunomodulatory efficacy of echinacea preparations concluded that while echinacea preparations have been found to have an immunomodulatory effect in the body, data regarding which preparation and dose to use for a specific indication are not clear (Melchart, Linde, Worku, Bauer, & Wagner, 1994).

Studies Related to Immune Response

A clinical review of the literature of thirteen randomized, placebo-controlled, and blinded studies on the effect of oral echinacea extracts (either of the root, the herb, or the herb and root) in reducing the incidence, severity, or duration of acute upper respiratory illness (e.g., colds and flulike symptoms) in humans, supports the traditional use of echinacea at the early stage of upper respiratory infection. In the study by Hoheisel, Sandberg, Bertram, Bulitta, & Schafer (1997), 120 adult factory workers were given 20 drops of Echinacin, an *E. purpurea* preparation, every two hours the first day when respiratory symptoms were first noticed and then three times daily after that. Although this and other such reviewed studies showed a shorter duration for upper respiratory illness or a reduction in those who had signs of an oncoming cold actually getting a "real cold," none of the studies supported the use of echinacea as a preventive measure (Barrett, Vohmann, & Calabrese, 1999). A possible risk reduction of 10% to 20% was shown for preventing upper respiratory infection (Melchart, Walther, Linde, Brandmaier, & Lersch, 1998).

In a German, unblinded study of 203 women with recurrent vaginal yeast infections in which all of the women were treated with the standard medication, topical econazole cream, and some of the women also took oral doses of Echinacin (*E. purpurea* leaf juice extract) for ten weeks, the women who took the echinacea had a 16.7% recurrence rate, whereas those that did not had a 60.5% recurrence rate (Coeugniet & Kuhlnast, 1986 as reported in Blumenthal et al., 2000).

Animal and in vitro studies have shown that oral ingestion of ethanol extracts of *E. purpurea, E. angustifolia,* and *E. pallida* significantly stimulate phagocyte activity (Bauer et al., 1988). Ethanolic extracts of echinacea, *E. purpurea* being the most active, have been shown to increase phagocytosis in vitro by 20% to 30% (Awang & Kindack, 1991).

Studies Related to Other Health Patterns

Skin Care. One large uncontrolled German study of echinacea ointment in 4598 people found that the ointment was 85% effective in treating wounds, eczema, leg ulcers, burns, herpes simplex, and inflammatory skin conditions (Viehmann, 1978 as reported in McCaleb et al., 2000).

Restoration. Some preliminary animal studies have demonstrated that a highly purified polysaccharide called "arabinogalactan" from an *E. purpurea* cell culture has a significant ability to strongly and selectively activate macrophages against some tumors. Echinacea may present opportunities for those with symptoms associated with cancer in the future (Luettig, Steinmuller, Gifford, Wagner, Lohmann-Matthes, 1989).

Mechanism of Action

The immunostimulatory activity of echinacea is thought to be due to a combined action of several constituents (as reported in Awang & Kindack, 1991). The polysaccharides in echinacea, also thought to be immunologically active, are more present in fresh juice or in extracts prepared with large amounts of water and are not found in ethanol extracts because of their precipitability. Echinosides (often used as the biologic marker for the preparation of standardized extracts of echinacea) have a weak bacteriostatic action and have no immune stimulating effects (Foster & Tyler, 1999). Echinosides have been found to show slight antimicrobial activity against streptococci and *Staphylococcus aureus*. Echinacin extract has been found to have antiviral activity and the roots of *E. purpurea* and *E. angustifolia* have antifungal activity (Awang & Kindack, 1991). The antiviral activity of echinacea is said to in part be due to caffeic acid, chicoric acid, and echinacin (Duke, 1997).

It is not known exactly which constituents in echinacea have the immunologic effect, but a lipophilic substance, isobutylamide, is thought to be responsible for the tingling sensation on the tongue often associated with therapeutic effect (Bauer, Jurcic, Puhlmann, & Wagner, 1988). Preparations of echinacea are thought to be effective because they stimulate the lymphatic tissue in the mouth and therefore initiate an immune response (Foster & Tyler, 1999).

Echinacea's therapeutic effects on wound healing and upper respiratory infection are thought to be related to its ability to stimulate the production of properdin, a serum protein that neutralizes viruses and bacteria, and to inhibit microbes from secreting the enzyme hyaluronidase, which enables infection to spread throughout the body and breaks down the cells' hyaluronic acid (HA). HA exerts a protective effect, increases skin-forming cells, and helps lubricate joints. It also has been found to stimulate fibroblast production, which aids in wound healing (Haas, 1991 as reported in WHO, 1999).

USE IN PREGNANCY OR LACTATION:

One recent preliminary study of 412 women, 206 of whom took echinacea during pregnancy and 112 of whom took it during the first trimester, found that there was no significant difference between the women in the control group who did not use echinacea and those in the study group who did (Gallo et al., 2000).

Midwives recommend echinacea after birth for symptoms relating to mastitis, nipple fissures, *Streptococcus* and *Staphylococcus* infections, pneumonia, and puerperal fever (Duke, 1997; Weed, 1986). Nipple fissures may be associated with fungal infection (Bodley &

Powers, 1997) and therefore may respond well to the antifungal action of echinacea.

Herbal Caveat—Pregnancy or Lactation

Some herbs are contraindicated in pregnancy because of a risk of the herb or one of its constituents stimulating the uterus and therefore possibly promoting fetal loss. Many herbal practitioners do not recommend herbal remedies, in particular oral doses of herbs, during the first trimester of pregnancy and seek an alternative. However, herbs are successfully used during pregnancy, especially to prepare the body for the birth. Herbs are relatively unstudied in pregnancy and lactation, so patients need to be made aware through education of the potential benefits and risks of using herbs for health conditions that arise during pregnancy or lactation. The use of herbal remedies during pregnancy often warrants a referral to a knowledgeable herbal practitioner.

USE FOR CHILDREN:

Some herbalists recommend putting a few drops of *E. angustifolia* tincture on an infant's umbilical stump several times daily to encourage healing and discourage infection. If an infection is present in the stump, some midwives recommend giving the infant one drop of echinacea tincture per pound of body weight one time daily by mouth (Weed, 1986). Breastfeeding mothers may want to consider taking echinacea extract a few days before their baby's immunizations.

Herbal Caveat—Children

Children have special needs in regard to herbal therapies. They require lesser amounts of herbs and often respond well to mild teas and topical applications such as compresses and baths. The lowest dose of oral preparations should be tried first before increasing the amount given children. Caregivers should observe children closely for responses to herbal remedies. Younger children, particularly infants, have traditionally been given herbs either through their mother's breast milk or in the form of a homeopathic remedy because of their sensitivity to medicines and treatments and the immaturity of their liver. It is recommended that a person knowledgeable in the herbal treatment of children be consulted before the offering of any herb to a child for the first time.

CAUTIONS:

Echinacea should be avoided by those who experience allergic sensitivity to other plants in the Asteraceae family (Blumenthal et al., 2000). Possible allergic reactions from internal use could include shivering, fever, and headache (WHO, 1999). There was one report of a woman with atopy who experienced an anaphylactic reaction after taking dietary supplements and an echinacea extract. Skin and radioallergosorbent (RAST) testing has detected echinacea binding IgE in atopic patients; therefore, there is a possible risk for allergic reaction (Mullins, 1998). However, in all of the large clinical trials, only mild side effects have ever been reported (Barrett et al., 1999).

Because echinacea is an immune stimulant, and theoretically the body could adapt to the stimulation thereby showing a decline in the immune stimulant effects, many herbalists recommend resting periods during the use of echinacea. Echinacea is best taken only when needed (i.e., when coming down with a cold) and often is recommended not to be taken for more than six to eight weeks.

The oral use of *E. purpurea* juice for ten weeks had no adverse effects in 60 patients in a clinical trial. In another study, an aqueous extract of *E. purpurea* was taken four times daily for twelve weeks with no physical adverse effects or changes in leukocyte counts (Brinker, 1998).

Because of the potential for stimulating autoimmune processes (Schulz, Hansel, & Tyler, 1998), the internal use of echinacea is contraindicated in progressive systemic diseases such as tuberculosis, leukosis, collagenosis, multiple sclerosis, human immunodeficiency virus (HIV), and other autoimmune diseases (McGuffin et al., 1997). This recommendation is based on theoretic considerations and not on any reports of adverse results (Blumenthal et al., 2000).

It has been noted that the metabolic condition of diabetics declines upon parenteral application. However, parenteral preparations are no longer approved in Germany (Blumenthal et al., 2000). Theoretically, echinacea may interfere with medical immunosuppressive therapy (Newall et al., 1996); therefore, practitioners and their patients may need to explore this possibility and make choices regarding the best modalities and the timing for the patient. Echinacea has not been shown to definitively prevent the onset of upper respiratory illness and is therefore not recommended as a preventive measure (Barrett et al., 1999).

It is important that echinacea be used judiciously because the roots can take up to three to four years to get to a harvestable size (Foster, 1991), and the demand for cultivated echinacea exceeds production. Sources of echinacea in the wild are dwindling, so health practitioners and consumers must do their part to help ensure that echinacea will continue to be available for medicinal purposes.

NURSING EVIDENCE:

Historical Nursing Use

No data are available at this time.

Potential Nursing Applications

Nurses may want to explore the possibility of researching and using echinacea clinically to reduce the length of experience of infections, in particular upper respiratory infections, such as colds and influenza. For example, occupational health nurses may want to consider tracking the results of patients' use of echinacea as related to absence from work during cold and flu season.

Because using echinacea in conjunction with vaginal antifungal cream has been shown to be highly effective in recurrent vaginal yeast infection, nurses may want to consider recommending that women consider taking echinacea as part of their self-care regimen.

Nurses also might want to consider using echinacea in patients with discomfort related to oral ulcers or sore throat. Echinacea has antimicrobial acitivity, is able to numb and heal the mucous membranes.

Integrative Insight

An herb teacher of mine once told me that herbs can be "irritants." This was not meant to be derogatory of herbs but was simply a descriptive statement of the action of some herbs in the human body. Echinacea is an irritant in a sense. Its prickly nature is represented in the bristles of its cone and how it tingles or prickles the tongue. It irritates the body's immune system to act against bacteria, viruses, or fungus. Biomedical evidence has some idea how the plant accomplishes its stimulating work, but as is true for several herbs, the action of echinacea cannot be ascribed to one constituent. It is probable that a synergy of constituents and activities occurs that enables echinacea to cause its response in the human immune system.

Echinacea also may represent irritation in another way. Echinacea was well known among indigenous North American Indians. The information about the plant's medicinal benefits was shared with those who settled in North America. Eclectic physicians described echinacea as having "extraordinary powers" (Felter & Lloyd, 1983, p. 674). They claimed that echinacea was a drug that "from start to finish was an Eclectic medicine" (Felter & Lloyd, 1983, p. 671). This statement could be construed to mean that there was perhaps a claiming of the remedy as belonging to the Eclectics. Native Americans gave the knowledge of echinacea to the early settlers just as many traditional healers have in other cultures. Traditional healers share their knowledge and wisdom of a plant in good faith. Echinacea reminds us of the "prickles" that sometimes can form between biomedical and traditional healers when proprietary notions get involved. Herbs and their health benefits do not "belong" to one person or group of healers or practitioners. Herbs provide an opportunity for healing that is open to everyone.

Another way echinacea irritates is through its tingle in the mouth. Echinacea is a wonderful plant to introduce to people who may be very critical of the use of medicinal herbs. I have seen many a skeptical colleague with cold or flu symptoms change their minds because of echinacea and because of the tingle. They experience the plant's action very specifically in their mouth and then they experience the effect on the discomfort they feel with cold or flu symptoms. Not all herbs are so fast acting and poignant!

Oral

Echinacea should be taken so that it can be tasted as the immune-stimulating activity starts in the mouth. It is best to swish and swallow. Echinacea preparations may contain more than one *Echinacea* species.

Infusion. Use 0.3 ounce (0.9 g) root in 5 ounces (150 ml) boiled water. Take several times daily as a tea (Blumenthal et al., 2000).

Tincture. (1:5 [g/ml], 55% alcohol): Take 30 to 60 drops three times daily (Blumenthal et al., 2000).

Fluid Extract. 1:1 (g/ml): Take up to ½ teaspoon (1 to 2 ml) three times daily (Murray, 1995).

Juice of Aerial Part of Plant in Ethanol. Take approximately ½ teaspoon (2 to 3 ml) three times daily (Murray, 1995).

Freeze-dried Plant. Take 325 to 650 mg three times daily (Murray, 1995).

Standardized Extract. Often *E. angustifolia* products are standardized to their echinoside content. It is questionable as to whether or not this biologic marker for standardization is helpful (Foster & Tyler, 1999).

Topical

Poultices, compresses, and creams have been used for skin conditions including burns, infections, decubiti, and inflamed areas related to eczema or psoriasis. Clinical herbalists may recommend topical use be accompanied by internal use.

Environmental

The Plains Indians have used *E. angustifolia* in the smoke treatment for headache (Vogel, 1970). Purple cone flower is a beautiful ornamental plant to have in the garden while you are waiting for the roots to get large enough for harvest.

Herbal Caveat—Therapeutic Applications

In traditional and conventional herbal medicine, amounts of herbs given to patients are based on individual needs. The amounts or "doses" recorded here are provided so that the health practitioner has a general idea of the amounts recommended for an adult patient. Dosing in herbalism not only refers to amount of plant used but also includes when, where, and how to take a plant medicine. These dosages should not be used as guidelines for indiscriminate intervention without proper assessment, critical thinking, and patient education on the part of the practitioner.

Note: Please see chapter 5 for detailed descriptions of how to prepare various applications.

PATIENT INTERACTION:

For many reasons, echinacea should be used judiciously. It is best to use it at the onset of cold or flu symptoms, not to prevent a cold or flu from happening. Echinacea stimulates the immune system. The body, when overstimulated, may actually turn off its response, so most practitioners recommend that echinacea only be taken when symptoms occur. When taking echinacea internally, it may be best to take it as a tea or liquid extract. The tingling sensation you will feel in your mouth shows that the echinacea is working. This numbing action can be very soothing for sore throats and mouth ulcers that often accompany colds or flu. The benefits of echinacea may best be experienced if it is gargled and swished before swallowing. Echinacea is also very helpful used topically for healing wounds and other troublesome skin conditions. Do not use echinacea if you have a known allergy to plants in the Asteraceae family or have a diagnosed autoimmune disorder without discussing it with a knowledgeable health practitioner.

Herbal Caveat—Patient Interaction

Patients considering the use of an herb or formula of herbs in self-care benefit from education about the plant itself and the use of the plant in healing. This education can come through many sources, including local herbalists; plant specialists such as botanists; health practitioners such as nurses, nutritionists, naturopaths, and other physicians; and various written references including the scientific literature. Patients need to remember that their unique health care needs are not necessarily represented in any literature they may encounter. Therefore, it is recommended that a knowledgeable mentor be consulted before initiating self-care with any herb being used for the first time.

NURTURING THE NURSE-PLANT RELATIONSHIP:

Note: You may want to keep a journal of your experiences with the herb.

Echinacea causes a characteristic tingling sensation when taken in the mouth. The tingle surprises quite a few people at first, but it is really helpful for sore throats and mouth sores and may even start the systemic immune response. To get to know echinacea, experience the tingle. Try putting some liquid extract of *E. angustifolia* or *E. purpurea* in a very small amount of water and then holding it in your mouth for two minutes. Gargle, swish, and swallow and then sit quietly and notice if you have an unusual sensation in your mouth. This can be a very powerful experience!

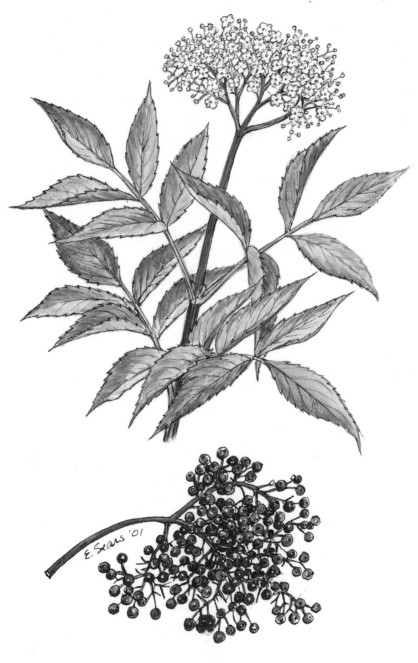

Sambucus nigra

Elder

- **LATIN NAME:** *Sambucus nigra*

- **FAMILY:** Adoxacaeae

- **COMMON NAMES:** Elder, black elder flower and berries, European elder flower and berries, sambucus, sweet elder, common elder, American elderberry

- **HEALTH PATTERN:** Immune response

- **PLANT DESCRIPTION:**

Elder is a commonly cultivated, ornamental shrub used along lawns and in gardens. It also can grow as large as a small tree and is found throughout Europe, Asia, North Africa, and the United States (Blumenthal et al., 2000). It is found in damp grounds, thickets, and waste places. Elder grows from 5 to 12 feet (1½ to 4 meters) high and has stems that are filled with a porous pith, especially when young. The stems are covered with a rough, pitted gray bark, but the central stems are smooth. The numerous small white flowers are star-shaped and about ¼ inch (6 mm) across. They appear in June and July in large, level-topped clusters approximately 8 inches (20 cm) across. From September through October, the fruit ripens into numerous purplish-black berries that are in clusters (Felter & Lloyd, 1983; Hutchens, 1992).

- **PLANT PARTS USED:** Flowers, berries, leaves, and bark

- **TRADITIONAL EVIDENCE:**

Cultural Use

Asian. In TCM, a related species of elder *(Sambucus williamsii)* is used. The flowers are used to promote sweating and urine. The twigs, leaves, and roots are used for treating the symptoms of rheumatoid arthritis and other conditions. The plant is usually used in the form of a decoction and taken internally (Leung & Foster, 1996).

North American Indian. North American Indians use several species of elder for medicine, as a food, and to make toys and musical instruments. The Algonquin use an infusion of the bark scraped upward as an emetic and the bark scraped downward as a laxative. The Cherokee use an infusion of the berry for rheumatism. The leaves are used to wash sores to prevent infection. Creek women use a poultice of pounded roots to apply to swollen breasts. The Iroquois use a poultice of the bark to apply for headache pain. The berries are used for fevers. They infuse the pith and drink it for heart disease. The Seminole use the bark of the root as a purification emetic after funerals (Moerman, 1998).

As a food source, the Cherokee use the berries to make wine, pies, jellies, and to dry for winter use. The Iroquois dry the berries and use them to take as a food on long hunting trips. The fresh berries are mashed, made into small cakes, and dried for future use. Dried berries are soaked in water and made into a sauce during the winter. Boys use the larger stems of elder to make popguns or blowguns. Some tribes use the hollow twigs to make flutes, pipes, arrow shafts, whistles, clappers, and tobacco containers (Moerman, 1998).

The Tepehuan make a tea of the flowers of their native elder species to be used for fever and heart trouble. They use crushed, young leaves in a poultice for cuts. The Pima make a hot tea from the flowers and use it internally for colds. It is used as a warm drink for fevers. The Mountain Pima prepare a strong drink from elder leaves to be used for fever and stomach problems. The crushed leaves are applied to the head for headaches (Kay, 1996).

Hispanic. Elder flowers are used as a skin wash, for colds, and for fevers. The berries are made into a cough syrup with onion and garlic, and the leaf is used in a bath with peppermint for arthritis. One of the main uses of elder by Mexican Americans is in a tea for children. Mexican Americans use tea made of elder flowers, spearmint, chamomile, or basil for the relief of infant colic. It is given to bring out the rash of chicken pox and to cause sweating that will lower fevers. The flowers and leaves are brewed into a tea for high blood pressure, whooping cough, as an enema for hemorrhoids, and as a douche for vaginal infections, or the tea is poured over the head for sunstroke or sunburn. The berries are used in corn gruel for those recovering from illness (Kay, 1996).

East Indian. Traditional Ayurvedic medicine practice in India includes the use of elder as a cathartic and for epilepsy. The flowers are used to promote sweating and as a laxative. The berries increase the output of urine (Nadkarni, 1976).

Middle Eastern. Israelis have done extensive research on the use of elderberry in the successful treatment of influenza and other viral illnesses (Elliman, 1994).

European. The people of Denmark believed that a spirit lived in the branches of the elder and watched over it. If anyone cut down the tree and made furniture out of the wood, the spirit was supposed to follow the wood into the home and haunt the owners! Others thought that elder would ward off evil influences and drive off bad spirits. Some would bring a stick of elder to be used in wedding ceremonies for good luck. In England, it was thought that elder was never struck by lightning, and that a sprig of it carried in the pocket was a charm against rheumatism. Elder leaves were placed in windows and doors to prevent evil from entering the house. Others grew elder trees by their doors for the same purpose (Grieve, 1971).

Elder flowers are used in Germany as a standard medicinal tea for fevers associated with the common cold. The flowers are combined with other herbs for the treatment of symptoms of colds and flu (Blumenthal et al., 2000). Elder is commonly used throughout the United Kingdom and in Belgium, Yugoslavia, Bulgaria, Hungary, and Romania. The British Herbal Compendium lists the use of elder flowers for the common cold and fever and as a diuretic (Bradley, 1992).

Culinary Use

Elder flowers are used as a flavoring in numerous food products such as alcoholic and nonalcoholic beverages, frozen dairy desserts, candy, gelatins, puddings, and baked goods (Leung & Foster, 1996). The berries are an excellent source of vitamin C (Duke, 1985). They are never eaten raw, only cooked.

Elder flower fritters can be made by dipping the entire flower cluster into batter and then frying them in a deep pan of hot fat. The new shoots have been cooked and served like asparagus (Duke, 1985). Elder flowers also can be sprinkled onto pancakes as they are grilling.

Use in Herbalism

Elder was one of the oldest known medicines in the Old World and its uses can be traced back to ancient Egypt (Kay, 1996). Much traditional lore, romance, and superstition has been created about elder. Shakespeare in *Cymbeline* refers to it as a symbol of grief. A common medieval belief was that the apostle Judas was hanged on an elder tree. Others believe that Christ's cross was made of elder wood. As a consequence of these old stories, the elder became a symbol of sorrow and death. Many other superstitions grew out of these legends.

In 1875, physicians recommended the use of elder for epilepsy. Scrapings from the outer bark were used to make an infusion. This was given to the patient by mouth every fifteen minutes when a seizure was approaching (Hutchens, 1992). The leaves of elder, which have an unpleasant odor, were prepared as a topical application and used to repel mosquitoes and other biting insects.

The first spring shoots of the plant or the later leaves and stalks are boiled in fat broth to be taken as an expectorant. The berries are used for the same purpose and also for edema in the lower extremities. The juice of the root is used as an emetic, for snakebites, and the bites of rabid dogs. The juice of the green leaves can be applied to skin inflammations. Berry juice is boiled with honey, cooled, and dropped into the ears for symptoms of ear pain. The berries are simmered in wine and taken internally as a diuretic. A floral water made from the flowers is used topically for sunburn, freckles, and to take away headaches and the first symptoms of colds by bathing the head. This same preparation also is used to bathe old sores and ulcers of the lower extremities to help them heal. The floral water was used as a wash to take away redness of the eyes and shaking of the hands. It was believed that if a woman with delayed menses would sit upon elder, her monthly bleeding would occur (Culpeper, 1990).

Elder was used by American Eclectic physicians as a stimulant to increase secretion of various bodily functions. A warm infusion of elder flowers was used as a diaphoretic and a gentle stimulant. A cold infusion was used for its cooling properties in treating symptoms of childhood liver problems and erysipelas. The juice of the berries prepared as a syrup was used as an alterative and as a mild laxative. The inner green bark was used as a cathartic. Other preparations were used specifically for edema of the lower extremities (Felter & Lloyd, 1983). Infusion of elder flowers and peppermint is believed to be an infallible remedy taken at the first signs of a cold or flu. It is said that this preparation promotes sweating and sleep (Grieve, 1971).

Externally, elder has been used for eruptions of the skin that occur on edematous extremities, especially if accompanied by discharge of serum. It is used on burns, eczema, and on old ulcers (Felter & Lloyd, 1983). The berries also can be made into a wine that can be taken for symptoms at the beginning of a cold such as shivering and sore throat. The berries were used for colic, diarrhea, and epilepsy. Green elderberry ointment was used for hemorrhoids (Grieve, 1971).

Current herbal uses of elder are for its diaphoretic action and its increased bronchial secretion activity. It has demonstrated anti-inflammatory, antiviral, and diuretic activity in in vitro studies (Blumenthal et al., 2000). Elder berries are used to promote sweating, but the berries are not as effective as the flowers in this regard.

Buckle recommends the use of elder flower in the form of a distilled floral water applied topically to assist wound healing (Buckle, 1997). Elder flowers have been used in many cosmetic preparations to remove skin spots, decrease irritation, remove freckles, and soften and preserve the skin if used regularly (Hutchens, 1992).

Cosmetic Use. Elder flower water was a common ingredient in cosmetic lotions, medicines, and eye preparations (Grieve, 1971).

BIOMEDICAL EVIDENCE:

Studies Related to Immune Response

A double-blind clinical trial was conducted after the results of an in vitro study demonstrated the antiviral activity of Sambucol, a standardized elderberry extract in syrup form. Twenty-seven people with at least three of the following symptoms participated in the study: fever more than 38°C, myalgia, nasal discharge, and cough. Children received 2 and adults 4 tablespoons of Sambucol each day or placebo. A significant improvement in flu symptoms, including fever, was demonstrated within two days of receiving Sambucol in 93.3% of the treatment group, whereas 91.7% of the placebo group showed improvement within six days. Most participants had confirmed cases of influenza B and some had both A and B antibodies. Investigators conclude that elderberry extract seems to significantly enhance the immune response to influenza (Zakay-Rones et al., 1995).

Studies Related to Other Health Patterns
No data are available at this time.

Mechanism of Action
Elder has demonstrated antiviral activity in vitro and in vivo (Zakay-Rones et al., 1995). It prevents influenza virus from entering respiratory tract cells and is being studied for activity against HIV (Duke, 1997). After ingestion of 25 g of elderberry extract, antioxidants called "anthocyanins" present in elderberry have been detected in human serum (Cao & Prior, 1999).

USE IN PREGNANCY OR LACTATION:
There are no known contraindications to the use of elder flowers during pregnancy (Blumenthal et al., 2000). One traditional remedy used by midwives is an herbal oil made from elder flowers and olive oil that is applied to sore nipples and breasts during lactation. It is claimed that this will relieve the pain and sensitivity (Weed, 1986).

Herbal Caveat—Pregnancy or Lactation
Some herbs are contraindicated in pregnancy because of a risk of the herb or one of its constituents stimulating the uterus and therefore possibly promoting fetal loss. Many herbal practitioners do not recommend herbal remedies, in particular oral doses of herbs, during the first trimester of pregnancy and seek an alternative. However, herbs are successfully used during pregnancy, especially to prepare the body for the birth. Herbs are relatively unstudied in pregnancy and lactation, so patients need to be made aware through education of the potential benefits and risks of using herbs for health conditions that arise during pregnancy or lactation. The use of herbal remedies during pregnancy often warrants a referral to a knowledgeable herbal practitioner.

USE FOR CHILDREN:
In Germany, elder flower is indicated for colds and to increase bronchial secretions in cases of congestion. The recommended maximum daily dose is 3 tablespoonfuls of the infusion (Schilcher, 1992).

Weed (1986) recommends elder blossom tincture to reduce infant's fevers. She believes that it brings balance to the mechanism that regulates body temperature and will reduce very high fevers without fail. Recommendations are to use 1 drop of tincture per pound of body weight by placing it directly under the infant's tongue.

Herbal Caveat—Children
Children have special needs in regard to herbal therapies. They require lesser amounts of herbs and often respond well to mild teas and topical applications such as compresses and baths. The lowest dose of oral preparations should be tried first before increasing the amount given children. Caregivers should observe children closely for responses to herbal remedies. Younger children, particularly infants, have traditionally been given herbs either through their mother's breast milk or in the form of a homeo-

---

pathic remedy because of their sensitivity to medicines and treatments and the immaturity of their liver. It is recommended that a person knowledgeable in the herbal treatment of children be consulted before the offering of any herb to a child for the first time.

CAUTIONS:

There are no known drug interactions with elder flowers or berries and no known side effects when used appropriately (Blumenthal et al., 2000; McGuffin et al., 1997). Elderberries are not to be eaten raw. They should be ripe (purple-black in color) when harvested and must be cooked. The raw and unripe fruit, seeds, bark, and leaves of *S. nigra* and related species contain the cyanogenic glycoside, sambunigrin, the ingestion of which can cause nausea, vomiting or severe diarrhea (McGuffin et al., 1997).

It has been reported that children using peashooters made from elder stems have experienced cyanide poisoning and severe diarrhea. It is not known specifically which species of elder caused the poisoning (Kay, 1996). The recommended treatment was for cyanide poisoning (Duke, 1985).

I also recommend that people observe their bowel habits while taking elderberry. Some berries can be very astringent (drying) and the last thing someone with cold or flu needs is to be constipated. Although no side effects have been noticed in the studies that have been reported, this is my clinical observation. Therefore, I usually recommend taking an elderberry tea or taking the standardized extract syrup in warm water and making sure to drink plenty of fluids throughout the day.

NURSING EVIDENCE:

Historical Nursing Use
No data are available at this time.

Potential Nursing Applications
In the United States influenza epidemics occur nearly every year and are responsible for significant morbidity and mortality, including approximately 20,000 deaths per year (Brammer et al., 2000). Other countries around the globe have similar concerns about influenza. Influenza outbreaks have a significant impact on productivity. Business and service industries suffer tremendously when the numbers of staff and customers dwindle during peak outbreaks. Respiratory viruses have a pattern of causing longer term illness that can weaken the body and make it more susceptible to bacterial infections such as pneumonia. Nurses may want to consider recommending elderberry. This is especially important when flu vaccine shortages occur and the healthy in the workforce may be asked to allow the elderly and infirm to get their shots first.

Elderberry extract has been shown to significantly reduce the time a person experiences flu symptoms to days rather than weeks. Public health nurses might consider conducting larger clinical studies of the impact of elderberry on their influenza statistics, keeping in mind that present studies show that elder does not necessarily influence incidence but duration of symptoms.

Nurses also may wish to explore the clinical use of elder flowers in promoting sweating. For instance pediatric nurses may wish to study the effects of elder tea and rest in children with cold symptoms and perhaps compare the children receiving elder tea with other children receiving antibiotics and/or antipyretics in terms of length of illness and sequelae. Distilled elder flower water also might be researched for its skin, wound, and burn healing properties.

Integrative Insight

Biomedical and traditional evidence supports the use of elder in the care and treatment of people with influenza and other viral illnesses. While there may be no "cure" for the common cold or influenza, elder has been shown to support the body in moving through the illness in a shorter period of time. The concept of moving through an illness is important in health care. People develop immunity when they experience the diseases that occur around them. Some might even say that those who live through an infectious disease can be strengthened by the experience because they then have acquired primary immunity to the disease. An infectious illness, such as a cold or flu, becomes more serious when it continues to produce symptoms that go on for weeks and even months. The viral illness gradually weakens the body and the spirit, because the person may feel exhausted just from feeling sick for so long. Bacterial illness, weakness, fatigue, and anorexia can then become complications of what was originally a viral illness.

One goal of nursing care during viral illness must be to help the patient maintain their strength and ability to move through the illness as quickly as possible so that the viral illness does not weaken the patient and allow other complications to occur. Elder flowers assist in moving the virus through the body by opening the pores and increasing perspiration. This also helps with regulation of fever. Elderberries, although the mechanism is not exactly clear, are able to help the person move through their illness more quickly. This is considered beneficial in herbalism so that the patient is not overcome by the illness and can experience it at a manageable level.

In the biomedical paradigm, the goal of preventing disease from occurring in the first place might be very appropriate for some who are weak and invalid already. But for many, experiencing disease on occasion can be a way of allowing the body to cycle through part of a natural adaptation response to environmental stimuli such as viruses. Using elder to promote a potentially positive adaptation response in sustaining viral illness might be a more appropriate choice of approach to care for some patients.

Oral

Infusion. Use 1 teaspoon dry berries or flowers (3 to 4 g) in 5 ounces (150 ml) water. Take 1 to 2 cups several times daily as hot as can be sipped safely (Blumenthal et al., 2000).

Unless otherwise prescribed, use 10 to 15 g of the whole flower daily in divided doses (Blumenthal et al., 2000).

It is recommended that elder flower tea be taken hot while in bed because the diaphoretic effect is best experienced when physically warm. It is thought that diaphoretic tea has no effect in the morning, but should be taken in the afternoon when the natural diurnal pattern of the body creates a rise in temperature. When taken during this time, it will produce prompt sweating (Schulz et al., 1998).

Tincture. 1:5 (g/ml): Take $\frac{1}{2}$ to $1\frac{1}{2}$ teaspoons (2.5 to 7.5 ml) three times daily (Blumenthal et al., 2000).

Standardized Extract/Syrup as per the Zakay-Rones Study. Take 4 tablespoons (60 ml) per day for adults and 2 tablespoons (30 ml) per day for children.

Topical

Elder flower distilled water can be sprayed in wounds, burns, and skin inflammations to promote healing.

Environmental

Elder is often grown as an ornamental shrub.

Herbal Caveat—Therapeutic Applications

In traditional and conventional herbal medicine, amounts of herbs given to patients are based on individual needs. The amounts or "doses" recorded here are provided so that the health practitioner has a general idea of the amounts recommended for an adult patient. Dosing in herbalism not only refers to amount of plant used but also includes when, where, and how to take a plant medicine. These dosages should not be used as guidelines for indiscriminate intervention without proper assessment, critical thinking, and patient education on the part of the practitioner.

Note: Please see chapter 5 for detailed descriptions of how to prepare various applications.

Elder flowers and ripe berries (must be cooked) have been shown to support the immune system during colds and flu. It is often recommended by herbalists that herbs be taken at the first sign of discomfort during cold and flu season rather than waiting until the virus has weakened the body. Elder flower tea can be considered to promote sweating and elderberries to support the immune system during a bout of influenza. There are no known drug interactions with elder, but studies may not have been conducted that describe the results of taking over-the-counter cold and flu remedies and elderberry at the same time. It may be best to choose to try one at a time, rather than take the two together.

Herbal Caveat—Patient Interaction

Patients considering the use of an herb or formula of herbs in self-care benefit from education about the plant itself and the use of the plant in healing. This education can come through many sources, including local herbalists; plant specialists such as botanists; health practitioners such as nurses, nutritionists, naturopaths, and other physicians; and various written references including the scientific literature. Patients need to remember that their unique health care needs are not necessarily represented in any literature they may encounter. Therefore, it is recommended that a knowledgeable mentor be consulted before initiating self-care with any herb being used for the first time.

NURTURING THE NURSE-PLANT RELATIONSHIP:

Note: You may want to keep a journal of your experiences with the herb.

There is nothing sweeter than a little elder flower or elderberry tea or syrup with its rich, sweet, warming, and somewhat astringent taste. If you know of a shrub that hasn't been sprayed and can harvest the flowers or berries yourself, try putting some flowers on a pancake before flipping it over. Or make a syrup from the cooked berries. First press out the juice from the berries and strain into a saucepan. Add honey or natural sweetener and then simmer and reduce until thickened. Refrigerate. Nurses are often highly exposed to influenza and respiratory viruses. Try taking the syrup as soon as you feel upper respiratory symptoms coming on during flu season. Keep a journal record of the number of viral illnesses you have and how long your symptoms last.

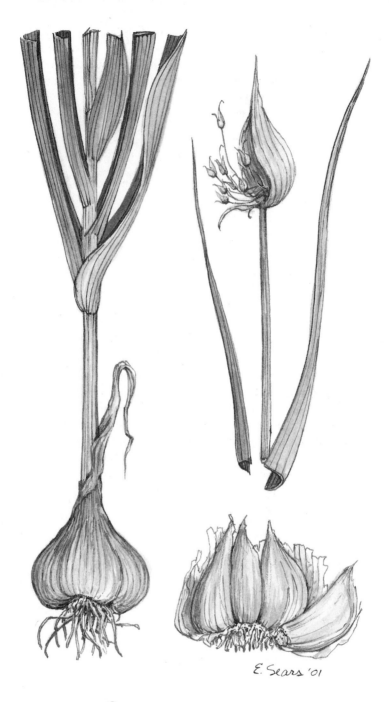

Allium sativum

Garlic

🌿 **LATIN NAME:** *Allium sativum*

🌿 **FAMILY:** Liliaceae

🌿 **COMMON NAMES:** Garlic, garlic clove

🌿 **HEALTH PATTERN:** Immune response

🌿 **PLANT DESCRIPTION:**

The garlic plant has a stem that grows up to 2 feet (0.7 meter) high. The leaves are long, narrow, and flat like grass (Grieve, 1971). The flowers appear in July and are in the form of pink, red, or white umbrella-shaped clusters at the ends of the stems. The underground bulb is the medicinal part and is formed of about eight wedge-shaped compressed bulblets arranged circularly around a central stem. The smaller bulblets are succulent and fleshy with a strong pungent odor and taste. Some experts think that garlic is native to Sicily, but others disagree. It has been around for so long that it is difficult to trace its origin. It is found in Asia and is cultivated in gardens in the United States and Europe (Felter & Lloyd, 1983).

🌿 **PLANT PART USED:** Fresh or dried garlic bulb with its secondary cloves

🌿 **TRADITIONAL EVIDENCE:**

Cultural Use

Asian. In TCM, garlic, "da suan," has been used for many years to treat diarrhea, dysentery (amebic and bacterial), tuberculosis, diphtheria, bloody urine, hepatitis, scalp ringworm, and vaginal trichomoniasis (Leung & Foster, 1996). It is classified as an herb that expels parasites and has been used for treating food poisoning from shellfish and to prevent influenza. It is not recommended for those with yin deficiency with heat signs. Garlic is considered an irritant to the skin and is not applied long term or taken internally by those with problems of the mouth, tongue, or throat. Topical applications to the perianal area and enemas are not recommended during pregnancy (Bensky & Gamble, 1993).

In Japanese macrobiotic tradition, a topical garlic plaster to the heel is used when a person is feeling cold (Kushi, 1993).

North American Indian. North American Indians use garlic species that grow wild near their homes. The Cherokee use it as an agent to rid the intestines of gas, as a diuretic, and an expectorant. It also has been used to increase the output of urine and eliminate edema. The Cherokee also use garlic for the treatment of asthma, and for croup in children, intestinal worms, and colic. Other tribes use garlic topically for protection from the bites of poisonous snakes, scorpions, and spiders. As a food source, tribes use it cooked with other seasonings in soups, relishes, and flavorings or dried for winter use (Moerman, 1998). The Mountain Pima insert a clove of garlic into the rectum to treat fevers (Kay, 1996).

Hispanic. Mexican Americans apply fresh garlic, "ajo," to scorpion stings and snakebites and to their feet during a cold. Garlic is used to build the immune system and the heart. It is used as an internal remedy for high blood pressure and diabetes (Kay, 1996). Garlic tea is used for breaking up mucus that is difficult to expel and for sore throat. It is also used topically in olive oil for earache and other body pain.

African. Garlic was introduced into Africa many years ago. It is used in the treatment of respiratory infections and as an agent that destroys intestinal worms. In Nigeria, it is applied topically for certain skin conditions. In Chad, fresh garlic bulbs are used to prepare tonics for diabetics (Iwu, 1993).

East Indian. Traditional medicine in India uses garlic, "lasuna," to expel round worms from the intestines. It is used topically to apply to the abdomen to treat gastrointestinal complaints. It is applied as a liniment for convulsions, nervous and spasmodic conditions, general paralysis, gout, sciatica, and skin diseases such as leprosy. Garlic is used internally to prevent typhus, typhoid, and diphtheria. It also is used to treat pneumonia, bronchitis, and tuberculosis. Garlic is used extensively in the diet in India as a spice to flavor chutneys, vegetables, curries, and pickles (Nadkarni, 1976).

Russian/Baltic. Hundreds of years ago, the Russians believed that wearing amulets made of garlic would protect them from evil spirits that caused infectious diseases. Garlic continues to be well respected today for its antiparasitic, antibacterial, and virucidal properties. Russian doctors during World War II used garlic in the field to treat wounds. It was reported to have prevented gangrene and sepsis and came to be known as "Russian penicillin." Russian traditional healers have long advocated eating one clove of raw garlic every day. It is added to salads or mixed with salt and chopped tomatoes and spread on dark rye bread. Current Russian medicine recognizes garlic to be effective for treating poor intestinal tone, poor digestion, colitis, and putrefactive bacteria in the intestines. It is used to expel intestinal parasites and stimulate the function of the liver and gallbladder. Russian doctors recommend the use of garlic to those who have been exposed to lead poisoning. It is used to strengthen the heart, for arteriosclerosis, high blood pressure, bronchitis, and diabetes. The traditional herbalists of Russia use garlic to prevent colds, flu, and other viruses. They use it for migraines and insomnia. They treat corns on the skin by applying raw garlic cloves for twelve to eighteen hours (Zevin, 1997).

European. The German Commission E approves the use of garlic to support attempts to decrease serum lipids and to prevent vascular changes due to aging (Blumenthal et al., 2000). Garlic is used in Norway and middle Europe for diabetes (Augusti, 1996). Garlic was used in England as a vinegar that was taken internally to prevent being infected with the plague.

Culinary Use

Garlic is widely used as a culinary ingredient throughout the world. Garlic oil is used as a flavoring in most food products such as nonalcoholic beverages, frozen dairy desserts, candy, gelatins, baked goods, meat products, relishes, fats, oils, snack foods, and gravies (Leung & Foster, 1996).

Use in Herbalism

Garlic has been used historically to protect against the plague, promote the flow of urine and menstruation, to treat bites from dogs and poisonous insects, to kill intestinal worms in children, as an expectorant, to decrease lethargy, for skin sores and ulcers, and for earaches. It was used as a treatment when sickness occurred from drinking polluted water or overdosing on highly active plants such as henbane, wolfbane, and hemlock. It also has been used for the treatment of jaundice, cramps, convulsions, hemorrhoids, and a condition known as "melancholy" (Culpeper, 1990).

Garlic has been used specifically for leprosy. It also was used for smallpox by chopping it and applying it to the feet bound in a linen cloth. Other uses of garlic included cough syrup for asthma, hoarseness, and difficult breathing. It was claimed that a clove of garlic pounded with honey and taken two or three nights in succession was good for rheumatism. It also was used for edema of the lower extremities. Garlic juice boiled in milk and taken internally was used to expel intestinal worms (Grieve, 1971).

American Eclectic physicians used garlic in cases of coughs, pertussis, hoarseness, and intestinal worms. Poultices of garlic were used topically along the spine and on the chests of infants suffering from pneumonia. A mixture of garlic juice, sweet almond oil, and glycerin was dropped into the ears to treat deafness (Felter & Lloyd, 1983).

Currently, garlic is one of the most popular herbs used in Western Europe and the United States to reduce certain risks associated with cardiovascular disease. Current uses of garlic include its ability to lower serum lipids, decrease blood pressure and blood sugar, and its antimicrobial activity (Blumenthal et al., 2000). Garlic also is used for preventing and alleviating the symptoms associated with bacterial, parasitic, and fungal infections and viral infections such as colds and influenza. Garlic is an excellent expectorant. Garlic with purple skin is thought to demonstrate the most effective action against microbes and amoebic infection (Bensky & Gamble, 1993).

There are many stories of the mystical power of garlic. One European superstition claims that if a man chews a bit of garlic before running a race, his competitors will not be able to outrun him (Grieve, 1971). Garlic also was believed to be able to ward off vampires, demons, and other harmful beings (Foster & Tyler, 1999).

BIOMEDICAL EVIDENCE:

Garlic has been the focus of numerous studies, some of which have studied the traditional use of garlic for infection (its antimicrobial effects). In general, little *clinical* research seems to address the traditional use of garlic in preventing infectious disease in humans by strengthening their immune response in some way. Many published studies have been written regarding the cardiovascular and anti-cancer effects of garlic (Foster & Tyler, 1999).

Because of the many forms in which garlic can be used, it is imperative that studies about garlic's effects not only clarify the form of garlic being studied, but also that the investigators make their conclusions from the research relate to the particular form of garlic that has been studied. For example, a garlic study published in the *Journal of the American Medical Association* in 1998 concluded that "There is no evidence to recommend garlic therapy for lowering serum lipid levels" (Berthold, Sudhop, & von Bergmann, 1998, p. 1902). This study specifically looked at Tegra, a steam-distilled garlic oil that does not contain allicin, the constituent known for lowering cholesterol (American Botanical Council, 1998). It would have been best had the conclusion been written so as not to generalize the findings of the study to all other forms of garlic.

Studies Related to Immune Response

Although garlic *extract* has been found to inhibit *Helicobacter pylori* in vitro (Sivam, Lampe, Ulness, Swanzy, & Potter, 1997), investigators for a human trial have concluded that whole sliced garlic did not have a significant effect in vivo on *H. pylori* in 12 adult participants. The investigators write, "Caution must be used when attempting to extrapolate data from in vitro studies to the in vivo condition" (Graham, Anderson, & Lang, 1999, p. 1200). This is another example of equating studies in which two different garlic forms were used—whole sliced garlic (in vivo) and garlic extract (in vitro). The investigators state that their research does not support the in vitro data and that in vitro data on traditional remedies should not be released to the public before in vivo testing because of the possibility of misleading the public. Although this may be a reasonable and prudent suggestion, they make reference to two very different substances. Garlic extract may be effective in vivo for *H. pylori* infection. In another study of garlic and *H. pylori*, garlic *oil* also was found to be ineffective against *H. pylori* in a study of twenty patients (Aydin, Ersoz, Tekesin, Akcicek, & Tuncyurek, 2000).

In a study, 34 men with diagnosed *Tinea pedis* received an ajoene cream (the organic trisulfur compound in garlic), Acuagel, for seven days. After the seven days, 79% were completely symptom free, and the other 21% were symptom free after an additional seven days of Acuagel application (Ledezma et al., 1996).

Animal studies have shown that mice fed a garlic extract fifteen days before influenza infection were protected from illness (Duke, 1999).

Studies Related to Other Health Patterns

Mobility. The studies presented here relate to the mobility of the blood, and in this case, the movement of lipids or cholesterol in the blood and their relationship to heart disease.

Garlic powder tablets, 800 mg taken orally every day for four weeks by 60 participants in a randomized, double-blind, controlled parallel group study, significantly reduced the participants' ratio of circulating platelet aggregates by 10.3% and spontaneous platelet aggregation by 56.3% (Kiesewetter et al., 1993).

Aortic stiffness is a part of human aging whether or not the individual has a history of heart disease. One epidemiologic, cross-sectional study of 101 subjects who had been taking amounts greater than or equal to 300 mg of standardized garlic powder for greater than or equal to two years compared with 101 control subjects demonstrated that the garlic powder seems to have a protective effect on the elasticity of the aorta (Breithaupt-Grogler, Ling, Boudoulas, & Belz, 1997).

Hormone Balance. One German study had found that garlic powder tablets (Kwai) did reduce cholesterol levels significantly in patients with hypercholesterolemia, but some have questioned the findings in relation to the perceived limitations of the study, namely that the diets of the subjects and the lipid measurements were not controlled (Mader as reported in Blumenthal et al., 2000). In a later study in which these limitations were addressed, American researchers concluded that there was no significant difference in the ability of garlic powder to lower cholesterol levels. This conclusion applied to both the control and treatment groups in one multicenter, randomized, placebo-controlled trial of 50 patients, 28 of whom received garlic powder (Kwai) tablets, 300 mg three times a day, equivalent to 2.7 g or 1 clove of fresh garlic per day (Isaacsohn et al., 1998). However, a 1993 metanalysis of the literature, which included five studies ($N = 365$) adhering to inclusion criteria of being published, randomized, and placebo-controlled studies, found that garlic, in supplements approximating ½ to 1 clove per day, did exhibit a significant reduction on total cholesterol levels by at least 9% and sometimes up to 15%. One limitation of the metanalysis is that in three of the five studies, Kwai garlic tablets were used; in one study spray-dried powder was used; and in the fifth study, garlic aqueous extract was used. None of the studies placed dietary restrictions on participants (Warshafsky, Kafer, & Sivak, 1993).

The issue according to Isaacsohn et al. (1998) is that although animal studies seem to show an effect of garlic on cholesterol levels in animals fed a high-fat diet, if humans who participate in garlic studies receive a modified, low-cholesterol diet, there seems to be no significant effect. "In all studies in which the expected lipid effect is modest, dietary stabilization becomes a crucial factor in establishing the true lipid-lowering capacity of the treatment under investigation" (Isaacsohn et al., 1998, p. 1193). It may be significant that studies that have found no effect of garlic powder on cholesterol levels often report some dietary control, such as an American Heart Association Step 1 diet, as part of the methodology (Superko & Krauss, 2000).

Mechanism of Action

The biologic action of garlic, as with all *Allium* species, is related to its organosulfur compounds. The antibiotic principle in garlic, allicin (which is effective against numerous gram-negative and gram-positive bacteria), is also known as "Russian penicillin." An in vitro study demonstrated that Fraction 4, a protein isolated from aged garlic extract, is an efficient immunopotentiator (Morioka, Sze, Morton, & Irie, 1993). Garlic or its constituent allicin is also effective against certain multidrug-resistant strains of bacteria. Most bacteria are unable to develop resistance to it because its mechanism of action is not like other antibiotics. The parent substance of allicin, alliin, is a sulfur-containing amino acid derivative that does not have antimicrobial activity. According to Foster & Tyler (1999), alliin becomes allicin when the garlic bulb is ground and the alliin comes in contact with an enzyme in the bulb that converts the alliin to allicin.

The active principles in fresh garlic are released through grinding as in chewing; however, many people do not like the after-effects of chewing fresh garlic cloves. Fresh garlic extracts with the constituent allicin also have demonstrated antifungal, antiparasitic, and antiviral activity in vitro (Ankri & Mirelman, 1999). Fresh garlic has been shown to be have greater antifungal activity against *C. albicans* than nystatin in vitro (Arora & Kaur, 1999).

The antithrombotic and significant antifungal action of garlic is related to its ajoene consitutent (Augusti, 1996). Dried garlic preparations are said not to contain allicin or ajoene. Dried preparations do contain alliin, both allicin's and ajoene's precursor. The enzyme that converts the alliin to allicin and ajoene is very unstable in the presence of acids and is said to be destroyed by gastric secretions (Foster & Tyler, 1999). Therefore, enteric-coated, dried garlic preparations may be more effective.

USE IN PREGNANCY OR LACTATION:

In general, ingestion of therapeutic amounts of garlic is not recommended during pregnancy or lactation because of its emmenagogic effects (Blumenthal et al., 2000; Brinker, 1998; McGuffin et al., 1997).

Some infants demonstrate sensitivity to the odor of garlic in the mother's milk, and some experience colic symptoms related to the sulfur compounds. Garlic oil in capsules was found to increase the odor of amniotic fluid in the five women given the supplement in a small study of 10 pregnant women. In utero experience of garlic, as well as other foods, may affect postnatal food preferences (Mennella, Johnson, & Beauchamp, 1995).

Some knowledgeable midwives recommend the internal use of garlic, either raw or as oil capsules, to reduce elevated blood pressure during pregnancy (Weed, 1986). Weed also recommends a garlic treatment for hemorrhoids that occur during pregnancy (Weed, 1986).

Herbal Caveat—Pregnancy or Lactation

Some herbs are contraindicated in pregnancy because of a risk of the herb or one of its constituents stimulating the uterus and therefore possibly promoting fetal loss. Many herbal practitioners do not recommend herbal remedies, in particular oral doses of herbs, during the first trimester of pregnancy and seek an alternative. However, herbs are successfully used during pregnancy, especially to prepare the body for the birth. Herbs are relatively unstudied in pregnancy and lactation, so patients need to be made aware through education of the potential benefits and risks of using herbs for health conditions that arise during pregnancy or lactation. The use of herbal remedies during pregnancy often warrants a referral to a knowledgeable herbal practitioner.

USE FOR CHILDREN:

Some caution that oral administration of therapeutic doses of fresh garlic to children is dangerous and possibly fatal (as reported in McGuffin et al., 1997). Schilcher (1992) does not report any contraindications in children.

Herbal Caveat—Children

Children have special needs in regard to herbal therapies. They require lesser amounts of herbs and often respond well to mild teas and topical applications such as compresses and baths. The lowest dose of oral preparations should be tried first before increasing the amount given children. Caregivers should observe children closely for responses to herbal remedies. Younger children, particularly infants, have traditionally been given herbs either through their mother's breast milk or in the form of a homeopathic remedy because of their sensitivity to medicines and treatments and the immaturity of their liver. It is recommended that a person knowledgeable in the herbal treatment of children be consulted before the offering of any herb to a child for the first time.

CAUTIONS:

It is not recommended that large amounts of garlic be consumed for ten to fourteen days before surgery because it may prolong bleeding time. Garlic is contraindicated in those who have a known allergy to it (Blumenthal et al., 2000). Rare side effects of the ingestion of garlic may include gastrointestinal symptoms, allergic type reactions, and an odor of garlic on the skin and breath (Blumenthal et al., 2000).

There are no known interactions between garlic and prescription drugs; however, garlic is known to substantially increase the anticoagulant effect of warfarin and therefore could increase bleeding times. It has been reported that blood-clotting times have doubled in patients who are taking warfarin when taking garlic *supplements* (Blumenthal et al., 2000).

Garlic also is contraindicated in those with acute or chronic inflammation of the stomach or other gastrointestinal surfaces because certain constituents of garlic can cause gastroenteritis. When high levels of purified constituents of garlic are used on a regular basis, iodine uptake by the thyroid is reduced. It also has been suggested that insulin dosages may need to be adjusted because of the blood-sugar-lowering effects of garlic in rat experiments (Brinker, 1998). People who have kidney problems should avoid garlic because it may irritate the kidneys (Zevin, 1997).

NURSING EVIDENCE:

Historical Nursing Use

Nurses mixed garlic juice with sugar and made it into a syrup for use with babies who had cough or pulmonary problems (Felter & Lloyd, 1983).

Potential Nursing Applications

As the list of resistant strains of microorganisms grows, nurses may need to deal with a public that is restless for suggestions for dealing with infection. Garlic has been shown to be capable of inhibiting viruses, fungi, and gram-negative and gram-positive bacteria, without resistance developing. Nurses may want to consider researching the addition of garlic to the diet of some patients as a preventive measure against infectious disease. Nurses also might consider integrating the use of garlic and onion syrup back into the domestic self-care guidelines given to patients dealing with cough and cold symptoms. Nurses also might consider performing ethnographic and/or historical studies on the traditional medicinal uses of garlic and the support of the immune system.

Integrative Insight

Both biomedical and traditional evidence demonstrate garlic's versatility in dealing with infection. It has been shown to have broad-spectrum effects against a number of bacteria and has significant antifungal, antiparasitic, and antiviral properties. It has been successfully used during serious infectious diseases such as plague and leprosy, and it is used for the more common upper respiratory infections as well. Some of the constituents in garlic, such as allicin and ajoene, which contribute to its ability to support the body through infection, have been identified. Yet more data is needed to understand how garlic stimulates the human immune response system and how that effect may influence overall health. Many people who eat garlic regularly claim to have fewer or perhaps no viral illnesses sometimes for years.

Garlic's signature odor, as with the odor of many plants, may be responsible for attracting or repelling pathogenic substances. In the case of garlic, many things such as plague have historically steered clear of garlic eaters. Biomedical evidence does seem to point, however, to the most effective form of garlic as being the chewing of the fresh cloves. I have an eighty-year-old friend who tucks a big clove in her cheek every time she feels that she has been exposed to a cold or flu and she stays healthy. How can eating garlic hurt, especially if people that come in close contact with each other are all indulging in the same garlic preventive?

Heating garlic can limit the odor and taste of garlic. Although heating garlic has been shown to destroy the enzyme that converts alliin to allicin, people still receive health benefits from cooked garlic. This may be due to the other constituents in garlic. Duke (1999) says that there is more to the beneficial effects of garlic than the sulfur compounds affected by the destruction of the enzyme. I always recommend that if a person must cook garlic, then it be cooked just a little so as to preserve the "bite" as much as possible. It may be the bite, like the tingle of echinacea, that stimulates immune response.

THERAPEUTIC APPLICATIONS:

Oral

Whole Herb. Use approximately 0.14 ounce (4 g) daily of fresh garlic bulb (Blumenthal et al., 2000).

Infusion. Use about 0.14 ounce (4 g) in 5 ounces (150 ml) of water daily (Blumenthal et al., 2000).

Tincture. 1:5 (g/ml): Take 4 teaspoons (20 ml) daily in divided doses (Blumenthal et al., 2000).

One beneficial way to take garlic is to use two or three raw cloves each day in food preparation. Leave the thin peel on when cooking garlic for the extra antioxidant action such as occurs from the quercetin in the peel.

Topical

Garlic Oil. See Nurturing the Nurse-Plant Relationship.

Garlic Plaster for the Heel (to warm a patient who is shivering). Grate some garlic and wrap it in cheesecloth. Apply this to the heel. Remove it when the heel feels hot (Kushi, 1993).

Poultice or Paste. Chop garlic clove finely, place in fine gauze, and apply to the skin for treating parasitic infestation, such as applying to the perianal area for pinworms. This may be irritating to the skin.

Hemorrhoid Application. Wrap a peeled clove of garlic in one layer of gauze, oil it, and insert it into the rectum overnight to reduce swelling (Weed, 1986).

Environmental

Some people find the odor of garlic highly offensive. The skin and breath of people who eat garlic can exude the odor of the herb. Odorless garlic capsules are one solution, but some people like to eat their medicine. If you cook or eat Chinese food, you may have noticed that lots of garlic is used in many dishes. Have you also noticed that you do not get the odor problem? This may be related to the ginger and other herbs and spices that are used in the cooking. If you have been using whole garlic for medicinal purposes, perhaps without the ginger, you can try adding ginger to your food or you can try an old remedy for garlic breath. Try chewing roasted coffee beans or parsley leaves and seeds (Felter & Lloyd, 1983).

Herbal Caveat—Therapeutic Applications

In traditional and conventional herbal medicine, amounts of herbs given to patients are based on individual needs. The amounts or "doses" recorded here are provided so that the health practitioner has a general idea of the amounts recommended for an adult patient. Dosing in herbalism not only refers to amount of plant used but also includes when, where, and how to take a plant medicine. These dosages should not be used as guidelines for indiscriminate intervention without proper assessment, critical thinking, and patient education on the part of the practitioner.

Note: Please see chapter 5 for detailed descriptions of how to prepare various applications.

PATIENT INTERACTION:

Garlic is an old medicinal remedy that has been used for thousands of years. It is known as "Russian penicillin" for its antibacterial, antiparasitic, antifungal, and antiviral effects. It has been shown to be effective in lowering cholesterol. Many people in many cultures swear by the immune system and heart strengthening effects of their daily "dose" of two cloves of garlic in mashed potatoes, vegetable, or pasta dishes. Some evidence suggests that garlic may be most effective if chewed fresh or pounded first or taken in a dried, tablet form that has been coated with a substance to protect the active substances in garlic from being destroyed by acid juices in the stomach. Medicinal amounts of garlic can significantly thin the blood, so let your health practitioner know if you are taking a medication with blood-thinning action.

Herbal Caveat—Patient Interaction

Patients considering the use of an herb or formula of herbs in self-care benefit from education about the plant itself and the use of the plant in healing. This education can come through many sources, including local herbalists; plant specialists such as botanists; health practitioners such as nurses, nutritionists, naturopaths, and other physicians; and various written references including the scientific literature. Patients need to remember that their unique health care needs are not necessarily represented in any literature they may encounter. Therefore, it is recommended that a knowledgeable mentor be consulted before initiating self-care with any herb being used for the first time.

NURTURING THE NURSE-PLANT RELATIONSHIP:

Note: You may want to keep a journal of your experiences with the herb.

Garlic is not hard to get to know. Try chopping some of the cloves, breathing in the fresh aroma, and then putting it in your next batch of mashed potatoes during cold season. Chop the garlic into fine pieces or use a garlic press. Sauté the garlic in butter or ghee on medium heat for 30 to 60 seconds—leave as much of the bite in the garlic as you can tolerate. Add the garlic to the mashed potatoes.

One other way to get to know the medicinal benefit of garlic is to make and use a garlic ear oil for ear pain that often accompanies head congestion and ear infection. The protocol in one clinic I worked in was to check the eardrum, and if it was intact and was only pink and not severely inflamed (i.e., it was early on in the infection), garlic-mullein flower ear oil drops were given. Pharmaceutical antibiotics were not the first choice of treatment for our team. The ear oil is so easy to make that children can learn to make it. I used to teach the girl scouts how to make their own ear oil.

Garlic-Mullein Flower Ear Oil. Peel and thinly slice the cloves of one garlic head. If you have access to fresh mullein flowers *(Verbascum thapsus)*, use equal parts flower and garlic. There is no need to wash the flowers and the tap water will contaminate your oil. If you do not have flowers just make garlic oil. Put the herbs in a wide-mouthed jar and cover the herbs with olive oil. Place a piece of cheese-cloth over the jar opening and secure it with a rubber band. Let the oil stand in a warm place for approximately two weeks. Swirl the oil gently occasionally during the extraction period. Strain and press the oil out of the herbs into small medicine bottles with glass droppers.

To use the oil, start by warming the bottle of oil in a small pan of warm water. Test a drop of oil on your wrist. When it is warm, take a few drops of the oil and massage gently in a circular and downward motion behind the ear and along the neck (following the eustachian tube). Then gently massage in front of the ear.

Tip your head, pull the earlobe to open the ear canal and drop the oil in the ear until you can feel it fill (about 4 drops). Place a cotton ball gently in the ear. This remedy can be very helpful when the ear is sore or stuffy during colds and flu. It is not to be used internally if the eardrum has ruptured and/or the ear is draining, but it can still be massaged externally behind the ear.

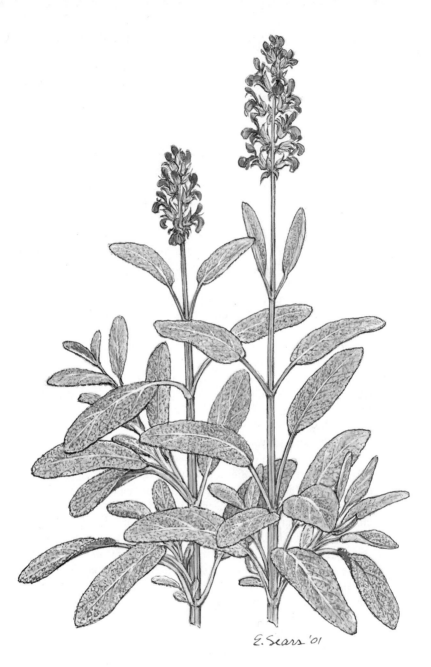

E. Sears '01

Salvia officinalis

Sage

@ **LATIN NAME:** *Salvia officinalis*

@ **FAMILY:** Lamiaceae

@ **COMMON NAMES:** Sage, broad-leaf sage, common sage, dalmation sage, garden sage, true sage

@ **HEALTH PATTERN:** Immune response

@ **PLANT DESCRIPTION:**

Sage is an evergreen, shrublike plant that is native to the Mediterranean area and is widely cultivated in Turkey, Greece, Italy, France, and the United States (Blumenthal et al., 2000). It has a square (four-sided) stem with downy leaves that are opposite each other on the stem. The leaves are about 2 inches (5 cm) long and appear wrinkled. The whole plant is of a soft gray-green color and reaches about a foot (0.33 meter) in height. The blue to purple flowers appear in June and July in spikes. The sage plant has a characteristic aromatic odor, and a bitter, astringent, aromatic taste (Felter & Lloyd, 1983; Grieve, 1971). *Salvia officinalis,* or garden sage, is not the same plant as clary sage, which is *Salvia sclarea.*

@ **PLANT PART USED:** Leaves

@ **TRADITIONAL EVIDENCE:**

Cultural Use

Asian. TCM medicine practitioners use the root of *Salvia miltiorrhiza,* "danshen," grown in China to "invigorate the blood" and to "clear heat." It is used for dysmenorrhea, amenorrhea, palpable masses, and pain due to blood stasis. It also is used to soothe irritability, restlessness, palpitations, and insomnia (Bensky & Gamble, 1993).

The Japanese call *danshen* "tanjin," and use it similarly to the way it is used in Chinese medicine (Rister, 1999).

North American Indian. North American Indians have used several varieties of sage because many are found throughout North America. *S. officinalis* has been used by the eastern tribes. The Cherokee use a sage infusion for diarrhea, colds, sore throat, coughs, as a diaphoretic, and as a laxative. A syrup is made from the leaves by adding honey and then the syrup is taken for the symptoms of asthma. They use an infusion for nervousness. The Mohegans use sage tea to remove intestinal parasites from the body and chew the fresh leaves as a tonic (Moerman, 1998). Native Americans of the southwest use sage tea made from the leaves and flowers to alleviate stomach disorders and to reduce fever. Women also use it during childbirth (Kay, 1996).

Other species of sage are used by various Native American tribes. Those in California grind sage seeds and mix them with water to create a mucilaginous substance that is used to keep the mouth and throat moist. The Catawbas make a salve of the roots of a wild sage to apply to wounds (Vogel, 1970). The Navajo pour an infusion of sage and other herbs over burning coals to use as a steam for conditions such as headache and insomnia (Vogel, 1970).

Hispanic. Hispanics call sage "salvia." The old Hispanic culture used many varieties of sage that were found growing in their areas. The seeds were taken with water twice a day to protect against dysentery and fever. A poultice was made of the seeds and applied to the abdomen. Other uses of sage were for conditions involving the head, epilepsy, paralysis, convulsions, deafness, and fainting. It was used to promote menstruation and facilitate childbirth (Kay, 1996).

Currently, some Mexican Americans drink a tea made of sage and other herbs for discomfort associated with cold, sore throat, toothache, arthritis, insect bites, and skin conditions and to relieve nervousness.

East Indian. In India, sage is used for flatulence, poor digestive function, gingivitis, and inflammation of the pharynx and tongue (Blumenthal et al., 2000). Sage has been used to relieve fatigue and preserve the teeth and to procure immortality (Nadkarni, 1976). *S. officinalis* has been used in Europe and elsewhere, but no mention is made of this variety being specifically used in India. Many other varieties of sage are described, however. *Salvia plebeia*, which grows in India, is used as a stimulant, carminative, diuretic, expectorant, and others. It is used for symptoms relating to hemorrhoids; palpitations; problems of the liver, brain, and heart; and to induce abortion. The seeds are used to treat gonorrhea, excessive menstrual bleeding, and diarrhea (Nadkarni, 1976).

Russian/Baltic. Sage has been one of the most popular herbal remedies in Russia. It has been used to treat a wide variety of ailments. Hot sage tea is used as a gargle for sore throats in both adults and children. It also is used to reduce the secretion of milk in nursing mothers who were beginning to wean their babies. Sage tea is used to aid digestion and to treat inflammation of the gallbladder and urinary bladder. It is used for flatulence (Zevin, 1997).

European. The German Commission E has approved the internal use of sage leaf for poor digestion, excessive perspiration, and night sweats, and the external use for inflammations of the nose and throat. Germany has licensed sage infusion for inflammation of the gums and mucous membranes of the mouth and throat, as an aid in the treatment of gastrointestinal irritation, and for use on pressure areas of the skin (Blumenthal et al., 2000). Sage is taken internally to reduce the secretion of saliva (Foster & Tyler, 1999).

The Anthroposophical approach to healing regards sage as being able to support the warmth-creating process within the body. One of the ways it does this is to stimulate perspiration in those who sweat little and to stop perspiration in those who sweat heavily (Husemann & Wolff, 1982).

Culinary Use

Sage has been commonly used since medieval times as a culinary herb often served with meat. It has been used in stuffings for fowl and pork and was used as a preservative, most importantly for meat before the advent of chemical preservatives. The English used sage leaves minced with onion and other ingredients to make gravy. The leaves were added to a pint of claret with lemon peel and shallots and allowed to steep for two weeks. A tablespoon of this was then added to various foods as a flavoring (Grieve, 1971).

Sage oil is currently used to flavor a wide variety of foods, such as baked goods, meats, condiments, relishes, vegetables, soups, gravies, and others (Leung & Foster, 1996).

Use in Herbalism

In the first century C.E., the Greeks reported that sage decoction stopped bleeding from wounds and cleaned ulcers and sores. They also used sage juice in warm water for hoarseness and coughing and to enhance memory (Blumenthal et al., 2000). Early European herbalists recommended sage decoction to promote menstruation, "cause the hair to become black," stop bleeding from wounds, clean skin ulcers, and promote the passage of urine. It was claimed that sage was good for the liver. Some used three teaspoons of sage juice with honey on an empty stomach to help stop the pulmonary bleeding that accompanied tuberculosis. Sage was applied to sore joints to help decrease pain. Gargles made of sage with other herbs were used for sores in the mouth and throat (Culpeper, 1990).

The American Eclectic physicians in the late 1800s used sage specifically in cases when the patient had cold extremities, soft relaxed skin, poor circulation, and exhaustive sweats. Sage was reported to be effective in restoring gastric tone and decreasing flatulence. Sage tea was taken warm in order to destroy intestinal worms and to cause diaphoresis during fevers. Some considered sage an effective agent to calm excessive sexual desires. Sage was applied to the breasts of lactating women when it was thought necessary to stop the production of milk. The infusion was used as a gargle for sore throat. Sage oil was applied to rheumatism to decrease the pain (Felter & Lloyd, 1983).

Sage infusion is used in the treatment of delirious fevers and nervous excitement by giving it in small, repeated doses. It is used as a stimulant tonic in general debility of the stomach and nervous system and poor digestion. Sage is used for typhoid fever, abdominal bloating, liver complaints, kidney trouble, colds, sore throats, measles, joint pain, and excessive perspiration. A cup of strong sage infusion relieves headaches due to nervousness (Grieve, 1971).

Externally, sage infusion is used for skin abrasions and ulcers. It is applied to the scalp to darken the hair. The fresh leaves are rubbed on the gums to strengthen them. The dried leaves of sage were smoked in a pipe for the relief of asthma (Grieve, 1971). The powdered leaves are pounded with salt and vinegar and applied to tumors in the mouth and other areas (Duke, 1985).

In current herbalism, sage is reported to be antibacterial, astringent, secretion-stimulating, perspiration-inhibiting, and to have the ability to stop the growth of certain viruses and fungi. It is used as a tonic, antiseptic, antispasmodic, and astringent. It is used to reduce perspiration such as night sweats, to stop the flow of milk in lactating mothers, to treat nervous conditions such as vertigo, trembling, and depression. It is also used for diarrhea, gastritis, sore throat, insect bites, and dysmenorrhea. Sage is a source of antioxidants (Leung & Foster, 1996).

Sage essential oil (not to be confused with clary sage essential oil), has antispasmodic effects on tight muscles and is used for dysmenorrhea. It is recommended for topical use to kill lice. Sage essential oil also is used for estrogen support during menopause because of its estrogen-like action (Buckle, 1997).

Cosmetic Use. Sage oil is used as a fragrance in various creams, detergents, lotions, perfumes, and soaps (Leung & Foster, 1996).

BIOMEDICAL EVIDENCE:

No published clinical studies were found to support this long-used medicinal herb. Laboratory studies discussed here demonstrate that the antimicrobial action of this plant is primarily related to its tannins and essential oil content.

Studies Related to Immune Response

Pure sage essential oil has been shown in vitro to have antimicrobial action against *E. coli, Shigella sonnei, Salmonella sp., Klebsiella ozaenae, Bacillus subtilis, C. albicans, C. krusei, C. pseuditropicalis, Torulopsis glabrata*, and *Cryptococcus neoformans* (Jalsenjak, Peljnjak, & Kustrak, 1987).

Studies Related to Other Health Patterns

No data are available at this time.

Mechanism of Action

Sage essential oil contains the constituents thujone, cineole, and camphor. Thujone has been shown to be responsible for the antimicrobial activity of sage (Jalsenjak et al., 1987). These three constituents, all monoterpenes, are also known to be epileptogenic (Burkhard, Burkhardt, Haenggeli, & Landis, 1999). The flowers and leaves of sage have been found to inhibit the growth of *S. aureus* and *Streptococcus pyogenes* (Kay, 1996). Sage has been shown to have strong antioxidative activities, especially because of the labiatic and carnosic acids. The phenolic acids, salvin and salvin monomethyl ether, have antimicrobial activities, especially against *S. aureus* (Leung & Foster, 1996). Sage contains high levels of tannins, plant constituents that have an antimicrobial and soothing effect, which may explain its use for sore throat (Duke, 1997).

USE IN PREGNANCY OR LACTATION:

The use of therapeutic doses of sage during pregnancy and lactation is not recommended because of its reported ability to promote the onset of menstruation by the volatile oil thujone (Blumenthal et al., 2000; Brinker, 1998); however, normal culinary doses may be safe (McGuffin et al., 1997). Midwives often recommend avoiding sage during the first trimester (Weed, 1986).

Sage has traditionally been used to reduce lactation so it should not be used if breastfeeding is desired (McGuffin et al., 1997). Midwives recommend drinking sage leaf tea to help reduce excessive engorgement of breasts during lactation (Weed, 1986); however, I have not seen women helped by sage when trying to decrease milk production.

Herbal Caveat—Pregnancy or Lactation

Some herbs are contraindicated in pregnancy because of a risk of the herb or one of its constituents stimulating the uterus and therefore possibly promoting fetal loss. Many herbal practitioners do not recommend herbal remedies, in particular oral doses of herbs, during the first trimester of pregnancy and seek an alternative. However, herbs are successfully used during pregnancy, especially to prepare the body for the birth. Herbs are relatively unstudied in pregnancy and lactation, so patients need to be made aware through education of the potential benefits and risks of using herbs for health conditions that arise during pregnancy or lactation. The use of herbal remedies during pregnancy often warrants a referral to a knowledgeable herbal practitioner.

USE FOR CHILDREN:

All essential oils should be stored away from children for their safety. The lethal dose of sage essential oil for a three-year-old child is about 5 teaspoons (26 ml) (Buckle, 1997).

Sore throats may be safely treated with sage leaf infusion or 1 to 2 drops of the essential oil in $3\frac{1}{2}$ ounces (100 ml) of water and used as a gargle (Schilcher, 1992).

Herbal Caveat—Children

Children have special needs in regard to herbal therapies. They require lesser amounts of herbs and often respond well to mild teas and topical applications such as compresses and baths. The lowest dose of oral preparations should be tried first before increasing the amount given children. Caregivers should observe children closely for responses to herbal remedies. Younger children, particularly infants, have traditionally been given herbs either through their mother's breast milk or in the form of a homeopathic remedy because of their sensitivity to medicines and treatments and the immaturity of their liver. It is recommended that a person knowledge-able in the herbal treatment of children be consulted before the offering of any herb to a child for the first time.

CAUTIONS:

It has been reported that after prolonged ingestion of sage tincture or of the pure essential oil, epileptic-like convulsions have occurred (Brinker, 1998; Burkhard et al., 1999). Breathing in the scent of the essential oil for prolonged periods has been reported to cause feelings of intoxication and giddiness (Duke, 1985).

Although not grounded in biomedical evidence, one nurse/aro-matherapist recommends that sage essential oil not be used by those with estrogen-dependent tumors because of its scareol content (Buckle, 1997). It is speculated that sage may interfere with hypo-glycemic and anticonvulsant therapies and may potentiate the seda-tive effects of some drugs (Newall et al., 1996).

NURSING EVIDENCE:

Historical Nursing Use

Sage tea has historically been used by caregivers such as the Ameri-can midwife Martha Ballard in the late 1700s and early 1800s, as a tea for the sick (Ulrich, 1990).

Potential Nursing Applications

Nurses may want to consider using sage clinically and studying its ex-tensive successful traditional uses, especially in relation to its effects on the mucous membranes of the mouth and throat and the discom-fort associated with sore throat, mouth sores, gum disease, and hali-tosis. Nurses also might want to research its strong antimicrobial ac-tions as in the case of slow-healing decubiti. Sage tea also might be considered by midwives in the suppression of lactation in women who choose not to breastfeed their infants or for women who give their ba-bies to adopting parents.

Integrative Insight

Although little biomedical evidence supports the traditional uses of sage, traditional evidence has been strong in the use of sage tea, es-pecially as a gargle during cold and flu to relieve and heal mucous membranes of the mouth and pharyngeal areas. Sage is highly effec-tive in reducing discomfort in the throat associated with viral and bacterial infection. Large doses of sage tea should not be taken. Sage tea gargles at the earliest feeling of the scratchy throat that accom-panies a cold or flu are often helpful in healing. It is best to recom-mend making the gargle with sage leaf rather than essential oil. Gar-gling stimulates the lymphatic system in the throat and, with the antimicrobial activity of sage, supports the overall immune response in the throat area.

Sage also helps regulate fever and perspiration of the skin during viral illness such as the common cold. Sage exhibits adaptogen activity in that it either increases or decreases the perspiration of the body, depending on the patient's need. Adequate perspiration is key to the illness being resolved without the virus lodging in one area of the body and weakening any particular organ. Excessive perspiration, however, such as occurs during many days of fever, can actually weaken the body. Sage also helps promote wound and skin healing not only in the mouth, such as with oral ulcers, but also with pressure sores and inflamed areas that occur anywhere on the body. Sage's aromatic, stimulating and anti-inflammatory activities help resolve the symptoms associated with cold and other infectious processes.

THERAPEUTIC APPLICATIONS:

Oral

Recommendations are to use about 4 to 6 g daily of sage leaf for infusions, tinctures, and topical applications.

Infusion. Use 1 to 3 g dried leaf in 5 ounces (150 ml) of water, three times per day (Blumenthal et al., 2000).

Fluid Extract. 1:1 (g/ml): Use ½ teaspoon (1 to 3 ml) three times a day (Blumenthal et al., 2000).

Essential Oil. 00.1 to 0.3 ml (Blumenthal et al., 2000)

Topical

Gargle or Rinse. Prepare a warm infusion of 2.5 g of leaf in 3½ ounces (100 ml) of water. Or use 2 to 3 drops of essential oil in 3½ ounces (100 ml) of water (Blumenthal et al., 2000). If this gargle is too astringent (tightening) to the mucous membranes of the throat, make a gargle with half chamomile and half sage instead.

Environmental

Sage infusion can be poured over hot coals in a steam bath for headache, insomnia, eye trouble, and arthritis.

Herbal Caveat—Therapeutic Applications

In traditional and conventional herbal medicine, amounts of herbs given to patients are based on individual needs. The amounts or "doses" recorded here are provided so that the health practitioner has a general idea of the amounts recommended for an adult patient. Dosing in herbalism not only refers to amount of plant used but also includes when, where, and how to take a plant medicine. These dosages should not be used as guidelines for indiscriminate intervention without proper assessment, critical thinking, and patient education on the part of the practitioner.

Note: Please see chapter 5 for detailed descriptions of how to prepare various applications.

PATIENT INTERACTION:

Many people recognize their early symptoms of coming down with a cold or flu. One symptom many people experience is a scratchiness in the throat, yet few people do anything about this warning symptom. Sage tea gargle is a very old remedy that could be used for soothing sore throat. Sage has natural antimicrobial properties and also can shrink the mucous membranes in the throat that become swollen by the cold virus.

Herbal Caveat—Patient Interaction

Patients considering the use of an herb or formula of herbs in self-care benefit from education about the plant itself and the use of the plant in healing. This education can come through many sources, including local herbalists; plant specialists such as botanists; health practitioners such as nurses, nutritionists, naturopaths, and other physicians; and various written references including the scientific literature. Patients need to remember that their unique health care needs are not necessarily represented in any literature they may encounter. Therefore, it is recommended that a knowledgeable mentor be consulted before initiating self-care with any herb being used for the first time.

NURTURING THE NURSE-PLANT RELATIONSHIP:

Note: You may want to keep a journal of your experiences with the herb.

Gargling with Sage. This is one herb to have in your medicine chest at all times. Nurses are exposed to so many viruses and bacteria and often because of their high stress work environment become highly susceptible to infection. Often those infections start in the nasopharynx. Sage tea gargles can be used at the earliest sign of sore throat, a discomfort that can be an alert that the immune system is working hard. Sage gargling has two benefits: (1) Gargling stimulates the lymph nodes in the neck. The lymph fluid only moves by muscle movement, so gargling provides the exercise to move out the bacteria that have "lost the battle" so that the nodes can keep up their immune function. (2) Sage has strong antioxidant, antimicrobial, and astringent properties. Sage gargles can be very soothing.

Purchase or pick from your garden 2.5 g of sage leaf and steep in $3\frac{1}{2}$ ounces (100 ml) of boiled water. Strain and add cool water until the gargle is warm but not hot. Gargle about $\frac{1}{2}$ cup (120 ml) of tea over at least five minutes every two hours when awake until the soreness subsides. Rest well.

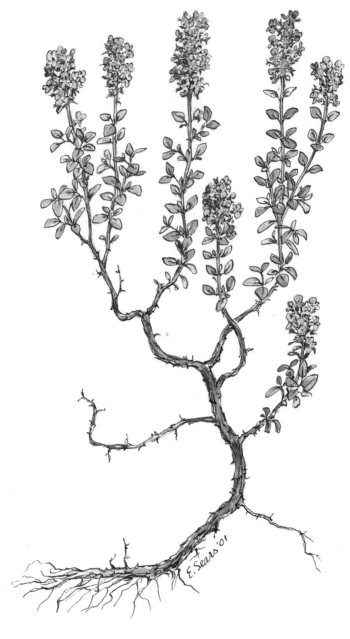

Thymus vulgaris

Thyme

🍃 **LATIN NAME:** *Thymus vulgaris*

🍃 **FAMILY:** Lamiaceae

🍃 **COMMON NAMES:** Thyme, common thyme, garden thyme

🍃 **HEALTH PATTERN:** Immune response

🍃 **PLANT DESCRIPTION:**

The name "thyme" is said have come from a Greek word meaning "to fumigate" or "rise into flames" because thyme was used as an incense. Thyme is cultivated throughout the world for its medicinal and culinary uses. It is easily grown in home gardens. Thyme is a small shrubby plant that grows from 6 to 10 inches (15 to 25 cm) tall. It has numerous branches with many tiny leaves that are only about ⅛ inch (about 4 mm) long and 1/16 inch (about 2 mm) wide. The small bluish-purple flowers appear during the summer on the terminal ends of spikes. The plant is best collected when in flower and carefully dried. The entire herb has a strong, pungent, spicy fragrance and taste (Felter & Lloyd, 1983).

🍃 **PLANT PARTS USED:** The aerial parts

🍃 **TRADITIONAL EVIDENCE:**

Cultural Use

North American Indian. The Delaware tribe uses thyme as an infusion for fever and chills (Moerman, 1998).

Hispanic. A tea is used for colds and sinus as well as inner infections.

East Indian. A distilled oil from the leaves of thyme is used in India for its antiseptic and deodorant properties. A decoction of the leaves is used for itching and other skin problems (Nadkarni, 1976).

Russian/Baltic. Thyme, known as "our lady's herb," does not grow well in the extreme north of Russia, but grows in other parts of the country. Thymol, the extract, has been used as an antiseptic and disinfectant. It has been combined with other herbs for chest congestion, bronchitis, whooping cough, worms, and skin conditions. The oil of thyme has been used for toothache, nerve pain, and swellings (Hutchens, 1992). Official Russian medicine approves thyme for spasms in the stomach, nerve pain, insomnia, and for respiratory and digestive infections. It also is used as a gargle for tonsillitis and laryngitis and as an expectorant for coughs, bronchitis, and asthma. Its use is recommended for childhood bed-wetting and diarrhea. Thyme extracts are applied topically for symptoms of headache, dandruff, and sore eyes. Infusions of thyme are taken for skin conditions such as itching, rashes, infections, and wounds (Zevin, 1997).

European. The German Commission E approves the use of thyme for treating symptoms of bronchitis, whooping cough, and other inflammation of the respiratory tract. It has been used to improve digestion and to treat bad breath and inflammation of the mouth (Blumenthal et al., 2000).

Practitioners in Anthroposophical medicine use thyme to affect the rhythmic system, to relax convulsive coughing, and strengthen the nervous system. Thyme also is used to treat rickets and diseases characterized by the oozing of fluids due to inflammation. It is used as a diuretic (Husemann & Wolff, 1982).

Culinary Use

Thyme is often used as a culinary herb in sauces, stuffing, pickles, stews, soups, and in the preservation process for olives (Grieve, 1971). Thyme was used in ancient Rome to flavor cheeses and alcoholic beverages.

Use in Herbalism

Thyme infusions have been used for whooping cough, shortness of breath, mild stomach pain, and gout. Thyme ointment has been applied topically for the treatment of abscesses and warts. Thyme oil was an ingredient in an herbal cigarette that was smoked for stomach upset, fatigue, and headache. Thyme also was used in embalming oils (Blumenthal et al., 2000; Grieve, 1971).

Thyme is used to strengthen the lungs and as an expectorant. It is given to children as a tea for coughs. Thyme also is used to eradicate intestinal parasites. Some women used it during childbirth to hasten delivery. An ointment made of thyme is used on swellings, warts, and to relieve low back pain and poor eyesight. It is also used for gout, stomach problems, and flatulence (Culpeper, 1990). Thyme is considered to be tonic, carminative, antispasmodic, and an emmenagogue. It can be taken in the form of a cold infusion for poor digestion, and warm infusion for dysmenorrhea, flatulence, colic, headache, and to promote perspiration. Thyme oil is applied locally to nerve and rheumatic pain. Thyme is prepared with other herbs and given to children for nervous and spasmodic conditions, whooping cough, and sore throat (Felter & Lloyd, 1983). Thyme flowers also have been used like lavender in sachets to keep insects away from linens and clothing (Grieve, 1971).

Thymol, a powerful antiseptic extracted from thyme, was used in the early 1900s as a local anesthetic, and to medicate gauze and wool for surgical dressings. Thymol was so popular as an antiseptic that it also was used in lotions and mouthwash and as a treatment for ringworm, eczema, psoriasis, and burns. Thymol was added to preparations for respiratory problems such as laryngitis, sore throat, bronchitis, and whooping cough. It was given internally to expel parasites and for diabetes (Grieve, 1971). Several species of thyme including *Thymus vulgaris* are used in treating cancer (Leung & Foster, 1996).

The essential oil of thyme has analgesic and antiaging properties and inhibits certain bacteria, fungi, and viruses. It also can stimulate the immune system. It has been found that many infections that are resistant to antibiotics can be eradicated with essential oils. This especially applies to sinus and respiratory tract infections. Thyme essential oil is often recommended for use in vaporizers for inhalation to help treat symptoms of respiratory infections (Buckle, 1997). Thyme oil is currently used in cough drops, liniments, mouthwashes, and in topical antifungal preparations.

Cosmetic Use. It also is used in toothpastes, soaps, detergents, creams, lotions, and perfumes (Leung & Foster, 1996).

BIOMEDICAL EVIDENCE:

Few clinical trials of the use of thyme whole herb preparations have been conducted. Studies have been performed to explore the antimicrobial effect of thyme essential oil because there has been a renewed interest in the use of essential oils as disinfectants and for the protection of livestock and the food supply from disease, pests, and spoilage.

Studies Related to Immune Response

One in vitro study analyzed the antibacterial activity of several volatile oils and found thyme oil to have the widest spectrum of antibacterial activity. Just a few of the bacteria that thyme was most active against include *Aeromonas hydrophila, Clostridium sporogenes, Flavobacterium suaveolens, Proteus vulgaris, Salmonella pullorum,* and *S. aureus.* It was also highly active against *E. coli, Klebsiella pneumoniae,* and *Pseudomonas aeruginosa.* It is suggested that essential oils such as those found in thyme may reduce the onset of spoilage of foods and decrease contamination of the food supply. In addition, although thyme and thymol, a main constituent in thyme, lack solubility, they still have been shown to be an important source of disinfectant (Dorman & Deans, 2000).

In another in vitro study, thyme was the essential oil that exhibited the lowest concentration needed to inhibit *E. coli* and *C. albicans* (0.03% v/v) (Hammer, Carson, & Riley, 1999). Essential oil extracted from the thyme plant in full flower demonstrated the most antimicrobial activity against the nine types of gram-negative and six types of gram-positive bacteria studied in vitro. Thyme oil was effective against both gram-positive and gram-negative bacteria but was more effective against gram-positive bacteria (Marino, Bersani, & Comi, 1999). *Thymus vulgaris* aqueous extract has been shown to significantly inhibit *H. pylori* in vitro and was more effective than some antibiotics (Tabak, Armon, Potasman, & Neeman, 1996).

In an in vitro study, an alcohol extract of thyme was found to be effective at killing head lice. It was most effective when the treatment was followed with a rinse of thyme essential oil, vinegar, and water (Veal, 1996).

Studies Related to Other Health Patterns

Digestion. Thyme, in particular thymol, has an extensive history of successful use in dentistry related to its antiseptic qualities. Thymol is the main ingredient in Listerine, an over-the-counter mouthwash. In vitro studies of the effect of thyme oil on bacteria commonly found in the mouth, such as *Streptococcus mutans,* one of the major etiologic agents of dental caries, and *S. aureus,* one of the major organisms associated with dental infection, showed that thyme oil has significantly effective germicidal action against these microbes (Meeker & Linke, 1988).

Mechanism of Action

The wide spectrum activity of thyme oil is thought to be due to the phenol component, thymol. Thymol can be bactericidal or bacteriostatic, depending on the concentration used (Dorman & Dean, 2000). Thymol has been found to contain isomers that are similar in chemical structure to certain morphinelike analgesics (Buckle, 1997).

USE IN PREGNANCY OR LACTATION:

The use of thyme is not recommended during pregnancy because of its ability to promote uterine and menstrual bleeding (Brinker, 1998; McGuffin et al., 1997; Weed, 1986). There are no known restrictions for its use during lactation (Blumenthal et al., 2000).

Herbal Caveat—Pregnancy or Lactation
Some herbs are contraindicated in pregnancy because of a risk of the herb or one of its constituents stimulating the uterus and therefore possibly promoting fetal loss. Many herbal practitioners do not recommend herbal remedies, in particular oral doses of herbs, during the first trimester of pregnancy and seek an alternative. However, herbs are successfully used during pregnancy, especially to prepare the body for the birth. Herbs are relatively unstudied in pregnancy and lactation, so patients need to be made aware through education of the potential benefits and risks of using herbs for health conditions that arise during pregnancy or lactation. The use of herbal remedies during pregnancy often warrants a referral to a knowledgeable herbal practitioner.

USE FOR CHILDREN:

Thyme has been used in Germany to reduce the congestion and severity of symptoms associated with whooping cough. (Schilcher, 1992).

Herbal Caveat—Children
Children have special needs in regard to herbal therapies. They require lesser amounts of herbs and often respond well to mild teas and topical ap-

plications such as compresses and baths. The lowest dose of oral preparations should be tried first before increasing the amount given children. Caregivers should observe children closely for responses to herbal remedies. Younger children, particularly infants, have traditionally been given herbs either through their mother's breast milk or in the form of a homeopathic remedy because of their sensitivity to medicines and treatments and the immaturity of their liver. It is recommended that a person knowledgeable in the herbal treatment of children be consulted before the offering of any herb to a child for the first time.

CAUTIONS:

The essential oil content of thyme can vary tremendously from species to species as well as within a certain species of thyme. Duke (1997) writes that the potency variations of the active compounds in thyme are even related to genetics and can vary as much as "ten thousand fold" within a single species of thyme (p. 10). Buyers and growers should beware.

Thymol, a constituent in thyme, is considered quite toxic. Toxic symptoms can include nausea, vomiting, headache, dizziness, convulsions, coma, and cardiac and respiratory arrest (Gosselin as reported in Leung & Foster, 1996). Undiluted red thyme oil has been shown to be very irritating to animal skin but not human skin (Leung & Foster, 1996). Thymol, the phenol in thyme, can be irritating to the skin (Veal, 1996).

Based on in vitro data, it is assumed that people with a sensitivity to birch pollen and celery may have a cross-reaction to thyme (WHO, 1999). Although no cases of anaphylaxis have been reported in the literature, one case of allergic reaction to thyme and oregano eaten in food has been reported. Skin prick testing was subsequently done and cross-reactivity within the plants of the Lamiaceae family was found in this person. There was no reactivity to birch or mugwort pollen in this individual (Benito, Jorro, Morales, Pelaez, & Fernandez, 1996).

Thyme essential oil is contraindicated in those with hypertension and epilepsy (Buckle, 1997). One source reports that excessive internal use of thyme may overstimulate the thyroid gland (Zevin, 1997), and Anthroposophical practitioners do not use thyme in patients with thyrotoxicosis because it is known that thyme acts like iodine (Husemann & Wolff, 1982).

NURSING EVIDENCE:

Historical Nursing Use
No data are available at this time.

Potential Nursing Applications
Many essential oils, including thyme oil, have been shown to have significant antimicrobial activity in vitro. Human clinical studies and

case studies are needed. Thyme oil with its broad range of antimicrobial activity may be very helpful in disinfecting wounds and decubiti, for instance. Thyme also may prove effective in disinfecting sick wards as the increase in antibiotic-resistant strains of bacteria mutation continues. Nurses also might want to consider the use of thyme baths in the care of those with upper respiratory conditions such as whooping cough and bronchitis. School nurses may want to consider developing head lice protocols that include thyme hair rinses.

Integrative Insight

Thyme has a long history of successful traditional use in the healing of those with upper respiratory discomfort, such as cough and bronchospasm, as well as inflammatory skin conditions. It is used both internally and externally and has been shown with biomedical evidence to have strong antimicrobial activity, mostly because of its thymol constituent. Using thyme can be a powerfully stimulating experience. Its aroma is a key element of the plant's personality. Thyme's aroma is commanding. It commands healing within the chest.

In the second century, Galen gave the thymus gland in the chest its name because it reminded him of a bunch of the thyme plant (Diamond, 1979). The thymus gland is considered by some healers to be the seat of life energy and is therefore the first organ to be affected by stress. Thyme and the thymus have a connection in that thyme has the potential to clear (i.e., disinfect) the chest area where the thymus gland does its work—the development of the immune response in the newborn and later on, the development of a healthy immune system and maturation of T cells (*Tabor's Cyclopedic Dictionary,* 1997).

Clearing the chest also means clearing the area around the heart. The heart and lungs are vital organs of survival. Some healers use thyme to stimulate the immune response of the whole chest area, including the heart. "Chinese medicine has long asserted that there is a subtle energy flow through the heart and on to the thymus gland and thus to and throughout the body's immune system. These ancient healers knew that what we feel in our heart is conveyed to our immune system" (Pearsall, 1998, p. 224). Thyme reminds us to take the time to connect with our heart as the center of discernment and healing to recognize that which invades our healthy world and causes us excessive stress and inharmony. Out of that heart connection is the opportunity for a greater and more effective immune response.

THERAPEUTIC APPLICATIONS:

Oral

Infusion. For adults, use about 1 to 2 g of herb for one cup of tea. Take orally several times daily as needed (Blumenthal et al., 2000). Children up to one year should use 0.5 to 1 g of the dried herb in an infusion taken several times daily (WHO, 1999).

Fluid Extract. 1:1 (g/ml): Use up to about ½ teaspoon (1 to 2 ml) taken orally one to three times daily (Blumenthal et al., 2000).

Tincture. (1:10 g/ml, 70% ethanol): Take 40 drops in a small amount of water up to three times per day (WHO, 1999).

Topical

Compress. Prepare a 5% infusion to be used as a compress (Blumenthal et al., 2000).

Gargle. Use a 5% infusion as a gargle or mouthwash (WHO, 1999).

Massage. Add 2 drops of thyme essential oil into 2 tablespoons (30 ml) of almond oil and use this for massage (Lawless, 1998).

Environmental

Bath. See Nurturing the Nurse-Plant Relationship for whole herb directions or add up to 5 drops of thyme essential oil to the morning bath to help alleviate symptoms of physical and mental fatigue, depression, lethargy, hangovers, and headaches (Lawless, 1998).

Using thyme essential oil in a vaporizer is reported to help clear the mind and alleviate nervous headaches, anxiety, worry, and mental chatter. It is purifying to the atmosphere in the home (Lawless, 1998).

The burning of thyme can repel insects (Duke, 1985).

Herbal Caveat—Therapeutic Applications

In traditional and conventional herbal medicine, amounts of herbs given to patients are based on individual needs. The amounts or "doses" recorded here are provided so that the health practitioner has a general idea of the amounts recommended for an adult patient. Dosing in herbalism not only refers to amount of plant used but also includes when, where, and how to take a plant medicine. These dosages should not be used as guidelines for indiscriminate intervention without proper assessment, critical thinking, and patient education on the part of the practitioner.

Note: Please see chapter 5 for detailed descriptions of how to prepare various applications.

🍃 PATIENT INTERACTION:

Thyme is great in food and it is also one of the oldest medicinal remedies. Thyme baths are easy to prepare and are very helpful with the discomfort of the common cold and respiratory tract as well as for inflammation. Thyme has natural antibiotic properties and can be used to disinfect your mouth, throat, and lungs where germs like to hide. Gargling with the original Listerine (thymol is the first ingredient) and taking an aromatic bath in a thyme infusion can be considered. Thyme essential oil should be used under the guidance of a knowledgeable caregiver. Drinking excessive amounts of thyme tea is not recommended.

Herbal Caveat—Patient Interaction

Patients considering the use of an herb or formula of herbs in self-care benefit from education about the plant itself and the use of the plant in healing. This education can come through many sources, including local herbalists; plant specialists such as botanists; health practitioners such as nurses, nutritionists, naturopaths, and other physicians; and various written references including the scientific literature. Patients need to remember that their unique health care needs are not necessarily represented in any literature they may encounter. Therefore, it is recommended that a knowledgeable mentor be consulted before initiating self-care with any herb being used for the first time.

NURTURING THE NURSE-PLANT RELATIONSHIP:

Note: You may want to keep a journal of your experiences with the herb.

To experience thyme, try Listerine with a thyme bath with a thymus tap (see explanation below) after a workday when you have been exposed to an onslaught of bacteria.

Begin by gargling three times with Listerine to begin the disinfecting of the throat and mouth. Make sure that you gargle way back in the throat because many germs like to incubate in the back of the nasopharynx.

For the bath, prepare a strong infusion of thyme using 2 cups (227 g) of dried thyme and 2 quarts or liters of boiled water. Cover and steep for ten minutes. Strain and pour into a filled tub (98°F). Immerse yourself and breathe deeply. Plan to be in the tub for twenty minutes. People with strong hearts can submerge themselves so that the water level is above the heart; otherwise the water level should be below the heart. While in the tub, gently tap your sternum with your finger tips, alternating hands. This is called a "thymus tap" and is thought to stimulate the thymus and decrease stress (Diamond, 1979). After the bath, wrap yourself in two big towels and a blanket and let yourself perspire for thirty to sixty minutes. I don't recommend doing this in bed unless you plan to change the sheets, because the body is shedding the toxins and virus/bacteria through the pores. Do not reuse the towels after this process without washing them first. Your heart may beat slightly fast as you go through this very important second part of the thyme bath experience. Do not skip this step. When your heart rate is back to normal and you are no longer perspiring, sponge off a little with a warm wash cloth and dress warmly. Remember to put on socks. Get into bed and rest well.

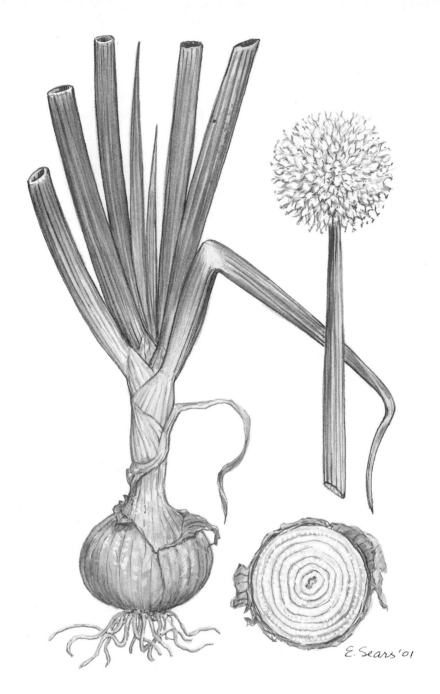

Allium cepa

Onion

🍃 **LATIN NAME:** *Allium cepa*

🍃 **FAMILY:** Liliaceae

🍃 **COMMON NAMES:** Onion

🍃 **HEALTH PATTERN:** Immune response

🍃 **PLANT DESCRIPTION:**

The name *Allium* comes from the Celtic word "all," meaning pungent. The common onion is a garden plant having an underground bulb covered with a thin papery reddish, yellow, or white membrane. The bulb has many juicy, concentric layers. The above-ground leaves are shiny green, hollow, and upright. They can reach a height of more than 3 feet (1 meter). The bulb tastes less pungent than garlic and has some degree of sweetness.

🍃 **PLANT PART USED:** Underground bulb

🍃 **TRADITIONAL EVIDENCE:**

Cultural Use

Asian. Two onions are used in TCM that are a different species from *A. cepa. Allium pstulosum L.*, called "cong bai," is an herb used to release the exterior and induce sweating such as during the early stages of a cold. It is used externally as a poultice for toxic abscesses. The other onion used in Chinese medicine is *Allium macrostemon,* "xie bai." This onion is used to regulate or move "qi" and blood to alleviate pain, especially of the chest and abdomen (Bensky & Gamble, 1993).

In Japanese macrobiotics, cooked onions are eaten to calm the nervous system, relieve irritability, and reduce muscle soreness after heavy work. A cut raw onion is put under the pillow in cases of insomnia (Kushi, 1993).

North American Indian. Many varieties of onion that grow wild were used by Indians throughout North America. *A. cepa*, the garden onion, has been used as both food and medicine by several tribes. The Mohegan make a syrup of onion to be taken for colds. The Shinnecock also make an onion cold syrup and also use onion as a disinfectant because of its aromatic essential oil. They place the heart of an onion in the ear to cure earaches. The Havasupai of the Southwest use the bulbs for food. The Navajo also use the onion as a food source and store them for winter use. Other tribes eat them raw, roasted, or boiled. The Iroquois use peelings from the bulbs to make fabric dye (Moerman, 1998). The Cheyenne apply a poultice of onion bulbs and stems to carbuncles (Lewis & Elvin-Lewis, 1977).

Hispanic. Onion, "cebolla," cough syrup is used as an expectorant. Heated pieces of onion are cooled and then applied to corns on the toes. Onion also is sliced and put in the sick room of the ill. It is believed that the onion absorbs the sickness from the room.

Pacific Islander. In Hawaii, onion, "akaakai," is used traditionally in the treatment of the common cold, tuberculosis, venereal diseases, and otitis media (Kaaialamanu & Akina, 1922 as reported in Farbman et al., 1993).

East Indian. *A. cepa* is cultivated throughout India as a food and medicine. Both the bulbs and seeds are used. The bulbs are eaten raw by flavoring them with lemon juice, salt, and pepper. They are used medicinally for edema, fever, bronchitis, colic, and scurvy. Onions are eaten twice daily with black pepper for malaria. Roasted onions are applied to boils, bruises, and wounds to bring relief and healing. Onion juice is used like smelling salts for fainting, infantile convulsions, headache, and epileptic seizures. Onion juice also is dropped into the ears to help earache, and sniffed up into the nostrils for nosebleeds. It helps heal insect bites and scorpion stings and certain skin diseases. Onions have been used in the treatment of enlarged spleen, sore throat, jaundice, dyspepsia, rheumatism, coughs, and hemorrhoids (Nadkarni, 1976). Ayurvedic medicine uses onion in the form of a decoction, infusion, and fresh juice. It also may be used in its raw form or cooked or roasted. The juice is combined with honey; ginger juice; and ghee, clarified butter (Blumenthal et al., 2000).

European. The German Commission E recommends the use of onion for loss of appetite and the prevention of atherosclerosis (Blumenthal et al., 2000). In Italy, onion has been used traditionally to repel parasites and insects. For instance, cutting an onion in half and putting it on the windowsill or rubbing it on the skin is used to repel mosquitoes. People with parasitic infection macerate an onion in white wine and drink it in the morning on an empty stomach. Also, a cataplasm of onion with garlic and absinth is applied externally to the abdomen (Guarrera, 1999).

Culinary Use

Onion oil is used as a flavor ingredient in many processed foods such as beverages, baked goods, gelatins, meat and meat products, condiments, relishes, salad dressings, soups, gravies and snack foods (Leung & Foster, 1996). When cooking ground beef, adding onion has been shown to reduce the mutagenicity associated with the beef (Kato et al., 1998).

Use in Herbalism

The onion bulb has been used as a food and medicine for thousands of years, especially for cough and common cold (Crellin & Philpott, 1990). Onions also have been eaten as a protective agent against infection. Onions have been used to promote the appetite, treat bites from rabid dogs and other creatures, and to bring on menstrual bleeding. Onions are steeped in water overnight and given to children to drink on an empty stomach to kill intestinal parasites. They are sometimes roasted in the fireplace and eaten with honey or sugar and oil. This is said to be a good expectorant for tough phlegm. Onion juice has been snuffed up into the nostrils to clear the sinuses and get rid of lethargy. Onions have been prepared as a salve or in vinegar for topical application to a variety of skin problems (Culpeper, 1990). Onions are cooked in milk and taken internally to help clear lung congestion (Schulz et al., 1998).

The American Eclectic physicians used onion during the nineteenth and early twentieth centuries much as they used garlic, although they recognized that the actions of onion were milder. Onion was made into a syrup with sugar and used for the treatment of coughs and bronchial conditions. It also was given as a tincture for kidney gravel and generalized edema (Blumenthal et al., 2000; Grieve, 1971). A roasted onion was said to be helpful if applied directly to skin tumors or to the ear in cases of otitis media. A cataplasm of onion pounded with vinegar and applied for three days and changed three times a day has been known to cure bunions and corns (Felter & Lloyd, 1983; Grieve, 1971). Onions also are mashed and applied as a poultice to burns, and the skins can be boiled gently and applied to the skin for conditions such as scabies (Duke, 1997).

Currently, onion is used to dispel intestinal gas, promote urinary output, increase bronchial secretions, improve digestion, and help destroy parasitic intestinal worms (Leung & Foster, 1996). It is recommended to eat raw onions daily to help veins maintain or regain their elasticity to prevent varicosities (Weed, 1986). Onion also is indicated for its antibacterial actions, ability to lower lipids and blood pressure, and action against platelet aggregation (Leung & Foster, 1996).

BIOMEDICAL EVIDENCE:

There is very little clinical research on the traditional uses of onion, especially regarding its long history in stimulating the immune response to infectious disease. Some of the in vitro data is included here describing the microbes onion has been shown to be effective against.

Studies Related to Immune Response

In vitro studies have shown that fresh onion extract demonstrates antibacterial activity against *S. mutans, S. sobrinus, Porphyromonas gingivalis,* and *Prevotella intermedia*, all known to be responsible for dental caries or adult periodontis. The onion extract had no antibacterial activity if the onion was steam processed or left at 37°C for two days after grating (Kim, 1997). Gram-positive bacteria are more sensitive to Egyptian onion oil than are gram-negative bacteria. In vitro studies showed that onion oil significantly inhibited *Bacillus anthracis, Bacillus cereus, Micrococcus luteus, S. aureus,* and gram-negative *E. coli* and *Klebsiella pneumoniae* (Zohri, Abdel-Gawad, & Saber, 1995). Another in vitro study reports that even though historically onion has been used in the treatment of infection, onion extract has no antibacterial effect except in high doses with *Streptococcus pneumoniae* and *Moraxella catarrhalis* (Farbman, Barnett, Bolduc, & Klein, 1993).

Studies Related to Other Health Patterns

Skin Care. One case study reported the significant pain relief and wound healing effects of the direct application of a half bulb of onion to a stingray bite. A local fishing family in the Northern Territory of Australia treated a severe stingray bite to the foot by stopping bleeding, emersing the foot in hot water, and then applying the onion. The wound healed without incident (Whiting & Guinea, 1998).

Restoration. In a retrospective study of 564 patients with stomach cancer, a significant reduction in risk of stomach cancer exists among those who consume onion and other *Allium* vegetables. Onion extracts also have been found to inhibit tumor growth in animal and in vitro studies (You et al., 1989).

In a study of 5 participants, ingestion of 225 g of fried onion after an overnight fast was shown to significantly increase quercetin (flavonoids) levels and increase overall antioxidant plasma concentrations (McAnlis, McEneny, Pearce, & Young, 1999).

Mobility. Aqueous extracts of fresh onion given to rats orally or intraperitoneally in high doses of 500 mg/kg significantly lower thromboxane B2 levels. Boiled onion had little antithrombotic activity (Bordia, Mohammed, Thomson, & Ali, 1996).

Hormone Balance. Animal studies have shown that onion extract, the equivalent of 2 g/kg of dry onion, significantly prevents the rise in serum cholesterol and triglyceride levels caused by eating an atherogenic diet (Lata et al., 1991).

Mechanism of Action

This plant's pungent personality and its therapeutic effects are related to its sulfur content. Onions contain allicin (diallylsulfide oxide), a constituent with a mild stimulating action that can cause a counterirritant reaction (Crellin & Philpott, 1990). The onion allicins and cepaenes, organosulfur compounds, have a wide range of therapeutic activities including antiasthmatic effects. The anti-inflammatory effects of onion are thought to be related to the cepaenes constituents (Augusti, 1996). The sugars released when cooking onion and, to a lesser extent, the antioxidant action of quercetin have been shown to reduce the mutagenicity of ground beef (Kato, Michikoshi, Minowa, Maeda, & Kikugawa, 1998).

The skin of onions can contain as much as 3% quercetin, a flavonoid that has a known skin soothing and anti-inflammatory action (Duke, 1997).

USE IN PREGNANCY OR LACTATION:

There are no known contraindications for the use of onion during pregnancy and lactation (Blumenthal et al., 2000).

Herbal Caveat—Pregnancy or Lactation

Some herbs are contraindicated in pregnancy because of a risk of the herb or one of its constituents stimulating the uterus and therefore possibly promoting fetal loss. Many herbal practitioners do not recommend herbal remedies, in particular oral doses of herbs, during the first trimester of pregnancy and seek an alternative. However, herbs are successfully used during pregnancy, especially to prepare the body for the birth. Herbs are relatively unstudied in pregnancy and lactation, so patients need to be made aware through education of the potential benefits and risks of using herbs for health conditions that arise during pregnancy or lactation. The use of herbal remedies during pregnancy often warrants a referral to a knowledgeable herbal practitioner.

USE FOR CHILDREN:

No precautions have been reported for the use of onion by children (WHO, 1999).

Herbal Caveat—Children

Children have special needs in regard to herbal therapies. They require lesser amounts of herbs and often respond well to mild teas and topical applications such as compresses and baths. The lowest dose of oral preparations should be tried first before increasing the amount given children. Caregivers should observe children closely for responses to herbal remedies. Younger children, particularly infants, have traditionally been given herbs either through their mother's breast milk or in the form of a homeopathic remedy because of their sensitivity to medicines and treatments and the immaturity of their liver. It is recommended that a person knowledgeable in the herbal treatment of children be consulted before the offering of any herb to a child for the first time.

CAUTIONS:

There are no known drug interactions associated with the oral intake of onion (Blumenthal et al., 2000). Eating large, therapeutic amounts of onions over a long period of time may interfere with hemoglobin production and may lead to red blood cell lysis (Augusti, 1996). Reactions such as asthma, contact dermatitis, and eye irritation with tearing have been reported (Valdivieso et al., 1994).

Historical Nursing Use

Caregivers have used onions for most ailments. They have been used as poultices and compresses and were often applied to the feet (Ulrich, 1990). Nurses have used onion poultices applied externally to areas of inflammation, especially to the chest.

Potential Nursing Applications

With the increase in lung disease, asthma, and tuberculosis (some report related to increases in air pollutants), the lungs are often weakened through repeated viral and bacterial infections. The risk for infection such as pneumonia is greater. Preventive care, including lifestyle and dietary changes, can be recommended, especially at the beginning of cold and flu season. Nurses may want to consider adding onion as part of their recommendations. Nurses may want to suggest that patients increase their intake of onion in foods and learn to make an onion syrup to be taken when congestion, cold, or flu begin to cause discomfort. Nurses also might consider clinical research to explore the traditional use of onion poultices applied to the feet or chest in the care of people with upper respiratory discomfort or the external application of onion skin to promote wound and skin healing.

Integrative Insight

Onion has traditionally and biomedically been shown to be able to address challenges to the immune system, especially upper respiratory conditions. Most people are aware of the powerful odorous effects of onions. Part of the onion's personality and its therapeutic effects involves causing the eyes to tear and the sinuses to run when preparing the onions for use. The nose runs when a person is coming down with a cold to help the body shed the virus. Onions help by assisting this process of keeping secretions moving and therefore are often used in breaking up mucus in the head and chest. Onion is warming, stimulating, and penetrating, and it doesn't have to be eaten to do its work. Onions are often applied externally. When used externally, their pungency can be inhaled and felt. Local heat from the onions increases the "fever" to the area, bringing with it all the benefits of localized fever in terms of controlling the spread of infection.

For the immune system to do its work, it has to be able to send its messengers to the place of infection or inflammation. Onions help break up or clear mucous and other substances that block the immune system from doing its work. Pungent substances like onions gently but diligently clear the way for the immune system. Onions also introduce their own antibacterial, antiviral, or antiparasitic substances. Pharmaceutical antibiotics have only the ability to address the exact bacteria they were designed to destroy. Antibiotics, energetically speaking, are cooling and therefore may not have the ability to penetrate mucus and other secretions as do other warming pungent substances. Onions, especially fresh chopped or lightly cooked, perform multiple actions at one time; at the very least they increase heat, provide an antimicrobial action, and break up mucus. Accepting that a substance has the ability to perform multiple actions at the same time may make it difficult to understand the substance fully from a biomedical perspective, but it also makes the substance less likely to fail as a healing agent as the environment changes and bacteria and viruses mutate.

THERAPEUTIC APPLICATIONS:

Oral

Eating. Eat about 2 ounces (50 g) per day of the fresh bulb or about 1 ounce (20 g) per day of the dried bulb.

Infusion. Steep 1 to 2 teaspoons in 4 ounces (120 ml) water.

Succus. Use 1 teaspoon (5 ml) of the pressed juice from the fresh bulb three to four times daily.

Tincture. Use 1 teaspoon (5 ml) three to four times daily (Blumenthal et al., 2000).

Syrup. See Nurturing the Nurse-Plant Relationship.

Topical

Poultice. Chop one onion into small pieces and place it in the center of flannel fabric. Fold over the edges and secure them so that the onion will not spill out. Place the poultice over the inflamed area, such as the chest, a sore joint, the feet, or on or behind the ear for ear infection, and leave in place for one to two hours, but do not secure the poultice in place because this could lead to skin irritation. Check the skin every fifteen to thirty minutes. (You can use a slurry of either chopped raw or lightly cooked onion.)

Cataplasm. Pound onion in vinegar and apply to bunions and corns for three days, changing the cataplasm three times a day (Felter & Lloyd, 1983).

Environmental

The odor of onion is remarkable in its ability to permeate a house and cause people's eyes to tear and noses to run.

Herbal Caveat—Therapeutic Applications

In traditional and conventional herbal medicine, amounts of herbs given to patients are based on individual needs. The amounts or "doses" recorded here are provided so that the health practitioner has a general idea of the amounts recommended for an adult patient. Dosing in herbalism not only refers to amount of plant used but also includes when, where, and how to take a plant medicine. These dosages should not be used as guidelines for indiscriminate intervention without proper assessment, critical thinking, and patient education on the part of the practitioner.

Note: Please see chapter 5 for detailed descriptions of how to prepare various applications.

PATIENT INTERACTION:

Onion is a readily available remedy for discomfort associated with upper respiratory conditions such as the common cold. Onion skin is also effective in the care of various skin conditions. Onion can be eaten, taken as a syrup, and applied externally to the chest, ears, feet, skin, and inflamed areas. Eating onion in highly excessive amounts is not advisable, but moderate amounts have been known to be beneficial in supporting the body's ability to deal with challenges to the immune system.

Herbal Caveat—Patient Interaction

Patients considering the use of an herb or formula of herbs in self-care benefit from education about the plant itself and the use of the plant in healing. This education can come through many sources including local herbalists; plant specialists such as botanists; health practitioners such as nurses, nutritionists, naturopaths, and other physicians; and various written references including the scientific literature. Patients need to remember that their unique health care needs are not necessarily represented in any literature they may encounter. Therefore, it is recommended that a knowledgeable mentor be consulted before initiating self-care with any herb being used for the first time.

NURTURING THE NURSE-PLANT RELATIONSHIP:

Note: You may want to keep a journal of your experiences with the herb.

One of the first lengthy novels I read as a child was *Christy,* by Catherine Marshall. I think my interest in healing with plants was really piqued when I read about Christy and a local healer in the Appalachian Mountains applying an onion poultice to the chest of a person who was very ill with a respiratory disease that was probably tuberculosis. The poultice's success is vividly described as it caused the person to cough up copious amounts of green phlegm. The onion is a great domestic medicine and can be used inside and outside the body. Two of my favorite onion recipes for colds, flu, and bronchial conditions follow.

Onion Cress Soup

> Two large yellow or white onions chopped into small pieces but not minced
>
> 4 cups (960 ml) vegetable or onion stock
>
> Two large bunches of watercress *(Nasturtium officinale).* The leaf is used in many countries to relieve symptoms associated with respiratory illness and catarrh. In therapeutic amounts, it is contraindicated in pregnancy.
>
> Liquid Aminos to season and add minerals (if available). If not, use sea salt.

Cook the onions in the stock on medium low heat until the onions are very tender. Do not boil. Add the liquid aminos or sea salt to taste.

Trim the leaves from the cress stalks and before serving the soup add the cress to the onion soup. Cook for two minutes. (The cress is best if it is still green when served so only add as much as you plan to eat at one time.) Enjoy and rest well after eating.

Onion Syrup

    1 to 2 large yellow or white onions thinly sliced (Experience the onion's effects on your tear ducts!)

    ¾ to 1½ cup (180 to 360 ml) of honey (or any sugar)

In a large container, alternately layer the onion slices and then the honey. Let it stand for three days in a dark corner of the kitchen and then strain the syrup into a colored glass bottle. Store in the refrigerator. The syrup can be taken on a spoon just like any cough syrup or can be added to a tea. Rest well after taking.

CHAPTER 10

Skin Care

INTRODUCTION

ONE OF THE MOST IMPORTANT HEALTH-PROMOTING
activities of nursing care is the care of a patient's skin. Nurses promote
healthy skin by bathing patients to help the skin in its excretory activity.
They aid patients' skin in temperature regulation by providing warm blankets or cooling measures when needed. Nurses help keep the skin moist by
providing fluids and applying skin creams and ointments. When skin integrity is damaged in some way, nurses specialize in caring for the wound.
Nurses use a host of techniques, including bandaging and topical applications, in supporting the healing of skin tissue.

The skin as an organ is different from the rest of the body's systems
because it is not located in a specific area. It is generalized throughout
the body, inside and out. Skin and mucosa define or create the boundaries between one organ and the next and the entire body and its environment. The skin is an organ that defines the individual, where they exist in space or where they "end" and where another person or object
"begins." The skin is also a highly developed organ in that it has the potential to regenerate itself all the time. This is a special quality of skin because most organs in the body, once damaged, do not regenerate at all or
at least not as quickly as does skin. In caring for the skin, nurses work
with the regenerative energy in skin to promote healing.

Skin care is part of the art and the science of nursing. Nurses wash wounds to help the body shed old damaged tissue and bring forth new, stronger tissue. They anoint the skin with moisturizers to help hydrate the skin and use scented creams in massage of the skin to bring comfort and relaxation to patients who are stressed and ill. Nurses apply direct pressure to injured skin to stop bleeding, and they apply cold or warm dressings or ointments when tissues swell or are damaged in some way. Finally, nurses touch the skin of their patients to reassure, comfort, and demonstrate connection. Nurses touch sometimes to demonstrate caring without the intent of providing a skin care intervention. At other times, nurses touch the skin and provide an intervention such as wound care. Although the outcome of wound care may be measurable, the effects of the interpersonal connection that occurs with skin care of any kind may not be. Many nurses consider the interpersonal part of skin care as important to the success of the care as the actual intervention (e.g., wound care) (Papantonio, 1998).

Herbs have been used for centuries in the care of the skin. Herbs can soothe and calm inflamed skin, stop pain, help control bleeding, regulate temperature through promoting perspiration, astringe and/or hydrate the skin. Herbal remedies for the skin include compresses, poultices, oil, salves, floral waters, and baths to name a few. Caregivers experience the unique healing properties of plants when using them. Plant remedies extend the connection between caregiver and patient to connection with nature as well. Connection with nature and nature's remedies can be soothing, calming, and healing for many patients. Using them in patient care also can be soothing for caregivers because they touch and apply the plant material themselves.

The herbs in this chapter—calendula, aloe, yarrow, rose, and witch hazel—are used to support normal skin activities and to correct imbalances in skin condition. For example, they may increase perspiration or hydration of the skin. They may astringe the tissues or calm inflammation. These are different actions than nurses have experienced with the use of steroid medications. Steroids, although clearly effective for skin conditions, have serious potential adverse effects. "These include numerous local and systemic reactions, varying from mild to life-threatening. Skin atrophy and suppression of the hypothalamic-pituitary-adrenal axis are the most feared actions" (Korting, Schafer-Korting, Hart, Laux, & Schmid, 1993). This is one of the reasons why herbal therapies are considered for use by patients and practitioners alike. Herbs can provide alternatives to the use of stronger medications, especially when medications may not be necessary or desired, such as in the skin care of an infant. Some herbal skin products have been found to contain steroid drugs as well as herbs (Keane, Munn, DuVivier, Taylor, & Higgins, 1999). These remedies are not included in this book.

The herbs in this chapter have been shown through many centuries in many cultures to promote healthy skin function. In herbalism, healthy skin also is considered to be a measure of the health of the whole body. Skin conditions are not just treated topically. Herbal support for other excretory organs such as the liver, kidneys, and colon are considered as well. Some conditions such as acne are considered a sign of excessive stress (from overload of toxins) on the immune system and excretory organs. Herbal alteratives, such as red clover or burdock, would be considered in helping the body deal with the excessive toxin load.

In herbalism, as in nursing care for the skin, the patient's diet also is assessed carefully. The goal of nutritional care for patients with wounds is to promote collagen synthesis. Patients need a healthy balanced diet with proper amounts of carbohydrates; protein; copper; iron; zinc; and vitamins such as A, K, and C to promote healthy skin from within. As with any skin care regimen, healing is rarely a result of the topical intervention alone. The successful use of herbs in the care of the skin includes attending to the patient's diet and the environmental stressors that can potentially have a negative effect on the immune system and the skin's ability to regenerate and heal itself in the first place.

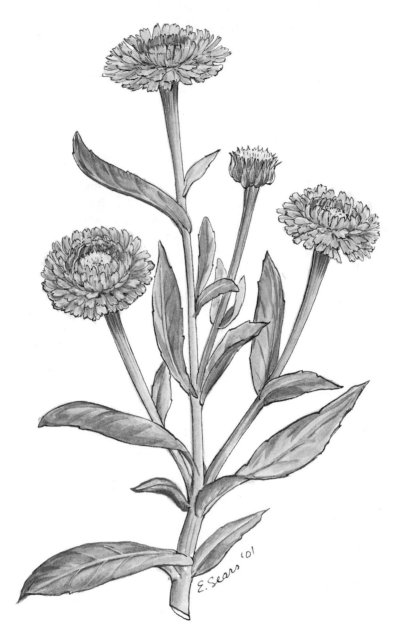

Calendula officinalis

Calendula

🍃 LATIN NAME: *Calendula officinalis*

🍃 FAMILY: Asteraceae

🍃 COMMON NAMES: Calendula, marigold, pot marigold, poet's marigold, Mary gowles, golds, holigold, marybud

Note: Do not confuse with the ornamental variety of marigold (*Tagetes* spp.).

🍃 HEALTH PATTERN: Skin care

🍃 PLANT DESCRIPTION:

Calendula is native to the Mediterranean area. Its name refers to the plant's habit of blooming throughout the calendar year in warm climates. In some areas it blooms every month, or during the new moon. Calendula is often confused with ornamental marigolds of the genus *Tagetes* that are commonly planted in pots and gardens. Calendula is a medicinal plant with light green leaves and golden orange to yellow flowers. Each daisylike flower has a central orange disk with numerous yellow-orange florets.

Calendula flowers open in the morning and close in the afternoon. If the flowers are closed after 7 A.M., it is said that there will be rain. Calendula was a rain indicator plant in early times. It grows from 12 to 20 inches (30 to 50 cm) high and has hairy stems and leaves. The plant blooms throughout the summer. If the flowers are to be used medicinally, they should be harvested from June to October in the morning before the flower heads open up. Flower heads can be dried intact and then the florets removed before use.

🍃 PLANT PART USED: Flower petals

🍃 TRADITIONAL EVIDENCE:

Cultural Use

East Indian. Calendula is used as an astringent and styptic (Nadkarni, 1976).

Russian/Baltic. Calendula has been used for several hundred years in Russian folk medicine. It is cultivated extensively on farms in Russia, and its preparations are used to tonify the action of the heart, reduce blood pressure, and decrease edema. Russian women use calendula both to delay menstruation and to help relieve the pain of dysmenorrhea. It also is used to treat tonsillitis and other conditions of the mucous membranes of the mouth. It is used for its anti-inflammatory and antiseptic actions (Zevin, 1997).

European. Calendula has been a favorite medicinal plant of the German people for cancer, wound healing, gastrointestinal complaints such as stomach cramps, fungal infections such as athlete's foot, and varicose veins. Many renowned physicians and healers, including Hildegarde of Bingen, Abbe Kneipp, and Maria Treben have used calendula as a remedy for symptoms related to the skin such as impetigo, bedsores, and malignant growths. The German Commission E approves the internal and topical use of calendula flowers for inflammation of the oral mucosa. It is approved for external use for poorly healing wounds, including bedsores, ulcerations, and swelling (Blumenthal, Goldberg, & Brinckman, 2000; Treben, 1980).

Historically, the French *Pharmacopoiea* from 1840 described five preparations from the leaves, seed, and whole herb of calendula that were used to cure some cancers (Boucaud-Maitre, Algernon, & Raynaud, 1988). Calendula also is used in Europe for sunburn and other mild burns, and as an immunostimulant for skin inflammations and herpes zoster infections (Leung & Foster, 1996). Bulgarians use calendula as an anti-inflammatory, antipyretic, and antitumor agent (Kalvatchev, Walder, & Garzaro, 1997). Calendula ointment is the first choice for the treatment of wounds (Schilcher, 1992).

Culinary Use

Calendula florets (petals) are edible. Calendula often was used as a soup starter during the Middle Ages. The fresh florets can be included in salads to add color. The flowers are used in cooking as a mildly salty flavoring and as a yellow coloring agent. Some people use the dried florets as a substitute for saffron (Leung & Foster, 1996) in foods such as rice and chowders (Blumenthal et al., 2000). Powdered calendula blossoms are used to color butter, custards, and liqueurs. Some herb enthusiasts eat sandwiches made from calendula florets, mayonnaise, cheese, and liverwurst (Duke, 1985).

Use in Herbalism

The medicinal use of calendula can be traced back to ancient Greece where, as with many yellow-flowered members of the Asteraceae family, it was used to treat gallstones and liver diseases (Zevin, 1997). Yellow color in a plant is a signature usually associated with the liver (bile) in herbalism. Calendula was used in early England to strengthen the heart. The flowers were dried and powdered, mixed with turpentine and lard, and used as a topical application (Culpeper, 1990). American Eclectic physicians used calendula as a stimulant and diaphoretic.

Calendula possesses antispasmodic, diaphoretic, anti-inflammatory, wound-healing, and antiseptic properties (Newall, Anderson, & Phillipson, 1996). It is used internally for spasmodic conditions, suppressed menstruation, typhoid fever, and jaundice. It is applied topically to cancerous tumors and ulcers. Calendula is an excellent topical application to prevent gangrene, infection, and tetanus. It is used on the skin of infants to prevent or heal chafing, excoriation, and diaper rash. Preparations of calendula are used to wash abscesses, eczema, burns, and skin ulcers. It has been used postoperatively on the surgical wound to aid healing. Calendula not only improves wound and skin healing but also can help prevent scar tissue formation and has been used historically in healing wounds created by herbal escharotics in the treatment of tumors (Naiman, 1999). Some report that the hydroalcoholic extracts of calendula have the greatest wound-healing capabilities (Schulz, Hansel, & Tyler, 1998) and some report that carbon dioxide preparations of calendula are best.

Calendula has been used for sore throat, conjunctivitis, sore nipples, vaginitis, nasal congestion, and varicose veins (Felter & Lloyd, 1983). It has been used "primarily in domestic practice as a mild aromatic and diaphoretic" (Cook & Lawall, 1926, p. 1010). It was recommended to rub a fresh flower of calendula onto the skin in cases of bee or wasp stings to reduce pain and swelling. A lotion made from the flowers can be used on sprains. A decoction is used internally to "throw out" the rash of measles and smallpox (Grieve, 1971). Calendula has been used traditionally to heal skin cracks and sores and for the treatment of impetigo, acne, burns, and frostbite (Buckle, 1997). Internally, calendula also is recommended for stomach disorders, gastric and duodenal ulcers, and dysmenorrhea (Wren, 1988). It is also helpful when taken in sips by patients with nausea and vomiting related to stomach virus or by patients with anorexia due to physiological or psychological illness.

Cosmetic Use. Calendula is used in skin care products such as lotions, creams, ointments, and shampoos (Leung & Foster, 1996).

BIOMEDICAL EVIDENCE:

The published studies on calendula have dealt primarily with the constituents of the plant. The active principles responsible for the plant's wound-healing and anti-inflammatory properties, "remained unknown until the mid-1980's" (Foster & Tyler, 1999, p. 85). No published human clinical trials that examine the traditional uses of calendula were found. Studies of the whole flower's use in humans are needed.

Studies Related to Skin Care

One controlled study in rats compared the wound healing effects of calendula ointment with allantoin, allantoin alone, and the ointment without calendula or allantoin. The calendula allantoin ointment produced significantly more epithelization of wounds than was found in the other control groups. Changes in the wounds were found as early as twenty-four hours after application of the calendula allantoin ointment (Kloucek-Popova, Popov, Pavlova, Krusteva, 1982).

Another study of Wister rats found that calendula tincture (1:10) made from the leaves and flowers applied topically to wounds significantly increased wound contraction rate and granuloma breaking strengths and decreased the time necessary for the eschar to fall off. This indicates that calendula tincture facilitates the collagen maturation and the epithelization phases of wound healing in rats (Rao et al., 1991).

Studies Related to Other Health Patterns

Immune Response. Traditional medicine in many countries contains accounts of the ability of calendula to deal with many types of infection. In vitro studies have recently demonstrated the ability of an organic extract of calendula flowers to inhibit the reverse transcriptase activity of human immunodeficiency virus (HIV) by 85% after thirty minutes (Kalvatchev et al., 1997).

Mechanism of Action

A single active principle that promotes wound healing has not been identified in calendula. "One hypothesis is that this action is based on synergistic effects of the volatile oil and the relatively high concentrations of xanthophylls that are present in the herb" (Schulz et al., 1998, p. 259). The anti-inflammatory and wound healing effects of calendula may be related to the triterpene flavonoids and saponins (Brown & Dattner, 1998).

The bright yellow-orange color of the flower is due to the presence of carotenoids. Carotenoids are soluble in fat, not water, which is why calendula is extracted in oil, fat, or carbon dioxide for many of its applications. Flavonoids are water soluble and calendula tea is used as well. In a study of freeze-dried calendula flowers, the water-soluble flavonoids from the flowers increased the rate of neovascularization and induced the deposition of hyaluronan, a polysaccharide associated with the formation of new capillaries (Patrick, Kumar, Edwardson, Hutchinson, 1996).

USE IN PREGNANCY OR LACTATION:

There are no known contraindications for the use of calendula during pregnancy or lactation (Blumenthal et al., 2000; McGuffin, Hobbs, Upton, & Goldberg, 1997). One source says that calendula is contraindicated during early pregnancy because of its potential to promote uterine bleeding (Brinker, 1998). Calendula can be used during lactation to heal cracked nipples and is nontoxic to the baby (Buckle, 1997; Weed, 1986).

Herbal Caveat—Pregnancy or Lactation

Some herbs are contraindicated in pregnancy because of a risk of the herb or one of its constituents stimulating the uterus and therefore possibly promoting fetal loss. Many herbal practitioners do not recommend herbal remedies, in particular oral doses of herbs, during the first trimester of pregnancy and seek an alternative. However, herbs are successfully used during pregnancy, especially to prepare the body for the birth. Herbs are relatively unstudied in pregnancy and lactation, so patients need to be made aware through education of the potential benefits and risks of using herbs for health conditions that arise during pregnancy or lactation. The use of herbal remedies during pregnancy often warrants a referral to a knowledgeable herbal practitioner.

USE FOR CHILDREN:

Calendula cream is helpful in the care of a baby's sensitive skin, especially in relieving symptoms related to diaper rash.

Herbal Caveat—Children

Children have special needs in regard to herbal therapies. They require lesser amounts of herbs and often respond well to mild teas and topical applications such as compresses and baths. The lowest dose of oral preparations should be tried first before increasing the amount given children. Caregivers should observe children closely for responses to herbal remedies. Younger children, particularly infants, have traditionally been given herbs either through their mother's breast milk or in the form of a homeopathic remedy because of their sensitivity to medicines and treatments and the immaturity of their liver. It is recommended that a person knowledgeable in the herbal treatment of children be consulted before the offering of any herb to a child for the first time.

CAUTIONS:

There are no known side effects or drug-drug or herb-drug interactions associated with the internal use of calendula (Blumenthal et al., 2000; Schulz et al., 1998).

NURSING EVIDENCE:

Historical Nursing Use

European, in particular Anthroposophical, nurses use calendula cream or oil for promoting healthy skin integrity such as in the prevention of bedsores.

Potential Nursing Applications

Nurses may want to consider using calendula compresses for patients with decubitus ulcers and other wounds and calendula ointment for burns, diaper rash, and wound care. Nurses also might consider giving sips of calendula tea to people who are very nauseated and have stomach cramps and using the tea as a mouthwash for inflamed mucous membranes. Nurses also might try adding a diluted calendula tincture to their conjunctivitis protocols to use as an eyewash for those with itchy, red eyes.

Integrative Insight

Calendula applications are very safe and have years of effective use as a traditional remedy for skin conditions, gastrointestinal discomfort, wounds, and conjunctivitis to name a few. There is little clinical research on the use of the plant, and although there has been more phytochemical research, few biomedical studies have been conducted that support the traditional uses of calendula. Some might reject the use of calendula because no biomedical evidence supports its use, yet others agree that, as is true of many plants, the secret of the medicinal action of the plant lies in the whole plant and the synergy of dozens of therapeutic constituents, which is not understood at the present time. Until calendula is understood from a biomedical perspective, nurses can explore the extensive safe traditional use of calendula flowers. I have seen numerous cases of conjunctivitis clear up with the use of calendula eyewash, and the skin cream is outstanding in wound and rash care.

Gentle calendula is an excellent plant to consider using when teaching children about herbs that they can use in self-care. The flowers are easy to grow. The seeds are somewhat unusual in that they are shaped like crescent moons with jagged edges. Children like to plant the seeds in paper cups and then care for the calendula seedling until it is big enough to transplant outside. They can be shown how and when to harvest the beautiful flower heads, dry them, and make them into an oil that they can rub on skin scrapes or sores.

When teaching children the simple steps of growing and harvesting calendula and making it into a medicament, one would never guess that the reasons for its healing properties have been eluding scientists. Perhaps one of the children we teach to grow calendula will one day find a way to unlock the mystery of the synergy involved in the flower's ability to heal human skin.

THERAPEUTIC APPLICATIONS:

Oral

Infusion. 1 to 2 g dried flower petals in 5 ounces (150 ml) water (Blumenthal et al, 2000).

Tincture. 1:5 (g/ml): 1 to 2 teaspoons (5 to 10 ml) (Blumenthal et al, 2000).

Fluid Extract. 1:1 (g/ml): Up to ½ teaspoon (1 to 2 ml) (Blumenthal et al., 2000)

Topical

Infusion for Compresses and Wound Care. Use 1 to 2 g of dried flowers in 5 ounces (150 ml) water.

Tincture for External Use. Use either the tincture 1:10 g/ml from flowers or a tincture 1:20 g/ml to 1:30 g/ml from the flowering herb. These may be dabbed undiluted onto the wound. For compresses, dilute the tincture in three parts of freshly boiled water (Schilcher, 1992).

Eyewash. For discomfort related to conjunctivitis, wash both eyes three times a day with 1 to 2 ounces (30 to 60 ml) of lukewarm water with 5 to 10 drops of homeopathically prepared calendula tincture.

Mouthwash. Use 2 teaspoons (10 ml) of tincture in 1 cup (240 ml) of water.

Ointment. Use the dried flower petals to prepare a salve or ointment (see chapter 5).

Environmental

No environmental uses for calendula are known.

Herbal Caveat—Therapeutic Applications

In traditional and conventional herbal medicine, amounts of herbs given to patients are based on individual needs. The amounts or "doses" recorded here are provided so that the health practitioner has a general idea of the amounts recommended for an adult patient. Dosing in herbalism not only refers to amount of plant used but also includes when, where, and how to take a plant medicine. These dosages should not be used as guidelines for indiscriminate intervention without proper assessment, critical thinking, and patient education on the part of the practitioner.

Note: Please see chapter 5 for detailed descriptions of how to prepare various applications.

PATIENT INTERACTION:

Calendula flowers can be steeped to make a tea for gastrointestinal discomfort and for use as a compress to heal burns and wounds. Calendula petals also can be used to make an oil or ointment for use in healing wounds or diaper rash. Calendula flowers are edible, but be sure to know the difference between the edible/medicinal flower and the ornamental garden variety of marigold (genus, *Tagetes*).

Herbal Caveat—Patient Interaction

Patients considering the use of an herb or formula of herbs in self-care benefit from education about the plant itself and the use of the plant in healing. This education can come through many sources, including local herbalists; plant specialists such as botanists; health practitioners such as nurses, nutritionists, naturopaths, and other physicians; and various written references including the scientific literature. Patients need to remember that their unique health care needs are not necessarily represented in any literature they may encounter. Therefore, it is recommended that a knowledgeable mentor be consulted before initiating self-care with any herb being used for the first time.

NURTURING THE NURSE-PLANT RELATIONSHIP:

Note: You may want to keep a journal of your experiences with the herb.

You can make your own calendula oil from start to finish. Begin by purchasing calendula seed and sowing it according to the directions. The seed is shaped like a half moon and is somewhat jagged. Wait to harvest the flowers until there are at least twenty large blossoms. Early in the morning, when the sun has risen and the flowers are about to open all the way, collect the flowers and put them in a small paper bag to dry. You can also cut the stems with the flowers and hang them in a dry dark place instead of using the paper bag technique. When fully dry, put the crushed flower petals in a medium-sized wide-mouthed bottle (approximately 12 ounces [360 ml]). Cover the flowers with cold-pressed vegetable oil, such as canola or safflower oil. Seal the jar and leave it for four to eight weeks. Shake the jar once a day. The oil should be a deep yellow color when the extraction is complete. When this occurs, press the oil out of the flower petals and strain the oil into a dark bottle. This oil will keep refrigerated for approximately one year.

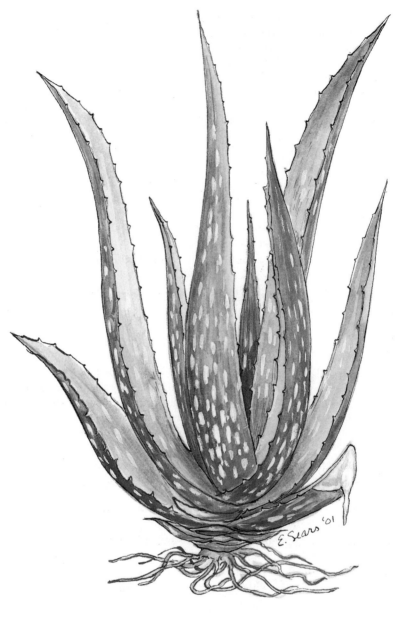

Aloe vera

Aloe

- **LATIN NAME:** *Aloe vera* (syn. *Aloe Barbadensis Miller, Aloe perfoliata L.* var. *vera*)

- **FAMILY:** Aloeaceae

- **COMMON NAMES:** Aloe, aloe vera, burn plant, medicine plant, bitter aloes

- **HEALTH PATTERN:** Skin care

- **PLANT DESCRIPTION:**

Aloe vera is a succulent plant similar in appearance to cacti, but they are not botanically related. It is a perennial with strong, fibrous roots and numerous fleshy, light green leaves that proceed upward from the soil. The leaves are narrow, tapered, and succulent, with small spines like teeth at the edges. Aloe is native to Africa and there are over 360 species (Leung & Foster, 1996).

- **PLANT PARTS USED:** Leaf and occasionally the root

- **TRADITIONAL EVIDENCE:**

Cultural Use

Asian. Aloe vera leaf juice is used in Traditional Chinese Medicine (TCM) in a powdered form as a purgative herb that clears heat and removes fire from the liver energy system. It is used for symptoms of epigastric discomfort, dizziness, headache, irritability, fever, constipation, and tinnitus. It is not given in cases of rectal bleeding, during menstruation and pregnancy, or for deficiency of the spleen or stomach (Bensky & Gamble, 1993).

The bitter aloe latex has been used in traditional Japanese herbalism since the fourth century B.C. It is used for the same symptoms as in Chinese medicine, signs of liver heat such as red eyes, emotional excesses, and tension below the rib cage. In addition, it is used to kill parasites, especially roundworms in children, and to improve digestion (Rister, 1999).

North American Indian. North American Indians of the southwestern United States apply aloe juice to skin boils, bedsores, burns, and diabetic ulcers to aid healing. They use the juice by cutting off a leaf of the plant, warming it briefly over the kitchen stove, and then squeezing the inner leaf gel onto the area to be treated (Kay, 1996).

Hispanic. Aloe, known as "savila" among Hispanics, is most often used for burns and ulcers but also is used for acne, cuts, wounds, arthritis, diabetes, balding, constipation, and diarrhea (Trotter, 1981). Mexican Americans in Las Cruces are reported to recommend 3 tablespoons (45 ml) of aloe juice in orange juice each morning for joint pain. They apply the gel to age spots on the skin to help them fade. Others claim that drinking the gel helps relieve the symptoms of colitis and other gastrointestinal disturbances. Others have cured dermatitis with a mixture of aloe, avocado pulp, and vitamin E cream (Kay, 1996). Some Mexicans use aloe with cactus for a cleansing of the body of any ailment.

African. Aloe species are native to Africa. It was regarded as a sacred plant by the Egyptians. Preparations made from the leaf are used to care for those with skin and eye disorders (DeSmet, 1999).

East Indian. East Indian practitioners use aloe vera root for colic, the fresh juice for fevers, and the pulp is used on the uterus (Nadkarni, 1976).

Middle Eastern. Arabs have used aloe leaf in the treatment of wounds for many centuries (Zawahry, Hegazy, & Helal 1973). There is reference in the Bible to the use of aloe. The aloe of the Old Testament is actually a type of lemon-scented wood known as *Aloexylon*. One source suggests that it is possible that the Israelites may have learned of the African plant aloe with thick leaves when they were in exile and that the aloe in John 19:39 is indeed the aloe used today in wound healing (de Waal, 1980).

Russian/Baltic. Aloe vera has been used for many years in Russia to treat various symptoms. The people have grown aloe in their homes since at least the 1930s. The plant is used for treating cuts, minor burns, scrapes, cold sores, sunburn, and other types of skin problems. The leaf is cut off of the plant, split down the middle, and the gel from the center is applied to the affected area of the skin. At times a bandage may be placed over the leaf to hold it in place on the wound, but some believe that aloe works best when the skin is exposed to the air (Zevin, 1997).

Russian medical practitioners recommend the use of Aloe vera for the treatment of frostbite, burns, wounds, boils, sunburn, wrinkles, and insect bites. Internally, the fresh juice is used to treat stomach and intestinal ulcers, diseases of the digestive tract, and excess stomach acid. It also has been used to stimulate appetite, to stimulate the immune system during the treatment of ulcers, and to treat respiratory illnesses (Zevin, 1997).

European. Aloe was in use in Britain by as early as the tenth century (Grieve, 1971). English physicians used various species of aloe as a source of juice that was made into an oral preparation. It was used as an energetic laxative that could cause cramping. Germans use dried aloe leaf juice to promote ease of defecation after rectal surgery and for hemorrhoids, anal fissures, and refractory constipation (Leung & Foster, 1996).

Culinary Use

Highly diluted aloe extracts are used to impart a subtle bitter flavor to certain beverages and candies. Many health food stores carry aloe juice products that are normally produced from aloe gel diluted with water and mixed with citric acid and preservative. Pure aloe juice is rarely sold in the marketplace (Leung & Foster, 1996).

Use in Herbalism

Aloe has been used in healing for centuries. It has been used internally for delayed menstruation, rectal prolapse, chronic constipation, atony of the large intestine, and to purge intestinal worms (Felter & Lloyd, 1983). It is often given with other herbs to decrease the cramping effects of the aloe (Grieve, 1971). Currently, the only "officially" recognized use of aloe is as an ingredient in tincture of benzoin (Leung & Foster, 1996).

Fresh aloe vera gel that is expressed from the leaves is a well-known traditional medicine. Aloe leaf yields two different medicinal substances, each from different parts of the plant. Aloe vera gel is contained in the center part of the succulent leaves. The bitter, yellow-colored latex from the plant is derived from cells that line the inner surface of the leaf skin. The latex is used as a harsh laxative and is known as the drug "aloe" or "aloes." The latex is obtained by cutting the leaves and allowing the bitter sap to drip out. It is then processed into the drug form. Aloe vera gel is obtained by pressing the leaves or through solvent extraction with chemicals (Leung & Foster, 1996). The gel does not have laxative properties (McGuffin et al., 1997).

Aloe vera is popularly known as the "burn," "first aid," or "medicine" plant. The fresh gel from the leaf can be immediately applied topically to burns, sunburns, insect bites, and wounds to promote healing. Aloe vera gel is currently used as a demulcent, wound healing agent. It is also given internally for healing gastrointestinal problems such as ulcers.

BIOMEDICAL EVIDENCE:

Although significant past evidence confirms the traditional use of aloe for improving the health of the human skin, some studies over the past few years appear to contradict these findings. It has been suggested that, "the inconsistency and nonreproducibility of various reports concerning the effects of prostaglandin and thromboxane synthetase inhibitors (it is hypothesized that aloe inhibits thromboxane A_2) on the healing process of experimental partial-thickness burns could be attributed to the fact that different investigators do not use identical burn wound models, nor do they employ the same modalities of treatment" (Kaufman, Kalderon, Ullmann, & Berger, 1988, p. 159). To be able to fully evaluate the results of research on aloe, the wound models and the form of aloe (product) used must be clearly specified. The quality of aloe vera gel, which is often used in studies, can vary greatly. The principle component in aloe gel is a glucomannan, similar to guar and locust bean gums. "These gums are frequently mixed with aloe gel to increase its viscosity and yield. Currently there is no meaningful assay method that distinguishes genuine liquid gel products from adulterant mixtures" (Leung & Foster, 1996, p. 28).

Studies Related to Skin Care

Human clinical trials of the effect of topical application of either aloe vera gel (ALOECORP) or Dremaide Aloe (Dermaide Research Corporation) to partial thickness burns ($N = 50$), frostbite ($N = 56$ in the treatment group), or the skin of patients with inadvertent intra-arterial drug abuse ($N = 25$), demonstrated significant improvement in healing of tissue with less tissue loss, complications, and morbidity than those treated with conventional methods. Animal studies that compared the use of aloe to methylprednisolone acetate, aspirin, U38450, and Carrington wound gel demonstrated that aloe either produced significantly more improvement or was comparable to other medications in healing burns, frostbite, and tissue injury related to drug abuse or electrical injury (Heggers, Pelley, & Robson, 1993).

Two case studies presented by a clinical nurse specialist and enterostomal therapist report the use of water-based aloe gel (Carrasyn Gel) in the care of patients with necrotizing fasciitis. The aloe gel used in the treatment of the wounds provided the moist environment needed in the wound care and decreased the number of dressing changes needed so that patient comfort was increased (Ardire & Mrowczynski, 1997). Another nurse reported noticing the beginning of the granulation of a pressure sore after ten days of direct application of aloe juice directly from the leaf. The sore was completely healed in four weeks (Cuzzel, 1986).

Case study reports also demonstrate that aloe gel, extracted from the fresh leaves after draining them of the yellow bitter sap for forty-eight hours (also after being homogenized, filtered, and adding a preservative), significantly improved the healing of chronic lower limb ulcers, seborrheic alopecia, and acne vulgaris. The only untoward effect occurred in people with leg ulcers, who experienced increased pain at the start of the treatment, which the investigators equate with the improvement in circulation to the area (Zawahry et al., 1973). Another case study demonstrated the successful use of stabilized aloe gel 2% in the care of a 52-year-old woman with lichen planus (Hayes, 1999).

In a placebo-controlled trial, aloe vera extract 0.5% in a cream base of castor and mineral oils significantly resolved skin plaques in 60 patients with slight-to-moderate chronic psoriasis. In the aloe cream group, 83.3% of patients were said to have been cured as compared with placebo (2%). The aloe cream healed 82.8% of the chronic plaques as compared with placebo (7.7%) (Syed et al., 1996).

In an animal study, aloe gel, prepared from fresh leaf (lyophilized and reconstituted with water before application), 30 mg given orally or topically twice a day, resulted in increased collagen contents of granulation tissue as compared with controls (Chithra, Sajithlal, & Chandrakasan, 1998).

In a controlled trial of 194 breast cancer patients receiving radiation therapy, there were no significant differences between those patients who received aloe vera gel (98% pure gel from the *Aloe Barbadensis Miller* plant) topical applications before radiation and those who did not in regard to radiation-induced dermatitis (Williams et al., 1996).

One animal trial of 14 guinea pigs found that aloe vera gel from a crude extract from the center of the leaves of the plant impaired the wound healing of second-degree burns as compared to silver sulfadiazine cream (Kaufman et al., 1988). In vitro studies have demonstrated that aloe vera in concentrations greater than 70% (for gram-positive bacteria) and 60% (for gram-negative bacteria) has an antimicrobial effect similar to silver sulfadiazine (Robson, Heggers, & Hagstrom, 1982).

Aloe vera gel (85%) dressings significantly improved the healing time in 27 patients with partial thickness burns (11.89 days as compared with 18.19 days; $p < 0.002$) as compared with Vaseline gauze. The two dressings were applied to either ends of the same wound and were changed twice daily. The wounds treated with aloe were shown to have early epithelialization. The subjects treated with aloe did experience slight discomfort and pain (Visuthikosol, Sukwanarat, Chowchuen, Sriurairatana, & Boonpucknavig, 1995).

Studies Related to Other Health Patterns

Immune Response. Acemannan, a polysaccharide in aloe vera, currently is being used in the treatment of HIV and acquired immunodeficiency syndrome (AIDS) at oral dosages of 800 to 1000 mg per day. It is believed to possess significant immune enhancing and antiviral activity. Acemannan is used as an adjunct to other AIDS therapies such as zidovudine (AZT). Approximately ½ to 1 quart (½ to 1 liter) of aloe vera gel is required to provide the daily recommended dose of acemannan. No clinical studies are referenced (Werbach & Murray, 1994).

Digestion. Three physicians reported that 12 patients with peptic ulcer experienced complete recovery, confirmed by radiology, after being given an emulsion of 2½ drams of cellulose-free aloe gel in mineral oil daily for approximately one year. The physicians report numerous patients, after healing from acute peptic ulcer disease, had no recurrences after 18 months of taking 1 tablespoon of aloe emulsion each night (Blitz, Smith, & Gerard, 1963).

Mechanism of Action

Aloe vera is known to penetrate and anesthetize tissue; it is bactericidal, virucidal, and fungicidal and has anti-inflammatory properties similar to those of a steroid (Robson et al., 1982). Although the composition of aloe vera gel is not clearly defined, it is known that the active constituents of aloe are cathartic anthraglycosides, particularly aloin (barbaloin), which is a glucoside of aloe-emodin (Leung & Foster, 1996). Aloe "penetrates injured tissue, relieves pain, is anti-inflammatory and dilates capillaries and increases the blood supply to the injured area by inhibiting thromboxane A_2 and maintaining the PGE_2 and PGF_{2a} ratio without causing a collapse of the injured blood vessels" (Heggers et al., 1993, p. S52).

It is suggested that the significant improvement in psoriasis patients due to aloe vera extract is related to the plant gel's ability to act in an occlusive manner by penetrating the dermis and deeper tissues (where psoriasis occurs), keeping the skin moist, and directly inhibiting the psoriatic plaques by suppressing proliferation and stimulatory differentiation of the cells in the epidermis (Syed et al., 1996).

Animal studies demonstrate that aloe vera gel seems to improve wound healing by increasing collagen content of granulation tissue. Aloe-treated wounds have a higher content of aldehydic groups, which may indicate that aloe-treated wounds may undergo a higher degree of cross-linking, which results in an increase in the tensile strength of the wound. Aloe-treated wounds also synthesize greater amounts of type III collagen as compared with controls, indicating the possibility for early wound healing and better organization of the type I collagen in the final scar (Chithra et al., 1998).

USE IN PREGNANCY OR LACTATION:

Midwives recommend using aloe vera gel for topical application to a torn perineum after birth. Because the bottled gel may contain preservatives that may irritate sensitive skin, it is suggested to use the fresh gel directly from the leaves. Express the gel onto a gauze pad or a menstrual pad and fix it in place. Replace it as often as necessary. The gel is reported to be remarkably healing and cooling when used in this manner (Weed, 1986).

Midwives recommend the use of fresh aloe vera gel topically to aid in healing sore nipples. The gel should be rinsed off with water before the baby nurses because it tastes quite bitter (Weed, 1986). Aloes or the purgative principle (for internal use) from the aloe leaf is contraindicated during pregnancy (McGuffin et al., 1997).

Herbal Caveat—Pregnancy or Lactation
Some herbs are contraindicated in pregnancy because of a risk of the herb or one of its constituents stimulating the uterus and therefore possibly promoting fetal loss. Many herbal practitioners do not recommend herbal remedies, in particular oral doses of herbs, during the first trimester of pregnancy and seek an alternative. However, herbs are successfully used during pregnancy, especially to prepare the body for the birth. Herbs are relatively unstudied in pregnancy and lactation, so patients need to be made aware through education of the potential benefits and risks of using herbs for health conditions that arise during pregnancy or lactation. The use of herbal remedies during pregnancy often warrants a referral to a knowledgeable herbal practitioner.

USE FOR CHILDREN:

Aloe vera gel should not be used on infants because of the bitter taste that may come into contact with the mouth (Schilcher, 1992). The oral use of aloes is contraindicated in children under ten to twelve years old (World Health Organization [WHO], 1999).

Herbal Caveat—Children

Children have special needs in regard to herbal therapies. They require lesser amounts of herbs and often respond well to mild teas and topical applications such as compresses and baths. The lowest dose of oral preparations should be tried first before increasing the amount given children. Caregivers should observe children closely for responses to herbal remedies. Younger children, particularly infants, have traditionally been given herbs either through their mother's breast milk or in the form of a homeopathic remedy because of their sensitivity to medicines and treatments and the immaturity of their liver. It is recommended that a person knowledgeable in the herbal treatment of children be consulted before the offering of any herb to a child for the first time.

CAUTIONS:

Presently, no commercial preparation of aloe vera gel has proven to be chemically stable during storage. It is believed that many of the active constituents in the gel deteriorate during its shelf life, so it is recommended to use the fresh gel directly from the leaf (WHO, 1999). Aloe vera gel (not the dried leaf latex) used internally has been found to improve the hypoglycemic effect of certain pharmaceutical medications when given to those with diabetes. Because of the antihyperglycemic action of aloe vera gel, it is suggested that those with blood sugar irregularities use it cautiously when taking it internally (Brinker, 1998).

It is best to apply fresh aloe gel to wounds right after the wound occurs. Aloe is not recommended for puncture wounds because its ability to penetrate the skin may carry puncture contaminants deeper (Sturm, 1999). One case of a severe reaction, including redness and swelling, to the application of aloe juice directly from the leaf has been reported in a woman who had just had a perioral chemical peel (Hunter & Frumkin, 1991). It is not clear that the woman drained the leaf before applying it to the wounds on her face so that she was using only the gel. It is important to cut the spines off the sides of the leaf before attempting to use the gel from the inner pulp because much of the yellow latex is stored under the spines and the peel. The yellow sap must be drained from the leaf before using it for open wounds.

The mechanical process that is used to separate the aloe gel from the bitter latex may not be entirely effective in some cases. Sometimes aloe gel is contaminated with the laxative principle. Those who consume the gel may have an unwanted laxative effect (Foster & Tyler,

1999). The dried leaf latex with the laxative properties (not aloe vera gel) is contraindicated internally during profuse menstruation, pregnancy, lactation, gastrointestinal inflammation, ulcerative colitis, Crohn's disease, colitis, and irritable bowel syndrome. It is not to be given to children under twelve years or used by anyone longer than eight to ten days. It is contraindicated in intestinal obstruction, kidney disorders, appendicitis and abdominal pain of unknown origin. Overuse or misuse can cause potassium loss leading to increased toxicity of cardiac glycosides and the reduced absorption of oral drugs. Overuse aggravates potassium loss caused by diuretics (Brinker, 1998; Schulz et al., 1998). The laxative preparation of aloe should be used only if no effect can be obtained through dietary changes or bulk-forming laxatives (WHO, 1999).

NURSING EVIDENCE:

Historical Nursing Use

Nurses use aloe gel topically for wound and burn care.

Potential Nursing Applications

Nurses may want to continue exploring the clinical use of aloe gel in wound, burn, and decubitus ulcer care. Nurses also might want to research the use of aloe in skin care, in healing peptic ulcers, and in aiding defecation postoperatively.

Aromatherapists recommend a compress of a base oil or gel and an appropriate essential oil in the care of wounds that are open and contaminated. Nurses may want to try using aloe vera gel as a base for the compress (Buckle, 1997) and adding an appropriate essential oil such as lavender in the case of burns.

Integrative Insight

There is a long history of traditional use and extensive research regarding the use of aloe gel for the promotion of healing of burns and wounds. Although there is some controversy in the literature, it is clear that aloe gel is worthy of consideration in the skin care practice of nurses. Nurses have to perform so many treatments and interventions that are uncomfortable for patients. Applying fresh aloe gel is not one of those interventions. It can be cooling, soothing, and healing inside and out.

Like the physicians in the study described above (Blitz et al., 1963), my grandfather also used to tap his aloe plants every time a friend told him that they had an ulcer. They would drink the gel in some water and be pain free. It is common sense that people would consider drinking the gel for burning sensation in their belly, especially if they know the plant as the "burn plant" and they have seen it soothe sunburns. Using herbs such as aloe on the skin and mucous membranes often gives dramatic results that people can see and feel.

THERAPEUTIC APPLICATIONS:

Oral

Most of the oral dosages given in plant medicine resources old and new are for the drug aloes rather than aloe gel.

Aloe Latex (Laxative): The correct oral dose is the smallest amount required to produce a soft-formed stool. For adults and children over ten years old, use 0.04 to 0.11 g of Curacao or Barbados aloe or use 0.06 to 0.17 g of Cape aloe dried latex. These dosages correspond to 10 to 30 mg of hydroxyanthraquinones per day (WHO, 1999).

For those who want to drink aloe gel or juice, it is best to find out as much as possible about the actual aloe content and then decide how much to drink. One source reports that HIV patients receiving acemannan took 800 to 1600 mg per day, which may be equivalent to ½ to 1 quart (½ to 1 L) of juice (Werbach & Murray, 1994).

Topical

Aloe vera gel, either commercially produced or acquired from one's own plants, may be applied liberally to the skin as often as desired. Leaves up to 1 foot (approximately 30 cm) long can be removed from the plant without damage. It is best to harvest a leaf during the afternoon when the plant has had time to move the maximum amount of sap up into the leaves (Rister, 1999). It is recommended to wash the leaf in water and a mild chlorine solution. Remove the outer layers of the leaf, taking care to not tear the green rind, which could result in contamination of the leaf gel with the leaf latex (WHO, 1999). Cut the spines off first and then slice the leaf down the middle to have the best access to the gel. Use the fresh gel or preparations containing 10% to 70% fresh gel (WHO, 1999). The aloe latex product is not used topically.

Environmental

Aloe vera is cultivated as a houseplant. It does not grow well outside if the temperature drops below 41°F. It grows well in both sun and shade. The leaves may be cut off as needed for burns and other skin problems.

Herbal Caveat—Therapeutic Applications

In traditional and conventional herbal medicine, amounts of herbs given to patients are based on individual needs. The amounts or "doses" recorded here are provided so that the health practitioner has a general idea of the amounts recommended for an adult patient. Dosing in herbalism not only refers to amount of plant used but also includes when, where, and how to take a plant medicine. These dosages should not be used as guidelines for indiscriminate intervention without proper assessment, critical thinking, and patient education on the part of the practitioner.

Note: Please see chapter 5 for detailed descriptions of how to prepare various applications.

When considering the use of aloe vera, it is very important to know a little about the structure of the leaf of the plant. A yellow sap inside the green skin of the leaf has a purgative effect on the bowels. The translucent pulp inside the spongy leaf is what aloe gel is made from. It is possible to get some sap in the gel, so if taking the gel internally watch for any unwanted laxative effects. Because the aloe has such a limited and questionable shelf life, it is best to purchase an aloe plant and prepare your own gel from the plant's leaves. Larger amounts of juice are often recommended by practitioners who may or may not understand that the juices and gels on the market can be very low in actual aloe gel content. Care should be taken not to inadvertently cut across the outside of the leaves during preparation to avoid getting the sap in the gel. When using aloe leaf externally for burns and wounds, cut off the spines and then cut the leaf down the middle and lay the leaf with the slippery cooling gel face down on the skin. The gel also can be collected and then put on the skin without the whole leaf effect. Do not take aloe internally if you are pregnant or under the age of twelve.

Herbal Caveat—Patient Interaction

Patients considering the use of an herb or formula of herbs in self-care benefit from education about the plant itself and the use of the plant in healing. This education can come through many sources, including local herbalists; plant specialists such as botanists; health practitioners such as nurses, nutritionists, naturopaths, and other physicians; and various written references including the scientific literature. Patients need to remember that their unique health care needs are not necessarily represented in any literature they may encounter. Therefore, it is recommended that a knowledgeable mentor be consulted before initiating self-care with any herb being used for the first time.

NURTURING THE NURSE-PLANT RELATIONSHIP:

Note: You may want to keep a journal of your experiences with the herb.

Purchase a large leafed aloe vera plant. The leaves should be spongy and healthy looking. Prepare the leaf as previously described and place the leaf on the back of your arm. Feel the cool and moist properties of the plant as you use the leaves to soothe your skin. After the gel dries, your skin may feel slightly tight. Apply a mild moisturizer if needed. To try aloe as a drink, drain the yellow sap from a leaf and then scoop out the pulp from the center of a leaf. Chop finely and then mash in a dish so that the gel is collected in the dish. Put all of the gel and the pulp in a glass, add a few ounces of water, stir vigorously, and drink. This soothing aloe drink tastes slightly bitter.

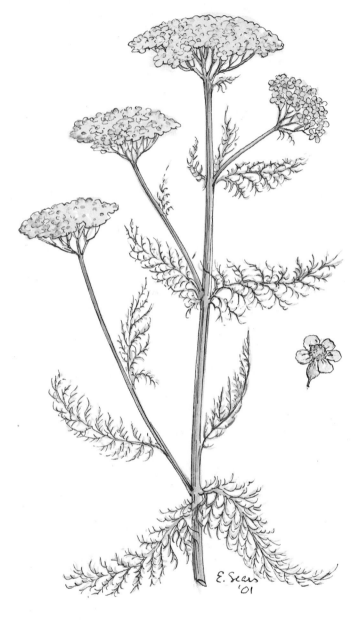

Achillea millefolium

Yarrow

- LATIN NAME: *Achillea millefolium*

- FAMILY: Asteraceae
     Note: Do not confuse *A. millefolium* with *A. tomentosa* or *A. micrantha* (golden yarrow), an ornamental garden plant.

- COMMON NAMES: Yarrow, achillea, milfoil, millefolium, noble yarrow, sanguinary, soldier's woundwort, thousandleaf, bloodwort, knight's milfoil, nosebleed.

- HEALTH PATTERN: Skin care

- PLANT DESCRIPTION:
     The genus name *Achillea* comes from the Greek name of the hero Achilles, who according to legend, stopped the bleeding from the battle wounds of his fellow soldiers by using yarrow leaf. The species name *millefolium* (thousand leaves) refers to the many segments in its foliage. Yarrow is a common herb found in pastures, fields, and waste places throughout the temperate zones of North America and Europe. It is a perennial that can grow 12 to 24 inches (30 to 60 cm) in height. The stem is angular rather than round, and feels rough. The leaves are lanceolate and alternate on the stem, 3 to 4 inches (7.5 to 10 cm) long, and approximately 1 inch (2.5 cm) wide. Each leaf is divided into many segments, giving the leaves a feathery appearance. The minute daisylike flowers are clustered in flat-topped heads at the ends of the stalks and can be white or light pink. The pink yarrow has been favored traditionally for medicinal use, and it is unclear if the pink is another species or is just a product of the environment in which it is grown. The flowers bloom from May to October and are best harvested during July. The entire plant is rather downy, with white silky hairs. The plant has an aromatic fragrance and a bitter and astringent taste (Felter & Lloyd, 1983).

- PLANT PARTS USED: The fresh or dried aerial parts harvested during the flowering season are used. Hildegard of Bingen used the root.

- TRADITIONAL EVIDENCE:
Cultural Use
     Asian. In ancient China, yarrow was considered a sacred plant. The plant was thought to perfectly embody the balance between the principles of yin and yang, the two main principles found in nature (Lawless, 1998). Its stems continue to be used to make the divination sticks of the I Ching. Fresh yarrow herb is mashed into a poultice for topical application on wounds and sores. The dried herb is recom-

mended for internal bleeding, especially for menstrual disorders and hemorrhoids (Leung & Foster, 1996).

North American Indian. Yarrow is widely used by Native American tribes throughout North America for a variety of symptoms. The Navajo use yarrow to treat fevers, headaches, and sores. It is used as a cold remedy, for fevers, respiratory disorders, stomach disorders, diarrhea, hemorrhoids, tuberculosis, menstrual hemorrhage, chest pain, and heart problems. External use includes application to boils, burns, swellings, wounds, and sores; for bronchitis, earache, toothaches, and sore throat; and it can be added to the bath for arthritic pain (Moerman, 1998). The flowers are burned to release smoke that assists in breaking a fever, warding off evil spirits, and reviving those who are comatose. The flowers also are used as a ceremonial smoke (Vogel, 1970).

Hispanic. The ancient Aztecs used yarrow as an emetic to cure coughs. It was used by women during childbirth. It was said to heal genital ulcers and skin sores if applied topically. Yarrow infusion has been taken internally for stomach complaints, flatulence, and diarrhea (Kay, 1996). Today, Hispanics of the southwestern United States use yarrow, "plumajillo," as an anti-inflammatory, for wounds and burns, and to stop heavy bleeding such as nosebleeds. It is used for colds, skin problems, and discomfort associated with a weak stomach, and to increase the flow of urine. Mexican Americans drink a preparation of yarrow for anemia, colds, and painful and bloody urination (Kay, 1996).

East Indian. Yarrow has been used in India as a bitter and in medicated vapor baths for fevers (Fleter & Lloyd, 1983). The powdered leaves and flower heads are used to dispel intestinal gas and cramps and as a tonic. A hot infusion of the leaves is used to promote timely menstrual bleeding (Nadkarni, 1976).

Russian/Baltic. Russians call yarrow the "herb of a thousand leaves." Its use is recorded in Russia as far back as the fourteenth century, but it was undoubtedly used before then in folk medicine. During the eighteenth and nineteenth centuries, Russian doctors used yarrow to treat hemorrhage and dysentery (Zevin, 1997). Russian herbalists use yarrow to stop internal bleeding, including bleeding from the lungs, stomach, nose, and hemorrhoids. It is the herb of choice to treat excess menstrual bleeding because it both helps blood clot and also strengthens the uterine muscles. Yarrow is given to nursing mothers who want to increase their milk supply. The herb acts as a relaxant to the muscles of the intestines and urinary tract and is recommended for gastritis, stomach and duodenal ulcers, and to stimulate the appetite and dispel flatulence. It is given to reduce high blood pressure, stimulate the flow of bile from the liver and gallbladder, and guard against the formation of kidney stones and gallstones (Zevin, 1997).

European. In early Great Britain, yarrow was highly regarded as a wound-healing agent, as its names, soldier's wound wort and knight's milfoil, demonstrate. Yarrow has been called "herba militaris," the "military herb." In Sweden, it was called "field hop" and was used in the making of beer. Some believe that beer made with yarrow is more intoxicating than that made with hops (Grieve, 1971).

German traditional medicine includes the use of yarrow for discomfort related to menstruation, menopause, gastrointestinal complaints, bedwetting in the young or old, prolapsed uterus, migraine, rheumatic pain, bleeding, angina, and hemorrhoids. Yarrow is known as the "cure of all ills" and has been used for medically hopeless situations with success. "That yarrow works on the bone marrow and thus stimulates blood renewal is not well known" (Treben, 1980, p. 50). The German Commission E approves the use of yarrow internally for symptoms such as loss of appetite, poor digestion, and gastrointestinal spastic conditions. It is approved for external use in sitz baths for female pelvic pain and cramps (Blumenthal et al., 2000; Schulz et al., 1998). The British Herbal Compendium lists yarrow as an oral remedy for fevers, common cold, and digestive problems. It recommends the external use for application to slow-healing wounds and for skin inflammation (Bradley, 1992).

Yarrow is used in Italy for intermittent fevers and in Scotland as an ointment for wounds (Felter & Lloyd, 1983). In Germany, yarrow preparations are used instead of iodine for children's minor scrapes. Yarrow has been found to have bacteriostatic and anti-inflammatory actions. The tincture is diluted 1:1 or 1:2 with water so it won't sting infants and young children (Schilcher, 1992). It also is used in Germany for depression and moodiness (Lawless, 1998).

For serious insomnia during the summer, the German mystic/ herbal healer Hildegard of Bingen recommended two parts yarrow and one part fennel. The two herbs are cooked and then placed on the temples and around the head. Powdered green sage is mixed with a small amount of wine and placed over the heart and around the neck. In winter, fennel seed and yarrow *root* can be used instead. The heat of the fennel induces sleep, the heat of the sage slows the heart and dilates the neck veins to invite sleep, and the heat of the yarrow makes the sleep sound (Flanagan, 1996). Hildegard of Bingen also recommended yarrow before surgery and after internal injury. She also had a yarrow beverage that she gave for preventing metastasis that included "3 pinches of yarrow powder in fennel tea at first and then 3 pinches of yarrow powder in warm wine" (Naiman, 1999, p. 187).

Culinary Use

Yarrow is used in bitters and vermouths. The flowers are used in herb teas (Leung & Foster, 1996). The Council of Europe states that yarrow can be added to foods and beverages for flavoring purposes provided that the thujone content of the finished product does not exceed 0.5 mg/kg (Newall et al., 1996). In the United States, yarrow is approved for use only in alcoholic beverages as a flavoring and the finished product must be thujone-free (Newall et al., 1996). Thujone is a potentially toxic chemical if consumed in large amounts.

Use in Herbalism

Yarrow has been used externally as an ointment for wounds, skin inflammation, ulcers, and fistulas. A decoction can be made of yarrow and applied to the scalp to prevent hair loss. Internally, yarrow is used in the treatment of gonorrhea, leukorrhea, bladder complaints, and diarrhea. The leaves have been chewed to ease toothaches (Culpeper, 1990).

In the late 1800s, yarrow was recommended specifically for chronic diseases of the urinary tract. It was thought to tonify the circulatory system and mucous membranes. It was used for sore throat, hemoptysis, blood in the urine, and other instances of mild bleeding. Yarrow also was used to treat urinary incontinence, diabetes, hemorrhoids, dysentery, and cancer. It was given in cases of amenorrhea, flatulence, and spasmodic conditions. Yarrow was used as a douche for leukorrhea (Felter & Lloyd, 1983).

Yarrow tea was and still is considered one of the best remedies for the fevers associated with the common cold. It is given to induce perspiration in the early stages of a cold, in measles, and in other diseases characterized by skin eruptions. But one herbalist cautions not to use yarrow by itself internally if one's fever is greater than 102°F because it may temporarily increase the fever (Weed, 1986). The whole plant also is decocted and used for hemorrhoids and kidney disorders (Grieve, 1971).

Yarrow tincture often is used as a topical agent to stop bleeding by astringing the tissues. Yarrow is used for poor appetite, stomach cramps, gas, gastritis, coughing up blood, nosebleed, hemorrhoidal bleeding, bloody urine, wounds, sores, and rashes (Leung & Foster, 1996). Yarrow tea or infusion is recommended for use in cases of persistent bladder infections (Weed, 1986). Yarrow is regarded as a nerve tonic that can rejuvenate the entire system. Aromatherapists recommend yarrow essential oil in the bath or a massage for symptoms of menopause. It is claimed to be able to help one maintain emotional equilibrium as changes occur in the body (Lawless, 1998).

BIOMEDICAL EVIDENCE:

Although there are centuries of recorded use of yarrow for wound healing and stopping the bleeding associated with injury to skin and body tissues, published clinical research was not found. Some research on the plant constituents has been done (see Mechanism of Action).

Studies Related to Skin Care

No data are available at this time.

Studies Related to Other Health Patterns

Hormone Balance. Some researchers are exploring yarrow's traditional use as a contraceptive. Preliminary animal studies have demonstrated that yarrow extract given intraperitoneally or orally has an antispermatogenic action in mice (Montanari, de Carvalho, & Dolder, 1998). Yarrow was once classified as an oral contraceptive that causes temporary sterility and as an emmenagogue, an agent that affects menstruation (de Laszlo & Henshaw, 1954).

Mechanism of Action

Miller and Chow (1954) found the alkaloid in yarrow, achilleine, to be an active hemostatic agent (as reported in Chandler, Hooper, & Harvey, 1982a) which may explain the plant's use in stopping bleeding. Yarrow contains sesquiterpene lactones, the precursors of azulenes that have known antimicrobial, anticancer, and antipruritic activity. The anti-inflammatory activity of sesquiterpene lactones may account for the effectiveness of yarrow in providing relief for the discomfort associated with many skin conditions, including wounds. Yarrow's traditional use to treat the discomforts associated with illness of women's reproductive system may be related to its thujone content. The spasmolytic activity of yarrow is attributed to the presence of flavonoids and thujone, a known abortifacient (Chandler et al., 1982a).

Among the four sterols and four triterpenes present in yarrow, beta-sitosterol is the major sterol and alpha-amyrin is the primary triterpene (Chandler et al., 1982b). Alpha-peroxyachifolid, a sesquiterpene lactone in yarrow, has been identified as the main sensitizer to those who experience allergic reaction to yarrow. This sesquiterpene lactone is present in other plant species in the Asteraceae family and may explain why there is cross reactivity in sensitive individuals (Hausen, Breuer, Weglewski, & Rucker, 1991).

USE IN PREGNANCY OR LACTATION:

The internal use of yarrow is not recommended during pregnancy (Blumenthal et al., 2000) because of its ability to stimulate the uterine musculature and promote menstrual bleeding (McGuffin et al., 1997). However, there are no known restrictions for its use during lactation (Blumenthal et al., 2000).

Midwives recommend the external application of yarrow compresses or poultices to the legs during pregnancy for symptoms related to varicose veins. It also is recommended to use an ointment made from yarrow and plantain to help shrink hemorrhoids and to relieve the associated pain. Yarrow leaf poultice or ointment is recommended for use on cracked and sore nipples to aid healing and decrease pain during lactation (Weed, 1986).

Herbal Caveat—Pregnancy or Lactation

Some herbs are contraindicated in pregnancy because of a risk of the herb or one of its constituents stimulating the uterus and therefore possibly promoting fetal loss. Many herbal practitioners do not recommend herbal remedies, in particular oral doses of herbs, during the first trimester of pregnancy and seek an alternative. However, herbs are successfully used during pregnancy, especially to prepare the body for the birth. Herbs are relatively unstudied in pregnancy and lactation, so patients need to be made aware through education of the potential benefits and risks of using herbs for health conditions that arise during pregnancy or lactation. The use of herbal remedies during pregnancy often warrants a referral to a knowledgeable herbal practitioner.

USE FOR CHILDREN:

Because of its bacteriostatic and anti-inflammatory actions, yarrow tincture can be used instead of iodine for children's minor scrapes. The tincture is diluted 1:1 or 1:2 in water so it won't sting infants and young children (Schilcher, 1992). Teas do not need to be diluted.

Herbal Caveat—Children
Children have special needs in regard to herbal therapies. They require lesser amounts of herbs and often respond well to mild teas and topical applications such as compresses and baths. The lowest dose of oral preparations should be tried first before increasing the amount given children. Caregivers should observe children closely for responses to herbal remedies. Younger children, particularly infants, have traditionally been given herbs either through their mother's breast milk or in the form of a homeopathic remedy because of their sensitivity to medicines and treatments and the immaturity of their liver. It is recommended that a person knowledgeable in the herbal treatment of children be consulted before the offering of any herb to a child for the first time.

CAUTIONS:

There are no known side effects associated with using yarrow, except in those individuals who are allergic to other plants in the Asteraceae family, such as arnica, calendula, and chamomile (Blumenthal et al., 2000; Brinker, 1998). In these individuals, yarrow may cause contact dermatitis (Leung & Foster, 1996). There are no known drug/herb interactions pertaining to yarrow (Blumenthal et al., 2000).

NURSING EVIDENCE:

Historical Nursing Use

Yarrow was used in colonial America by midwives for stopping bleeding and healing wounds (Ulrich, 1990).

Potential Nursing Applications

Nurses might want to use yarrow because it has been used historically as a hemostatic given preoperatively to prevent excessive bleeding during and after surgery. There are a number of ways nurses might want to consider using yarrow clinically in skin care. The two examples described here have to do with bleeding skin and promoting skin perspiration. First, yarrow can be considered for stopping bleeding by using compresses with patients who have bleeding hemorrhoids or using tea for women with excessive menstrual bleeding.

Yarrow also makes an excellent sitz bath for the discomfort women have with fibroids and pelvic pain.

Secondly, it can be used to help increase perspiration in people who have viral illness such as cold or flu. Nurses know that there is no cure for the common cold. Practitioners often wonder why people continue to see their physicians when they are coming down with a cold. Scientists may have identified that the common cold is caused by a virus, but there still is no cure. In the past, how quickly a person moved through an illness such as a head cold was important. There are remedies involving the use of yarrow that exemplify the value in supporting the body by helping it move through the illness quickly.

Yarrow opens the pores and encourages sweating. In many traditions, the concept of sweating an illness out of the body is well known. In TCM, the herbs that have this action are said to "release the exterior" of the body. Native Americans use the sweat lodge. A classic sweating tea recommended by herbalists includes yarrow, peppermint, and elder flower. This release, or sweat, enables the body to shed the virus much as it does when the nose drips, shedding the virus through excess secretions. An old remedy for the common cold (and many chronic discomforts) in herbalism was to "take a pint of yarrow tea made strong, on going to bed, and put a hot brick to thy feet wrapped in a cloth wet with vinegar" (Coffin, 1849, p. 158). Today, people coming down with a cold can still benefit from a hot water bottle at their feet and a cup of yarrow tea before going to bed with lots of warm blankets. In the morning, they should bathe, dress warmly, and change the bed linen.

Nurses help patients learn home remedies and self-care practices, especially for illnesses like the common cold for which there is no cure. Nurses may want to explore the use of herbal teas such as yarrow in the self-care practices they teach and perhaps study the effects on groups of patients. For example, occupational health nurses may want to teach the use of yarrow as part of a "sweat out the common cold" technique to employees and record any changes in absenteeism.

Integrative Insight

Although there is little biomedical support of the traditional uses of yarrow, the potential is great. Yarrow has been used extensively not only in wound care and stopping bleeding but also in care of people with viral illness and cancer. In a sense, the modern Achilles heel of health care has been the inability to find the cure for viral illness such as the common cold. Some scientists and healers believe, as did Hildegard of Bingen, that cancer is also a microbial (viral) illness. The extensive traditional evidence surrounding the use of yarrow may provide nurses information and perhaps a new perspective on providing care that can support the body in healing during viral illness and maybe even how to prevent viral illness from finding the weakness or Achilles heel in a person in the first place.

Oral

Infusion. Use up to ½ teaspoon (1 to 2 g) in 5 ounces (150 ml) of freshly boiled water. Steep for ten to fifteen minutes. Drink three times daily between meals (Blumenthal et al., 2000).

Fluid Extract. 1:1 (g/ml): Take up to ½ teaspoon (1 to 2 ml) three times daily between meals (Blumenthal et al., 2000).

Tincture. 1:5 (g/ml): Take 1 teaspoon (5 ml) three times daily between meals (Blumenthal et al., 2000).

Topical

Massage. Add 2 drops of yarrow essential oil to 1 tablespoon (15 ml) of a carrier oil for massage (Lawless, 1998).

Environmental

Sitz Bath. Use 4 ounces (100 g) of yarrow in 5 gallons (20 L) of warm to hot water, or just enough to cover the hips with the knees bent up. Wrap the upper body in towels and soak for ten to twenty minutes. Rinse (Blumenthal et al., 2000).

Full Bath. Add 5 drops of yarrow essential oil or a bath infusion to the bath for symptoms of premenstrual tension, insomnia, nervousness, and other stress-related conditions.

The flowers can be burned to release smoke that, in the tradition of Native Americans, assists in breaking a fever, warding off evil spirits, and reviving those who are comatose (Vogel, 1970).

Herbal Caveat—Therapeutic Applications

In traditional and conventional herbal medicine, amounts of herbs given to patients are based on individual needs. The amounts or "doses" recorded here are provided so that the health practitioner has a general idea of the amounts recommended for an adult patient. Dosing in herbalism not only refers to amount of plant used but also includes when, where, and how to take a plant medicine. These dosages should not be used as guidelines for indiscriminate intervention without proper assessment, critical thinking, and patient education on the part of the practitioner.

Note: Please see chapter 5 for detailed descriptions of how to prepare various applications.

● PATIENT INTERACTION:

Yarrow has been used for centuries in wound healing, stopping bleeding (not replacing the first-aid technique of direct pressure), women's discomforts, and gastrointestinal problems. It is taken internally as tea and used externally in baths, sitz baths, oils, and tinctures. Yarrow may cause an allergic reaction in those who are allergic to plants in the daisy family. It is helpful during the early stage of the common cold and is taken as a tea before bed to help the body sweat, thereby facilitating the virus's exit from the body. Do not to use yarrow internally if your fever is greater than 102°F unless you are under the care of a knowledgeable herb practitioner because it may temporarily increase the fever.

Herbal Caveat—Patient Interaction
Patients considering the use of an herb or formula of herbs in self-care benefit from education about the plant itself and the use of the plant in healing. This education can come through many sources, including local herbalists; plant specialists such as botanists; health practitioners such as nurses, nutritionists, naturopaths, and other physicians; and various written references including the scientific literature. Patients need to remember that their unique health care needs are not necessarily represented in any literature they may encounter. Therefore, it is recommended that a knowledgeable mentor be consulted before initiating self-care with any herb being used for the first time.

NURTURING THE NURSE-PLANT RELATIONSHIP:

Note: You may want to keep a journal of your experiences with the herb.

Sweating It Out With Yarrow. Herbalists find that when someone is coming down with a cold, their pores often close and they do not perspire, which traps the illness (virus and/or bacteria) inside. Next time you feel like you are coming down with a cold, and you have no fever, try a "sweat" with yarrow. First fill your hot water bottle, burp it, and place it under the covers at the foot of your bed. If your feet are cold to the touch, soak them in a warm footbath (adding rosemary bath oil is very warming and the essential oil is antimicrobial too). After the footbath, put on some warm cotton, silk or wool socks. Do not wear socks or clothes that are made from unnatural fibers because your skin and clothes need to breathe during the sweat. Make a cup of yarrow tea, either plain or add equal parts peppermint and elder flowers. Get into bed and sip it while you relax your body. Ask your heart the question, "Do I want to or need to be ill right now and if so why? What do I need to learn from this illness?" Wait and listen closely for the answer. Going through a sweat experience is not only a physiologic process, it is a mental, emotional, and spiritual process and a time for reflection. Yarrow is a time-honored assistant to this important healing process.

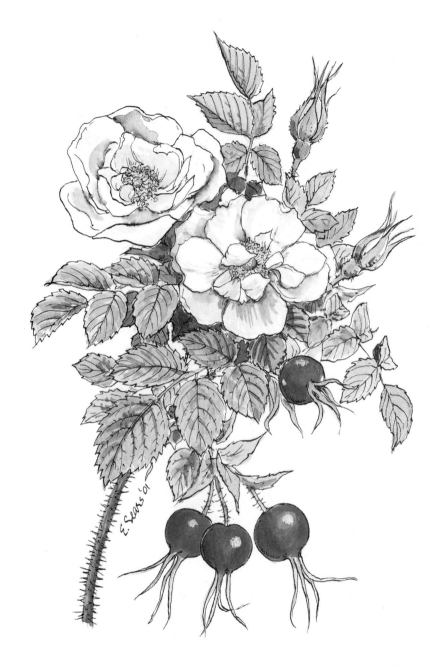

Rosa gallica

Rose

🍃 **LATIN NAME:** *Rosa damascena, Rosa centifolia, Rosa gallica*

🍃 **FAMILY:** Rosaceae

🍃 **COMMON NAMES:** Rose, damask rose *(R. damascena),* cabbage rose *(R. centifolia),* French rose *(R. gallica)*

🍃 **HEALTH PATTERN:** Skin care

🍃 **PLANT DESCRIPTION:**

The rose is cultivated throughout the world as a garden ornamental for its rare beauty. It is an erect shrub 3 to 6 feet (1 to 2 meters) in height. Its branches have numerous sharp prickles. The shiny green leaves are oblong or oval. The blossoms are large, showy, colorful, and usually fragrant with many overlapping petals. Wild roses have only five petals that are usually pale red or pink (Felter & Lloyd, 1983). If the rose blossoms are to be used for medicinal purposes, they should be harvested before they are fully open and air-dried (Felter & Lloyd, 1983). In the autumn, the seed-pod called the rose-hip ripens, turns red, and can be harvested. Roses today are highly cultivated for their visual beauty and not necessarily for their scent. "The 'true old rose scent' is the property of that famous trinity that once constituted the chief Rose wealth of the western gardening world—*Rosa centifolia*, the cabbage rose; *Rosa damascena*, the damask rose; *Rosa gallica*, the French rose. . . . The true old rose scent, the scent that has charmed humanity from time immemorial, is assuredly the most exquisite and refreshing of all floral odours— pure, transparent, incomparable—an odour into which we may burrow deeply without finding anything coarse or bitter" (Wilder, 1974, pp. 74-75).

🍃 **PLANT PARTS USED:** Flower and rosehip

🍃 **TRADITIONAL EVIDENCE:**

Cultural Use

Asian. The blossom or hip of the Chinese rose, *R. chinensis,* called "yue ji hua," is used to invigorate blood, especially of the liver. It is used for irregular menstruation, premenstrual breast tenderness, menstrual pain related to blood stagnation, and to reduce swelling, especially of the neck. *R. rugosa,* "mei gui hua," invigorates "qi" and blood and is used for liver-stomach disharmony (Bensky & Gamble, 1993). Rose hips are used in TCM for conditions relating to urinary incontinence, involuntary loss of semen, and vaginal discharge. It is used as an astringent for prolapsed rectum and uterus and excessive uterine bleeding. Rose is often used as medicinal wine and externally as a paste (Bensky & Gamble, 1993).

Rose hips are a traditional Japanese remedy for memory loss associated with aging. Other traditional Japanese uses of rose hips include treatment of irregular menses, abdominal or chest pain and swelling, swollen lymph glands, abdominal pain, emotional stress, and constipation (Rister, 1999).

North American Indian. The Paipai use roses to treat fever, menstrual problems, eye infections, and stomachache. Rose is used as a laxative and as a birth aid (Kay, 1996). North American Indian tribes use a decoction of the roots of the rose plant as a cough remedy and to treat eye problems. An infusion of the bark and leaves is used as eyedrops for blindness. An infusion of the twig bark is taken in cases of difficult birth and women in labor chew the rose hips to hasten the delivery. A poultice of the chewed leaves is applied to bee stings. The rose leaves are placed into moccasins for athlete's foot. Tribes in Alaska cook the rose hips to extract the juice as a source of vitamin C and then use the juice to make jellies, jam, and marmalades. Sometimes the hips are strung together to make a necklace (Moerman, 1998).

Hispanic. Mexican Americans recommended the application of rose oil to mothers whose breasts are inflamed. A tea made of rose petals is given to infants for fever. Rose also is used as a gentle laxative and to ease children's coughs. Dry rose petals are powdered and applied to diaper rash, and rose petal tea is given to the infant orally also to help cure diaper rash. In addition, it is given for infant colic (Kay, 1996).

In the 1700s, Hispanics used roses for numerous complaints, including hemorrhage, depression, paralysis, scurvy, fainting, loose teeth, vomiting, worms, and heat in the stomach (Kay, 1996). In the southwestern United States, a wild rose called "rosa de Castilla" is used to ease the discomfort related to kidney stones and sore throat and as an eyewash. Dry rose petals, ground and mixed with lard, are applied to cold sores.

East Indian. Rose water from the blossoms of *R. centifolia* is listed in the *Pharmacopoeia* of India as an official medicine. The rose is used as a mild laxative and carminative. *R. damascena* also is used for the distillation of rose water and rose oil. The petals are used to make a syrup that is used as a laxative and for sore throat and enlarged tonsils, uterine hemorrhage, and cold sores. It is given to those who need to gain weight (Nadkarni, 1976).

European. *R. gallica* flowers are officially allowed in Germany for the treatment of symptoms of mild inflammation of the oropharyngeal mucosa (Leung & Foster, 1996). Rose has been used traditionally for women's discomforts and to strengthen the heart and beautify the skin. Anthroposophical practitioners apply rose oil to the skin of newborn babies to help them adjust to extrauterine life.

Culinary Use

Roses are edible and a traditional ingredient in the foods in the Middle East, especially in desserts. In addition to sprinkling rose water on desserts, it is sprinkled on guests as a sign of welcome before the meal. Rose water is a popular flavoring for drinks, rice pudding, and yogurt desserts. Rose petal jam and cordial are still popular in Europe. One drop of rose oil is wonderful in chocolate milk, ice cream, pudding, and whipped cream. Rose petals can be added to salads, but be sure they are pesticide free (Green, 1999). Rose blossoms and petals are a popular strewing flower (as at weddings) and ingredient in fragrant potpourris. The petals can be crystallized and eaten as a candy.

The petals are used in the making of rose butter. Fragrant petals are placed into the bottom of a covered dish. Butter that was wrapped in wax paper is placed on top of the petals. More petals are then added to completely cover the butter. The lid is put on the dish, and then the butter is allowed to sit overnight. The next day, the butter should have absorbed the fragrance of the roses. It can be spread on bread with a few rose petals (Grieve, 1971). Rose hips are a rich source of vitamin C (Brinker, 1998) and can be made into a conserve or jam (Culpeper, 1990).

Use in Herbalism

The use of rose in healing has such a long and beautiful history that entire books have been written on the flower.

> "The Rose distills a healing balm,
> The beating pulse of pain to calm."
>   (Wilder, 1974, p. 80)

It is believed that the origin of the cultivated rose was Northern Persia. From there it spread across Mesopotamia to Palestine, Asia Minor, and Greece and then on to southern Italy. The Romans and Greeks cultivated the red rose. Their legend says that the flower sprang from the red blood of Adonis. The Romans used the rose quite lavishly at their banquets. They used them for decoration and to strew upon the floors. Rose petals were floated in their wine during the winter! Brides and grooms were crowned with roses. The blossoms were scattered in the paths of victors and adorned the prows of their war vessels. Sappho, the Greek poetess, declared about 600 B.C. that the rose was the "queen of flowers" (Grieve, 1971). History records that in 220 A.D. rose petals were strewn 8 inches deep upon the ground when Cleopatra first met Mark Antony. Nero was supposed to have used vast quantities of rose petals in his chambers. Christian mystics have associated the rose with the Virgin Mary and divine love. Rose is still associated with love today. The Rosicrucian Order adopted the rose as their symbol. The Islamic Sufis adopted the rose as a symbol of mysticism.

Avicenna is said to have been the first to produce rose water. In Persia between 1582 and 1612, oil of rose was discovered. At the wedding feast of a princess and emperor, a canal that circled the whole gardens was filled with rose water for the couple to row their boat upon. As the sun heated the water, the bridal pair noticed that an oil was forming on the top. It was skimmed off and discovered to be an exquisite perfume. The manufacture of Otto (or Attar) of roses was begun. The process was introduced into Europe by way of Asia Minor. Otto of roses began to be produced in France, the French roses having the reputation of being superior to any grown in England. Bulgaria also began distilling the oil and became a major world supplier. Even today, Bulgarian rose oil (often from *R. damascena auct. non-Mill.* and harvested from May to July) is considered the finest in the world.

Many traditions are associated with the rose. It was once a British custom to suspend a rose over the dinner table as a sign that all confidences were to be held sacred. In later years, the plaster ornament in the center of a ceiling was known as "the rose." Early English physicians used rose petals for their medicinal qualities. The blossoms were thought to have different actions according to their color, with the white and red roses being the ones that were mainly used. Rose is considered tonic, slightly laxative, and astringent (Wood & Bache, 1839). Rose decoction continues to be used today to relieve headache and pain in the eyes, ears, throat, and gums. A poultice is made of the blossoms and applied to the area of the heart to soothe inflammation in the chest. Rose petals are used in various conditions to cool the heat of inflammation, both internally and externally (Grieve, 1971). Roses are used for excess menstrual bleeding, digestive problems, gonorrhea, and for liver symptoms. Delicious medicinal preparations can be made from rose petals, including syrup of roses, honey of roses, sugar of roses, and vinegar of roses. These are used for fevers, headache, jaundice, joint pain, fainting, weakness, "trembling of the heart," poor digestion, and infection (Culpeper, 1990). Roses are tonic and astringent. They stop bleeding and excessive mucous discharge and ease the discomfort related to bowel disorders and eye complaints (Felter & Lloyd, 1983).

The fruit of the wild rose, called the "rosehip," can be picked when ripe and then dried and powdered. It has been used for leukorrhea, to increase urinary output, and ease diarrhea. Rose hips are used in treating symptoms related to stress, diarrhea, thirst, infection, and gastritis. Rose hips are used commercially as a source of vitamin C and bioflavonoids. Vitamin C and bioflavonoids have the ability to strengthen capillaries and connective tissue (Pedersen, 1998). They are very nourishing to the skin when taken internally. Rose essential oil is reported to have analgesic and relaxing effects when applied topically. Rose oil is not red, but an orange-green color. It takes about 700 kg of roses to produce 1 kg of rose absolute, a compound that is extracted through the use of petrochemicals. Absolutes are not the same as essential oils. Essential oils can be water or steam-distilled. Seven hundred kilograms of roses also produces a quantity of essential oil that is about one-sixth the amount of absolute that can be produced (Green, 1999). Much of the rose absolute on the market is produced in Morocco, may have some benzene residues because of the extraction process, and is best used for perfuming rather than for medicinal use.

Some women dilute rose essential oil in a spray that can be applied to the face during menopausal hot flushes. The essential oil also has been used to relieve nausea, premenstrual depression, and as a sedative for insomnia (Buckle, 1997). In aromatherapy, rose essential oil is used as a general tonic, especially for the heart. It is used to soothe the nerves and as an aphrodisiac. It is thought to be especially useful for women who lack confidence in their own sexuality. The scent of roses can increase concentration and act as a sedative and antidepressant. It is used for emotional shock, bereavement, and grief. Some use it to treat depression, to regulate the appetite, and for obesity (Lawless, 1998).

Rose oil can reduce high blood pressure and decrease cholesterol and help in the treatment of heart arrhythmia. It also has been used in the treatment of gallstones. Rose has been discovered to have antispasmodic properties and can protect against gastrointestinal ulcers (Green, 1999).

Some experts think rose water's medicinal value is almost equal to rose oil's. It can be used in the bath to soothe the skin. It contains acids that restore proper pH and are beneficial when applied to the skin. It is believed that these acids are responsible for its ability to soften, hydrate, and act as an anti-inflammatory on the skin. Rose water is especially good for soothing dry, delicate, and mature complexions. It is also a remedy for headaches and for hangover (Green, 1999).

Cosmetic Use. Rose oil is used as a fragrance component of perfumes, creams, lotions, soaps, and detergents (Leung & Foster, 1996).

BIOMEDICAL EVIDENCE:

Although the use of rose for skin care is well established based on centuries of traditional use, and it is well known for its soothing action to the skin and mucosa, there have been few studies of the effects of rose.

Studies Related to Skin Care

Rose ointment is reported in one study to have been helpful in the relief of symptoms in cancer patients with radiation burns and radiodermatitis and was effective in 154 cases for which antibiotics were ineffective in treating skin ulcers (Christov, 1969 as reported in Green, 1999).

In an animal study in which rats were starved and subjected to chemical irritation and stress, the treatment group got rose oil,

250 mg/kg in water, and the control group got plain water, 25% of the animals in the rose oil group died and 60% of the animals in the control group died. Seventy percent of the treatment group that died had gastric mucosa that demonstrated a significant protective reaction to ulceration. Even if diluted up to 1 μkg/ml, the rose solution demonstrates an extremely high spasmolytic reaction compared with the other drugs in the study, atropine and papaverine (Maleev, Neshev, Stoianov, & Sheikov, 1972).

Studies Related to Other Health Patterns

Immune Response. A methanol extract of dried rose petals demonstrated moderate anti-HIV activity in vitro (Mahmood et al., 1996).

Mechanism of Action

Rose has been found to act on the central nervous system, including the brain. In 1941, scientist P. Nikolov found that rose oil has hypnotic effects. Many people have used rose water traditionally because rose oil is overpowering. Science confirms that rose inhibits the reactivity of the hypothalamus and pituitary systems in rats and can suppress the reactivity of the central nervous system if used to a point of overstimulation. The mechanism of action in the hypothalamus and pituitary is not clear. Treatment for a long time with high doses of rose oil up to 50 mg/kg body weight can lead to stress readjustment and the ability of the brain to compensate by going into a steady state of exhaustion. In too high a dose or exposure, rose oil can cause the body to reject signals from the environment much like a psychoactive drug. In this study, the rats not only experienced a pathologic increase in reactivity but also were affected emotionally. The geraniol content of the rose is thought to be responsible for the change in bioelectric activity, especially in the limbic structures (Maleev, Atsev, Neshtev, Stoianov, & Avramova, 1971, p. 152).

Acid constituents in rose water, such as carboxylic acid, produce softening, hydrating, and anti-inflammatory effects on the skin (Portarska et al. 1989 as reported in Green, 1999). Rose essential oil applied topically is reported to have an analgesic effect thought to be due to the terpene constituent, myrcene (Buckle, 1997). The spasmolytic activity of rose, found to prevent damage to the stomach mucosa of rats, is thought to be due to its ability to block M-cholinoreactive biochemical systems in the smooth muscle and a direct myotropic action (Maleev et al., 1972).

Rosehips contain vitamin C, necessary to increase capillary circulation within the brain. Increased circulation can lead to more oxygen and glucose being taken into brain tissue. Rose hips contain four times as much vitamin C as oranges. However, it is best to use rose hips that are either very fresh or whole because powdered rose hip loses its vitamin C content within six months (Rister, 1999).

USE IN PREGNANCY OR LACTATION:

Rose petals and leaves can be used as an astringent tea for toning the uterus and healing the perineum after the birth. Essential oils, including rose oil, are, in general, contraindicated during the first twenty-four weeks of pregnancy (Buckle, 1997).

Herbal Caveat—Pregnancy or Lactation

Some herbs are contraindicated in pregnancy because of a risk of the herb or one of its constituents stimulating the uterus and therefore possibly promoting fetal loss. Many herbal practitioners do not recommend herbal remedies, in particular oral doses of herbs, during the first trimester of pregnancy and seek an alternative. However, herbs are successfully used during pregnancy, especially to prepare the body for the birth. Herbs are relatively unstudied in pregnancy and lactation, so patients need to be made aware through education of the potential benefits and risks of using herbs for health conditions that arise during pregnancy or lactation. The use of herbal remedies during pregnancy often warrants a referral to a knowledgeable herbal practitioner.

USE FOR CHILDREN:

Be sure to use pure rose or rose essential oil products with children. Some cultures, such as in Germany, anoint a newborn baby's skin with rose oil for the first week after it is born to help it adjust to the extrauterine environment. A decoction of rose can be given to children with diarrhea.

Herbal Caveat—Children

Children have special needs in regard to herbal therapies. They require lesser amounts of herbs and often respond well to mild teas and topical applications such as compresses and baths. The lowest dose of oral preparations should be tried first before increasing the amount given children. Caregivers should observe children closely for responses to herbal remedies. Younger children, particularly infants, have traditionally been given herbs either through their mother's breast milk or in the form of a homeopathic remedy because of their sensitivity to medicines and treatments and the immaturity of their liver. It is recommended that a person knowledgeable in the herbal treatment of children be consulted before the offering of any herb to a child for the first time.

CAUTIONS:

Roses can be safely consumed when used appropriately (McGuffin et al., 1997). Rose water that is old or unrefrigerated can have high bacteria counts and should not be used (Green, 1999). Some people have allergic reactions to the scent of rose. Often the reaction is not felt when live roses or true essential oil of rose are encountered. When people report being sensitive to rose products, they also may be reacting to another chemical interacting with the rose such as can be found in absolutes.

Because rose is so common and is such a strong fragrance, most people have an opinion as to whether or not they like it. Sometimes people react negatively to rose for reasons other than allergic symptoms. If a person has an unhappy memory associated with roses, they may avoid rose and its fragrance. The smell of rose, like any fragrance, is perceived in the olfactory bulb and then proceeds to the olfactory center in the brain where it is linked to the limbic system, the part of the brain involved in memory. Nurse must be aware that although many people love roses, some do not because they do not have pleasant memories associated with the flower.

NURSING EVIDENCE:

Historical Nursing Use

Anthroposophical nurses use a prepared rose oil cream or pure essential oil diluted to 1% on the skin of newborns to protect them as they adjust to extrauterine life.

Potential Nursing Applications

There are numerous ways in which nurses might consider using rose petals, oil, water, or essential oil in the care of patients. First of all, the rose product used for therapeutic purposes must be pure and unadulterated. Nurses may wish to use rose for the protection of the sensitive skin of elderly and infant patients. The rose has been associated with the heart. Nurses might consider using rose essential oil to massage patients with hypertension and arrhythmias. Aromatherapists recommend the use of rose essential oil during the postoperative period following open heart surgery. It may reduce symptoms of postpump depression. It has been used topically to reduce erythema and tenderness after radiation therapy and as an inhalation to reduce the negative emotional impact of hospitalization (Buckle, 1997). Nurses also may try suggesting rose to women who are transitioning through menopause. Rose oil baths and face sprays may help with discomfort related to menopause. Labor and delivery nurses may want to explore having women chew rose hips when labor becomes difficult.

Integrative Insight

Rose is a very common traditional remedy for nourishing the skin and relieving discomfort related to menopause, menstruation, headache, and heart conditions. Although there is little biomedical evidence, there is extensive traditional data on the use of rose as a healing agent for all age groups. Rose is a good representative of the *art* of herbalism and how many remedies can be created from a single plant.

Rose water and oil are excellent for hydrating and massaging into the skin. The fragrance has a hypnotic effect on the central nervous system and can be sedating if perceived as pleasant. The hips can be eaten or decocted and are rich in vitamin C. Because the rose is a visual symbol of beauty and love, its very presence can stimulate warm feelings in people. The world can always use more love and perhaps more healing roses.

THERAPEUTIC APPLICATIONS:

Oral

Infusion. Add two pinches of petals to a pint (470 ml) of boiled water and steep three to five minutes (Beach, 1843).

Fresh Rose Hips. ¼ to ½ cup (2 to 4 oz) daily

Dried Rose Hips. 1 to 2½ teaspoons (1 to 12 g) daily

Extract of Rose Hips. 1½ teaspoons (9 g) of dried fruit in a cup of boiled water daily (Pedersen, 1998)

Topical

Massage. Add 1 drop of rose essential oil to 1 tsp (5 ml) almond oil for general body massage or 10 drops rose essential oil to 1 ounce (30 ml) carrier oil.

Ointment of Rose Water. Add 7 ounces (210 ml) of rose water and 8 minims of essential oil to 9 ounces (270 ml) almond oil and 1½ ounces spermaceti and white wax (Grieve, 1971).

Rose water spritzed on the face or applied to the temples is good for the complexion, stimulating to the spirits, and good for headaches, dizziness, and faintness.

Environmental

Bath. Add a few drops of rose essential oil to the evening bath to soothe and relax. Add it to the morning bath to ease hangovers.

As the following quote describes, roses can be very healing just by their presence. "A bowl of roses in the living room on a distressingly hot day does far more than please the eye and regale the nose; it distinctly enlivens the atmosphere and revives the occupants of the room. Even one fragrant rose in a slender glass vase will make a whole room sweet and fresh" (Wilder, 1974, p. 80).

Diffuser. Rose essential oil allowed to diffuse into the air of the home creates a romantic atmosphere or aids relaxation after a stressful day. Rose essential oil also is used as an antiseptic agent (Lawless, 1998). Rose petals also are used in potpourris to lightly scent the home, sheets, and clothing (Lawless, 1998).

Herbal Caveat—Therapeutic Applications

In traditional and conventional herbal medicine, amounts of herbs given to patients are based on individual needs. The amounts or "doses" recorded here are provided so that the health practitioner has a general idea of the amounts recommended for an adult patient. Dosing in herbalism not only refers to amount of plant used but also includes when, where, and how to take a plant medicine. These dosages should not be used as guidelines for indiscriminate intervention without proper assessment, critical thinking, and patient education on the part of the practitioner.

Note: Please see chapter 5 for detailed descriptions of how to prepare various applications.

PATIENT INTERACTION:

Rose petals and rose water are edible in moderate amounts. Be sure the roses or rose water taken internally are fresh and from a pure source. Rose water, compresses, ointment, and oil have been used extensively throughout history in the care of the skin. Rose is an astringent and is antimicrobial and anti-inflammatory. Pure rose essential oil can be used for therapeutic purposes. It can be analgesic and relaxing when applied to the skin.

Herbal Caveat—Patient Interaction

Patients considering the use of an herb or formula of herbs in self-care benefit from education about the plant itself and the use of the plant in healing. This education can come through many sources, including local herbalists; plant specialists such as botanists; health practitioners such as nurses, nutritionists, naturopaths, and other physicians; and various written references including the scientific literature. Patients need to remember that their unique health care needs are not necessarily represented in any literature they may encounter. Therefore, it is recommended that a knowledgeable mentor be consulted before initiating self-care with any herb being used for the first time.

NURTURING THE NURSE-PLANT RELATIONSHIP:

Note: You may want to keep a journal of your experiences with the herb.

Each week for one month, bring a single rose in a small vase to work for YOU! Pick roses of different colors, smell the differences between them, and see how they change your stress levels and your work environment. To encourage the rose to open fully after cutting, immediately place the stem of the cut flower in warm water. If possible, with the stem under water, cut off the bottom inch or so of the stem at an angle. This keeps air from getting into the stem. Remove all foliage that remains under water or it will decay. Recut the stem underwater every day if possible. Some people add a small amount of bleach to the water to keep down fungus and bacteria. Sugar, soda, or a commercial floral preservative can be used for food. Use this historic symbol of beauty and love as a reminder throughout the day that to heal there must be a connection with the love of the heart.

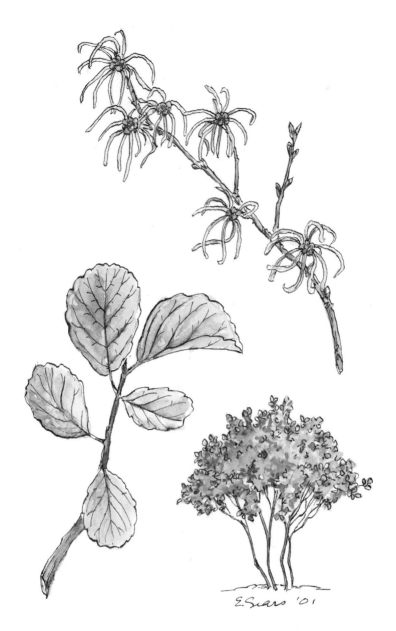

Hamamelis virginiana

Witch Hazel

🌿 **LATIN NAME:** *Hamamelis virginiana*

🌿 **FAMILY:** Hamamelidaceae

🌿 **COMMON NAMES:** Witch hazel, hamamelis, winterbloom, snapping hazel, spotted alder

🌿 **HEALTH PATTERN:** Skin care

🌿 **PLANT DESCRIPTION:**

Witch hazel is a shrub that grows in the southeastern United States, especially in areas of damp woods. It flowers from September to November when the leaves are falling. The seeds mature the following summer. "Witch," also spelt "Wych," is an Old English word for a tree with pliant branches. Witch hazel has several crooked branching trunks arising from the same root that are from 4 to 6 inches (10 to 15 cm) in diameter. They reach 10 to 12 feet (3 to 4 meters) in height and are covered with a smooth gray bark. The leaves are oval with toothed margins. The flowers are yellow with four $\frac{3}{4}$-inch-long (2 cm) linear, curled, or twisted petals. The seed is nutlike.

🌿 **PLANT PARTS USED:** Leaf, twig, and bark

🌿 **TRADITIONAL EVIDENCE:**

Cultural Use

North American Indian. Witch hazel has been highly valued and used by several North American Indian tribes. The Cherokee used an infusion of the twig for pain, fevers, sore throat, tuberculosis, and colds. The infusion also was used as a wash for sores and abrasions. The Chippewa use an infusion of the inner bark as a wash for skin problems and sore eyes. Witch hazel twig bark has been made into an infusion by the Iroquois and taken for bloody dysentery. They apply a poultice of the branches to body parts affected by cold. The plant was used internally as a blood purifier; for rheumatism, colds, coughs, and cholera; and to stimulate appetite and prevent hemorrhage after childbirth (Moerman, 1998). The Potawatomis use witch hazel twigs in their sweat lodges to create steam for the relief of sore muscles (Vogel, 1970).

European. The German Commission E approves the use of witch hazel preparations for the treatment of minor skin injuries, hemorrhoids, varicose veins, and local inflammation of skin and mucous membranes. Germany has licensed the use of witch hazel leaf and/or bark infusion for internal use in treating diarrhea and as a mouthwash for inflammation of the gums and mucous membranes of the mouth. In France, witch hazel extracts and tinctures are approved for use in oral and topical applications in treating symptoms related to venous insufficiency and hemorrhoids. Local applications are allowed for the relief of eye irritation and for oral hygiene (Blumenthal et al., 2000).

Culinary Use

The leaves of witch hazel are sometimes used as an ingredient in tea (Leung & Foster, 1996).

Use in Herbalism

Witch hazel water is obtained commercially by soaking (macerating) the twigs in twice their weight of water for twenty-four hours. The water is then distilled and alcohol (16% to 20%) is added, making it different than floral hydrosols. This is the bottled "witch hazel" found in most medicine cabinets (Leung & Foster, 1996). Witch hazel has been historically used as a tonic and astringent. Some also regard it as sedative. A decoction of the bark has been used for expectoration of blood, vomiting of blood, other hemorrhages, diarrhea, dysentery, and excessive mucus discharge. A poultice of witch hazel has been used for swellings; tumors; skin ulcers, including bed sores; and external inflammation, especially of the eyes. The decoction may be used as a wash for mouth sores, as an enema for bowel complaints, prolapsed anus, as a douche for prolapsed uterus, leukorrhea, and as an eyewash for ophthalmic problems.

Witch hazel has been used extensively in treating varicosities, hemorrhoids, hemorrhages, and other conditions due to relaxation of venous structures. Witch hazel is a popular remedy for sprains, bruises, wounds, sore muscles, and swellings. It also is used to make a topical treatment for burns, scalds, cuts, abrasions, and crushed fingers. It is used as a gargle for sore throat and tonsillitis. It is often used as a facial wash for dilated capillaries and freckles. Witch hazel is used in the treatment of inflamed breasts and has been applied hot to the abdomen and pelvis following childbirth (Felter & Lloyd, 1983). A strong decoction also has been injected into the vagina for prolapsed uterus (Beach, 1843). Witch hazel extract can be applied to insect and mosquito bites to relieve pain and swelling (Grieve, 1971).

🌿 BIOMEDICAL EVIDENCE:

Few clinical studies have been conducted on the use of witch hazel. Some studies explore the use of topical agents that may include witch hazel as one of their ingredients. Although this herb is highly regarded in many cultures, some biomedical investigators do not believe that it has medicinal value.

Studies Related to Skin Care

One study of 30 volunteer subjects demonstrated that a pH 5 Eucerin after-sun lotion with 10% witch hazel distillate exhibited an anti-inflammatory action of 20% at seven hours and 27% at forty-eight hours on erythema, whereas other control lotions had an effect of 11% to 15% (Hughes-Formella et al., 1998).

A study of witch hazel–phosphatidylcholine cream was found to exhibit a mild anti-inflammatory effect on the skin of healthy volunteers, almost as strong as 1% hydrocortisone (Korting, Schafer-Korting, Hart, Laux, & Schmid, 1993). However, a subsequent study, comparing the effect of witch hazel distillate cream (5.35 g distillate with 0.64 mg ketone per 100 g) to 0.5% hydrocortisone cream and a drug-free cream in 72 patients with atopic eczema, found that witch hazel was no more effective than the drug-free cream and significantly less effective in reducing discomfort than the hydrocortisone cream (Korting et al., 1995).

Studies Related to Other Health Patterns
No data are available at this time.

Mechanism of Action
Witch hazel leaf and bark have been reported to have astringent and hemostatic properties that have been attributed to the tannins present in the shrub. The leaves contain 8% and the bark from 1% to 3% tannins (Foster & Tyler, 1999). Astringent tannins coagulate surface proteins of cells, forming a protective layer of skin and reducing secretions and permeability (Brown & Dattner, 1998). Tannins have strong astringent properties. When applied topically, they cause proteins to precipitate out of cells, causing the superficial cell layers to tighten and shrink. This produces local capillary vasoconstriction or hemostyptic action. This decrease in vascular permeability results in an anti-inflammatory effect. The tightening, or astringent, action on the tissues deprives bacteria of a growth medium and is helpful for people with hemorrhoids, for example. This produces an indirect antibacterial action. Tannins also have a mild topical anesthetic action that soothes pain and itching (Schulz et al., 1998). Witch hazel *water*, which is usually the product sold over the counter, does not contain tannins so it is not known what is responsible for its actions (Leung & Foster, 1996).

USE IN PREGNANCY OR LACTATION:
Some midwives recommend 10 to 20 drops of witch hazel tincture (not the drugstore water) under the tongue to control uterine bleeding until the placenta is delivered. Witch hazel does not constrict the os and does not help expel the afterbirth (Weed, 1986).

Witch hazel water may be applied to varicose veins of the legs during pregnancy by spraying it on with a spray bottle or a saturated cloth. It helps tighten the skin and reduce pain and swelling. It can be applied to hemorrhoids during pregnancy also. Witch hazel water can be used in sitz baths after birth to soothe perineal tears, aid healing, and prevent infection (Weed, 1986).

USE FOR CHILDREN:

In Germany, witch hazel baths are recommended for children and infants who are immobilized, confined to bed, or have fecal or urinary incontinence. It is believed that the astringent action forms a protective layer on the sensitive skin (Schilcher, 1992). Some midwives recommend rubbing witch hazel onto the heads of infants with cradle cap, a condition caused by overactive sweat or oil glands that produces a crust on the scalp. It is believed that the tannins in witch hazel slow down the production of oil (Weed, 1986). Witch hazel water can be used topically for care of the umbilical stump of the newborn. Applied with a cloth, it will help the stump heal and dry quickly (Weed, 1986).

CAUTIONS:

There are no known contraindications to the use of witch hazel. There are no known herb-drug interactions with the use of witch hazel (Blumenthal et al., 2000), although the type of use (internal or external) was not specified.

Certain individuals may experience stomach irritation and, rarely, liver damage (McGuffin et al., 1997). Some people may experience allergic reactions such as contact dermatitis with the use of cosmetics or other topical agents that include witch hazel. One 31-year-old woman reacted to an eye gel she was using, but on patch test, she was reactive to the eye gel itself, the cucumber in the gel, and the witch hazel (Granlund, 1994).

NURSING EVIDENCE:

Historical Nursing Use

Nurses continue to use witch hazel in the care of postpartum women. Witch hazel compresses are applied to the perineum for the healing of hemorrhoids and soothing the tissues injured during the birth. One study of fifty maternity units in Britain found that although ice and oral analgesics were the first choice treatments for perineal pain management and although no controlled studies of its use for perineal pain have been conducted, witch hazel was still popular for use, particularly in general practitioner units (Sleep & Grant, 1988). The study was focused on perineal pain and not healing of perineal tissues.

Potential Nursing Applications

Nurses may want to consider researching the clinical application of witch hazel as a topical astringent in the care of wounds, hemorrhoids and other skin disorders, and irritation of the eyes. Nurse also might consider gently patting witch hazel onto the legs of people who are bedridden or must wear supportive stockings.

Integrative Insight

Witch hazel was dropped from the National Formulary in the United States in 1955 because it was believed to be without any medicinal virtues (Osol & Farrar, 1947). The Formulary states that Witch Hazel water is an "embrocation which appeals to the psychic influence of faith" (Osol & Farrar, 1947, p. 529). Foster and Tyler (1999) write that because red wine contains some tannins, it might have more therapeutic value than witch hazel. This is one perspective that focuses on the constituents of witch hazel.

Traditional evidence must not be overlooked, however. Witch hazel has a history in North American Indian medicine as a valuable healing herb. In the United States in 1744, many people doubted the use of witch hazel among other native medicines used by Indians of North America. But then they saw the Native Americans prepare and apply the plant. They saw a "cataplasm of the inner rind of the bark remove painful inflammation of the eyes" and blindness was averted (Vogel, 1970, p. 395). Witch hazel leaf and bark were eventually added to the National Formulary only to be removed later.

Nurses must decide whether witch hazel has healing value in their caregiving practices. It is possible that as technology develops, biomedical scientists may be able to identify and describe the mechanism of action of witch hazel. Witch hazel challenges us to find out how it works. Often herbs "work" because of the synergy of constituents rather than because of one particular substance. Perhaps in continuing to work with witch hazel, nurses will discover the secret of its healing action.

THERAPEUTIC APPLICATIONS:

Oral

Infusion. Steep 2 to 3 g leaf or bark in 5 ounces (150 ml) boiled water for ten to fifteen minutes. Strain and drink two to three times daily between meals (Blumenthal et al., 2000).

Fluid Extract. 1:1 (g/ml), 15% ethanol: Take ½ to about 1 teaspoon (2 to 4 ml) three times daily (Blumenthal et al., 2000).

Tincture. 1:5 (g/ml), 25% ethanol: Take ½ to about 1 teaspoon (2 to 4 ml) three times daily (Blumenthal et al., 2000).

Topical

Decoction of Bark for Topical Use. Boil about ¼ to ½ oz (5 to 10 g) of the bark in 1 cup (250 ml) water for ten to fifteen minutes. Strain and use.

Local Application. Use witch hazel water without a preservative, either undiluted or diluted 1:3 with water. Apply several times daily.

Compress. Semisolid or fluid preparations that contain 5% to 10% decoction or distillate are applied to linen, folded, and placed on the affected area. Hemorrhoid pads with witch hazel are commercially available. When applying witch hazel to the eyes to relieve irritation and swelling, apply the compress to the exterior lid of the eye.

Gargle. Use the strained decoction several times daily.

Ointment, Gel, or Salve. These semisolid preparations containing 10% decoction in a base of lanolin and yellow soft paraffin are applied locally.

Poultice. A semisolid paste containing 20% to 30% decoction is applied locally.

Tincture. 1:5 (g/ml): Tincture of witch hazel is available for use as an ingredient in an ointment, gel, or salve (Blumenthal et al., 2000).

Environmental

Full Bath. Make a decoction by simmering approximately ½ oz (10 g) of witch hazel leaves or bark in 1 cup (250 ml) of water for ten minutes. Strain and add the liquid to the bath water.

Sitz Bath. Add 3 tablespoons (45 ml) of commercial witch hazel water to the sitz bath (Schilcher, 1992), or you can make own witch hazel decoction and add it to the bath.

PATIENT INTERACTION:

Witch hazel has been used for centuries as a tonic and astringent to relieve the discomfort associated with such conditions as varicose veins, wounds, hemorrhoids and other skin disorders and irritation of the eyes. It is easy to make your own witch hazel decoction for topical use and you may want to consider this as opposed to buying the over-the-counter product, which has alcohol in it. The alcohol can sting and dry the skin. There are no known contraindications to using witch hazel, but some scientists have concluded from their research that the traditional use of witch hazel is unsupported, and they therefore believe that there is no real medicinal value in using it. One study did find that a lotion with 10% witch hazel had an anti-inflammatory action on the skin.

NURTURING THE NURSE-PLANT RELATIONSHIP:

Note: You may want to keep a journal of your experiences with the herb.

Set aside thirty minutes for this witch hazel immersion treat after a long day at work when your legs and eyes are very tired.

Purchase 2 oz (50 g) of witch hazel leaf, steep it for ten minutes in approximately 5 cups (1200 ml) of boiled water, and strain. Set aside 1 cup (240 ml) of the decoction and add ice cubes to it until it is cool to the touch. Take the remaining 4 cups (960 ml) of decoction and put it in a warm bath. Take four oval cotton pads and put them beside the tub next to the cup of cool witch hazel water. After getting in the bath, rinse and pat your face dry and then dip the cotton pads in the cool decoction. Wring them out gently and apply them to both closed eyes. Lie back and relax in the comforting presence of witch hazel.

CHAPTER 11
Sleep and Rest

INTRODUCTION

RESTLESSNESS AT BEDTIME AND SLEEP DISORDERS are on the rise. In the United States, a Gallup Organization survey found that 49% of American adults have difficulty sleeping five nights per month on average. Difficulty sleeping is even more prevalent in the elderly, affecting more than half of those over the age of 65 (Wagner, Wagner, & Hening, 1998). Some people believe that the only way to get a good night's sleep when they have insomnia is to take a sleeping pill. The public, as well as nurses, is very aware of the potential for addiction to sleeping pills. Pharmaceutical sleep aides actually suppress needed rapid eye movement (REM) sleep (Wagner et al., 1998), without which a person awakens in the morning feeling tired as if having not slept. Those who don't want to take sleeping pills often just suffer in silence. Many patients may never be informed that there are alternatives.

This chapter is about plant therapies that assist the body not only to sleep but also to have more restful sleep and even to be able to experience brief periods of rest throughout the day. Rest is different from sleep in that the person retains awareness of their surroundings. Rest is important for good health. Some herbal remedies help the body and mind retain a more restful state, and some remedies actually allow certain internal organs to rest. Rest is not necessarily a complete cessation of activity; nor is sleep, although it can be. Rest is defined in relation to a person's other activities. Periods of rest are pauses during the day. Periods of rest for the internal organs are times when the organ does not have to work as hard as it might normally. For example, *resting* the digestive tract can occur during fasting. *Resting* the kidneys can occur during a sauna when the skin takes over as a primary excretory organ.

Many people do not know how to calm or soothe themselves. They do not know how to rest. The nervous systems of people who do not have periods of rest can become overstimulated, especially in a high tech, industrial society. When people do not rest, their respirations become shallow and their heart rate and/or blood pressure accelerates. When moments of rest are used to deep breathe and relax muscles, people become rested *and* energized. Think of a cat on a sunny windowsill. The cat is resting, purring, and its eyes are closed. Yet at any moment the cat can spring up from its resting position to escape the grasp of a playful child. The cat is reserving energy for when it is needed. This is constructive rest.

Some herbs can help the body, mind, and internal organs rest. Some of the herbs discussed in this chapter not only help calm the nerves and allow more satisfying rest periods but also have qualities such as being antispasmodic to the colon, allowing the colon to rest. In addition, the very process of preparing herbal remedies allows a person a period of calmness and rest, if they choose to take it. Nurses are in a good position to remind people of the benefits to taking time for self-care. Preparing the remedies as discussed in this chapter can be restful. Taking a sleeping pill may address an underlying chemical imbalance in a person that causes them to sleep poorly, but how did the pattern of discomfort begin in the first place? How does a person restore the health pattern of sleep and rest? Lifestyle changes, not just biochemical changes, are usually in order.

Sleep patterns are part of one's overall lifestyle. How much and how well a person sleeps is critical to life and health. Hormone balance and neurotransmitters in the brain are affected by poor or nonexistent sleep. In *Lights Out,* by Wiley and Formby (2000), short nights and long work hours are shown to be major causes of heart disease, diabetes, and cancer. "The biggest problem with short nights year round, beyond appetite derangement, is that insulin will stay higher during the dark, when it should be flat, and cortisol falls so late it won't come up normally in the morning. This is a reversal of the normal hormonal rhythms" (p. 91). Wiley and Formby (2000) show that not sleeping well, especially since the invention of artificial light, is a major health crisis in the United States.

The herbs profiled in this chapter—valerian, chamomile, hops, lemon balm, and oat—have the potential to gently promote sleep; however, the herbs do not work on their own. The patient must establish a nighttime ritual of preparing to hibernate. The person must be committed to sleep and must change a lifestyle that emphasizes the wake state and the need for five to six hours of sleep per night. The patient must first be able to rest long enough to stop and tune into when they are sleepy. For numerous reasons, many people override the natural urge or need for sleep and just keep going until they get very sick. Expecting an herb to work when the person will not change sleep and rest habits is a setup for failure.

In any brilliant score of music, there are periods of rest and repose. Sleep and rest are part of the rhythm of all life forms. Flower petals close at night and animals go to their dens for the night or for an entire winter. Humans need to harmonize with the rhythms in nature associated with light and dark cycles. Rest and sleep are important parts of the pattern of health. The herbs discussed in this chapter provide an opportunity to help reestablish the rhythms of sleep and rest necessary for a happier, healthier existence.

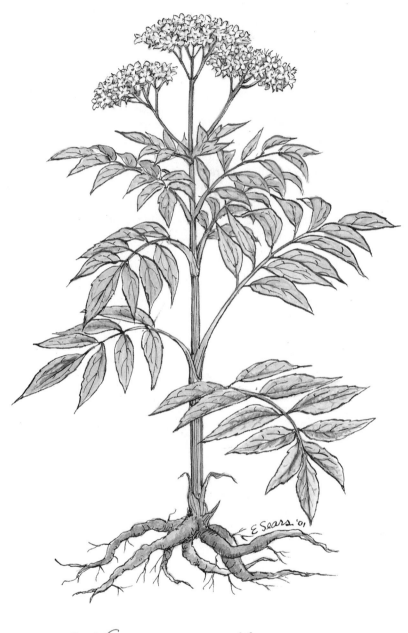

Valeriana officinalis

Valerian

🍃 **LATIN NAME:** *Valeriana officinalis*

🍃 **FAMILY:** Valerianaceae

🍃 **COMMON NAMES:** Valerian, common valerian *(V. officinalis),* Mexican valerian *(V. edulis),* garden heliotrope *(V. officinalis),* Pacific valerian *(V. sitchensis),* Indian valerian *(V. wallichi),* great wild valerian, amantilla, setwell, capon's tail

🍃 **HEALTH PATTERN:** Sleep and rest

🍃 **PLANT DESCRIPTION:**

The name "valerian" is derived from the Latin *valere,* meaning "to be well." Valerian is a perennial and likes to grow in moist environments and is often found along streams, in damp meadows, and woodlands. Valerian can grow to a height of 2 to 5 feet (0.6 to 1.5 meters). Its leaves are opposite each other on the channeled, hollow stem. Each leaf is deeply grooved with seven to ten pairs of lance-shaped leaflets. Valerian has flat clusters of tiny white-to-pink flowers that bloom from June through September. They have a sweet and somewhat peculiar smell. The roots are well known for their powerful odor, which some describe as a "dirty sock" fragrance. This smell develops naturally as the root dries and is not present in the fresh root. I once harvested a large row of Valerian in one day. At first, as I separated and washed the fragrant rhizomes I became very relaxed and sedate just from the smell of the roots. However, after a few hours I began to be forgetful and nauseated!

🍃 **PLANT PARTS USED:** Rhizomes and roots

🍃 **TRADITIONAL EVIDENCE:**

Cultural Use

Asian. Spikenard, a precious, aromatic oil used in Egyptian and Eastern civilizations in spiritual practices such as anointing, comes from a plant *(Nardostachys jatamansi)* that is a close relative of valerian.

North American Indian. Numerous North American Indian tribes have used various species of valerian. The root of *V. edulis* has been used as a poultice for wounds and lacerations. *V. sitchensis* root has been decocted and drunk by those with pain, colds, and diarrhea (Moerman, 1998). North American Indians have been said to believe that if a person with epilepsy does not respond to valerian, that patient cannot be cured (Lawless, 1998).

Hispanic. In Guatemala, valerian is used with other herbs to lower blood pressure. In Argentina, a tea made from valerian root is given to unruly children (Pedersen, 1998). Valerian is recommended for calming the nerves, for stomachache and times of extreme stress, and occasionally for pain. The Aztecs used mashed valerian root to promote urination and for kidney disease (Kay, 1996). The Incas used valerian leaves combined with sea algae in an ointment used in massage (Vogel, 1970).

East Indian. *V. wallichii,* known as *tagar* in Hindi, is used as a calmative and sedative. The valerianic oil is thought to decrease irritability in the brain and spine. Indian researchers have found that the sedative effect of valerian depends on the activity of many constituents found in the root (Nadkarni, 1976).

Russian/Baltic. According to legend, valerian was discovered by St. Panteleimon and has been well known in Russia for its calming properties for two thousand years (Zevin, 1997). It is also used for headache, hysteria, epilepsy, diarrhea, tapeworm, and fever. Valerian is used in vapor baths with children who have trouble sleeping (Hutchens, 1992).

European. Valerian has been a popular medicinal herb in Great Britain and much of Europe from the Middle Ages to the present day. Valerian preparations are a widely used nonprescription hypnotic and daytime sedative. The root was highly regarded for its healing properties by ancient Greeks and Romans, who considered it a powerful sedative. The Greeks hung bunches of valerian leaves on doors and in windows as protection from wicked spirits. It was thought to have magical properties and the ability to protect a person from thunder and lightning. Valerian was often used in love charms and was considered sacred to the Virgin Mary (Lawless, 1998).

One of valerian's many uses in European folklore has been as a homemade cough syrup in which the root is boiled with licorice, raisins, and aniseed. This expectorant is for those who are short winded and have a cough. It helps to open the passages and to expectorate phlegm easily (Culpeper, 1990). Valerian also has been used as a sedative for nervous unrest, neuralgic pains, and to promote sleep (Grieve, 1971). In addition to being used to relieve flatulence, village wise women recommended crushing the fresh green plant and applying it to the head to ease the "pains and prickings there" (Culpeper, 1990, p.187). It is not known if they were using valerian for common headaches or to ease other types of pains occurring in the head, such as toothache or neuralgia.

Culinary Use

In the Middle Ages, valerian root was used not only as a medicine but also as a spice and a perfume. Valerian extract and essential oil are used to flavor many food products, including but not limited to liquor, beer, root beer, baked goods, candy, and meat products (Leung & Foster, 1996).

Use in Herbalism

In the early 1600s, the British brought European valerian to the American colonies where it was easily cultivated. By 1820, *V. officinalis* was listed as an official therapeutic herb in *The United States Pharmacopoeia* and was later listed in *The National Formulary.* Valerian was well known and often used during this time by the Eclectics, a group of physicians who treated their patients primarily with herbal preparations. They used valerian to ease symptoms of nervousness, anxiety, difficulty sleeping, and digestive complaints (McCaleb, Leigh, & Morien, 2000). Valerian also was used to relax patients who were showing signs of the agitation that precedes seizures and to relieve symptoms of epilepsy (Felter & Lloyd, 1983).

Currently, because people are finding the fast pace of modern life stressful at times, valerian is gaining popularity as a relaxing nervine, an agent that relieves nervousness and anxiety. In addition to being taken as a single herb, valerian works synergistically with chamomile *(Matricaria recutita),* hops *(Humulus lupulus),* and lemon balm *(Melissa officinalis)* to produce a calming effect.

In addition to being a sleep aid, valerian also is used as an antispasmodic, carminative, stomach tonic, and sedative. It is regarded as a central nervous system (CNS) depressant and tranquilizer. It lowers blood pressure and has mild pain-relieving qualities. Conditions for which it is used include migraine, insomnia, fatigue, stomach cramps that cause vomiting, nervous tension, stress, restlessness, and anxiety (Leung & Foster, 1996; Felter & Lloyd, 1983). It does not promote addiction and can be used during withdrawal from benzodiazepines with the guidance of health practitioners.

Cosmetic Use. Valerian roots were laid among clothes as a perfume and insect repellent. Himalayan and Asian valerians were used for this purpose because of their pleasant and aromatic fragrance (Grieve, 1971).

BIOMEDICAL EVIDENCE:

Studies Related to Sleep and Rest

Valerian was shown to have a mild sedative effect and significantly improve sleep quality and sleep latency without hangover symptoms in a study of 128 subjects, in which participants received either 400 mg of valerian aqueous extract (coarsely ground *V. officinalis* root in capsule), a commercial Swiss preparation (60 mg valerian extract and 30 mg hops flower in a capsule), or placebo one hour before going to sleep (Leathwood, Chauffard, Heck, & Munoz-Box, 1982).

No significant effects with valerian were noted in another study by the same investigators, in which a very small sample of 10 patients was used and in which an objective measure, electroencephalographic (EEG) changes, was used to measure the effectiveness of valerian upon sleep (Leathwood et al., 1982). Leathwood et al. suggest that although no actual comparative studies have been conducted, the subjective results from individual studies of the effects of valerian 400 mg, benzodiazepines, or barbiturates on sleep latency seem to suggest that valerian may be at least as effective as small doses of the pharmaceutical sleep aides.

A significant improvement, or decrease in sleep latency compared with placebo was demonstrated in a double-blind, placebo-controlled trial in which 8 patients with mild insomnia received 450 mg of *V. officinalis* ground root in capsules. The subjects also were tested with 900 mg, and the higher dose did not improve results (Leathwood & Chauffard, 1985).

In addition to studies performed on valerian alone, several studies that examine a combination of valerian with hops, another herbal sleep aide, have been conducted. In one double-blind study, 150 mg each of valerian and hops were given to a group of 20 healthy subjects. Flunitrazepam was given to another group of 20 healthy people. The test substances were taken as a single morning dose and, that afternoon, a series of vigilance and reaction tests were administered. No impairments were established in the group that had taken the valerian/hops combination. Many significant impairments, based on a decline in vigilance, were found in the group that had taken the flunitrazepam (Gerhard et al., 1996 as reported in Schultz et al., 1998).

Twenty-four of twenty-seven patients participating in a double-blind, crossover study comparing the effect of a standardized tablet preparation containing *V. officinalis* 400 mg, hops flower extract 375 mg, and lemon balm extract 160 mg with another standardized product containing valerian 4 mg and "full" doses of hops and lemon balm reported improved sleep from the herbal sleep aide. Forty-four percent of these subjects reported "perfect sleep" without side effects the following day; no nightmares, which occurred when the subjects took conventional medications, were reported (Lindahl & Lindwall, 1989).

Studies Related to Other Health Patterns

No data are available at this time.

Mechanism of Action

From the 1960s to the 1980s, comprehensive research was conducted on the nature of the active constituents in valerian. In general, authorities agree that the herb's sedative effects are due to a combination of elements contained in the roots and rhizomes known as valepotriates and volatile oils (Foster & Tyler, 1999). Substantial data oppose this conclusion. Valepotriates are highly unstable compounds that deteriorate rapidly when in solution or exposed to oxygen. They are not well absorbed by the gastrointestinal tract after ingestion; are water insoluble; and according to some researchers, "are not present in aqueous or alcohol extracts of valerian root" (Leathwood et al., 1982, p. 65). Researchers have been puzzled about why the water extracts that contained no valepotriates and little volatile oils have proved to be effective in promoting sleep. Currently, the identity of the responsible constituents remains a mystery. Their effectiveness may be due to a combination of volatile oils and their derivatives and some as yet unidentified water-soluble constituents. Duke (1997) writes, "Valerian presents another opportunity for me to reiterate my belief that the whole herbal extracts used in natural medicines often make more sense than the 'magic bullet' herbal derivatives that the drug industry favors" (p. 295). Valepotriate-containing valerian products may be helpful in withdrawal from benzodiazepine drugs (Brinker, 1998).

Although the exact mechanism through which valerian exerts its sedative actions has not yet been established, it is suggested that it causes CNS depression and muscle relaxation. Research suggests that the hypnotic effects may be due to an interaction of the unknown constituents with central gamma-aminobutyric acid (GABA) receptors (Wagner et al., 1998). The monoterpene bornyl acetate, the sesquiterpene valerenic acid, as well as other sesquiterpene acids have a direct action on the amygdaloid body of the brain and "valerenic acid inhibits enzyme-induced breakdown of GABA in the brain resulting in sedation" (Houghton, 1999, p. 505). Valerian does not adversely affect REM sleep (WHO, 1999). In appropriate doses, it acts to gently relax and does not produce overly strong sedative or hypnotic actions. In one small pilot study of 14 elderly subjects with poor sleep, polysomnography seems to indicate that valerian has a mild tranquilizing effect and induces an increase of slow-wave sleep and reduces stage 1 sleep (Schulz, Stolz, & Muller, 1994). It may be that a combination of constituents is responsible for the sedative action or that the in vivo breakdown by-products could play a role in the effects. It also has been suggested that the relaxing properties could be due to a peripheral effect rather than a central effect (DeSmet, 1997).

USE IN PREGNANCY OR LACTATION:

All valerian species contain volatile oils that can affect smooth muscle in various internal organs, such as the uterus. For this reason, some nurse-midwives I have worked with have successfully used *V. officinalis* (whole herb in capsule) to stop premature contractions and threatened miscarriage. For hypertension during labor, 10 to 20 drops each of valerian and skullcap tinctures in a cup of warm water or herb tea have been effective. The effectiveness of this dose gradually diminishes over several hours. For a sustained effect, the tinctures are placed in hops tea or the dose is repeated periodically (Weed, 1986).

One source says that, "The use of valerian during pregnancy and lactation has not been established and should, therefore, be avoided" (Newall, Anderson, & Phillipson, 1996, p. 261). One species, *V. wallichi*, is reported to be an abortifacient and is said to affect the menstrual cycle (Newall et al., 1996).

USE FOR CHILDREN:

Although some have suggested not giving valerian to children because of its sedative effects, valerian can indeed be used by children for general nervousness, restlessness, anxiety, problems going to sleep, difficulty staying asleep all night, excitation, and stomach pain due to nervousness. If valerian is ever given to a child under 12 years of age, the child should be monitored closely by a health care provider (WHO, 1999). The goal of many practitioners is to avoid the use of pharmaceutical sedatives and tranquilizers in children; however, children often refuse the alternative of valerian tea or tincture because of its strong smell. They may be more likely to accept valerian capsules, tablets (Schilcher, 1992), or footbaths. Other relaxing herbs—catnip *(Nepeta cataria L.)*, chamomile *(Matricaria chamomilla)*, lemon balm *(Melissa officinalis)*, and lavender *(Lavandula angustifolia)*—are often more appropriate for pediatric use. Before using sedative herbs, it is important to extend a warm, caring approach to the child as the first step in addressing the health concern.

CAUTIONS:

There are no known contraindications for the use of valerian (Bradley, 1992). Because of the similarity in spelling, consumers often confuse valerian and Valium. Valium is the synthetic drug diazepam and has no relation to the herb. Valerian is a much milder sedative derived directly from the living green or dried root of the plant. Many herbalists recommend that valerian not be used for longer than three to four weeks at a time. Some recommend limiting use of valerian orally to two months per year (Zevin, 1997). Because valerian affects the CNS, it should not be taken with benzodiazepine derivatives (Ottariano, 1999) because they could potentiate each other. The CNS depressant activity of valerian may potentiate other sedatives. The depressant activity of valerian is not synergistic with oral alcohol intake (Newall et al., 1996); however, caution should be exercised with the administration of any herbal or pharmaceutical sedative in combination with alcohol use.

Using valerian preparations on the same day as pharmaceutical antihistamines may enhance the sedative effects of both. These effects can potentially endanger the user by impairing cognitive, somatic, or sensory function. Reduced alertness and reaction time can be dangerous to the user and to others when operating a motor vehicle or working with machinery (Brinker, 1998; McGuffin, Hobbs, Upton, & Goldberg, 1997).

In many herbalists' experience, including my own, some patients report that valerian causes a paradoxical effect in that it seems to act as a stimulant instead of a relaxant. It usually poses no health threat, just minor discomfort similar to strong coffee. Some traditional texts do identify valerian as a cerebral stimulant even while recognizing its sedative effects (Felter & Lloyd, 1983; Nadkarni, 1976).

Herbal preparations, such as valerian, that contain volatile oils could in theory cause an allergic reaction. Anaphylaxis and allergic reactions have never been reported for *Valeriana* species (DeSmet, 1997). Minor side effects have been reported with chronic, long-term use of valerian root. These include headaches, excitability, sense of uneasiness, and insomnia. Very large doses may result in arrhythmias and bradycardia, headaches, mental excitement, delusions (Lawless, 1998), and decreased intestinal motility. Another report stated that oral amounts up to 20 times the recommended dose caused only mild symptoms that resolved within one day. Four cases of liver damage have been associated with herbal preparations containing valerian root in combination with other herbs. Because research does not show valerian root to be toxic to the liver, it is doubtful that the hepatic damage was due to the valerian but rather to the other herbs, such as skullcap (WHO, 1999; De Smet, 1997).

There has been some concern about the possible carcinogenic properties of chemical compounds called valepotriates found in valerian root. Valepotriates are broken down rapidly in the body and pose very little concern. It also has been found that valerian preparations made by a water extraction contain no valepotriates. Valepotriate-free preparations include valerian tea, and any powders in tablet or capsule form that were made by water extraction. It is important in pediatrics to give only valepotriate-free preparations (Schilcher, 1992).

The U.S. Food and Drug Administration has declared valerian generally recognized as safe (GRAS) and approves its use.

NURSING EVIDENCE:

Historical Nursing Use

No data are available at this time.

Potential Nursing Applications

Valerian is the leading sleep aide in Europe, and many patients use it in their self-care practices. Nurses may want to consider either the oral, topical, or environmental clinical use of valerian with those patients who have health concerns related to sleep and/or rest.

Integrative Insight

Herbal sleep aides such as valerian cannot replace the comfort and rest patients often experience as a result of genuine caring and concern demonstrated through the science and art of nursing. Valerian is an effective sleep aide, yet nurses who suggest valerian for patients must follow the nursing process and critically explore the benefits and risks of the use of valerian for the individual patient as well as all other possibilities for improving sleep. Patients must be encouraged to examine their lifestyle and not simply expect that a dose of valerian is going to fully address their health concern, especially if it is chronic.

Nurses have historically used environmental interventions such as the use of hydrotherapies (i.e., footbaths), music, and relaxation practices to help promote sleep and rest. Nurses may effectively teach patients a relaxation program coupled with the use of valerian as a nonpharmacologic method to enhance rest and sleep. Some suggestions are described below.

I. Sleep and rest instructions
   A. Maintain a regular bedtime each night.
   B. Allow time to unwind each night for a few hours before bed.
   C. Use the bed and bedroom only for sleep, rest and sexual activity. Ideally there should be no TV, phone, or computers.
   D. Avoid stimulants and alcohol before bed.
   E. Create a nice environment in the bedroom that is free of noise and clutter, is a pleasant temperature, and has a comfortable bed.
   F. Refrain from eating heavy meals before bed.
   G. Avoid excessive exercise or stimulating activity in the late evening.
II. Relaxation training
   A. Progressive muscular relaxation teaches muscle groups to release tension by focusing awareness on them one by one.
   B. Focusing one's attention on slow, deep breathing relaxes the body and mind.

III. Use of valerian (choose one)
  A. After the evening meal
  B. One hour before bedtime
  C. At bedtime

These instructions can be taught to anyone who is willing to learn. The patient with chronic insomnia or inability to rest should be assessed fully either by an advanced practice nurse or physician to determine if there are any medical or psychiatric reasons for their insomnia. Referral to a sleep specialist may be indicated, especially for those patients with chronic or long-standing insomnia (Wagner et al., 1998). In any case of sleep difficulty, it is helpful to keep a sleep diary in which the patient records the effect of the therapy on their sleep patterns. The diary will help the patient and the nurse become aware of the effectiveness of the sleep and rest instructions, the relaxation training, and the use of valerian or other herbs or pharmaceuticals.

THERAPEUTIC APPLICATIONS:

Oral

Adults can use valerian as a tea, tincture, capsule, or tablet. When valerian is used to improve sleep, most practitioners recommend taking the herb no more than 30 to 60 minutes before bed. When using valerian during the daytime for restlessness, the dose is often divided in half (McCaleb et al., 2000). In some individuals, it takes 2 to 4 weeks for valerian to improve sleep patterns (Schultz et al., 1998). The following dosages are for adults:

Tea. 1 to 5 cups per day of tea with 2 to 3 g of dried root per cup (WHO, 1999)

Tincture. $\frac{1}{2}$ to 1 teaspoon per day (1 to 3 ml) once to several times daily (WHO, 1999)

Liquid Extract. Amount equivalent to 2 to 3 g taken once to several times daily (Blumenthal, Goldberg, & Brinckman, 2000)

Capsule/Tablet. (Dried ground root) 300 to 500 mg per day (McCaleb et al., 2000)

Standardized Extract. 300 to 500 mg per day. Because plant scientists have not agreed which constituent of valerian is most appropriate for standardization, the product may be standardized to 0.8% to 1% valerenic acid, 1% to 1.5% valtrate, or 0.5% essential oil (McCaleb et al., 2000).

Topical

Although Valerian may not be an herb of first choice in the making of ointments, it has been used topically for calming and anointing the body.

Environmental

A strong infusion—3.3 oz (100 g) of dried root in a tea (infusion)—can be added to a full bath for external use (WHO, 1999).

Valerian flowers can be added to bouquets of wild flowers. They have a subtle sweet fragrance that I have found can be very calming when used in a room of people with excessive stress and anxiety.

Herbal Caveat—Therapeutic Applications

In traditional and conventional herbal medicine, amounts of herbs given to patients are based on individual needs. The amounts or "doses" recorded here are provided so that the health practitioner has a general idea of the amounts recommended for an adult patient. Dosing in herbalism not only refers to amount of plant used but also includes when, where, and how to take a plant medicine. These dosages should not be used as guidelines for indiscriminate intervention without proper assessment, critical thinking, and preparation of patient education on the part of the practitioner.

Note: Please see chapter 5 for detailed descriptions of how to prepare various applications.

PATIENT INTERACTION:

Valerian is the leading sleep aid in Europe. It is not habit forming. You can get to know valerian by purchasing the plant from local greenhouses that carry herbs. Valerian likes to grow in moist, rich soil and is an attractive addition to the flower garden. Clusters of fragrant, small white flowers appear in the summer. In the fall, the roots can be harvested and used to make a relaxing tea. The whole dried roots of valerian can be taken orally as tea, tinctures, or capsule and can be used in the evening when it is time to prepare for sleep. Because of its sedative effects, it is not recommended to use valerian when alertness is required. On occasion, some people have found valerian to be stimulating rather than sedating.

Herbal Caveat—Patient Interaction

Patients considering the use of an herb or formula of herbs in self-care benefit from education about the plant itself and the use of the plant in healing. This education can come through many sources, including local herbalists; plant specialists such as botanists; health practitioners such as nurses; nutritionists, naturopaths, and other physicians; and various written references including the scientific literature. Patients need to remember that their unique health care needs are not necessarily represented in any literature they may encounter. Therefore, it is recommended that a knowledgeable mentor be consulted before initiating self-care with any herb being used for the first time.

NURTURING THE NURSE-PLANT RELATIONSHIP:

Note: You may want to keep a journal of your experiences with the herb.

To become more familiar with valerian's ability to promote sleep and/or rest try a cup of tea combined with conscious relaxation of the body. Set aside a quiet time at home that will be free from distractions. Prepare a cup of tea from the dried roots by using 1 teaspoon (3 to 5 g) of herb per 6 ounces (180 ml) of hot water. Let it steep for

15 minutes, strain, and sweeten if desired. Sit in a comfortable chair that fully supports the body in a relaxed position. While sipping the tea, consciously allow the mind to let go of any busy thoughts and intense feelings associated with the day. Slow, deep breathing facilitates the process of relaxation. Tense, squeeze, or contract your toes and feet and then let the energy go, imagining that your toes and feet are becoming very soft and malleable. Let your toes and feet rest. Gradually progress up your body to your legs, thighs, torso, arms, neck, and head, tensing and then resting each body part. Allow the face and jaw muscles to tense, then rest and let go of the tension. Coupled with the use of valerian tea, this can be a powerful and effective method to experience relief from nervous tension that often leads to inadequate rest and sleep. It is best to practice resting and preparing for sleep a few times each week until it becomes a comfortable and familiar process. Preparing valerian tea and experiencing its unique aroma and taste can become a signal to the body that a shift in lifestyle, a rest period, is about to occur. Proper amounts of sleep and rest can improve the body's ability to handle stress and increase energy throughout the day.

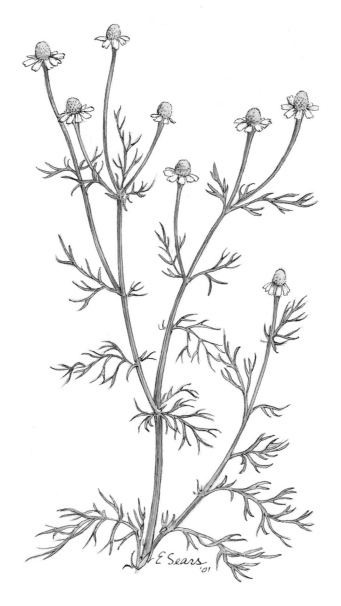

Matricaria recutita

German Chamomile

- **LATIN NAMES:** *Matricaria recutita, Chamomilla recutita,* and *Matricaria chamomilla* all refer to German or Hungarian chamomile.

- **FAMILY:** Asteraceae

  Note: *Anthemis nobilis* or *Chamaemelum nobile* refers to Roman or English chamomile, which are not included in this profile.

- **COMMON NAMES:** German chamomile, chamomile, camomile, Hungarian chamomile, wild chamomile, pinheads

- **HEALTH PATTERN:** Sleep and rest

- **PLANT DESCRIPTION:**

  The botanical name *Matricaria* is derived from the Latin word for womb, *matrix*. German chamomile is a low-growing annual. It is native to Europe, Asia, and India, but it is also found in Australia and is widely cultivated in the United States (Wren, 1988). It likes to grow in sunny areas with sandy, well-drained soil. The plant has delicate leaves and grows to a height of about 2 feet (0.6 meter). The flower heads are daisylike, about ¾ inch (2 cm) across with a hollow, yellow conical center surrounded by about fifteen white petals. The plant has an aromatic, applelike fragrance and a slightly bitter taste. The essential oil of the flowers is blue in color. Currently, chamomile flowers are acquired throughout the world by cultivation of select species. Argentina is the main supplier and produces about 5000 tons every year, with 3000 tons exported to Germany.

  Although German chamomile is profiled here, the following description of Roman chamomile is provided so that the two varieties can be better differentiated. Roman chamomile is also a low-growing plant, but it is a perennial. It has creeping, trailing stalks that are horizontal and lie along the ground. Vertical, erect stems sprout up from the horizontal ones with blooms that are about 1 inch (2.5 cm) across. The flowers have a yellow center and about eighteen white petals. The stems are covered with finely branching, threadlike leaves that give the plant a feathery appearance. The flowers appear from the end of July to September and are on singular drooping, erect stalks (Grieve, 1971). The plant is strongly fragrant with a bitter taste.

- **PLANT PART USED:** Flower head

- **TRADITIONAL EVIDENCE:**

  Cultural Use

  Asian. In China, the whole chamomile plant is taken as a tea for tumors of the digestive tract. The leaf is used for its cleansing properties and the flower is made into a plaster for indurations (Duke, 1985).

Hispanic. Chamomile, known as *manzanilla* in the Hispanic culture, is considered a panacea for many common illnesses, especially women's conditions. Chamomile flowers are taken as a strong tea for improving sleep and rest. The flowers are steeped and strained and the infusion is cooled and then used for an eye or skin wash, hair rinse, scalp conditioner, and as a compress for boils and abscesses. Pregnant women sip chamomile tea as soon as they feel labor pains. It is understood that chamomile tea will help the labor pains stop if the labor is false and continue if it is truly her time to deliver (Kay, 1996). A tea of chamomile, yerba buena (spearmint), and alhucema (lavender) has been used historically by Hispanic women for cleansing after childbirth. Chamomile tea is also taken for bronchitis, stomach problems, and as a blood purifier. Many people in the southwestern part of North America grow chamomile in their gardens.

Australian. Australians of British decent may use chamomile as described under the European section.

African. Chamomile grows well in Northern Africa and the cooler regions of the eastern and southern parts of Africa. Chamomile is used in tea form for its sedative, antiseptic, antispasmodic, and anti-inflammatory actions (Iwu, 1993).

East Indian. In Hindi, *M. chamomilla* is known as *babunphul* or *babuna*. Chamomile is cultivated in the Punjab in India. It is used for gastrointestinal spasms and as a nervine for health concerns such as irritability, colic, rheumatism, toothache, and false labor. Chamomile tea is applied to the genitals for a stimulating effect. Intravenous injections are used to lower blood pressure. Dried powder is used for skin that itches, eczema, impetigo capitis, and other open wounds (Nadkarni, 1976).

Middle Eastern. In Israel, chamomile is used to treat epilepsy and nervous conditions (as reported in Harris & Lewis, 1994). In Saudi Arabia, chamomile *(Matricaria aurea)* is known as *babunag* or *babunaj* (Ghazanfar, 1994). Chamomile grows throughout Saudi Arabia, Turkey, and Iran. Arabians often use chamomile in massage oils.

Russian/Baltic. Chamomile is known as *romashka* in Russia (Hutchens, 1992) and grows widely throughout the country. It is used for its relaxing, anti-inflammatory, and carminative properties. A tea of the flowers is often taken at bedtime to promote sleep. Russian folk dermatologists use chamomile infusions (1 tsp [5 g] of dried flower to 1 cup [250 ml] of water), taken internally to treat eczema, neurodermatitis, hives, and prurigo and externally for treating allergic dermatitis. Russian physicians use chamomile drops to treat ear infection (Zevin, 1997).

European. Europeans use a cool tea of chamomile flowers and ginger for cases of indigestion, intestinal colic and pain, gas, heartburn, diminished appetite, intestinal sluggishness, and as an appetite stimulant for the elderly and debilitated. German-Americans used chamomile as a *Schwitzgegreider,* or sweating herb (Vogel, 1970).

Chamomile is used in Polish children's hospitals as a sedative called Valupol (as reported in Harris & Lewis, 1994). Chamomile is used in Europe as a favorite herb to plant around homes. While strolling around the garden, the herb is purposefully walked on to cause it to release its fragrance. Since the Middle Ages, aromatic herbs used in this way have been called strewing herbs because they are strewn upon the floor to perfume the house.

Culinary Use

Chamomile is used to flavor a variety of foods and beverages, such as desserts, candies, liqueurs, baked goods, gelatins, and puddings (Duke, 1985).

Use in Herbalism

Both German and Roman chamomile, *Matricaria recutita* and *Anthemis nobilis*, are used medicinally. Because they are used for similar actions in the body related to the medicinal constituents they have in common, they have often been used interchangeably throughout history. German chamomile *(M. recutita)* is preferred in Europe and the United States, and Roman chamomile *(A. nobilis)* is used more often in other countries.

Chamomile has been used since antiquated times and was an important remedy in ancient Egypt, Greece, and Rome. Its name originated from the Greek *chamos* (ground) and *melos* (apple), alluding to its growing low on the ground and to the applelike scent of the fresh flowers (Blumenthal et al., 2000). The therapeutic uses of chamomile blossoms are recorded in the works of physicians such as Hippocrates, Dioscorides, Galen, and Asclepius. Wise men of Egypt consecrated chamomile as a sacred herb of the sun and considered it the only remedy for intermittent fevers (Grieve, 1971). Chamomile is used to the present day. Chamomile was so widely revered for its medicinal traits that the old herbalists agreed "it is but lost time and labour to describe it" (Grieve, 1971, p. 185).

Contemporary herbalists dry the flowers and make them into a tea for soothing nervous conditions. It is claimed that chamomile has a harmless, sedative effect for agitated states, even extreme conditions such as delerium tremens, especially if given in the early stages. Chamomile also has a positive effect in cases of intermittent fevers. The flower is used mainly for its anti-inflammatory, antispasmodic, nervine, and carminative actions. Chamomile tea is hypnotic (Duke, 1985). Chamomile essential oil has a calming effect on the emotions and is helpful for those who are hyperactive, who think too much, worry, or work excessively (Lawless, 1998).

Chamomile is one of the most popular ingredients used in medicinal herb teas, either singly or combined with other ingredients. In addition to tea, the flowers are used to make tinctures that are used as sleep aids, antispasmodics, and digestive remedies (Leung & Foster, 1996). Chamomile tea and tinctures are taken internally for restlessness and mild insomnia, gastrointestinal spasms, and inflammatory conditions of the gastrointestinal tract, including dyspepsia, epigastric bloating, poor digestion, and intestinal gas (WHO, 1999). Chamomile is used as a mouthwash for the treatment of canker sores (Ottariano, 1999). Chamomile has been used for premenstrual nervous irritability (Felter & Lloyd, 1983).

External preparations of chamomile such as salves are used for inflammation and bacterial diseases of the skin and mucous membranes (Schulz, Hansel, & Tyler, 1998), for inflammation of the genitals and perineal region, and as an inhalation for respiratory system inflammation (Leung & Foster, 1996). Other external applications include those for skin bruises, cracks in the skin, frostbite, and insect bites (WHO, 1999).

Cosmetic Use. Chamomile has long been used in cosmetic preparations. It is valued as a rinse to enhance the highlights in blond hair. The oil distilled from the flowers is used in perfumes, lotions, skin salves, hair dye, mouthwashes, soaps, and shampoos.

BIOMEDICAL EVIDENCE:

The following evidence on chamomile describes the effects of the flower related to the health patterns of sleep and rest as well as skin care, digestion, comfort, and pain relief. Although chamomile has been used to increase sleep and rest, few studies have explored this subject. Much of the biomedical literature has been devoted to discussing the mechanism of action of chamomile, but little clinical research has been reported.

Studies Related to Sleep and Rest

Chamomile tea has been shown to have a mild sedative effect in patients undergoing cardiac catheterization. In one study, in which a small sample of 12 adult, hospitalized patients underwent cardiac catheterization to provide constant measurements of cardiac output, oxygen consumption, and arterial pressure, while evaluating if chamomile tea taken orally (two tea bags in 6 oz of hot water) affected cardiac function, no significant cardiac effects were noted, with the exception of a small but significant increase in mean brachial artery pressure ($p < .05$); however, sedative effects of chamomile were demonstrated unexpectedly. Within 10 minutes after drinking the tea, 10 of the patients, although able to be aroused, fell into a deep sleep that lasted until the end of the catheterization procedure, which took about 90 minutes to complete (Gould, Reddy, & Gomprecht, 1973).

Studies Related to Other Health Patterns

Skin Care. In one controlled study, a chamomile ointment (Kamillosan, a German chamomile product on the market since 1921) was tested against a 0.25% hydrocortisone cream in the treatment of eczema in 161 patients, and the chamomile ointment was found to be comparable to hydrocortisone. Over a period of three to four weeks, the two preparations were administered topically to the patients' inflamed skin areas on their hands, forearms, and lower legs. The chamomile ointment proved to be comparable to hydrocortisone in reducing inflammation (Aertgeerts' study as cited in Blumenthal et al., 2000).

In a double-blind, placebo-controlled trial, a chamomile extract standardized to 3 mg chamazulene and 50 mg alpha-bisabolol was shown to significantly reduce the weeping wound area of 14 patients who had undergone dermabrasion of tattoos (Glowania, Raulin, & Swoboda, 1987).

Digestion. In a study in which a group of 165 chemotherapy patients receiving 5-fluorouracil (5-FU) were given either a chamomile mouthwash to treat oral mucositis or placebo, three times daily for fourteen days beginning on the first day of chemotherapy, there was no significant difference in oral ulceration scores between the two groups of patients. Unfortunately, the investigators do not give the specifics regarding the content of the chamomile mouthwash in the report of the study. There was no evidence that chamomile had any adverse affects in the patients who participated in this study (Fidler et al., 1996).

Comfort and Pain Relief. After seven days, in a double-blind study to determine the efficacy of herbal tea preparations on infantile colic, colic improvement scores were significantly better in those infants given an herbal preparation with chamomile than in the placebo group. Chamomile was one of the herbs included in the remedy given to the infants in the study. Criteria for choosing the infants for the study included presence of episodes of unexplained irritability, agitation, fussiness, or crying lasting more than 3 hours a day, for at least 3 days each week, and continuing for at least 3 weeks. Other symptoms of colicky infants included abdominal distention and tenderness, drawing up of the legs toward the abdomen, passage of gas, and explosive stools. During the seven-day study, the herbal preparation was given by the parents with every episode of colic, but not more than three times per day. It was determined that constituents in chamomile had antispasmodic effects on bowel contractility. No adverse effects from the herbal preparation were noted (Weizman, Alkrinawi, Goldfard, & Bitran, 1993).

Mechanism of Action

Current studies have examined many of the traditional uses of chamomile, including its anti-inflammatory, antispasmodic, antibacterial, and sedative actions, as well as antipeptic ulcer activity. Chamazulene, a major constituent in the essential oil of chamomile, acts as a pain reliever, helps with wound healing, has antispasmodic and anti-inflammatory properties, and has demonstrated antimicrobial activity. Data from in vitro studies seem to indicate that matricine, the actual constituent of chamomile blossoms, does not exhibit anti-inflammatory activity until transformed to chamazulene by exposure to heat during a water distillation process (Safayhi, Sabieraj, Sailer, & Ammon, 1994). The polysaccharides in chamomile are immunostimulating; they activate macrophages and B lymphocytes needed for the healing of wounds (Wagner, H. as cited in Wren, 1988).

Another constituent in chamomile oil, alpha-bisabolol, has been determined to be very effective in healing burns and decreasing the temperature of skin exposed to ultraviolet light (Wren, 1988). Alpha-bisobolol has anti-inflammatory, antimicrobial, and antipeptic activities (Leung & Foster, 1996). Another constituent, an ether, en-yn-dicycloether, has antispasmodic, antianaphylactic, antimicrobial, and anti-inflammatory properties (Leung & Foster, 1996).

One study exploring the sedative effects of chamomile determined that apigenin, a water-soluble constituent of the flowers, binds at the benzodiazepine receptor sites. This may provide a molecular reason for the weak CNS depressant effects of chamomile (as reported in Blumenthal et al., 2000).

Biochemical evidence seems to support the folkloric use of chamomile for anxiety, insomnia, nervousness, excessive stress, and for health concerns related to the skin. In vitro studies have confirmed that chamomile flowers have compounds that contribute to antibacterial and antifungal actions on the skin (Aggag & Yousef, 1972). The essential oil from the flowers has been reported to act against gram-positive bacteria such as *Staphylococcus aureus* and also against the fungus *Candida albicans* in concentrations above 0.05%, which may explain why topical applications of chamomile have been effective in wound healing. Chamomile flower liquid extract has been shown to prevent ulcer formation caused by ethyl alcohol, while bisobolol, a constituent of chamomile volatile oil, taken orally, has been shown to inhibit ulcer caused by indomethacin in rats (Brinker, 1998).

USE IN PREGNANCY OR LACTATION:

Chamomile has been used historically in small amounts during pregnancy to relieve nervous twitching and false labor pains that are accompanied by restlessness. The herb is recommended in small doses (Felter & Lloyd, 1983). If the pains go away after drinking chamomile tea, it is believed that the pain is false labor (Kay, 1996). Chamomile regulates uterine contractions. It has been suggested that internal use of excessive amounts should be avoided in early pregnancy because of the emmenagogic properties of the whole plant (not the flower). (Brinker, 1998).

Chamomile is useful during the latter months of pregnancy and during the birth process to decrease anxiety in the mother and family members. Chamomile cream or tea applied topically can be beneficial in decreasing inflammation and enhancing healing in those women who experience skin changes during pregnancy. Chamomile lotion is used topically to alleviate sore nipples in the nursing mother (Wren, 1988).

Herbal Caveat—Pregnancy or Lactation

Some herbs are contraindicated in pregnancy because of a risk of the herb or one of its constituents stimulating the uterus and therefore possibly promoting fetal loss. Many herbal practitioners do not recommend herbal remedies, in particular oral doses of herbs, during the first trimester of pregnancy and seek an alternative. However, herbs are successfully used during pregnancy, especially to prepare the body for the birth. Herbs are relatively unstudied in pregnancy and lactation, so patients need to be made aware through education of the potential benefits and risks of using herbs for health conditions that arise during pregnancy or lactation. The use of herbal remedies during pregnancy often warrants a referral to a knowledgeable herbal practitioner.

USE FOR CHILDREN:

Chamomile flowers have a long history of successful use both orally and topically for children's ailments. Children who benefit from chamomile are those who are restless, discontented, irritable, impatient, and always wanting to be held (Felter & Lloyd, 1983). Chamomile tea is given to children who are experiencing abdominal pain and colic because the flowers are antispasmodic to the intestinal tract (Ottariano, 1999). Historically, chamomile flowers have been used in tincture form for children's diarrhea. Chamomile tea is often given to children in spoonful doses as a sedative, especially during teething, for earache, stomach disorders, and infantile convulsions (Grieve, 1971).

Chamomile is a mild sedative for children that has no depressive effect. It is recommended as a tea for children who have difficulty sleeping or are irritable. Children often like the taste of chamomile tea. Chamomile tea is often given before bedtime to help relax the child who has difficulty sleeping for reasons such as teething pain (Bradley, 1992). Externally, a warm wet compress of chamomile can be used to soothe infant skin irritations such as eczema or diaper rash (Ottariano, 1999). The preparation is given orally as a carminative to dispel gas and relieve intestinal cramping. Chamomile has been tested for use in infant colic without adverse effects (Weizman et al., 1993).

Chamomile is also used to treat the minor eye problems of infants. A tea from the herb, strained carefully, is applied to the baby's eyes as a compress (Weed, 1986). Chamomile also is used for other childhood ailments such as colds, convulsions, earache, and measles (Hutchens, 1992). Caring for children's sensitive skin is very important in infants and children who are immobilized or bedridden, such as those with cerebral palsy and others who are chronically ill with fecal or urinary incontinence. An infusion of chamomile used for a full bath or a sitz bath can be considered in these cases. The use of some commercial bath products that claim to be made from chamomile is not recommended because the concentration of necessary anti-inflammatory constituents is minimal. Chamomile ointments and oils are excellent for use on children's dry or sensitive skin. These preparations are indicated for diaper rash, dermatitis, and seborrhea of the scalp. Inflamed areas with papules or itching and weeping scaling crusts on the cheeks and scalp are treated by applying a dilute tincture of chamomile flowers. Diaper rash is often treated with chamomile sitz or full baths or ointment. Chamomile also can be used for abrasions and other superficial wounds (Schilcher, 1992).

Sinusitis often can be overcome by the inhalation of steam that contains the volatile oils of chamomile. These oils are antibacterial and anti-inflammatory (Schilcher, 1992). Children should always be supervised during this procedure to avoid burns from the hot water or steam.

Herbal Caveat—Children

Children have special needs in regard to herbal therapies. They require lesser amounts of herbs and often respond well to mild teas and topical applications such as compresses and baths. The lowest dose of oral preparations should be tried first before increasing the amount given children. Caregivers should observe children closely for responses to herbal remedies. Younger children, particularly infants, have traditionally been given herbs either through their mother's breast milk or in the form of a homeopathic remedy because of their sensitivity to medicines and treatments and the immaturity of their liver. It is recommended that a person knowledgeable in the herbal treatment of children be consulted before the offering of any herb to a child for the first time.

CAUTIONS:

Chamomile has been reported to cause rare allergic reactions. Some individuals have experienced contact dermatitis from chamomile flowers and a few cases of anaphylactic responses have occurred due to the ingestion of preparations of chamomile (Subiza et al., 1989; WHO, 1999). However, a review of worldwide reports revealed a relatively low number of about fifty allergic responses to chamomile over a 105-year period from 1887 to 1992. Of the fifty, only five were actually traced to the use of *Matricaria recutita*. The rest were thought to have been induced by the *Anthemis* species. It was discovered that two of the individuals had a preexisting sensitivity to ragweed (member of the Asteraceae family, the same botanical family as chamomile) (Newall et al., 1996). Some herbalists suggest that persons with a known allergy to ragweed, asters, chrysanthemums, and other members of the Asteraceae family exercise caution when using chamomile preparations (Foster & Tyler, 1999).

Because instances of contact dermatitis have been reported from the use of topical preparations of chamomile, caution should be taken with any dermatologic condition that appears to worsen with use of the herb (Pereira, Santos, & Pereira, 1997). In these cases, the use of chamomile should be stopped. Chamomile tea used to wash the eye has in rare cases been shown to induce allergic conjunctivitis (Subiza et al., 1990).

Those who are taking CNS depressants or tranquilizers should be aware of the sedative effects of chamomile. The pharmaceutical drug and the herb hypothetically could potentiate each other (Ottariano, 1999). Chamomile oil has an LD50 of approximately 15 ml per kilogram in rats (Iwu, 1993).

NURSING EVIDENCE:

Historical Nursing Use

Nurses have used fomentations or hot stupes steeped in chamomile infusion and applied them to the abdomen to relive spasm in the internal organs (Weeks-Shaw, 1914). Senior nurses often recall putting small amounts of chamomile tea in baby's bottles to calm the symptoms of colic.

Potential Nursing Applications

Chamomile tea may prove beneficial for patients who are experiencing insomnia due to stress, anxiety, or nervousness, especially those who do not wish to use sedative drugs. Nurses may want to consider the clinical use and research of the internal use of chamomile tea and tincture for promoting sleep and rest. Nurses historically have attended the wounds of patients. Information and research on the benefits of topical uses of chamomile may be of benefit to future nursing protocols regarding the protection of skin integrity of patients. These protocols might include recommending the application of chamomile tea to abrasions, for example. Chamomile creams have been considered as effective as hydrocortisone for topical use on inflammation (Aertgeerts' study as cited in Blumenthal et al., 2000). Based on extensive evidence, pediatric and enterostomal nurses may wish to consider using chamomile topically for diaper rash, decubiti, and wounds.

Integrative Insight

Evidence from nursing and traditional sources as well as from the biomedical literature supports the use of chamomile for promoting sleep and rest and for the promotion of healthy skin and relief of pain. In Germany, chamomile is referred to as being *alles zutraut,* "capable of anything" (Berry, 1995). It is easy to grow, beautiful to have in the garden, and a readily available herbal remedy. Several reputable chamomile products already exist on the market that have been used and/or studied for years. Chamomile is one herb that can easily be integrated into nursing practice especially with children for a number of common health concerns. Some children's hospitals have already done so. Based on Israeli studies, nurses may want to consider creating protocols that include the use of chamomile for colic. Chamomile has no known side effects, as opposed to the pharmaceuticals being prescribed, which often have side effects in newborns with delicate digestive systems.

Many facilities now stock herbal teas in the patients' kitchens. Nurses may want to be sure that chamomile is one herb tea that is routinely available to all patients, especially before sleep at night or anxiety-producing procedures such as cardiac catheterization.

THERAPEUTIC APPLICATIONS:

Oral

Tea. ½ or 1 teaspoon of dried flowers in 1 cup (240 ml) of boiling water, taken by mouth three or four times daily. Most herbalists recommend that the flowers be steeped for no more than two minutes. Make sure the tea is prepared with the flowers and not the leaves and stems. For gastrointestinal concerns, use 3 g in 150 ml (5 oz) water three to four times daily (Blumenthal et al., 2000).

Tincture. (1:5 g/ml) 15 ml (1 Tbl) three to four times daily (Blumenthal et al., 2000)

Liquid Extract. (1:1 g/ml) 3 ml (½ tsp) three to four times per day (Blumenthal et al., 2000)

Topical

Poultice. When used as a poultice for swelling, inflammation, nerve pain, or to reduce swellings of the face due to abscesses, the flowers are placed into a cloth bag and then steeped in boiling water. The bag is placed on the skin as a hot application. A chamomile paste or plaster used for a poultice contains 3% to 10% m/m of the flower heads (Blumenthal et al., 2000).

Compress to the Stomach or Back. A small handful of flowers in 1 L (1 qt) of boiling water. The stomach compress can reduce intestinal spasm, and the back compresses (placed on the back of the shoulders and neck) are used for relief of headache.

Essential oil of Roman and German chamomile can be used topically for burns, eczema, and skin irritations (Keville & Green, 1995).

Environmental

Sitz Bath. Use about 4 oz (120 g) of dried flowers steeped in a quart (1 L) of hot water, then strain and use. For a full bath, steep about 4 oz (120 g) of dried flowers per gallon (3.5 to 4 L) of hot water, then strain and add to the rest of the bathwater (McCaleb et al., 2000).

Steam Inhalation for Colds and Sinus Spasm. A handful of flowers can be scattered in a large bowl and covered with 1 L (1 qt) of boiling water after which the patient can breathe the vapors for ten to twenty minutes.

Essential Oil Atomizer. The blue essential oil of German chamomile is an antidepressant and is used for patients experiencing extreme stress, hysteria, anxiety, insomnia, and suppressed anger.

Horticultural Therapy. The pale yellow essential oil of Roman chamomile also is used for depression and was used in medieval time by monks, who had their depressed patients actually lie on the chamomile flower beds in the healing garden (Keville & Green, 1995). Roman chamomile is still used in lawns today so that the fragrance, released when walked on, can be enjoyed.

Herbal Caveat—Therapeutic Applications

In traditional and conventional herbal medicine, amounts of herbs given to patients are based on individual needs. The amounts or "doses" recorded here are provided so that the health practitioner has a general idea of the amounts recommended for an adult patient. Dosing in herbalism not only refers to amount of plant used but also includes when, where, and how to take a plant medicine. These dosages should not be used as guidelines for indiscriminate intervention without proper assessment, critical thinking, and preparation of patient education on the part of the practitioner.

Note: Please see chapter 5 for detailed descriptions of how to prepare various applications.

🌼 PATIENT INTERACTION:

Dried, whole chamomile flowers are easily grown or can be obtained from a natural foods store that sells bulk herbs. Be sure to clearly identify any bulk herb you purchase. Become acquainted with the flowers' scent and taste by preparing a fresh cup of tea. Use 1 teaspoon (5 g) of the blossoms per cup, add hot water, and steep for two to three minutes before straining the tea into your favorite teacup or mug. The tea can be sipped during a time of relaxation, digestive upset, or just for enjoyment. Remember that one of this herb's qualities is that it can aid sleep and rest.

Be sure to test your own body's reaction to chamomile. There is some thought that those with ragweed allergies may experience cross-reactions to chamomile. Allergic reactions are rare, but you may want to consider an alternative herb or not use chamomile without the assistance of an herbal practitioner if you have a known allergy to ragweed.

Herbal Caveat—Patient Interaction

Patients considering the use of an herb or formula of herbs in self-care benefit from education about the plant itself and the use of the plant in healing. This education can come through many sources, including local herbalists; plant specialists such as botanists; health practitioners such as nurses, nutritionists, naturopaths, and other physicians; and various written references including the scientific literature. Patients need to remember that their unique health care needs are not necessarily represented in any literature they may encounter. Therefore, it is recommended that a knowledgeable mentor be consulted before initiating self-care with any herb being used for the first time.

🌼 NURTURING THE NURSE-PLANT RELATIONSHIP:

Note: You may want to keep a journal of your experiences with the herb.

Potted chamomile plants can be purchased from greenhouses in the spring and planted in the flower garden. It is enjoyable to watch them grow and begin to develop their small, daisylike flowers in the summer. The flowers can be picked to make a fresh tea when they are fully open. Chamomile flowers are receptors for sunlight. The petals open wide when the sun is shining and droop downward toward the earth when the sky is cloudy or evening approaches. It can be very satisfying to drink tea from a plant that is homegrown and full of the warmth of the sun.

If you don't want to wait a few months for the flowers to form, try making a tea with the dried blossoms purchased from health-food groceries that sell whole herbs. The delicate aroma and flavor of the tea may remind you of apples. If you find the tea enjoyable, try making a bath infusion and experiencing the relaxing effect of your home made chamomile spa at the end of a busy day.

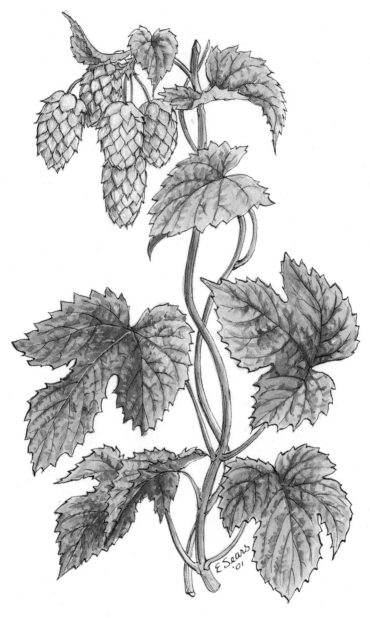

Humulus lupulus

Hops

🍃 **LATIN NAME:** *Humulus lupulus*

🍃 **FAMILY:** Cannabaceae

🍃 **COMMON NAMES:** Hops, European hops, common hops, hop strobile

🍃 **HEALTH PATTERN:** Sleep and rest

🍃 **PLANT DESCRIPTION:**

Hops is a perennial, climbing herb that has male and female flowers growing on separate plants. It is native to Europe, North America, and Asia (Blumenthal et al., 2000). Hops often grow on trees and fences, sometimes reaching a height of 24 feet (8 meters). The major countries that produce hops are the United States, Germany, and the Czech Republic. Most of the hops grown for commercial use are used to produce beer. The dark green leaves have heart-shaped lobes with finely toothed edges. They occur directly opposite each other on the stem. The flowers grow on a short stem that springs from the angle between the branch and the leaf. The male flowers occur in loose bunches, 3 to 5 inches (7.5 to 12.5 cm) long. The oblong female flowers appear June through September as yellow-green, leafy conelike structures with no petals. The flowers are known as *strobiles*. They measure about 1¼ inches (3 cm) long and release a yellow granular powder called lupulin from glands within the conelike structures. It is this golden powder that gives hops its medicinal value (Grieve, 1971). The powder, as well as the whole plant, has a very bitter taste and a characteristic aromatic odor.

🍃 **PLANT PARTS USED:** Female flowers that have the greenish leafy, conelike structures called strobiles

🍃 **TRADITIONAL EVIDENCE:**

Cultural Use

Asian. Hops tea has been used in relieving insomnia, restlessness, nervous diarrhea, intestinal cramps, lack of appetite, and other nervous conditions (Leung & Foster, 1996). Alcohol extracts of hops have been used in China to treat leprosy, tuberculosis, and acute bacterial dysentery, with varying degrees of success (Duke, 1985).

North American Indian. In North America, the Cherokee use hops as a pain reliever, a sedative, and for rheumatism and problems of the breast and uterus. They also use it for urinary stones and to decrease the inflammation in diseased kidneys (Blumenthal et al., 2000). The Delaware and Mohegan use hops in heated pouches and apply them for painful ears and toothache. The Meskwaki use the root for insomnia. The Shinnecock use hops for pneumonia (Moerman, 1998).

East Indian. Hops are used in East Indian cultures for nervous conditions, headache, and indigestion. The plant acts as a sedative and hypnotic (as reported in Blumenthal et al., 2000).

Russian/Baltic. Hops are used either alone or in combination with valerian, chamomile, and/or passion flower to relieve insomnia (Zevin, 1997).

European. Before the ninth century, hops was mainly used for making breads and beers in the Netherlands and England (Blumenthal et al., 2000). One of the favorite liquors of the Saxons and Danes was made from fermented malt and was called ale. After the introduction of hops to the brewing process, the drink was renamed *bier* or beer, but the liquor without hops retained the original name of ale (Grieve, 1971). Hops have been used traditionally in Europe as a tonic, diuretic, bitter, and more recently as a calmative (Schultz et al., 1998).

Culinary Use

Hops are used in the making of beer. The pharmacologic effects of hops may not survive the brewing process (Potters, 1988).

Use in Herbalism

The earliest written recordings of the use of hops are attributed to Pliny, who lived from 23 to 79 C.E. (Blumenthal et al., 2000). He said that the Romans enjoyed the young spring shoots of the plant as a vegetable dish. He documented that the species name, *lupulus,* was derived from the Latin name for wolf, *lupus,* because when the plant grows among certain trees, it chokes them with its embrace, just as the predator wolf chokes sheep with its strong bite. The genus name, *Humulus*, may have been derived from *humus,* the rich moist soil in which it grows, or the name may come from the Anglo-Saxon word *hoppan,* meaning to climb (Grieve, 1971). Hops are in the same botanical family as marijuana, Cannabaceae, and are thought to induce a mild euphoric effect when smoked (Foster & Tyler, 1999); however, hops are not usually smoked.

Hops have been used traditionally in small pillows. Dried hops are placed in a small cloth bag, or pillow. The pillow is gently warmed over heat and then used topically to relieve toothache, earache, and nervous conditions (Grieve, 1971). The therapeutic and sedative effects of hops have been observed over the years to be related to the inhalation of the aroma from the oil in the strobiles (Schulz, 1998). For example, hops pickers, who have prolonged exposure to the strobiles, often become tired easily as a result of the aroma and ingestion due to the transfer of hops resin from their hands to their mouths.

Traditionally, a small glass of hops tea is taken three times a day in the spring to stimulate a sluggish liver. In many forms of traditional herbalism, the health of the liver is considered of primary importance.

Certain plant therapies are often used in the spring to support the liver's natural tendency to become more active after the winter. The very bitter taste of the hops tea is thought to be the healing principle within the plant. A syrup made of the juice of the plant and sugar has been found to cure jaundice, ease headache, and cool sensations of heat in the stomach (Culpeper, 1990). Historically, hops juice has been considered a potent blood cleanser and was used for deposits of mineral salts found in hollow organs or ducts known as calculus trouble, (Grieve, 1971). Hops also have been used as an emmenagogue and a diuretic (Culpeper, 1990).

Hops compresses often are used in combination with chamomile and poppy flowers for swellings, skin inflammation, nerve pain, rheumatism, ringworm, bruises, and boils. Warm poultices of the moist, crushed hops strobiles are spread on a cloth and applied to the body for the same benefit (Grieve, 1971).

The traditional uses of hops include improving the appetite and promoting sleep and rest. Hops are used for the relaxing, diuretic, and pain-relieving properties of the strobiles. It is used in cases of nervousness, hysteria, and to induce sleep in instances of extreme agitation. Hops also are used in heart disease, nervous disorders, and neuralgia. It is used as a digestive tonic in jaundice, indigestion, liver complaints, and bladder irritation. It is also effective for delirium tremens.

In more recent herbal practice, hops strobiles are used in the form of tinctures, capsules, powders, dried extracts, tablets, and teas. Hops are used as a sedative, sleep inducer, antispasmodic, and aromatic bitter (Bradley, 1992). Hops are used topically for bacterial infection, too (Newall et al., 1996).

BIOMEDICAL EVIDENCE:

Hops strobile and hops extract were listed in the *National Formulary* in the United States from 1831 to 1910 (Blumenthal et al., 2000). Germany still allows hops extract to be labeled "for discomfort due to restlessness or anxiety and sleep disturbances" (Foster & Tyler, 1999, p. 216). The wording is based on a reasonable certainty of effectiveness, rather than on current controlled clinical studies. This is because studies cannot yet explain the tranquilizing effects of hops. The sedative effect is undisputed, but the reason for the action is not yet fully understood.

Studies Related to Sleep and Rest

A German randomized, double-blind, placebo-controlled study by Schmitz and Jackel, 1998 (as reported by Blumenthal, et al, 2000), assessing the quality of life of patients (sample size not reported) with exogenous sleep disorders, demonstrated that a hops-valerian preparation was equal to a benzodiazepine drug in terms of sleep quality, fitness, and quality of life.

None of the 15 participants in one study, treated with 250 mg of a lipophilic hops concentrate for five days, experienced any sleep-inducing effects (Stoker as reported in Schultz et al., 1998).

Hops usually are taken as tea or used in baths. Studies have shown that pharmacologically relevant concentrations of a sedative principle of hops, 2-methyl-3-butene-2-ol, can be found in both hops tea and hops bath preparations (Hansel, Wohlfart, & Schmidt, 1982).

Studies Related to Other Health Patterns

Elimination. An herbal extract containing hops and uva-ursi with alpha-tocopherol acetate (vitamin E) improved irritable bladder and urinary incontinence in 772 of 915 patients (Lenau et al., 1984 in German, as quoted in Newall et al., 1996).

Hormone Balance. For many years, hops were thought to have a powerful estrogenic effect on women. This belief occurred because, in earlier times when hops strobiles were picked by hand, the female pickers often developed menstrual irregularities. A study was done in which a carefully prepared hops extract was exposed to human endometrial cells in vitro. Although some studies have found the evidence to be inconclusive, this study confirmed estrogenic activity in the cells. It was determined that the activity was due to a phytoestrogen (plant chemical with estrogen-like effects) called 8-prenylnaringenin. This compound was seen to have greater estrogenic activity than the other well-known isoflavonoid phytoestrogens, genistein and daidzein, that are used to reduce menopausal symptoms. The question is whether 8-prenylnaringenin is of any importance to human health in the reduction of hot flashes and other menopausal indicators. Moderate intakes of isoflavonoid phytoestrogens have been associated with a decreased incidence of prostate and breast cancer, reduced heart disease, and a reduction in menopausal symptoms. The estrogenic activity of beer made with whole hops has been determined to be quite low, equivalent to only a few micrograms of estradiol (an estrogenic hormone). Results determined that drinking beer made from whole hops has minimal, if any, therapeutic or estrogenic value (Milligan et al., 1999).

Mechanism of Action

The sedative effect of hops is undisputed, but the reason for the action is not yet fully understood (Bradley, 1992). The effect may be due to the volatile alcohol, 2-methyl-3-butene-2-ol. The content of the volatile alcohol increases during storage (up to 0.15% in two years), suggesting that two constituents in hops, lupulone and humulone, might break down oxidatively, generating the sedative principle (Foster & Tyler, 1999). Lupulone, an antibiotic principle, is tuberculostatic (Duke, 1985).

The sedative action of hops may be due to 2-methyl-3-butene-2-ol, a chemical found in the plant, or it may be formed within the body as a by-product of the metabolism of alpha-acids after oral consumption (Hansel et al., 1982). Rats given 2-methyl-3-butene-2-ol have demonstrated 50% reduction in motility after being given this chemical found in hops. The onset of the depressant activity began within two minutes and peaked within two hours of being given to the rats (Wohlfart, Hansel, & Schmidt, 1983).

USE IN PREGNANCY OR LACTATION:

Hops are considered by some herbalists to be safe enough to drink nightly *if needed* during the last months of pregnancy. However, because of its phytoestrogenic properties, hops should be used with caution during the first trimester. It is contraindicated for regular use throughout pregnancy (Weed, 1986). Hops have been shown to have antispasmodic action on the uterine muscle (Newall et al., 1996) and to be helpful in relieving uterine afterpains following childbirth (Weed, 1986).

Some women traditionally have used hops tea to increase breast milk production. Some women have experienced that drinking beer has the same effect; however, some beers contain harmful chemical preservatives that pregnant or lactating women should avoid. Alcohol- and chemical-free brews of hops are available.

For hypertension during labor, some herbalists recommend that the midwife steep a handful each of dried hops, skullcap, and valerian in a quart (liter) of hot water for at least two hours and have the mother drink a cup of the tea as often as is necessary to maintain the desired blood pressure. The effect of one cup of the hops tea blend has been known to last about one to two hours. The mother can even sip the tea throughout labor, although the taste is quite bitter (Weed, 1986).

Herbal Caveat—Pregnancy or Lactation

Some herbs are contraindicated in pregnancy because of a risk of the herb or one of its constituents stimulating the uterus and therefore possibly promoting fetal loss. Many herbal practitioners do not recommend herbal remedies, in particular oral doses of herbs, during the first trimester of pregnancy and seek an alternative. However, herbs are successfully used during pregnancy, especially to prepare the body for the birth. Herbs are relatively unstudied in pregnancy and lactation, so patients need to be made aware through education of the potential benefits and risks of using herbs for health conditions that arise during pregnancy or lactation. The use of herbal remedies during pregnancy often warrants a referral to a knowledgeable herbal practitioner.

USE FOR CHILDREN:

Hops tea can be given to children who are experiencing restlessness, anxiety, and sleep disorders. Up to the age of 3, one cup per evening is usually sufficient. However, a tea made entirely of hops strobiles is often not very popular with children because of the bitter taste and the strong, aromatic smell (Schilcher, 1992). Children may be more likely to learn to tolerate the bitter, medicinal taste of hops tea if a small amount of sweet juice is added at first.

Another way to use hops with restless children is to make a hops pillow and give it to them to sleep with. A small decorative cotton or linen bag can be filled with a few ounces of dried hops strobiles. The filling may be used for about seven days before the aromatic principles evaporate.

Herbal Caveat—Children

Children have special needs in regard to herbal therapies. They require lesser amounts of herbs and often respond well to mild teas and topical applications such as compresses and baths. The lowest dose of oral preparations should be tried first before increasing the amount given children. Caregivers should observe children closely for responses to herbal remedies. Younger children, particularly infants, have traditionally been given herbs either through their mother's breast milk or in the form of a homeopathic remedy because of their sensitivity to medicines and treatments and the immaturity of their liver. It is recommended that a person knowledgeable in the herbal treatment of children be consulted before the offering of any herb to a child for the first time.

CAUTIONS:

Individuals with depression should not take hops orally (McGuffin et al., 1997). The sedative effect of the herb may exacerbate symptoms and create deeper depression. Brewery workers have been found to experience depression and nervous symptoms attributed to hops (Salvador, 1994). Contact dermatitis, often accompanied by conjunctivitis, has been observed in people who picked hops strobiles, possibly because of the allergenic properties of the pollen (Duke, 1985). The sedative action of hops may potentiate the effects of any tranquilizing pharmaceutical drugs or alcohol. The sedative activity of hops extract increases the sleeping time induced by pentobarbital in mice (Brinker, 1998). Based on current information, no toxicologic risk is associated with the intake of hops (Schulz, 1998). There are no known interactions with drugs (Blumenthal et al., 2000). Symptoms of overdose include severe diarrhea (Schilcher, 1992). Some recommend that people who are prone to allergic skin eruptions not use hops. In Germany, hops are not allowed in medicinal bath preparations (Leung & Foster, 1996).

Although female hops pickers have been known to experience menstrual changes during the hops harvest season, low levels of up to 300 nM of the phytoestrogen, 8-prenylnaringenin, present in beer made with whole hops, have had no apparent detrimental health effects when taken in moderate amounts. It is possible that the phytoestrogen in hops/beer may actually have health benefits when taken in moderate amounts, similar to the benefits (decreased incidence of cancer and heart disease and decreased discomfort related to menopause) observed with the ingestion of the phytoestrogens in soy (Milligan et al., 1999).

NURSING EVIDENCE:

Historical Nursing Use

Nurses historically have applied hops poultices to the chest and abdomen to relieve congestion during pneumonia and to relieve abdominal distention postoperatively; poultices also have been applied to wounds that are infected, painful, or inflamed (Harmer, 1924, p. 207). Hops also have been used as a compress on the abdomen to relieve spasms of the internal organs (Weeks-Shaw, 1914, p. 160).

Potential Nursing Applications

Hops tea might be considered for adults experiencing excitability, restlessness, sleep disorders, and lack of appetite or for children who are restless and agitated and having difficulty sleeping. A hops pillow can be given to patients to promote sleep. A warm bath with hops bath oil or infusion might be considered to promote the inhalation of hops' aroma, which is known to have sedative effects.

Integrative Insight

Hops are rarely recommended as a single herb to be taken for any medicinal purpose except in a bath or sleeping pillow to promote sleep. Consider combining hops with other relaxing herbs such as chamomile or valerian. Although the mechanism of action related to the sedative effects of hops remains unclear, it has been used for its calming and sedating effects for many years. Nurses who prepare patients for sleep may want to consider the traditional and nursing evidence suggesting that hops act as a gentle sedative without side effects.

THERAPEUTIC APPLICATIONS:

Oral

Tea. Pour 6 to 8 ounces of hot water over 1 to 2 teaspoonfuls of the dried hops strobiles. Allow it to infuse for 15 minutes, strain, and drink. The tea can be taken up to three times daily and before bed (Bradley, 1992).

Tincture. (1:5, 60% alcohol) 1 to 2 ml ($\frac{1}{4}$ to $\frac{1}{2}$ tsp) up to three times daily and before bed (Bradley, 1992)

Liquid Extract. (1:1 g/ml) 0.5 ml ($\frac{1}{10}$ tsp) in a single dose (Blumenthal et al., 2000)

Topical

Hops have been used traditionally in small pillows. Dried hops are placed in a small cloth bag or pillow. The pillow is gently warmed over heat and then used as a topical application to relieve toothache, earache, and nervous conditions (Grieve, 1971). External applications of hops are often used in combination either as a compress or poultice with chamomile and poppy flowers for swellings, skin inflammation, nerve pain, rheumatism, ringworm, bruises, and boils.

As a fomentation, hops are helpful for those with pneumonia, pleurisy, gastritis, and enteritis. An ointment made from hops and stramonium *(Datura stramonium L.)* leaf has been effective for eczema, ulcers, and painful tumors (Felter & Lloyd, 1983).

Environmental

Hops can be used as a bath infusion. Hops strobiles can be added to small pillows to improve sleep and rest in the user who inhales the aroma of the strobiles.

Herbal Caveat—Therapeutic Applications

In traditional and conventional herbal medicine, amounts of herbs given to patients are based on individual needs. The amounts or "doses" recorded here are provided so that the health practitioner has a general idea of the amounts recommended for an adult patient. Dosing in herbalism not only refers to amount of plant used but also includes when, where, and how to take a plant medicine. These dosages should not be used as guidelines for indiscriminate intervention without proper assessment, critical thinking, and preparation of patient education on the part of the practitioner.

Note: Please see chapter 5 for detailed descriptions of how to prepare various applications.

PATIENT INTERACTION:

Hops have been used for centuries as a calming medicinal herb. Dried hops flowers, called strobiles, can be used to make a relaxing and bitter-tasting tea. Although exact adult dosages are unknown, traditionally 1 teaspoon of the herb for each cup of hot water has been used to make a tea that is steeped for fifteen minutes. Hops also are used in hot compresses and poultices to relieve spasm in the abdomen or congestion in the lungs. Hops sewn into a small pillow with chamomile or valerian is also very relaxing. Beer contains hops. Drinking beer made from whole hops has minimal, if any, therapeutic value. It is recommended that people who are prone to allergic skin eruptions not use hops externally.

Herbal Caveat—Patient Interaction

Patients considering the use of an herb or formula of herbs in self-care benefit from education about the plant itself and the use of the plant in healing. This education can come through many sources, including local herbalists; plant specialists such as botanists; health practitioners such as nurses, nutritionists, naturopaths, and other physicians; and various written references including the scientific literature. Patients need to remember that their unique health care needs are not necessarily represented in any literature they may encounter. Therefore, it is recommended that a knowledgeable mentor be consulted before initiating self-care with any herb being used for the first time.

Note: You may want to keep a journal of your experiences with the herb.

To become better acquainted with hops, purchase several ounces of the dried strobiles. Using some soft fabric, sew a simple small bag or pillow. Stuff it with the hops and sew it closed. This hops pillow can be placed at the head of your bed, inside or under your regular pillow so that the aroma can lull you to sleep at night. If the odor of hops is too strong, just replace some of the strobiles with dried lavender or chamomile flowers.

Another way to experience the effect of hops is to make a tea from the dried strobiles. Place one or two teaspoons of the plant material into a tea ball or infuser. Put it into a cup and add boiling water. Let it steep for about 15 minutes. Sip it slowly and notice the effect in your body. The taste is bitter and cooling. Try comparing the taste and effects of fresh hops tea with the taste and effects of beer.

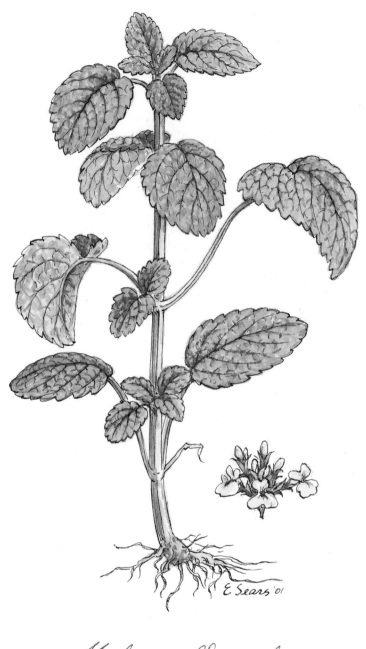

Melissa officinalis

Lemon Balm

- **LATIN NAME:** *Melissa officinalis*

- **FAMILY:** Lamiaceae

- **COMMON NAMES:** Lemon balm, sweet balm, cure-all, common balm, balm, Melissa, heart's delight

- **HEALTH PATTERN:** Sleep and rest

- **PLANT DESCRIPTION:**
  Lemon balm is an aromatic perennial of the Lamiaceae family that is native to the Mediterranean region and western Asia. It is widely cultivated in gardens throughout Europe and the United States. The plant grows 1 to 2 feet ($\frac{1}{3}$ meter) high and appears bushy, with many branching square stems. The leaves are opposite each other on the stems and are a broad oval or heart shape with toothed edges. The teeth are either sharp or rounded. The surface of each leaf is not smooth and shiny, but rough. The leaves can be either solid green or green with pale-yellow markings. The leaves emit a lemony fragrance when bruised and have a distinct but light lemony taste. The small yellow-to-white flowers appear from June to October, growing from the area where the leaf arises from the stem. Lemon balm dies down in winter but, being a perennial, appears again in spring from its rootstock. It will grow in a variety of conditions and soils. Harvest the plant just before it flowers or immediately after.

  The genus name *Melissa* is from the Greek word for "bee," alluding to the fact that bees cannot resist the sweet-smelling flowers (Grieve, 1971). The Greek nymph Melissa was the protectress of bees (Lawless, 1998). The word *balm* is an abbreviation of "balsam," which means fragrant oil.

- **PLANT PARTS USED:** The aerial or above-ground parts

- **TRADITIONAL EVIDENCE:**
  Cultural Use
  North American Indian. The Cherokee have used lemon balm for colds, fever, and as a stimulant. The Costanoan use it as a gastrointestinal aid (Moerman, 1998).
  East Indian. Healers in India have historically used lemon balm *(Melissa parviflora)* for its medicinal preparations similar to those used by the Greeks. They have used lemon balm for indigestion associated with anxiety or depression and as an antispasmodic, diaphoretic, and sedative (Nadkarni, 1976).

Middle Eastern. Balm oil is a favorite scent throughout the Middle East (Lawless, 1998).

Russian/Baltic. Lemon balm is very popular in Russia and is used in cooking and health care. The leaves are used in pillows to promote sleep. Commercial preparations of lemon balm used to lower blood pressure are common. Herbalists are studying the potential benefit of lemon balm for the treatment of attention deficit disorder (Zevin, 1997).

European. The ancient Greek and Roman physicians used lemon balm steeped in wine for both internal and external maladies. It was used topically for surgical wounds and to treat venomous bites and stings. Old European texts record the use of lemon balm to improve memory (Blumenthal et al., 2000).

In anthroposophical health practice, Melissa infusions or oil are used to bring about an airing through of the whole organism, to balance the relationship between water and air. Conditions associated with insufficient airing through are intestinal and menstrual disturbances and nervous disorders (Husemann & Wolff, 1982).

Culinary Use

The essential oil and extract of lemon balm are used in alcoholic (e.g., vermouth) and nonalcoholic beverages. The lemon-scented leaves make an aromatic beverage that is especially nice as a cool tea during warm weather. Victorian ladies enjoyed the fragrance of lemon balm leaves so much that they used it in potpourri to scent their homes. It was regarded as one of the most sweet-smelling herbs that could be grown in the garden. The leaves were considered invaluable for the permanence of their fragrance, which is brought out by touching or bruising the surface (Grieve, 1971). Because of its mild lemony taste, the fresh leaves are delicious added to salads and fish or chicken dishes, or chopped and added to stuffing and sauces.

Use in Herbalism

In the late 1600s, it was believed that lemon balm was of great benefit in all complaints stemming from a disordered nervous system. It was believed that people with this nervous condition could take lemon balm in wine and experience a renewal of vigor, strengthening of the brain, and relief from a sense of sluggishness and depression (Grieve, 1971). Some health practitioners, including Carl Jung, have used the fragrance of lemon balm to strengthen the memory and alleviate feelings of melancholy and sadness. In Paris in 1611, an early type of eau de cologne called "Carmelite water" was distilled from lemon balm, lemon peel, nutmeg, and angelica root. This special water has been known to be effective for the relief of nervous headache and radiating nerve pain (Grieve, 1971) and to improve the complexion (Keville & Green, 1995).

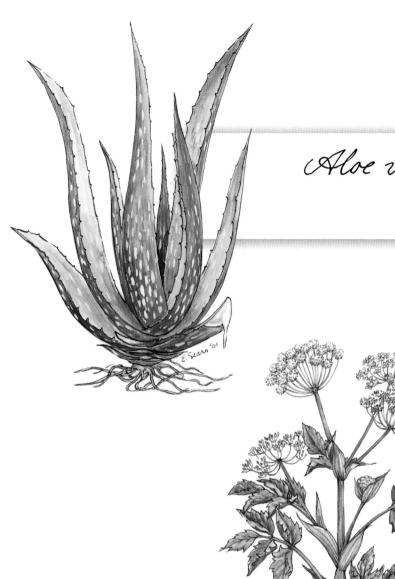

Aloe vera

aloe

Angelica sinensis

angelica

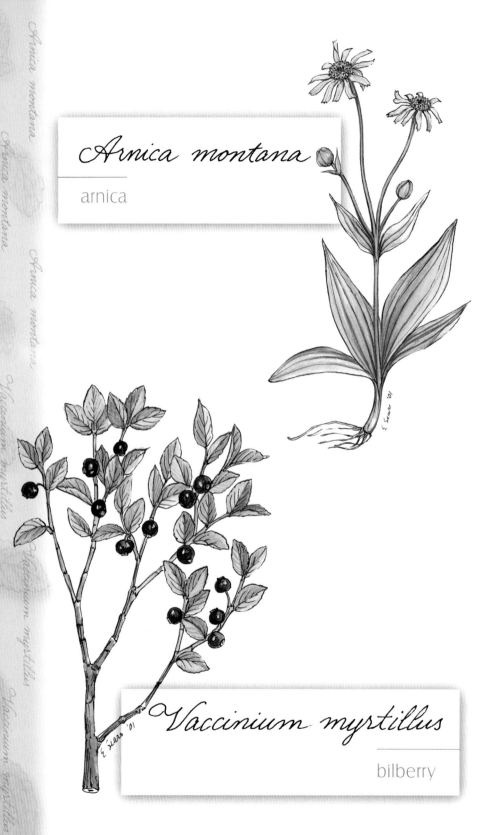

Arnica montana

arnica

Vaccinium myrtillus

bilberry

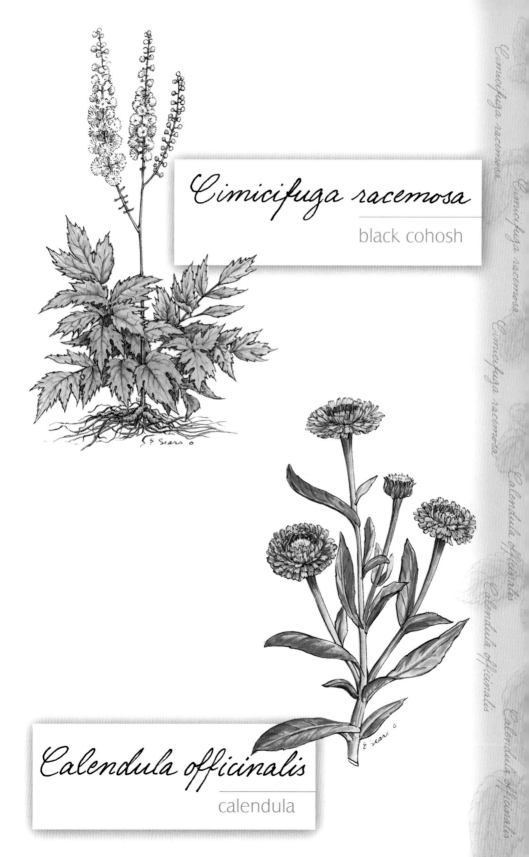

Cimicifuga racemosa
black cohosh

Calendula officinalis
calendula

Cascara sagrada
cascara sagrada

Capsicum frutescens
cayenne

E. Sears '01

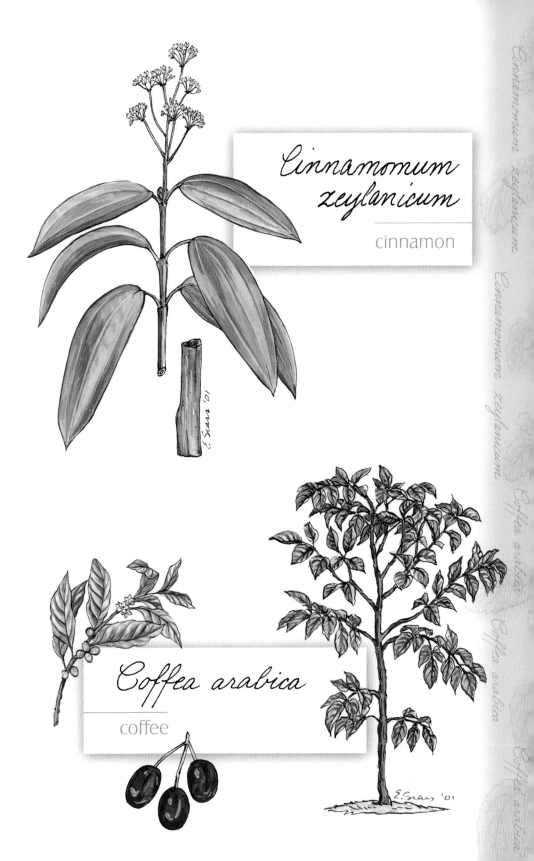

Cinnamomum zeylanicum

cinnamon

Coffea arabica

coffee

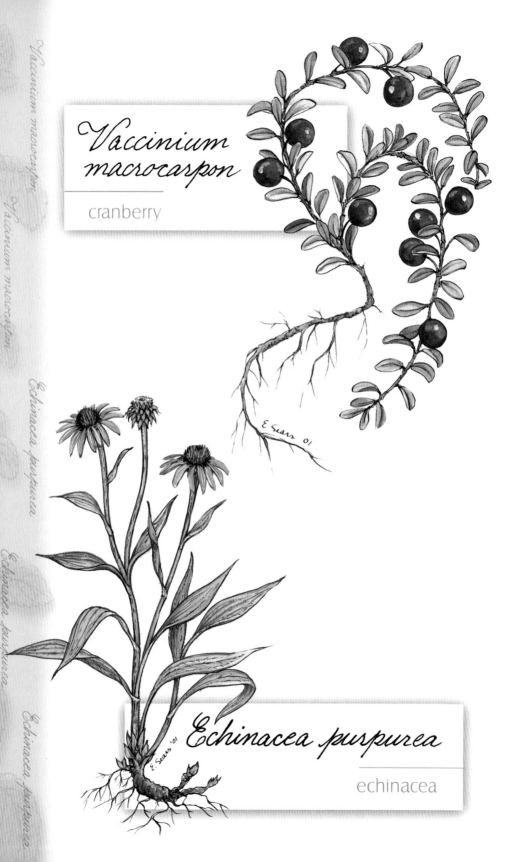

Vaccinium macrocarpon

cranberry

Echinacea purpurea

echinacea

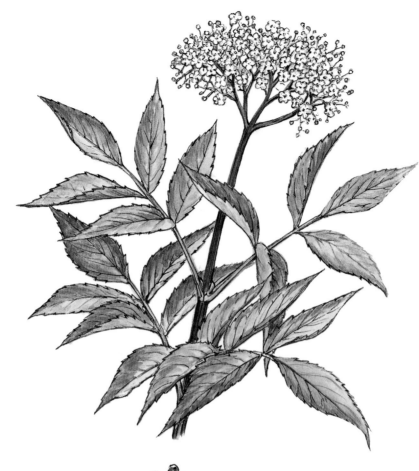

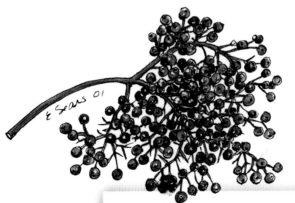

Sambucus nigra

elder

Ephedra sinica

ephedra

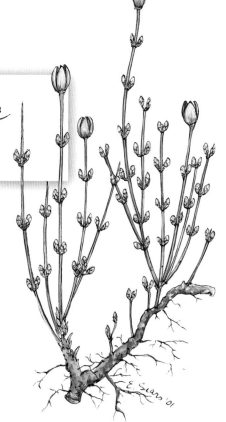

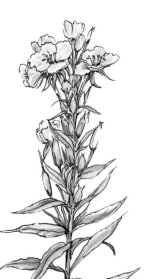

Oenothera biennis

evening primrose

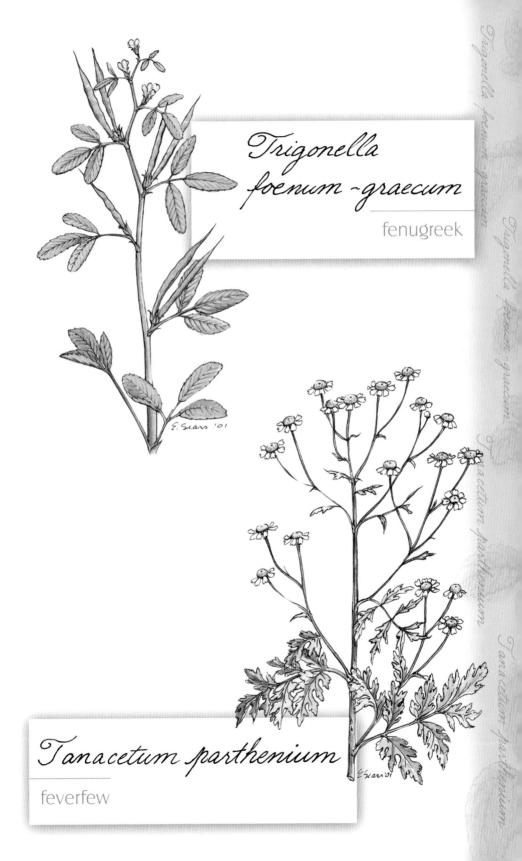

*Trigonella
foenum -graecum*

fenugreek

E. Sears '01

Tanacetum parthenium

feverfew

E. Sears '01

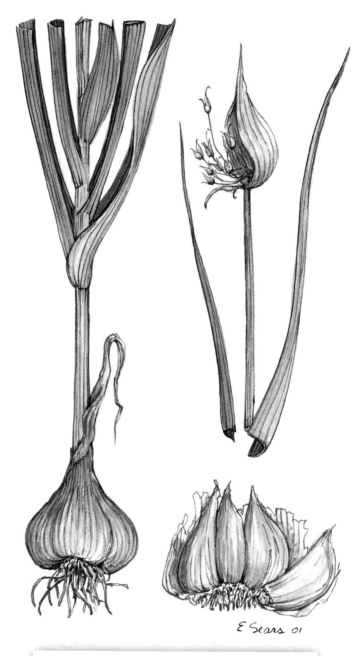

E Sears 01

Allium sativum

garlic

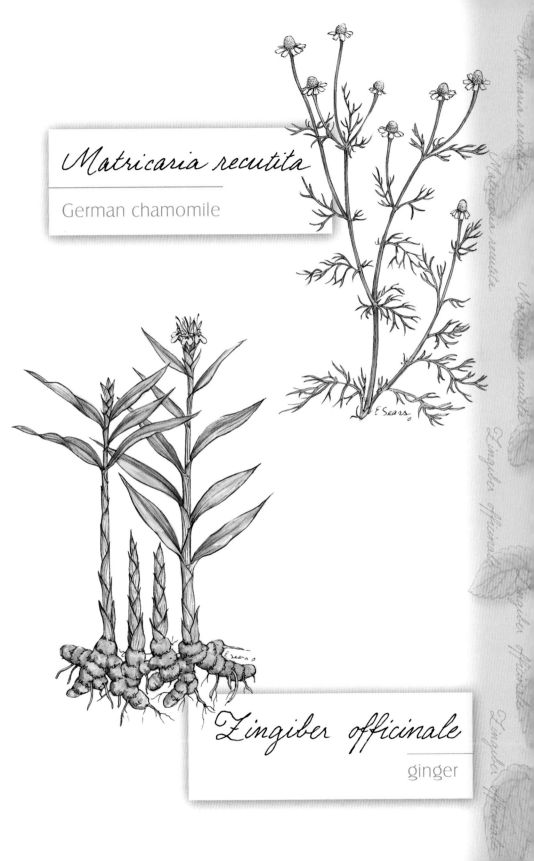

Matricaria recutita

German chamomile

Zingiber officinale

ginger

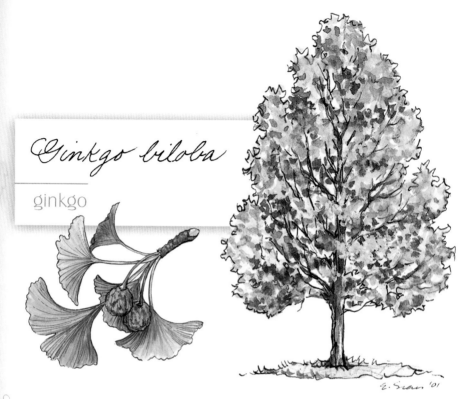

Ginkgo biloba

ginkgo

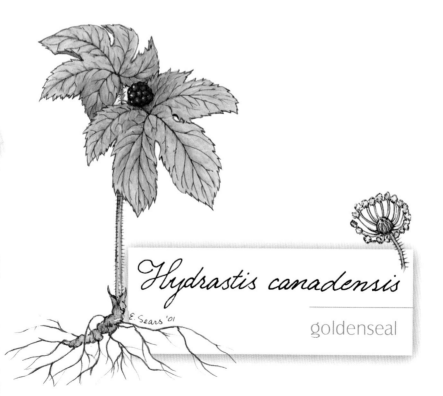

Hydrastis canadensis

goldenseal

E. Sears '01

E. Sears '01

Ginkgo biloba
Ginkgo biloba
Ginkgo biloba
Ginkgo biloba
Hydrastis canadensis
Hydrastis canadensis
Hydrastis canadensis
Hydrastis canadensis

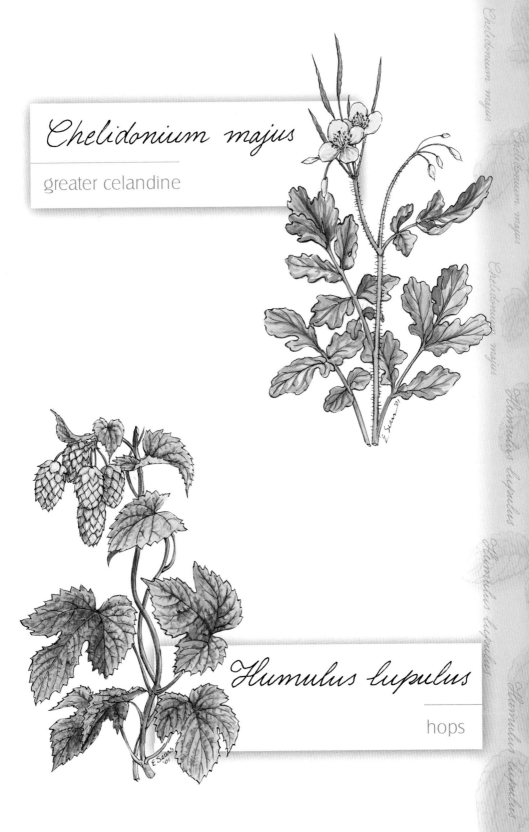

Chelidonium majus

greater celandine

Humulus lupulus

hops

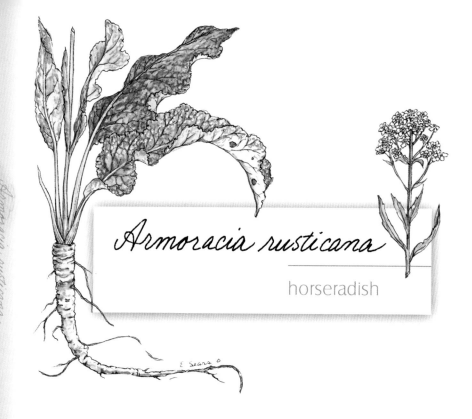

Armoracia rusticana

horseradish

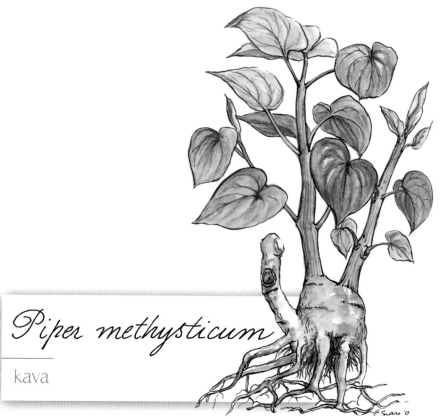

Piper methysticum

kava

Fucus vesiculosus

kelp

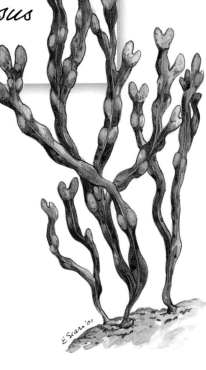

Pueraria lobata

kudzu

Lavandula angustifolia

lavender

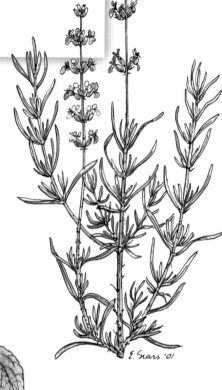

E. Sears '01

Melissa officinalis

lemon balm

E. Sears '01

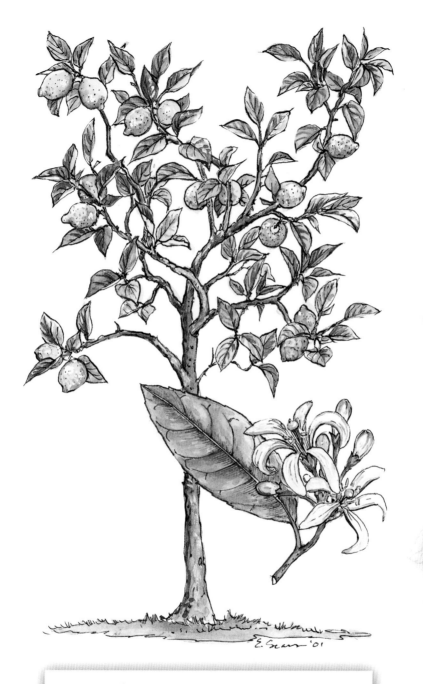

Citrus limon

lemon

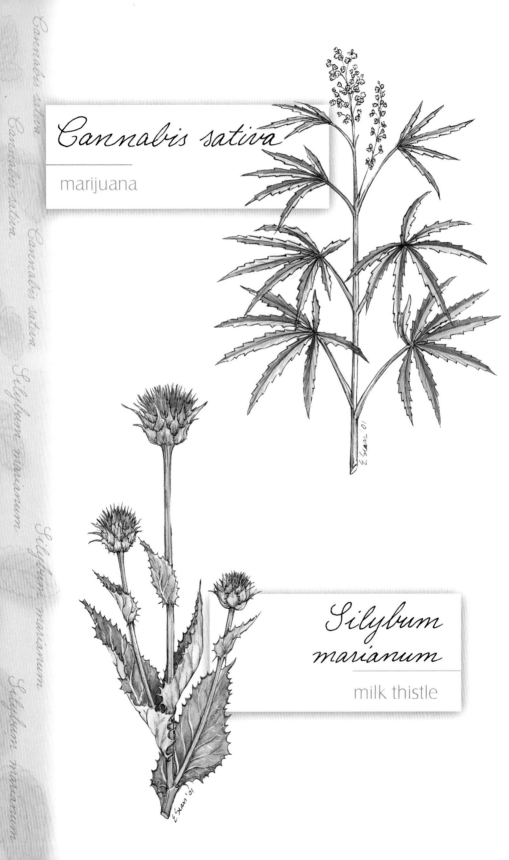

Cannabis sativa

marijuana

Silybum marianum

milk thistle

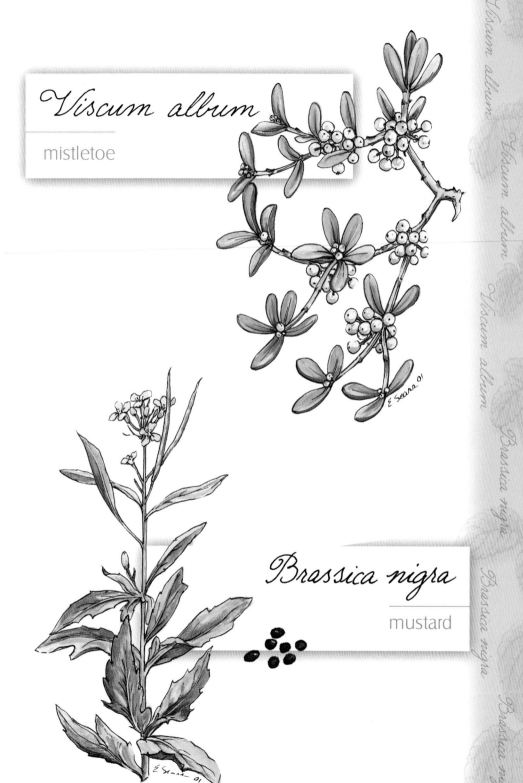

Viscum album

mistletoe

Brassica nigra

mustard

Viscum album
Viscum album
Viscum album
Brassica nigra
Brassica nigra
Brassica nigra

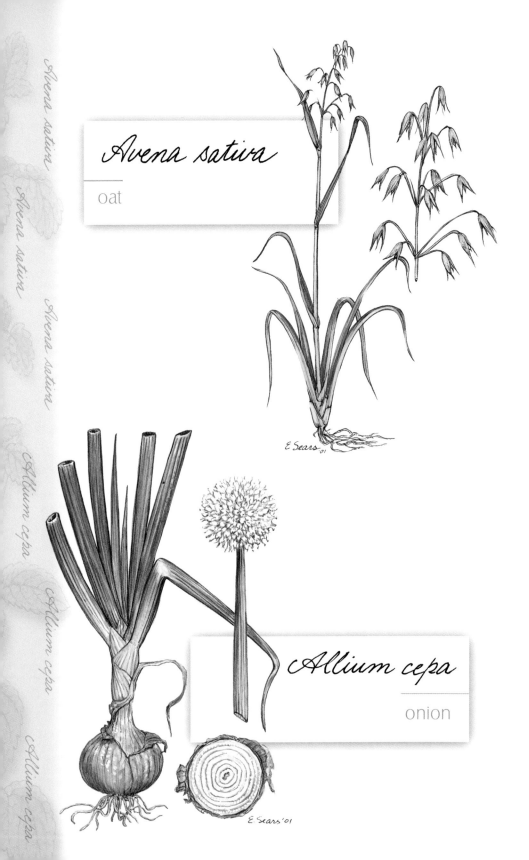

Avena sativa

oat

Allium cepa

onion

E. Sears '01

E. Sears '01

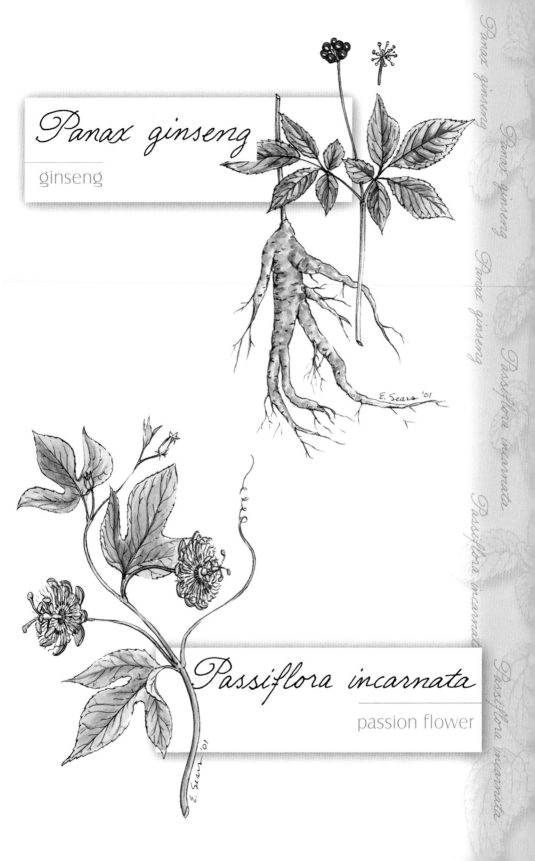

Panax ginseng

ginseng

E. Sears '01

Passiflora incarnata

passion flower

E. Sears '01

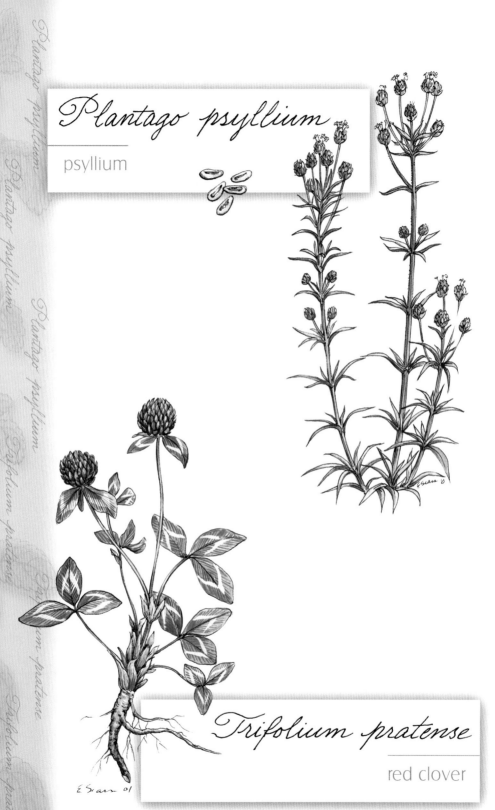

Plantago psyllium

psyllium

Trifolium pratense

red clover

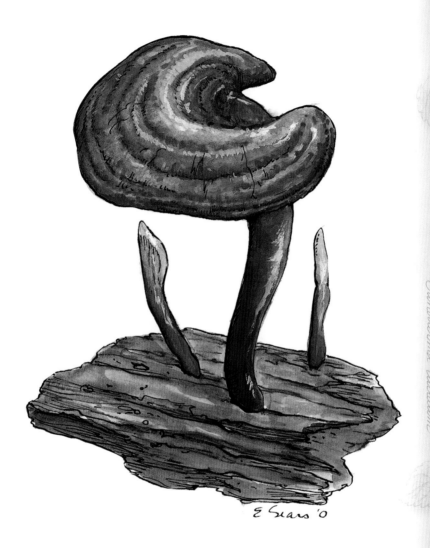

E Sears '0

Ganoderma lucidum

reishi

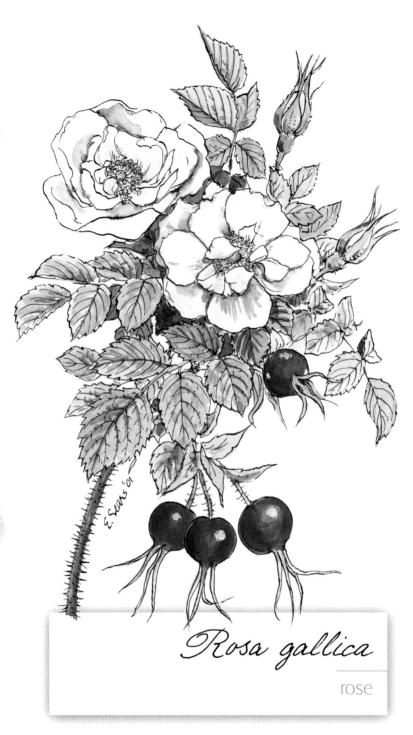

Rosa gallica

rose

Rosmarinus officinalis

rosemary

Salvia officinalis

sage

E. Sears '01

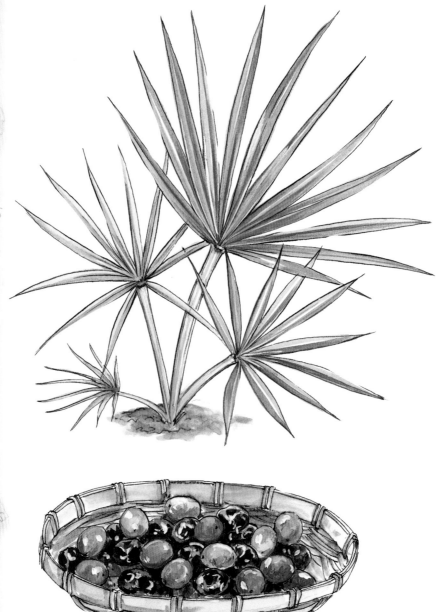

Serenoa repens

saw palmetto

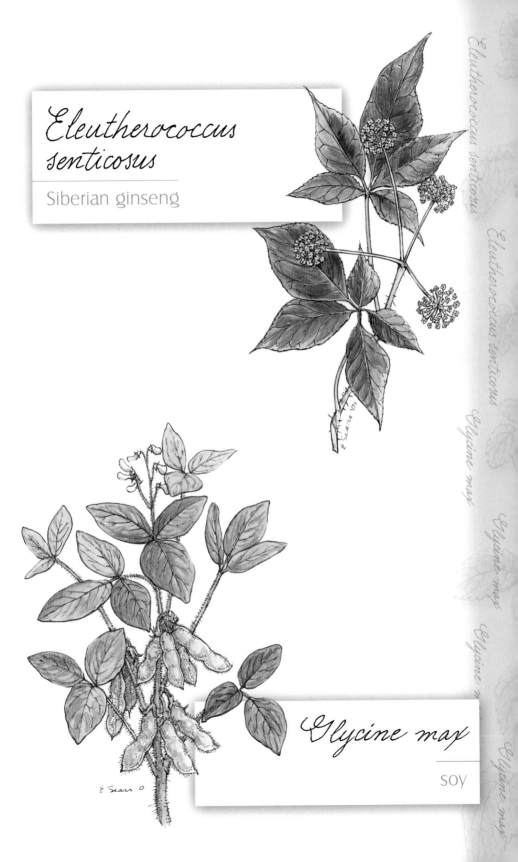

Eleutherococcus senticosus

Siberian ginseng

Glycine max

SOY

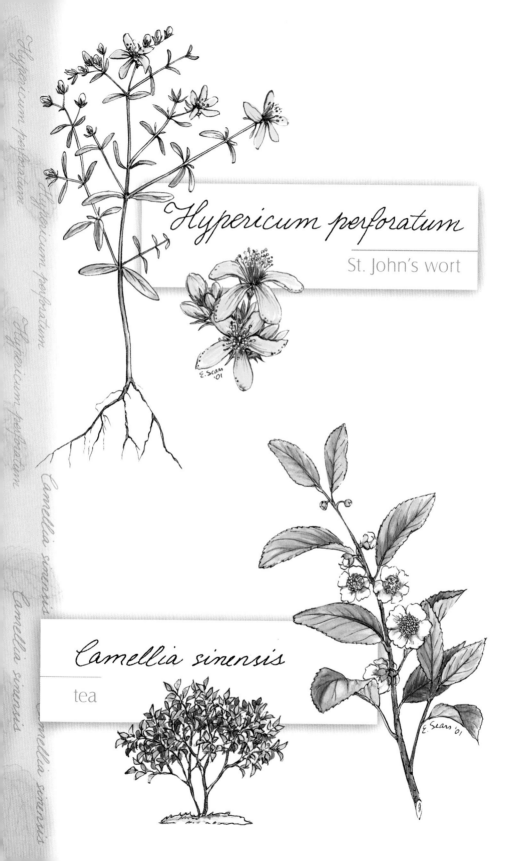

Hypericum perforatum

St. John's wort

E. Sears '01

Camellia sinensis

tea

E. Sears '01

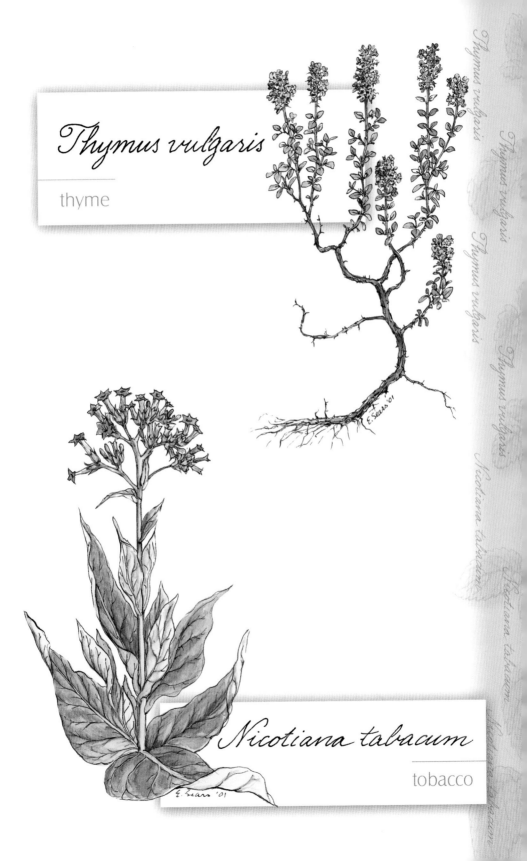

Thymus vulgaris

thyme

Nicotiana tabacum

tobacco

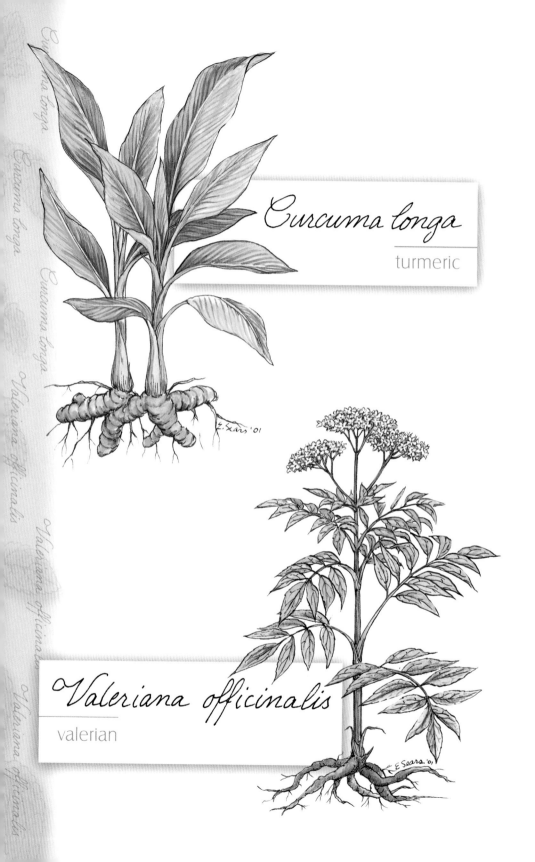

Curcuma longa

turmeric

Valeriana officinalis

valerian

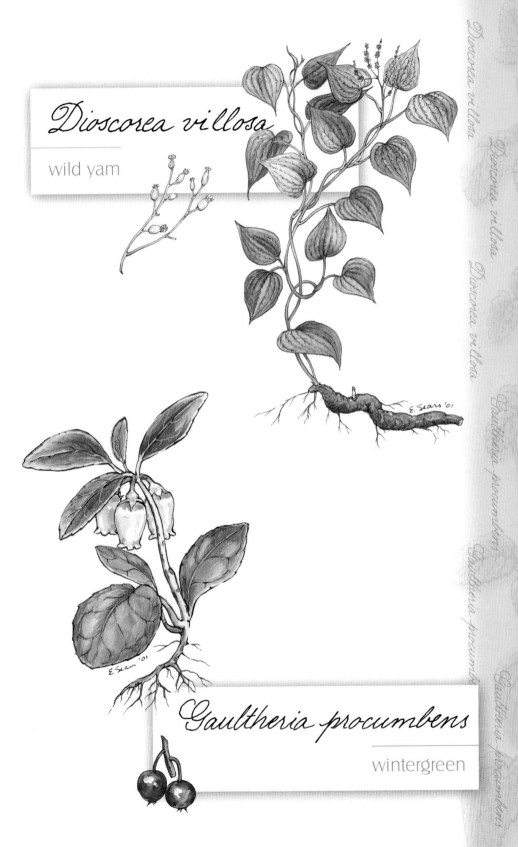

Dioscorea villosa

wild yam

Gaultheria procumbens

wintergreen

E. Sears '01

E. Sears '01

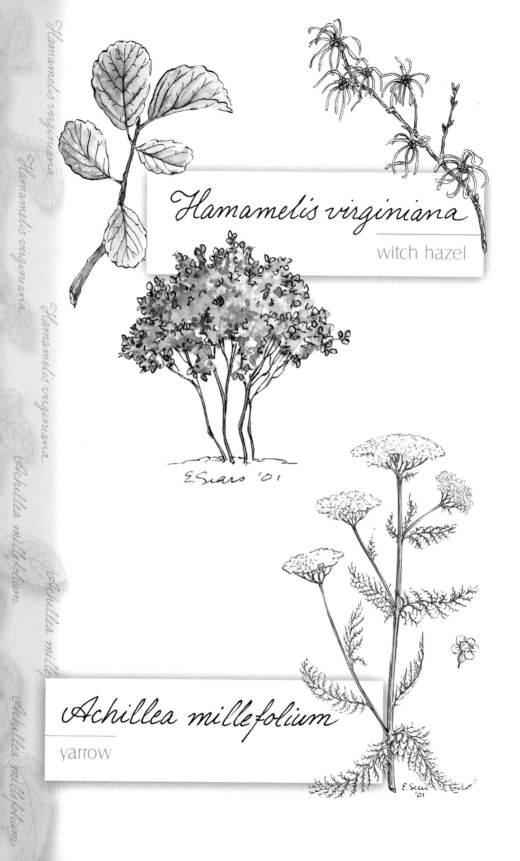

Hamamelis virginiana

witch hazel

E. Sears '01

Achillea millefolium

yarrow

E. Sears '01

In the late 1800s, lemon balm was frequently used as a tea to treat the discomfort of intestinal gas. The herb was used as a common remedy to induce sweating and to alleviate fever during colds and flu. The herb was reportedly used for female discomforts and to bring on the menstrual flow in cases of delayed menses. Some used lemon balm for cramps, headaches, and insomnia (Leung & Foster, 1996). It has been used to treat fever (Felter & Lloyd, 1983). Lemon balm also has been mixed with salt and applied topically to cysts in the skin. It is reported to be effective in cleansing sores and easing the pains of gout (Grieve, 1971).

More recently, lemon balm has been used in a dried form as tea, powdered in capsules, or as alcohol tincture. Lemon balm is well known among herbalists as a mild, but effective sleep aid as well as a tonic for the stomach in digestive problems (Leung & Foster, 1996). The German Commission E recognizes lemon balm for difficulty falling asleep related to nervous conditions (Blumenthal et al., 2000). It is used as a carminative, sedative, diaphoretic, and fever reducer. Lemon balm has been effective in improving symptoms of restlessness, excitability, palpitations, and headache in the treatment of certain psychiatric disorders (Wren, 1988).

In Germany, lemon balm is licensed as a standard medicinal tea for insomnia and digestive tract disorders. Alcohol extracts of the herb also are used in combination with sedative and hypnotic drugs and other sedative and carminative herbs. In the United States, lemon balm is often used as a mild sleep enhancer and digestive tonic (Blumenthal et al., 2000). It has often been recommended to treat psychological problems such as depression and neurosis (Zevin, 1997).

Fresh lemon balm leaves used in tea, tincture, or the bath can act as an emmenagogue (Weed, 1986). Balm is used to alleviate painful, delayed menstruation (Felter & Lloyd, 1983; Zevin, 1997).

Lemon balm has mild vasodilating properties so it can reduce heart rate and lower blood pressure. The tea is effective in relieving inflammation of the gums and mouth when used as a gargle or mouthwash (Zevin, 1997). Lemon balm is mildly stimulating, diaphoretic, and antispasmodic. It has an historical reputation for promoting longevity. The London Dispensary of 1696 reports that two men lived to be more than 105 years old by drinking lemon balm tea daily. This plant is also known as the scholar's herb because it helps the memory and clears the head (Lawless, 1998).

BIOMEDICAL EVIDENCE:

Published research is lacking supporting the use of lemon balm for improving sleep and rest.

Studies Related to Sleep and Rest

Published results of human clinical trials that support the traditional use of lemon balm for enhancing sleep and rest were not found.

Studies Related to Other Health Patterns

Immune Response. The antiviral properties of lemon balm have been confirmed by an in vitro clinical trial (Wren, 1988). The antiviral constituents, rosmarinic acid and other polyphenols, have been identified in lemon balm by chemical analysis. This has led to lemon balm being used in cases of viral infection. The effects of a cream containing extracts of 1% lemon balm (Lomaherpan) were studied in the treatment of skin lesions related to herpes simplex viral infection. Lemon balm was shown to be significantly effective in reducing recovery time from herpetic infection from the normal ten to fourteen days to four to eight days in a multicenter study of 115 people who applied the cream five times a day until the lesions were healed, but not exceeding 14 days (Wolbling & Leonhardt, 1994). In a second clinical trial of 116 patients by the same investigators, Lomaherpan was used 2 to 4 times daily for 5 to 10 days. The most significant finding of this study was that the lemon balm cream significantly reduced symptoms on day two after the lesion appearance—the time when the patients are most uncomfortable—as compared with placebo. In comparison with results of studies with other topical medications, such as acyclovir and idoxuridine, the lemon balm cream is adequate in the treatment of herpes simplex and does so without allergic reactions. The studies show that it is best to begin treatment at the early stages of infection (Wolbling & Leonhardt, 1994). Similar results were found in a study with 66 patients (Koytchev, Alken, and Dundarov, 1999).

Mechanism of Action

Lemon balm contains the monoterpenes citral and citronellal that have been reported to concentrate in the hippocampus (Mills, 1993 as reported in Perry, Pickering, Wang, Houghton, & Perry, 1999), a key area of the brain that is active in the storage of information or memory. The antiviral properties of lemon balm are due to the polyphenols (not caffeic acid) and the tannin present in the plant (Leung & Foster, 1996). In vitro studies have demonstrated that lemon balm extract seems to block virus entry into the cell (Wolbling and Leonhardt, 1994). Eugenol acetate in lemon balm oil is an effective antispasmodic substance (Leung & Foster, 1996).

Lemon balm has antithyroid properties that inhibit the normal metabolic effects of the thyroid gland. Freeze-dried extracts of the herb are found to reduce many of the effects of exogenous and endogenous thyroid stimulating hormone (TSH) on bovine thyroid glands. Lemon balm extract does this by inhibiting the proper binding of TSH to the plasma membranes and by inhibiting a required enzyme in vitro. It is debatable if the same activity occurs in the human body. However, in patients with Graves' disease, it was found that lemon balm extract inhibited certain antibodies (Wren, 1988).

There are no known restrictions for the use of lemon balm during pregnancy (Blumenthal et al., 2000). However, because of its traditional use as an emmenagogue, caution should be exercised if using lemon balm during the first trimester. Lemon balm tea could be used as a relaxing aid for the mother while in labor, as well as the father-to-be.

Herbal Caveat—Pregnancy or Lactation

Some herbs are contraindicated in pregnancy because of a risk of the herb or one of its constituents stimulating the uterus and therefore possibly promoting fetal loss. Many herbal practitioners do not recommend herbal remedies, in particular oral doses of herbs, during the first trimester of pregnancy and seek an alternative. However, herbs are successfully used during pregnancy, especially to prepare the body for the birth. Herbs are relatively unstudied in pregnancy and lactation, so patients need to be made aware through education of the potential benefits and risks of using herbs for health conditions that arise during pregnancy or lactation. The use of herbal remedies during pregnancy often warrants a referral to a knowledgeable herbal practitioner.

⬤ USE FOR CHILDREN:

The Cherokee Indians give a tea of lemon balm to infants for colic and stomachaches (Moerman, 1998). It is a mild sedative for children who are anxious, irritable, or experiencing difficulty sleeping. Children will probably find the taste of lemon balm tea pleasant, especially if sweetened with a small amount of juice at first. Studies are being conducted to investigate the therapeutic effects of lemon balm in children with attention deficit disorder (Zevin, 1997). Lemon balm could be applied topically for cold sores in children (Schilcher, 1992).

Herbal Caveat—Children

Children have special needs in regard to herbal therapies. They require lesser amounts of herbs and often respond well to mild teas and topical applications such as compresses and baths. The lowest dose of oral preparations should be tried first before increasing the amount given children. Caregivers should observe children closely for responses to herbal remedies. Younger children, particularly infants, have traditionally been given herbs either through their mother's breast milk or in the form of a homeopathic remedy because of their sensitivity to medicines and treatments and the immaturity of their liver. It is recommended that a person knowledgeable in the herbal treatment of children be consulted before the offering of any herb to a child for the first time.

⬤ CAUTIONS:

There are no known contraindications or side effects of the internal or external use of lemon balm (Blumenthal et al., 2000; McGuffin et al., 1997). However, because of its sedative effects, caution should be observed in taking lemon balm with other sedative herbs or drugs. These effects can potentially impair alertness or reaction time, especially when driving a motor vehicle or operating machinery.

Because of the controversy about the effects of lemon balm on the thyroid gland, it is suggested that those who have either hypothyroidism or hyperthyroidism should exercise caution if using this herb (Brinker, 1998).

Let the buyer beware—lemon balm has few essential oil glands, produces little essential oil, and therefore the essential oil is either very expensive or may be adulterated with citronella or lemon essential oil (Keville & Green, 1995).

NURSING EVIDENCE:

Historical Nursing Use

Nurses in early nineteenth century America used lemon balm infusion to cool fevers. Lemon balm was given warm to increase perspiration (Child, 1997).

Potential Nursing Applications

Lemon balm has long been used for all types of stressful conditions, traditionally being used as a remedy for a distressed spirit. It helps balance emotions and brighten one's mood. For this reason, lemon balm has been used to bring comfort to the bereaved family of one who is dying. It also has been given to the person who is dying and seems to bring solace to them with its relaxing, yet uplifting, properties (Lawless, 1998). Nurses, in particular hospice and psychiatric nurses, may want to consider lemon balm tea or bath for use in clinical practice/end-of-life care. Nurses may also want to consider further research on lemon balm as an aid to sleep and rest.

Integrative Insight

Fragrance when appropriately applied can have benefits for both practitioner and patient. Traditional evidence demonstrates that lemon balm fragrance and herb have the ability to calm the nerves, promote rest, and raise the spirits. They also may improve memory. Research is just beginning to demonstrate the benefits of this aromatic herb (as an antiviral). Perhaps the research will rekindle an interest in the medicine of this plant that was once used for psychiatric illness and digestive complaints among other discomforts. The delicate taste, as well as the fragrance, invites further exploration and research. The name "balm" also reminds nurses that herbs such as *Melissa* can be used as a soothing extension of the caring touch and nurturing spirit of the nurse when providing comfort.

THERAPEUTIC APPLICATIONS:

Oral

Tea. The fresh leaves make better tea than the dry (Grieve, 1971). Pour 6 to 8 ounces (180 to 240 ml) of hot water over 1 or 2 teaspoons of the dried herb. Let it steep and then strain. Drink up to 3 cups daily and a cup at bedtime.

To make a larger quantity of an infusion, put one ounce (30 g, or about two handfuls) of the dried leaves into a heat-proof quart jar. Fill the jar to the top with boiling water. Cover it tightly with the lid and let it infuse for up to four hours. After steeping, strain the leaves out and drink the infusion, one cup at a time. The remainder can be stored in the refrigerator for up to two days.

Liquid Extract. (1:1 g/ml) 1.5 to 4.5 ml ($\frac{1}{3}$ to 1 tsp) (Blumenthal et al., 2000)

Tincture. Ingest 30 to 60 drops three times daily and 30 to 60 drops before bedtime. The drops can be added to a small amount of warm water or herbal tea.

Topical

Lemon balm extract in a cream base is used topically to relieve symptoms associated with herpes simplex.

Environmental

The essential oil of lemon balm is very expensive but can be atomized for its calming and uplifting effects. For a less expensive experience, the fresh leaves can be infused and put into the bath.

Herbal Caveat—Therapeutic Applications

In traditional and conventional herbal medicine, amounts of herbs given to patients are based on individual needs. The amounts or "doses" recorded here are provided so that the health practitioner has a general idea of the amounts recommended for an adult patient. Dosing in herbalism not only refers to amount of plant used but also includes when, where, and how to take a plant medicine. These dosages should not be used as guidelines for indiscriminate intervention without proper assessment, critical thinking, and preparation of patient education on the part of the practitioner.

Note: Please see chapter 5 for detailed descriptions of how to prepare various applications.

PATIENT INTERACTION:

Lemon balm is a very pleasant tasting tea with a gentle, lemony fragrance. The leaves of this herb drunk as a tea have been known to promote rest, calm the nerves, and raise the spirit. Lemon balm has been known traditionally to help aid digestion; improve the memory; and promote a long, healthy life. Most of the biomedical research has been done in the area of the use of lemon balm cream on cold sores. The research demonstrates that lemon balm may be effective in reducing the length of discomfort associated with an outbreak of cold sores as well as decreasing the discomfort usually experienced on the second day of an outbreak. Do not self-medicate with this herb if you have a known or suspected thyroid condition.

Herbal Caveat—Patient Interaction

Patients considering the use of an herb or formula of herbs in self-care benefit from education about the plant itself and the use of the plant in healing. This education can come through many sources, including local herbalists; plant specialists such as botanists; health practitioners such as nurses, nutritionists, naturopaths, and other physicians; and various written references including the scientific literature. Patients need to remember that their unique health care needs are not necessarily represented in any literature they may encounter. Therefore, it is recommended that a knowledgeable mentor be consulted before initiating self-care with any herb being used for the first time.

NURTURING THE NURSE-PATIENT RELATIONSHIP:

Note: You may want to keep a journal of your experiences with the herb.

Getting to know lemon balm can be a truly uplifting experience. This plant is most aromatic in its fresh state, but also can be used dried, especially if whole leaf is available. The cut and sifted herb often loses its essential oils. Make enough fresh or dried infusion for a bath (see chapter 5). Run a warm, not hot, bath and prepare a cup of the lemon balm tea to drink while you are in the tub. Sample and smell the infusion before preparing the tub to be sure that you like it. Lemon balm can be soothing and calming and lift the spirit at the same time. How might you describe the herb to a patient?

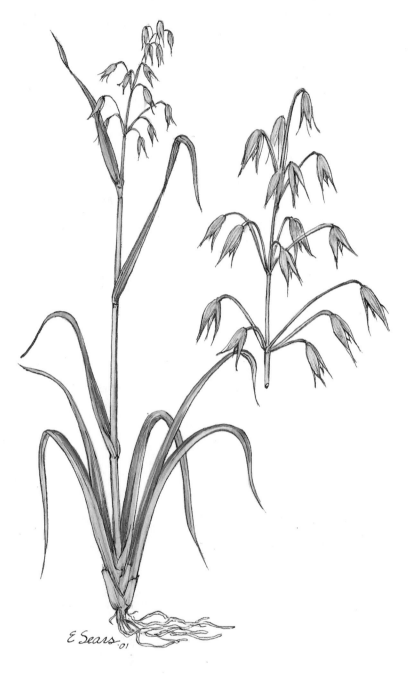

Avena sativa

Oat

🌿 **LATIN NAME:** *Avena sativa*

🌿 **FAMILY:** Poaceae

🌿 **COMMON NAMES:** Oats, wild oats, oat straw, groats, green oats, green tops, oatmeal, rolled oats

🌿 **HEALTH PATTERN:** Sleep and rest

🌿 **PLANT DESCRIPTION:**

Oats grow annually from seed and have a smooth stem that reaches heights of up to 4 feet (1.3 meters). The leaves are long, thin, and grasslike, emerging from the stem in a gently curving spiral. The top of the stalk bears drooping, greenish flowerlike seedpods that open in May. If allowed to fully mature, the seeds will develop into the common oat grain widely used as a food. Oatmeal is the ground grain. Oats are both wild and cultivated. The wild variety likes to grow in moist, shady places or grassy areas in woodlands. Oats are native to the warm Mediterranean zones of the world (Blumenthal et al., 2000). Oats have a slightly bitter taste and no odor.

🌿 **PLANT PARTS USED:** The immature, milky seed; dried oat stems (straw); dried and ground oat grain (seed) as oatmeal, cereals, or oat flour; the seed coat as oat bran

🌿 **TRADITIONAL EVIDENCE:**

Cultural Use

North American Indian. The Haisla, Karok, Kashaya, and Pomo have used oat as a food. The grain is the ground into a fine dry meal called pinole (Moerman, 1998).

Hispanic. Hispanics in the southwestern United States use oats medicinally for discomfort related to gout and lumbago, skin conditions, and as a nervine. Oats are used in the bath.

East Indian. A tincture of green oats is used for nervous system strain. A water-boiled extract of oat has been used successfully in India to cure people of their addiction to opium, and it reduced the desire for tobacco. Oat is not eaten for long periods of time without the inclusion of milk because it is thought to cause skin eruptions (Nadkarni, 1976).

European. In Europe, oats have a history of use as much more than a food staple. Cooked oats are eaten for the benefit to the nervous system, inflamed conditions of the stomach, and as a nutrient during feverish states, but they are avoided in cases of acidity of the stomach. The difference between "inflammation" and "acidity" of the stomach is not clear. Oats also are used as an easily digested food for the mother after childbirth. Cooked, strained oats are sometimes given as a demulcent enema, acting to soothe or protect the irritated mucous membrane of the bowel (Grieve, 1971).

Culinary Use

Oats have long been used as a food. The cultivation of oatmeal for nourishment dates back to at least 2000 B.C.E. (Blumenthal et al., 2000).

Use in Herbalism

A tincture of the oat seed when it is in its immature, milky stage of development is used as a nervous system restorative, to help with convalescence after an illness, and to strengthen a weakened constitution. Oats extract is a nervine and is used for those suffering nervous exhaustion and insomnia (Felter & Lloyd, 1983). It's often taken before bed with lemon balm and hops to promote calming of the nervous system and restful sleep. When oat is in its earliest stage and just flowering, the green grass is rich in avenin, a constituent considered a nutrient for nerve cells. The flowering oats are made into a drink that is taken regularly to calm and regenerate the nervous system (Vogel, 1991).

Oat is used to treat neurasthenia, an emotional and physical disorder characterized by fatigue, lack of motivation, feelings of inadequacy, and psychosomatic symptoms. It is used as a tonic to improve the heart muscle. Oat seed tincture has been used orally to treat multiple sclerosis, but the effectiveness of this application is not well researched (Blumenthal et al., 2000). It is reported to be used as an antidepressant, cardiac tonic, and to ease menopausal symptoms.

The colloidal (gelatinous) fraction of oatmeal is successfully used as a bath preparation to relieve the irritation of eczema and dry skin (Wren, 1988). External uses of oats included cooking the grain with vinegar and applying it to freckles and spots on the skin to cause them to fade. A poultice made of oatmeal and essential oil of bay leaf *(Laurus nobilis)* was used topically to relieve itchy skin, to treat leprosy and anal fistulas, and to help soften abscesses. Oats were often used topically to treat wounds and burns (Culpeper, 1990). Oat straw tea is used to treat shingles, herpes zoster, and herpes simplex. The German Commission E limits the use of oat straw to baths for reduction of inflammation and pruritus (Blumenthal et al., 2000). The saying, "he's sowing his wild oats," comes from the observation that horses fed oats become frisky. Oats may be a sexual stimulant for humans as well.

Historically, the dried roots of the oat plant were powdered and mixed with wine and vinegar. This formula was used to stimulate sweating in those who were infected with the plague. It was believed that the action of perspiring would drive the poisons that were causing the illness out of the body, and the oats would defend the spirit from danger (Culpeper, 1990).

veins. There are no known contraindications of this plant during pregnancy (Weed, 1986; Blumenthal et al., 2000).

Oatmeal that has been cooked as a cereal is very nutritive and moistening to the gastrointestinal tract. For this reason, it may be helpful if constipation occurs during pregnancy. It is not recommended to eat oats during times of dyspepsia or hyperacidity of the stomach (Felter & Lloyd, 1983).

Herbal Caveat—Pregnancy or Lactation

Some herbs are contraindicated in pregnancy because of a risk of the herb or one of its constituents stimulating the uterus and therefore possibly promoting fetal loss. Many herbal practitioners do not recommend herbal remedies, in particular oral doses of herbs, during the first trimester of pregnancy and seek an alternative. However, herbs are successfully used during pregnancy, especially to prepare the body for the birth. Herbs are relatively unstudied in pregnancy and lactation, so patients need to be made aware through education of the potential benefits and risks of using herbs for health conditions that arise during pregnancy or lactation. The use of herbal remedies during pregnancy often warrants a referral to a knowledgeable herbal practitioner.

USE FOR CHILDREN:

Oatmeal baths have been used for skin problems in children, such as for the itching that occurs with chicken pox. To make an oatmeal bath, fill a small cloth bag or clean stocking with dry oats. As the bathtub fills, allow the bag of oats to float in the warm water. Squeeze the bag to release the milky fluid from the oats and rub it across the skin to soothe rashes or itchy dry areas.

Oatmeal is a nutritious food for children and is soothing to the digestive tract after bouts of vomiting or diarrhea.

Herbal Caveat—Children

Children have special needs in regard to herbal therapies. They require lesser amounts of herbs and often respond well to mild teas and topical applications such as compresses and baths. The lowest dose of oral preparations should be tried first before increasing the amount given children. Caregivers should observe children closely for responses to herbal remedies. Younger children, particularly infants, have traditionally been given herbs either through their mother's breast milk or in the form of a homeopathic remedy because of their sensitivity to medicines and treatments and the immaturity of their liver. It is recommended that a person knowledgeable in the herbal treatment of children be consulted before the offering of any herb to a child for the first time.

CAUTIONS:

There are no known precautions to be taken with oats or oat extract (McGuffin et al., 1997). There are no known interactions with pharmaceutical drugs or other herbs. However, because of the mucilaginous properties of cooked oats, they may inhibit the absorption of medications from the gastrointestinal tract. High-fiber foods are known to slow or reduce the absorption of many medications, vitamins, and minerals. The water- soluble fiber in the oat grain can prevent or reduce the absorption of medications or food when the two are taken together (Brinker, 1998). It is recommended to take medications apart from oatmeal or oat bran.

NURSING EVIDENCE:

Historical Nursing Use

Nurses have used oatmeal poultices and baths to comfort those with dry and itching skin conditions.

Potential Nursing Applications

An oats bath can be recommended to patients with eczema; psoriasis; or infectious, itchy rashes, such as chicken pox. The soothing properties of oats can help decrease dry, itchy skin. Mothers may be encouraged to bathe their infants in oats water for diaper rash or other skin problems. Eating oatmeal can be recommended for people who have digestive problems, elevated cholesterol, or constipation. Nurses also may want to consider researching the nervine properties of oats, such as the effect of eating whole grain oatmeal on sleep patterns.

Integrative Insight

Oat is a tonic, or stimulant, for the nervous system and it also can promote restful sleep. It can stimulate the vitality of those who have suffered nervous exhaustion and calm those who are anxious. Oat seems to be able to create balance within the nervous system. The skin, as a peripheral and vital part of the nervous system, also is soothed and balanced by the demulcent nature of this herb. Looking at the actual plant, or a picture of the plant, one can sense its signature, or personality—strength and vitality as manifested in the straight stem and gentle repose and rest as demonstrated by the arching flowers. Clinically, oats have demonstrated an ability to soothe and comfort as well as nourish.

Oats are such a common food that they can easily be overlooked when searching for healing remedies. Informing people about the importance of giving their nervous systems a rest from the bombardment of various environmental stimuli by having quiet time at home and including whole grain oats as a regular part of their diet can be an important addition to the health promotion program of some patients, regardless of the person's blood cholesterol level.

THERAPEUTIC APPLICATIONS:

Oral

Tea. Pour 6 to 8 ounces (180 to 240 ml) of hot water over 1 to 2 teaspoons of the dried oat straw in a cup. Drink up to 3 cups (240 ml each cup) daily.

Tincture. Ingest 30 to 60 drops of the extract of the fresh, immature (green) milky seeds up to three times daily.

Liquid Extract. 0.6 to 2 ml (up to ½ tsp) (Wren, 1988)

Topical

Oats are used in baths to benefit the skin—see environmental section.

Environmental

Bath. Put 8 oz (225 g) of rolled oats into a cloth bag and hang it under the faucet as the bathtub fills. Use it to rub over the skin to release the emollient properties.

Herbal Caveat—Therapeutic Applications

In traditional and conventional herbal medicine, amounts of herbs given to patients are based on individual needs. The amounts or "doses" recorded here are provided so that the health practitioner has a general idea of the amounts recommended for an adult patient. Dosing in herbalism not only refers to amount of plant used but also includes when, where, and how to take a plant medicine. These dosages should not be used as guidelines for indiscriminate intervention without proper assessment, critical thinking, and preparation of patient education on the part of the practitioner.

Note: Please see chapter 5 for detailed descriptions of how to prepare various applications.

PATIENT INTERACTION:

Oats are a readily available home remedy. They can be very soothing to the nervous system and the skin, especially when the skin itches or is inflamed. Oatmeal baths can be taken to feel the calming effects of oats and promote restful sleep. Eating oats as a cereal is not only soothing to the intestinal tract but also may help lower serum cholesterol. An easy way to make a hot oat cereal is to first purchase some Irish oats. These are not the typical rolled oats that are commonly sold in stores. Irish oats are the cut whole grain. Toast ¼ cup (56 g) of the grain gently in a skillet. Put it into a thermos jar. Add 1 cup (240 ml) of boiling water. Let this sit overnight. Open it in the morning for a quick breakfast cereal. Add sweetener, nuts, or fruit only if the digestive system is strong. Traditional herbalists recommend that those recouperating from recent illness when the digestion has been weakened eat oats plain so that the grain does not ferment in the intestines.

Herbal Caveat—Patient Interaction

Patients considering the use of an herb or formula of herbs in self-care benefit from education about the plant itself and the use of the plant in healing. This education can come through many sources, including local herbalists; plant specialists such as botanists; health practitioners such as nurses, nutritionists, naturopaths, and other physicians; and various written references including the scientific literature. Patients need to remember that their unique health care needs are not necessarily represented in any literature they may encounter. Therefore, it is recommended that a knowledgeable mentor be consulted before initiating self-care with any herb being used for the first time.

NURTURING THE NURSE-PLANT RELATIONSHIP:

Note: You may want to keep a journal of your experiences with the herb.

Try eating oatmeal with the perspective of the grain's health benefits. Chew the grain thoroughly until the grain is mixed with saliva and becomes slightly sweet in your mouth. This helps stimulate digestion. Oats are one food that can be eaten regularly.

Get to know oat as a medicinal plant remedy by taking a bath in it. Oat baths are a great way to relieve stress on the sensitive nervous system. In the evening, fill the bathtub with warm water. For an oat bath, do not use water that is too hot. Hot baths are stimulating to the nervous system. Place about 8 oz (226 g) of oatmeal into a sock or nylon stocking and tie the top securely. Put the filled sock into the bath water, squeezing it to release the soothing properties of the oats. This bath also can be comforting for dry, itchy skin.

CHAPTER 12
Elimination

INTRODUCTION

M ANY HEALERS THROUGHOUT THE AGES HAVE REC-
ognized the importance of healthy elimination patterns. A person
must regularly excrete the by-products of the body's normal processes to
stay alive. When a baby is first born, one of the first things a nurse watches
for is the baby's ability to eliminate. Elimination occurs in five ways: through
the lungs as we exhale, through the liver as the blood is purified, through
the skin as we perspire, through the kidneys as the fluids of the body are filtered, and through the bladder, urethra, and bowels as the body's waste is
excreted. When any of these eliminatory processes is impaired, ill health
can ensue. The focus of this chapter is the elimination that occurs through
the urinary and intestinal tracts. Healthy urination and defecation are important to maintaining the vital energy levels of the body and a sense of
well-being.

Urinary and bowel elimination can be likened to the plumbing of a
kitchen sink. Imagine that you have washed the dishes and now want to
have the dirty water go down the drain but find that the drain is clogged.
The dirty water sits in the sink getting more fetid every hour. The problem with the lack of flow in elimination down the sink could be due to a
clogged drain way down deep in the pipes, but there could be other explanations for the problem. As you troubleshoot the problem, you realize

that the drain itself could be closed or too much dirty water might be going down the drain at one time, causing the sink to back up.

When a person's urinary and bowel elimination systems do not flow properly, they too can get backed up and become toxic. But just as the clogged sink may be due to more than one problem, the blockage of the flow of waste from the body is not limited to a problem in the kidneys, bladder, or intestines. The eliminatory actions of these organs—diuresis, urination, peristalsis, and defecation—are processes that are controlled by brain and hormonal activity as well as the kidneys, bladder, and intestines.

Herbs assist the body's eliminatory processes not just by "unclogging the drain." Herbs facilitate the flow of fluids in the body and the excretion of waste from the body in several different ways. Some herbs such as bearberry *(Arctostaphylos uva ursi)* and watermelon *(Citrullus lanatus)* have strong diuretic effects, increasing the amount of urine excreted from the body. Parsley *(Petroselinum crispum)* and juniper *(Juniperus communis L.)* are known for affecting kidney function. Some herbs, such as psyllium *(Plantago psyllium L.)*, soften and add bulk to the stool or restrain fluids in the case of diarrhea, while other herbs such as cascara sagrada *(Rhamnus purshiana)* are stimulating to the bowel and cause a purgative action.

Although it may be common for people to use a single herb to address the "plumbing" problem, this approach is not always effective in solving the matter for the long term. Concerns with elimination often involve more than one body system. For example, a patient who is excessively worried may have loose bowels every day until he or she is able to deal with worry and anxiety. Giving the patient herbs to astringe the fluids and bulk the stool would simply be a Band Aid action. This is why a holistic assessment is necessary to determine not only the proper herbs to be used for concerns about elimination but also whether or not herbs for elimination should be considered for use in the first place.

This chapter explores herbs that have a history of use as single-plant remedies in dealing with elimination issues related to the organs of elimination, the intestines, and the urinary tract. The herbs included are cranberry, psyllium, cascara sagrada, and saw palmetto. The first three herbs may be recognized as having been used or administered by nurses for some time. As you reflect upon the traditional, biomedical, and nursing evidence surrounding the use of these herbs, remember the sciences of anatomy and physiology because there is more to an elimination concern than the major symptoms initially presented by the patient. And remember the importance of water in the elimination process, because without lots of water flowing freely in the body, bathing the cells and helping to pull out the toxic waste from the body, no herb on the planet would be able to help.

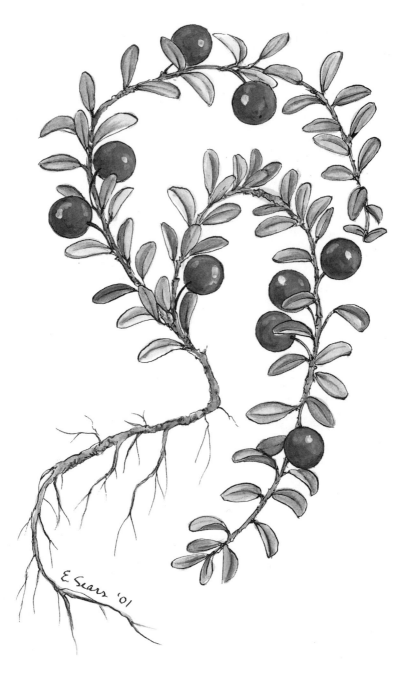

Vaccinium macrocarpon

Cranberry

- **LATIN NAME:** *Vaccinium macrocarpon*

- **FAMILY:** Ericaceae

- **COMMON NAMES:** Cranberry, low-bush cranberry, American cranberry

- **HEALTH PATTERN:** Elimination

- **PLANT DESCRIPTION:**

Cranberry is a trailing, evergreen shrub with slender stems that is found growing in bogs of North America, from Newfoundland to Manitoba and south through New England into Virginia, Ohio, and northern Illinois. A different species is found in northern and central Europe. The leaves are leathery and the flowers are white to pink. The fruit is round, glossy red, and approximately ½ inch (1 to 1.5 cm) in diameter with a very tart taste and astringent quality. Cranberries share the same plant family with blueberries, bilberries, huckleberries, and lingonberries.

- **PLANT PARTS USED:** Fruit, leaves

- **TRADITIONAL EVIDENCE:**

Cultural Use

Asian. Cranberry is used in current Japanese healing as an adjunct to treatments for bladder infection, which in traditional Japanese medicine is said to be a manifestation of "heat" that has moved into the lower part of the body manifesting as infection in the uterus or bladder (Rister, 1999).

North American Indian. North American Indians use several species of cranberry for food and medicine. *Vaccinium macrocarpon*, the North American cranberry, is used as food by the Quebec Algonquin. The Montagnais used an infusion of the branches to treat the symptoms of pleurisy. Other tribes dry the berries and store them for winter use. The Iroquois mash the berries and make them into small cakes that are dried for future food use (Moerman, 1998).

European. Cranberry has been used traditionally in Eastern Europe as a treatment for cancer (Leung & Foster, 1996).

Culinary Use

Cranberries are used to make cranberry juice, jelly, and sauce. The sauce is commonly eaten with poultry. Dried and fresh cranberries are also used in breads and pastries. The leaves of the plant are used as a tea substitute. The red pigment in the fruit pulp is used as a commercial food coloring (Leung & Foster, 1996).

Use in Herbalism

Cranberry has been used historically in topical applications for inflammatory swellings, skin infections, fever, tonsillitis, sore throat, swollen neck glands, and skin ulcers (Felter & Lloyd, 1983). Cranberry has been commonly used recently to comfort those with symptoms associated with urinary tract infections. Cystitis, or bladder infection, usually is caused by bacteria. Normally, urine is sterile as it is secreted from the kidneys. Bacteria can enter the bladder from the urethra and result in the symptom of burning pain during urination. Additional symptoms include the desire to urinate even if the bladder is empty; urine that is cloudy, dark, or foul smelling; low back pain; fever; and chills. Bladder infections are more common in women during pregnancy and menopause and in men who have prostate infections. Bladder infections are also more common in those who have diabetes and decreased immune system function and in those who have recently taken antibiotics. Cranberries also are used for relieving symptoms such as itching related to yeast infection.

Cranberry is used in capsule, fruit concentrate, dried fruit, and tablet form for the relief of urinary tract discomfort. The fruit juice also has been used traditionally as a diuretic, antiseptic, and as a home remedy for fevers and urinary tract infection (Leung & Foster, 1996).

BIOMEDICAL EVIDENCE:

Because so many anecdotal reports assert the cranberry's beneficial effects in regard to discomfort associated with urinary tract infection, its mechanism of action has been questioned. At first it was speculated that cranberries exert their beneficial effects by lowering urine pH, but data conflict. Cranberry's action is now thought to be due to its ability to prevent bacteria from adhering to the lining of the urinary tract.

Studies Related to Elimination

One study of 22 subjects compared the effects on urine acidification and bacterial adhesion of 15 oz (450 ml) per day of freshly prepared cranberry juice or concentrate with cranberry juice cocktail containing fructose and vitamin C. Measurements taken in the morning following nighttime ingestion of cranberry juice showed no effect, but measurements of bacterial adherence one to three hours after ingestion demonstrated significant results in 15 of 22 subjects ($p < .05$) for whom the urine tested before ingestion of the juice was used as a control (Sobota, 1984).

One study found that elderly women ($N = 153$) given either cranberry juice cocktail 300 ml (10 oz) per day for six months or placebo containing vitamin C, had significantly less bacteria with pyuria than controls. The major difference occurred between one and two months of treatment and continued throughout the study. The median pH levels of the cranberry group were actually higher than the control group (Avorn et al., 1994).

Cranberry, given as a daily supplement, one capsule of 400 mg cranberry solids, was shown in a six-month randomized, double-blind, crossover, placebo-controlled study of 19 sexually active women ages 28 to 44 with recurrent urinary tract infections, to be significantly more effective ($p < .005$) than placebo in reducing the occurrence of urinary tract infection (Walker, Barney, Mickelsen, Walton, & Mickelsen, 1997).

In a clinical study of 60 patients with urinary tract infection given 16 oz (480 ml) of cranberry juice per day for three weeks, 32 had a positive response, 12 were somewhat improved, and 16 had no improvement. Six weeks after discontinuing the cranberry juice, 27 of the 44 who had showed improvement during the study had recurrent infection (Prodromos, Brusch, & Ceresia 1968).

In a double-blind, placebo-controlled, crossover study of 15 children with neurogenic bladder who received cranberry concentrate, 2 oz (60 ml) per day for six months, no significant difference was noted in the acidification of the urine obtained by intermittent catheterization (Schlager, Anderson, Trudell, & Hendley, 1999).

In a double-crossover study in which the participants served as their own controls, cranberry juice, 118.3 ml of a 25% concentration, given three times a day with meals for four weeks to 21 male nursing home residents with a history of urinary tract infections, was shown to reduce significantly the pH of first morning urine during juice intake periods as compared with nonjuice periods. Analysis of variance for the individual juice and nonjuice periods was not statistically significant. Other positive effects noted during the study, although not studied directly, were decreased incidence of constipation, decreased urine odor and incontinence, and increased fluid intake (Jackson & Hicks, 1997).

Another small study of eight patients with multiple sclerosis showed that 6 oz of cranberry juice twice daily was significantly more effective in lowering urine pH than orange juice but was not able to produce or maintain an uninfected state (Schultz, 1984).

Studies Related to Other Health Patterns

Skin Care. The skin around urostomies can be particularly subject to injury from alkaline urine. In one study of 13 urostomy patients who received 160 to 320 g of cranberry juice daily for six months, the skin around the urostomy sites in 5 of the 6 patients who began the study with erythema, maceration, or pseudoepithelial hyperplasia showed significant improvement. The average pH of the urine *in the pouches* of the patients decreased significantly, but the pH of their *fresh urine* increased significantly. Although this study demonstrated that cranberry juice does not necessarily lower urine pH, it may be helpful in healing the skin at the stoma site, which is exposed to the patient's urine over time (Tsukada et al., 1994).

Digestion. Preliminary in vitro studies of the effect of a nondialyzable material derived from cranberry juice concentrate on dental plaque bacteria showed that the cranberry derivative was significantly effective in reversing and inhibiting the coaggregation of dental bacteria. Gram-negative bacteria that play a central role in periodontal disease are quite sensitive to cranberry. Cranberry juice, which often contains as much as 12% fructose and dextrose by weight, would be contraindicated for therapeutic use, however, because of the risk of increased plaque formation and dental caries due to the effects of the sugars in the juice (Weiss et al., 1998).

Mechanism of Action

The fact that cranberries contain fructose may partially explain their ability to inhibit some bacteria, in that it has been demonstrated that a 5% solution of fructose inhibits bacteria; however, cranberry juice inhibits bacteria that are not inhibited by fructose (Leaver, 1996). Cranberry juice contains a high molecular weight constituent that selectively inhibits mannose resistant adhesions produced by *E. coli* (Ofek, Goldhar, and Sharon, 1996). In vitro studies have shown that fructose and another nondialyzable constituent that has yet to be fully defined are thought to be responsible for cranberry's ability to inhibit adherence of bacteria to the urinary tract epithelial cells (Zafriri et al., 1989). An earlier study of cranberry found that hippuric acid produced from the benzoic acid in cranberries may be responsible for acidifying the urine (Blatherwick, 1914, p. 450). Cranberries contain arbutin, a chemical compound that is diuretic, antibiotic, and antifungal (Duke, 1997).

The plasma phenol and vitamin C concentrations of nine volunteers increased significantly after drinking 2 cups (500 ml) of cranberry juice, thereby raising the question about the potential antioxidant capacity of cranberry in preventing diseases known to be affected by dietary antioxidant intake such as heart disease and certain cancers (Pedersen et al., 2000). Low-density lipoprotein oxidation is inhibited by cranberry extracts in vitro in a way that is similar to red wine and grape juice (Wilson, Porcari, & Harbin, 1998).

USE IN PREGNANCY OR LACTATION:

Unsweetened cranberry juice or fresh pureed cranberries and water can be used by pregnant women. Weed (1986) recommends an 8-ounce (240 ml) glass every hour for ten hours for discomfort related to urinary tract infection.

Herbal Caveat—Pregnancy or Lactation

Some herbs are contraindicated in pregnancy because of a risk of the herb or one of its constituents stimulating the uterus and therefore possibly promoting fetal loss. Many herbal practitioners do not recommend herbal remedies, in particular oral doses of herbs, during the first trimester of pregnancy and seek an alternative. However, herbs are successfully used during pregnancy, especially to prepare the body for the birth. Herbs are relatively unstudied in pregnancy and lactation, so patients need to be made aware through education of the potential benefits and risks of using herbs for health conditions that arise during pregnancy or lactation. The use of herbal remedies during pregnancy often warrants a referral to a knowledgeable herbal practitioner.

USE FOR CHILDREN:

Cranberries are eaten as a food and may also be used therapeutically by children in moderation.

Herbal Caveat—Children

Children have special needs in regard to herbal therapies. They require lesser amounts of herbs and often respond well to mild teas and topical applications such as compresses and baths. The lowest dose of oral preparations should be tried first before increasing the amount given children. Caregivers should observe children closely for responses to herbal remedies. Younger children, particularly infants, have traditionally been given herbs either through their mother's breast milk or in the form of a homeopathic remedy because of their sensitivity to medicines and treatments and the immaturity of their liver. It is recommended that a person knowledgeable in the herbal treatment of children be consulted before the offering of any herb to a child for the first time.

CAUTIONS:

There is no known toxicity associated with the ingestion of cranberry. Patients at risk for oxalate and uric acid formation because of the potential for increasing the acidity of the urine (demonstrated in some studies) may be at risk when using medicinal amounts of cranberry. Patients with irritable bowel may experience diarrhea when ingesting medicinal amounts of cranberry. The high content of sugar found in some cranberry juices may lead to weight gain in some people (Leaver, 1996). Cranberry solids or extract supplements that contain no sugar might be more appropriate (than cranberry juice) for use in diabetic and hypoglycemic patients.

NURSING EVIDENCE:

Historical Nursing Use

Nurses have been recommending cranberry juice for a number of years for discomfort related to urinary tract infection. Nurses of the early nineteenth century recommended a poultice of stewed cranberries for cancer (Child, 1997).

Potential Nursing Applications

Nurses may want to consider recommending that certain patients drink occasional glasses of unsweetened cranberry juice or take a cranberry concentrate supplement as a preventive measure against urinary tract infection. The types of patients who could benefit from cranberry include those with indwelling catheters or patients who self-catheterize, patients with urostomies, persons who make urinary stones, patients with gram-negative-rod infections *(Proteus* and *Pseudomonas),* those who have had *E. coli* (Type I and Type P fimbriated) isolated from their urine, patients with foul smelling urine, and those who have excess mucus in their urine. Many women after vaginal delivery often like drinking cranberry juice. It is astringent (helpful after the loss of fluids and blood from an herbal medicine perspective) and also prevents bladder infections that are often an issue for pregnant and postpartum women. Nurses might want to consider continuing the research on the effectiveness of cranberry in caring for patients with skin breakdown related to urostomies.

Integrative Insight

Cranberry is one of the best examples of the interplay among disciplines that can occur in the development of understanding of a particular herb. Traditional herbalists, nurses, and other clinicians have recorded the medicinal effects of cranberry for many years. Science has examined how the cranberry "works" and has found that not only are the sugars in the berry helpful in healing the urinary tract of bacterial infection, but also that it contains a substance that keeps certain bacteria from adhering to the lining of the urinary tract and mucous membranes. With this knowledge more clinical and laboratory exploration can be done to further the understanding of the properties of cranberry and its effects in humans. The research on cranberry has been going on since 1914, if not before, reminding us that scientific understanding of plant medicines does not occur as a result of one study, nor does exploration end with one study.

THERAPEUTIC APPLICATIONS:

Oral

Cranberry juice: Drink 5 to 20 oz (150 to 600 ml) daily (Leung & Foster, 1996).
> Fresh fruit: ½ cup daily (120 ml).
> Dried fruit: 1 tablespoon daily (15 g) (Pedersen, 1987).
> Tablets: One or two 250-mg tablets three times daily (Rister, 1999).

Topical

Studies of the affects of cranberry, as in the study of patients with skin breakdown at their urostomy sites, show that sometimes the best therapeutic application for the skin may be to take the herb orally/systemically.

Environmental

The deep red color of cranberries can be enjoyed in home decorations.

Herbal Caveat—Therapeutic Applications

In traditional and conventional herbal medicine, amounts of herbs given to patients are based on individual needs. The amounts or "doses" recorded here are provided so that the health practitioner has a general idea of the amounts recommended for an adult patient. Dosing in herbalism not only refers to amount of plant used but also includes when, where, and how to take a plant medicine. These dosages should not be used as guidelines for indiscriminate intervention without proper assessment, critical thinking, and patient education on the part of the practitioner.

Note: Please see chapter 5 for detailed descriptions of how to prepare various applications.

Cranberry has been found in scientific studies to do just what people have said that it does—ease the discomfort associated with urinary tract infections. Just be careful not to drink too much of the juice because its high sugar content can lead to diarrhea and weight gain. Liquid and tablet cranberry concentrates can be taken instead of juice for those who may be sensitive to the sugar content. These supplements are stored in the refrigerator. Cranberry concentrates are quite tart, but a tablespoon or so of fruit juice can be added to make it palatable. It is best to take cranberry at the beginning signs of discomfort.

Herbal Caveat—Patient Interaction

Patients considering the use of an herb or formula of herbs in self-care benefit from education about the plant itself and the use of the plant in healing. This education can come through many sources, including local herbalists; plant specialists such as botanists; health practitioners such as nurses, nutritionists, naturopaths, and other physicians; and various written references including the scientific literature. Patients need to remember that their unique health care needs are not necessarily represented in any literature they may encounter. Therefore, it is recommended that a knowledgeable mentor be consulted before initiating self-care with any herb being used for the first time.

NURTURING THE NURSE-PLANT RELATIONSHIP:

Note: You may want to keep a journal of your experiences with the herb.

One way to get to know cranberries is to enjoy their flavor. The following is my family's recipe for cranberry sherbet. As a rule I do not recommend extremely cold foods, but on occasion this is one old family recipe that is fun to eat. It is unusual and tasty.

Ingredients:

4 cups cranberries

4 cups (960 ml) water

2½ cups (566 g) sugar or sweetener

1 cup (240 ml) orange juice

4 tablespoons (60 ml) lemon juice

2 tablespoons (30 ml) rose water

Simmer berries in water for fifteen minutes until mushy. Mash and strain. Add the sugar or sweetener and stir until dissolved. Add fruit juices and freeze in the bowl until mushy. Take out of freezer and beat with electric beater on low, then medium, then high until very frothy. Add rose water. Line a cupcake pan with cupcake papers and spoon frothy sherbet into the papers and freeze until hard. Usually makes 18 servings of sherbet. Decorate with fresh flower or candied violets, before serving.

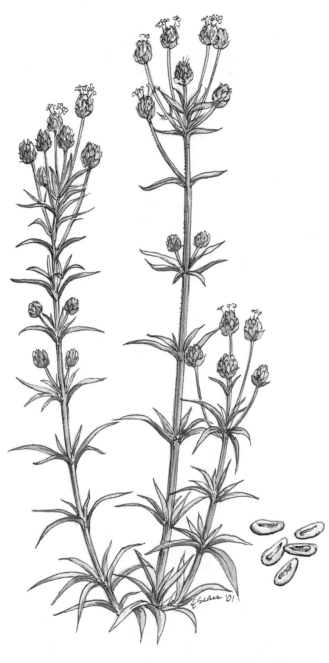

Plantago psyllium

Psyllium

- **LATIN NAMES:** *Plantago psyllium L., P. arenaria, P. ovata Forssk., P. afra L., P. indica L., P. asiatica L.*

- **FAMILY:** Plantaginaceae
  Note: The herb profiled here is plantago seed of the various species listed above. The herb known commonly as plantain leaf from P. lanceolata or P. major is not covered here.

- **COMMON NAMES:** Psyllium, psyllium seed, Indian plantago, pale psyllium, blonde psyllium, flea seed, ispagol, spogel, ispaghula

- **HEALTH PATTERN:** Elimination

- **PLANT DESCRIPTION:**

  Psyllium derives its name from the Greek *psylla* meaning "a flea." The ancient Greeks thought that psyllium seeds resembled fleas in some way, perhaps because of the small size of the seed or the color. *Plantago ovata* is a low-growing leafy plant native to Iran, Pakistan, and India, where it is cultivated. It produces small, white flowers. The seeds are smooth, pinkish brown ovals that range from $\frac{1}{16}$ to $\frac{1}{8}$ inch (approximately 1.5 to 3 mm) long. Each seed is enveloped in a husk that is a thin, white translucent membrane. The seeds do not have odor or taste. When soaked in water, they increase from eight to fourteen times their original size.

- **PLANT PARTS USED:** The seed and husk, a thin membranous layer on the seed coat.

- **TRADITIONAL EVIDENCE:**

  Cultural Use

  Asian. The seeds are prepared by frying them in saltwater before drying (Leung & Foster, 1996). Psyllium seed is known as *che qian zi* in Chinese. The species native to China are used to treat bloody urine, coughs, and high blood pressure and to drain damp heat, promote urination in cases of edema or painful urinary dysfunction, and for loose stools. Psyllium is used also for eye problems, such as dryness and cataracts, redness, swollen eyes, and sensitivity to light, and to treat lung disorders with copious phlegm and coughing. The entire plant is used to clear heat and toxicity. It is used both internally and externally for the reduction of abscesses and swellings (Bensky & Gamble, 1993).

  The Japanese traditionally use psyllium seed, *shazenshi,* to promote the descent of fluids in the body. This refers to the promotion of urination and the accumulation of moisture in the colon to relieve constipation. Psyllium is used in Japan much the same as in China (Rister, 1999).

  North American Indian. The Pima have used psyllium *(P. ovata)* as food and for diarrhea.

Hispanic. Hispanics in the southwestern United States primarily use plantain seed, which is known as *lanten*, not the psyllium profiled here.

East Indian. *P. ovata* seed is used in India to treat dysentery, diarrhea, urinary tract problems, digestive dysfunction, gonorrhea, and fevers. It is also used to treat coughs and colds and other respiratory complaints, especially in children. The powdered seeds are mixed with water and applied as a poultice to areas of the body affected by rheumatism, gout, and skin inflammation (Nadkarni, 1976).

European. Recent European reports have indicated the use of psyllium for habitual constipation and in cases when soft stool is desired such as anal fissures, hemorrhoids, and postrectal surgery. It has been indicated for use in irritable bowel syndrome, diverticulosis, as an adjunct to treatment for diarrhea, and in cases when an increase in dietary fiber is desired (Leung & Foster, 1996).

Culinary Use

The mucilage from the husk is used as a thickener or stabilizer in certain frozen dairy desserts (Leung & Foster, 1996). In 1989, psyllium was introduced into breakfast cereals with claims of being able to reduce cholesterol and produce health benefits associated with soluble fiber. Shortly afterward, the U.S. Food and Drug Administration declared that the products were "misbranded drugs" because of "insufficient evidence to support the labeling claims" (Leung & Foster, 1996).

Use in Herbalism

Psyllium has been used traditionally in the United States and Europe as a bulking laxative to treat the symptoms of chronic constipation. It also has been used topically as an emollient and demulcent. Psyllium is used in current herbalism for its ability to decrease bowel transit time, absorb toxins from the bowel, regulate intestinal flora, for its beneficial fiber, and its demulcent action on the digestive tract. Some recommend the use of bulk laxatives mainly for people over 50 who are sedentary and need something to stimulate the normal peristaltic action of the bowel. Psyllium also is recommended for use during chronic yeast *(Candida albicans)* infections. It is believed that psyllium can absorb the by-products of the yeast growth, thereby preventing the systemic reabsorption of the toxins (Pedersen, 1987). Psyllium also is used for the short-term treatment of diarrhea by its ability to absorb excess fluid in the intestinal tract (WHO, 1999). Various commercial preparations and over-the-counter laxatives contain psyllium, including Metamucil (G. D. Searle), Effersyllium (Stuart), Fiberall (Rydelle), and Naturacil (Mead Johnson).

✿ BIOMEDICAL EVIDENCE:

Studies Related to Elimination

One randomized, double-blind, multisite, two-week trial of 170 participants found that psyllium (Metamucil 1 teaspoon [5.1 g] twice daily) is significantly superior to docusate sodium, 100 mg twice daily, for softening stools, increasing stool water content, and decreasing discomfort associated with constipation in those with chronic idiopathic constipation. Both subjective and objective measures were assessed and subjects were instructed not to change their exercise or dietary habits during the study (McRorie et al., 1998).

A randomized, placebo-controlled study of 12 patients with Parkinson's disease demonstrated that psyllium (Metamucil 1 teaspoon [5.1 g] twice a day for four weeks) produced both objective and subjective improvements in constipation related to Parkinson's disease by increasing stool frequency and weight but not by affecting colonic transit or anorectal function (Ashraf, Pfeiffer, Park, Lof, & Quigley, 1997).

A study of 42 adults with constipation receiving either 1½ teaspoons (7.2 g) per day of psyllium alone or psyllium plus senna demonstrated a significant increase in stool frequency and stool weight that was somewhat better for the senna group. The psyllium alone laxative did not normalize bowel frequency or stool weight after one week in the chronically constipated adults. It is suggested that these results indicate that the use of psyllium-only laxatives in chronically constipated adults be used for more than one week or higher doses be used (Marlett, Li, Patrow, & Bass, 1987).

In a randomized, parallel group, twelve-month study of 102 patients with ulcerative colitis in remission who received either 10 g psyllium seed *(P. ovata)* by mouth twice a day, 1.5 g daily of mesalamine, or psyllium plus mesalamine, it was found that psyllium shows potential for being as effective as mesalamine in preventing relapse in patients with ulcerative colitis and therefore may be a viable alternative to the current treatment. According to the investigators, a larger study of 217 patients would be needed to test equivalence (Fernandez-Banares et al., 1999).

One human study of eight volunteers found that psyllium has been shown to significantly delay gastric emptying and reduce the acceleration of colon transit (Washington, Harris, Mussellwhite, & Spiller, 1998).

Studies Related to Other Health Patterns

Hormone Balance. A metanalysis of 8 studies with 384 participants who had received 2 teaspoons (10.2 g) of psyllium per day (Metamucil) for eight weeks or more demonstrated that psyllium supplementation significantly lowers serum total and low-density lipoprotein (LDL) cholesterol concentrations and ratios of serum LDL to high-density lipoprotein (HDL) cholesterol and of total cholesterol to HDL in participants consuming a low-fat diet beyond reductions achieved with diet only (Anderson et al., 2000a).

In a double-blind, placebo-controlled, parallel, multicenter trial of 163 participants who completed the study, psyllium 1 teaspoon (5.1 g) per day and dietary change were shown to reduce serum total cholesterol concentrations by approximately 5% and LDL cholesterol concentrations by 7% in adults as compared with placebo (Anderson et al., 2000b).

Mechanism of Action

In the presence of water, a plant constituent called mucilage, found in psyllium seed and husk (primarily), swells to form a slippery mass. When taken into the gastrointestinal tract, psyllium swells either because of the fluid in the gut or the fluids taken in with the psyllium. When the psyllium swells, it can cause a sense of fullness in the stomach. It ultimately becomes part of the feces. It adds bulk to the stool and keeps it hydrated and soft. The resulting bulk promotes more efficient peristalsis and evacuation of the bowel (Leung & Foster, 1996).

Psyllium's ability to decrease gastric emptying is thought to be due to its ability to increase the viscosity of the meal. More viscous meals only allow for shallower contractions associated with gastric emptying. "Psyllium may modify the response to rapidly fermentable, poorly absorbed dietary carbohydrates such as lactose, fructose, and sorbitol, which have been implicated in some studies of irritable bowel syndrome" (Washington et al., 1998, p. 320).

USE IN PREGNANCY OR LACTATION:

There are no known contraindications to the use of psyllium seed or husk during pregnancy or lactation if used within the recommended guidelines for the individual product (Blumenthal et al., 2000). One Chinese reference states that psyllium seed is contraindicated in pregnancy and the powder is used to treat malposition of the fetus at eight months of gestation (Bensky & Gamble, 1993).

Herbal Caveat—Pregnancy or Lactation

Some herbs are contraindicated in pregnancy because of a risk of the herb or one of its constituents stimulating the uterus and therefore possibly promoting fetal loss. Many herbal practitioners do not recommend herbal remedies, in particular oral doses of herbs, during the first trimester of pregnancy and seek an alternative. However, herbs are successfully used during pregnancy, especially to prepare the body for the birth. Herbs are relatively unstudied in pregnancy and lactation, so patients need to be made aware through education of the potential benefits and risks of using herbs for health conditions that arise during pregnancy or lactation. The use of herbal remedies during pregnancy often warrants a referral to a knowledgeable herbal practitioner.

USE FOR CHILDREN:

The recommended dose of psyllium for children 6 to 12 years old is half the adult dose. For children under 6 years, a health care practitioner should be consulted before using (WHO, 1999).

Herbal Caveat—Children

Children have special needs in regard to herbal therapies. They require lesser amounts of herbs and often respond well to mild teas and topical applications such as compresses and baths. The lowest dose of oral preparations should be tried first before increasing the amount given children.

Caregivers should observe children closely for responses to herbal remedies. Younger children, particularly infants, have traditionally been given herbs either through their mother's breast milk or in the form of a homeopathic remedy because of their sensitivity to medicines and treatments and the immaturity of their liver. It is recommended that a person knowledgeable in the herbal treatment of children be consulted before the offering of any herb to a child for the first time.

CAUTIONS:

A metanalysis of 19 clinical trials showed that psyllium is well tolerated in adults without serious adverse effects in oral amounts up to 4 teaspoons (20.4 g) per day (Anderson et al., 2000a). It is recommended to take psyllium seed or husk thirty minutes to one hour after taking other medications because intestinal absorption of the other medications may be delayed if taken simultaneously with psyllium seed or husk (Blumenthal et al., 2000). Insulin-dependent diabetics may need to reduce their insulin dosage while taking psyllium seed or husk (Brinker, 1998; McGuffin et al., 1997). In rare cases, allergic reactions to oral administration of psyllium seed or husk may occur (Blumenthal et al., 2000).

Psyllium seed or husk is contraindicated in cases of actual or threatened bowel obstruction, intestinal stenosis, and poor control of diabetes mellitus (Blumenthal et al., 2000; Brinker, 1998; McGuffin et al., 1997). As is common with all bulk laxatives, psyllium may temporarily increase flatulence and abdominal distention. Swallowing psyllium preparations dry may result in esophageal obstruction (Newall et al., 1996). Lots of plain water must be taken with psyllium to keep the stool moist so that the colon does not become impacted. Psyllium draws fluid from the moist mucous membranes of the gastrointestinal tract if there is not extra water in it. A patient who had been taking a psyllium powder product as part of an intestinal "cleansing" program once came into a clinic where I worked. She had abdominal pain, was admitted to the hospital, and ended up needing an appendectomy. When the surgeon opened her belly to remove the appendix, her bowel had perforated and psyllium was caked on her intestines. Part of her bowel had to be removed as well. She later admitted to not having read the label on the product and having no idea that she needed to drink lots of plain water with the psyllium. This is the only time I have seen a problem with psyllium. Elderly patients in particular should take psyllium with caution because they are often prone to dehydration.

It may be best not to chew psyllium seed. In a study in which dogs and rats were fed psyllium powder, it was found that a brownish-black pigment from the seed formed in proximal renal tubules. There was however, no associated kidney impairment (Schulz et al., 1998). The German Commission E and other authorities require a warning with psyllium products that if diarrhea persists for more than three to four days, a physician be consulted (Blumenthal et al., 2000).

To minimize the development of an allergic reaction to psyllium dust, health professionals who regularly dispense powdered psyllium seed should avoid inhaling the airborne dust while handling these products. To minimize the generation of airborne dust, the powder should be spooned directly from the container into the drinking glass and the liquid added immediately (WHO, 1999).

NURSING EVIDENCE:

Historical Nursing Use

Nurses have been administering psyllium products to patients for quite some time.

Potential Nursing Applications

When given a choice, as is done on postpartum wards for example, nurses may want to consider suggesting psyllium with the diet instead of docusate sodium to soften the stool. Cardiac rehabilitation nurses may want to consider the benefits of psyllium to decrease straining and also lower cholesterol.

Integrative Insight

Psyllium seems to be able to exhibit adaptogen action. It can regulate the fluids in the bowel, so if a person has diarrhea, psyllium helps retain fluids. Psyllium's ability to retain fluid also helps the person with constipation because the moistening, bulking action of the herb helps the person eliminate smoothly and comfortably. Although the biomedical diagnoses of diarrhea and constipation would seem to be on opposite ends of the spectrum, psyllium can work on either health concern with a similar action.

THERAPEUTIC APPLICATIONS:

Oral

Seeds: Take 5 to 10 g whole seeds three to four times daily. The seeds should be presoaked in 5 oz (150 ml) of warm water for several hours before ingestion. Each dose should be followed by drinking at least another 5 to 7 oz (150 to 210 ml) of water (Blumenthal et al., 2000).

Husk: Take 4 to 5 g of the whole seed husk one to four times daily. Stir it into 5 oz (150 ml) of water and drink immediately, followed by approximately 5 oz (150 ml) of water (Blumenthal et al., 2000).

Psyllium seed tea: Place 2 teaspoons of psyllium seed into a muslin cloth and tie securely. Put this into 1 cup (240 ml) of boiling water and steep for forty-five minutes. Remove the cloth and drink the tea while still warm (Rister, 1999).

Topical

Some cultures use a poultice of powdered psyllium seed mixed with water for skin irritations.

Environmental

None known.

Herbal Caveat—Therapeutic Applications

In traditional and conventional herbal medicine, amounts of herbs given to patients are based on individual needs. The amounts or "doses" recorded here are provided so that the health practitioner has a general idea of the amounts recommended for an adult patient. Dosing in herbalism not only refers to amount of plant used but also includes when, where, and how to take a plant medicine. These dosages should not be used as guidelines for indiscriminate intervention without proper assessment, critical thinking, and patient education on the part of the practitioner.

Note: Please see chapter 5 for detailed descriptions of how to prepare various applications.

PATIENT INTERACTION:

Through years of use, psyllium has been shown to be an excellent stool softener and bulking laxative, helpful for discomfort associated with constipation, irritable bowel, and ulcerative colitis. It also has been used traditionally for diarrhea and dysentery. Because psyllium can slow stomach emptying, be sure that you do not take your psyllium with other medications because it may affect your body's absorption of the other drugs. Although studies have shown this herb to be quite safe, even for long-term use, it is very important to drink adequate amounts of plain water (not juice or other liquids) with psyllium. Most people don't drink enough plain water anyway, so they must be extra careful when using psyllium.

Herbal Caveat—Patient Interaction

Patients considering the use of an herb or formula of herbs in self-care benefit from education about the plant itself and the use of the plant in healing. This education can come through many sources, including local herbalists; plant specialists such as botanists; health practitioners such as nurses, nutritionists, naturopaths, and other physicians; and various written references including the scientific literature. Patients need to remember that their unique health care needs are not necessarily represented in any literature they may encounter. Therefore, it is recommended that a knowledgeable mentor be consulted before initiating self-care with any herb being used for the first time.

NURTURING THE NURSE-PLANT RELATIONSHIP:

Note: You may want to keep a journal of your experiences with the herb.

To get to know psyllium, experience its slipperiness. Put two tablespoons (30 g) of psyllium powder in a bowl with one cup (240 ml) of tepid water and stir immediately. Let it sit. Then take the same amounts of water and psyllium and put them in a glass. Drink immediately after stirring and then drink another cup of plain water. Touch the psyllium in the bowl after a few minutes and experience the slipperiness of the mucilage from the seed and husk. Take psyllium internally for a few days and see if and how your elimination pattern changes!

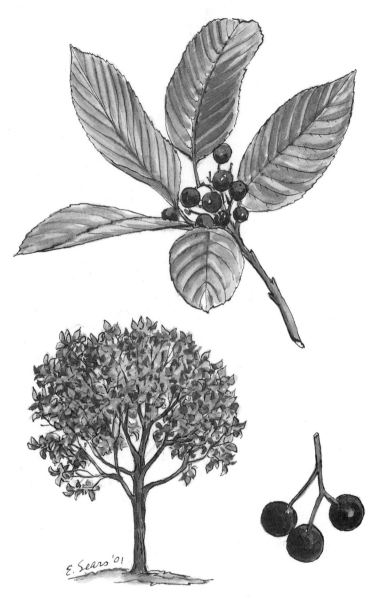

Cascara sagrada

CHAPTER 12

Cascara Sagrada

🍃 **LATIN NAMES:** *Frangula purshiana, Rhamnus purshiana*

🍃 **FAMILY:** Rhamnaceae

🍃 **COMMON NAMES:** Cascara sagrada, cascara, chittem bark, sacred bark, California buckthorn

🍃 **HEALTH PATTERN:** Elimination

🍃 **PLANT DESCRIPTION:**

Cascara sagrada is a tree that is native to the forests of the North American Pacific coast. It can be found from northern California to British Columbia and almost to the Alaskan panhandle. It prefers growing in moist areas below 1500 meters (4,500 feet) elevation. The tree also may be found in the Rocky Mountains in Idaho and Montana. The leaves, which have toothed edges, are from 3 to 5 inches (7.5 to 15 cm) long and about half as broad. When young, they are covered with fine hairs on the undersurface. As the tree ages, the leaves become bright green. Small, white clustered flowers appear after the leaves mature. The fruit is like a pea-sized black berry and is called a drupe (Felter & Lloyd, 1986).

🍃 **PLANT PART USED:** Aged, dried bark

🍃 **TRADITIONAL EVIDENCE:**

Cultural Use

North American Indian. North American Indians of the northwest coast used cascara sagrada and passed its use on to the settlers. A Spanish priest was so impressed with it that he christened it with a Spanish name that signifies "holy bark" (Vogel, 1970). Numerous North American Indian tribes in the Northwest use cascara bark as a laxative in various forms, including water decoctions and infusions, a cold macerate, and chewing the bark directly (Blumenthal et al., 2000).

East Indian. Several species of cascara sagrada have been used in Ayurvedic medicine. They have been used in treatments for the spleen, as an emetic and purgative, tonic, and astringent (Nadkarni, 1976).

European. The German Commission E approves the use of cascara sagrada bark for the treatment of constipation (Blumenthal et al., 2000). Germany has licensed the use of cascara bark tea for constipation and all disorders in which soft stools and easy evacuation are desired, such as in anal fissures, hemorrhoids, and following anorectal surgery. The British Herbal Pharmacopoeia recommends the use of cascara for similar conditions (Blumenthal et al., 2000).

Culinary Use

Only the bitterless extract of cascara is used as a flavor component in foods, beverages, frozen dairy desserts, candy, and baked goods (Leung & Foster, 1996).

Use in Herbalism

Cascara sagrada bark was introduced in 1877 into the United States by an eclectic physician, Dr. J. H. Bundy. Parke, Davis & Company created a fluid extract that became popular with the medical profession. It was used in cases of chronic constipation due to lack of intestinal tone (nervous or muscular) and some cases of indigestion. Cascara sagrada has been used to tone the entire intestinal tract. Ten drops of the fluid extract was often recommended after meals. Larger doses were used for certain types of headaches. Cascara also was used for hemorrhoids with loss of muscular tone of the rectum. The extract also has been used for rheumatism. It was sometimes used for diarrhea; jaundice; and problems of the liver, duodenum, and stomach (Felter & Lloyd, 1983).

Currently, cascara is used in commercial laxative preparations. It also is used in sunscreens. The crude aged bark is used in teas, capsules, tablets, and drinks (Leung & Foster, 1996). Cascara is often found in combination with other herbs to promote peristalsis, act as a purgative, and increase the flow of bile. Cascara is used to treat constipation, dyspepsia, liver congestion, gallstones, jaundice, intestinal parasites, and hemorrhoids (Pedersen, 1987).

BIOMEDICAL EVIDENCE:

Although cascara sagrada has been used for constipation for many years, little, if any, research on the herb has been published. Some studies have been conducted comparing the effectiveness of cascara and other laxatives in the preparation of patients for colonoscopy (Borkje, Pedersen, Lund, Enehaug, & Berstad, 1991; Hangartner, Munch, Meier, Ammann, & Buhler, 1989). Unfortunately, the studies were designed so that cascara was used only in conjunction with Golytely and not given by itself, making it difficult to estimate the effects of the cascara sagrada. More research on the laxative and possible purgative effects of cascara sagrada is needed.

Studies Related to Elimination

According to one British review of the literature on the effectiveness of laxatives with the elderly, few "good" comparative studies have been carried out regarding the main laxatives, including cascara, bran, psyllium, prucara, dioctyl sodium, lactulose, and lactitol. Based upon the review, Petticrew, Watt, and Sheldon (1997) recommend beginning care of constipation in the elderly with advice about dietary changes followed by "inexpensive" laxatives. They report that although they are used more often, there is "no evidence that expensive danthron laxatives are more effective than other laxative preparations and that further research comparing the different classes of laxatives is required" (p. iv).

Studies Related to Other Health Patterns
No data are available at this time.

Mechanism of Action
Many cascara sagrada species share the same anthraquinone derivative constituents that provide the laxative action (Blumenthal et al., 2000). Anthrone C-glycosides, the laxative constituents present in cascara, pass through the gastrointestinal tract unabsorbed after ingestion until they reach the colon where they are broken down by the colon's bacterial microflora. The anthrone exerts its action on the lining of the colon by affecting secretion and absorption and by increasing motility. It is not completely understood whether or not the bacterial reduction in the colon is necessary for the laxative effect to occur (deWitte & Lemli, 1990). The German Commission E states that the 1,8 dihydroxy-anthracene derivatives in cascara sagrada bark have a laxative effect because of their influence on the colon's motility. They inhibit stationary and stimulate propulsive contractions, resulting in accelerated intestinal passage and, therefore, a reduction in the absorption of liquid in the intestines (Blumenthal et al., 2000).

USE IN PREGNANCY OR LACTATION:
Cascara sagrada should not be used during pregnancy and lactation (McGuffin et al., 1997) because laxative effects can stimulate the uterus. One source states that the laxative-promoting constituents in cascara have been found to pass into breast milk, and it should not be used by nursing mothers because of the possibility of causing diarrhea with loss of water and electrolytes in the infant (Brinker, 1998). Another source reports that there have been only two reports of increased amounts of diarrhea in nursing infants whose mothers were given cascara sagrada. The American Academy of Pediatrics lists cascara as compatible with breastfeeding, but it may be better for lactating women to consider increasing the fiber in their diet and taking bulk-forming laxatives such as psyllium to help ease symptoms of constipation because bulking laxatives are not absorbed the way cascara is (Hagemann, 1998).

Herbal Caveat—Pregnancy or Lactation
Some herbs are contraindicated in pregnancy because of a risk of the herb or one of its constituents stimulating the uterus and therefore possibly promoting fetal loss. Many herbal practitioners do not recommend herbal remedies, in particular oral doses of herbs, during the first trimester of pregnancy and seek an alternative. However, herbs are successfully used during pregnancy, especially to prepare the body for the birth. Herbs are

relatively unstudied in pregnancy and lactation, so patients need to be made aware through education of the potential benefits and risks of using herbs for health conditions that arise during pregnancy or lactation. The use of herbal remedies during pregnancy often warrants a referral to a knowledgeable herbal practitioner.

USE FOR CHILDREN:

Possible causes of constipation in young children include poor quality food, bad eating habits, suppression of defecation reflex while at school or traveling, fear of pain if anal tears are present, and psychosomatic factors. Steps should be taken to determine the cause and increase dietary fiber before stimulant laxatives are used (Schilcher, 1992). The use of cascara is not recommended for children under 12 years of age (Blumenthal et al., 2000; McGuffin et al., 1997).

Herbal Caveat—Children

Children have special needs in regard to herbal therapies. They require lesser amounts of herbs and often respond well to mild teas and topical applications such as compresses and baths. The lowest dose of oral preparations should be tried first before increasing the amount given children. Caregivers should observe children closely for responses to herbal remedies. Younger children, particularly infants, have traditionally been given herbs either through their mother's breast milk or in the form of a homeopathic remedy because of their sensitivity to medicines and treatments and the immaturity of their liver. It is recommended that a person knowledgeable in the herbal treatment of children be consulted before the offering of any herb to a child for the first time.

CAUTIONS:

Most herbal clinicians suggest that cascara only be used if the desired effects cannot be obtained through dietary changes or the use of gentler bulk-forming laxatives. Laxatives, such as cascara, that act by stimulating the muscles of the intestinal tract should not be used over an extended period of time (one to two weeks) without supervision of a health practitioner. Extended use can result in chronic intestinal sluggishness and dependence.

The use of cascara is contraindicated in those with intestinal obstruction such as Crohn's disease, ulcerative colitis, appendicitis, and abdominal pain of unknown origin (Blumenthal et al., 2000; McGuffin et al., 2000). It is also contraindicated in individuals who are generally debilitated because of the possibility of loss of water and electrolytes (Brinker, 1998) and those who are known to abuse laxatives, such as those who have eating disorders.

The fresh bark contains a substance known as *"free anthrone,"* which may cause severe vomiting and gastrointestinal cramps. The fresh bark must be stored for one year or artificially aged by heat and aeration for the free anthrone to dissipate (Blumenthal et al., 2000). Long-term use or abuse of cascara can cause disturbances of electrolyte balance, especially potassium deficiency, that can lead to disorders of heart function and muscular weakness. This is of particular concern in those individuals who are also using cardiac glycosides, diuretics, corticosteroids, or licorice root. Potassium loss may result in an increased effectiveness of cardiac glycosides. Potassium deficiency can be made worse by the simultaneous application of thiazide diuretics, corticosteroids, or licorice root. Long-term use of cascara can also lead to albuminuria and hematuria. Cascara can sometimes cause harmless pigmentation of the intestinal mucosa that reverses upon discontinuation of the preparation (Blumenthal et al., 2000).

NURSING EVIDENCE:

Historical Nursing Use

Nurses have historically administered cascara sagrada to patients for short-term use.

Potential Nursing Applications

Cascara has potential for use in clinical nursing practice at times when a strong bowel purgative is necessary, such as when preparing the bowel for colonoscopy.

Integrative Insight

Cascara is a strong purgative herb that is not meant for everyday use. It is a stimulating laxative that also tones the intestinal tract. A nurse's best advice for patients is to have them try dietary and lifestyle changes first such as increasing mild exercise, water, and fiber in the diet. Both traditional and biomedical data point to saving cascara as a last resort and using bulking agents such as psyllium first in addition to diet and lifestyle changes.

THERAPEUTIC APPLICATIONS:

Oral

Bark (Must be dried and aged, not fresh): 0.3 to 1.0 g as a single daily dose.

Infusion: Steep 1 to 2 g of bark in 5 oz (150 ml) boiled water for ten to fifteen minutes.

Cold macerate: Steep 1 to 2 g of bark in 5 oz (150 ml) of cold water for several hours, then boil and strain. (Extraction with boiling water can prevent some of the chemical changes that occur during cold water maceration. Ninety percent of the hydroxyanthracenes in cascara sagrada are released after six hours in cold maceration [Blumenthal et al., 2000].)

Elixir: approximately ¼ teaspoon (1 to 2 ml) of the flavored and sweetened alcoholic fluid extract.

Fluid extract 1:1 (g/ml): approximately ¼ teaspoon (1 to 2 ml).

Tincture 1:5 (g/ml): ½ to ⅔ teaspoon (2 to 4 ml).

Topical

Not used topically.

Environmental

Not used environmentally.

Herbal Caveat—Therapeutic Applications

In traditional and conventional herbal medicine, amounts of herbs given to patients are based on individual needs. The amounts or "doses" recorded here are provided so that the health practitioner has a general idea of the amounts recommended for an adult patient. Dosing in herbalism not only refers to amount of plant used but also includes when, where, and how to take a plant medicine. These dosages should not be used as guidelines for indiscriminate intervention without proper assessment, critical thinking, and patient education on the part of the practitioner.

Note: Please see chapter 5 for detailed descriptions of how to prepare various applications.

PATIENT INTERACTION:

Cascara is a strong laxative herb that should be used under the guidance of a health practitioner. For occasional constipation or discomfort related to elimination, try increasing the amount of time you spend exercising and your water and fiber intake, try other gentler herbs such as psyllium next, and save cascara as a last resort.

Herbal Caveat—Patient Interaction

Patients considering the use of an herb or formula of herbs in self-care benefit from education about the plant itself and the use of the plant in healing. This education can come through many sources, including local herbalists; plant specialists such as botanists; health practitioners such as nurses, nutritionists, naturopaths, and other physicians; and various written references including the scientific literature. Patients need to remember that their unique health care needs are not necessarily represented in any literature they may encounter. Therefore, it is recommended that a knowledgeable mentor be consulted before initiating self-care with any herb being used for the first time.

NURTURING THE NURSE-PLANT RELATIONSHIP:

Note: You may want to keep a journal of your experiences with the herb.

Cascara is strong medicine. It has a strong purgative action on the intestines and therefore is not recommended for casual use. Nurses have given cascara as a laxative over the years but now recognize, as have other health practitioners, that constipation is best addressed by a "stepped-care" approach, the first step being to change the diet and include regular walking. Nurses too can benefit from regular habits, which lead to regular elimination cycles. You can try a small amount of cascara tea to experience its taste. Also try increasing the fiber in your diet. Eat a bran muffin rather than a piece of white bread for breakfast. Once a week, try eating a plate of steamed vegetables with some drops of dark sesame oil, fresh lemon juice, and a little sea salt. Food does not have to be raw to increase fiber in the diet and if digestion and elimination are sluggish, cold raw foods are not necessarily recommended. As for walking, nurses who work in the community or in a hospital ward often do lots of that, but it is still best to do some walking that is solely for improving your health.

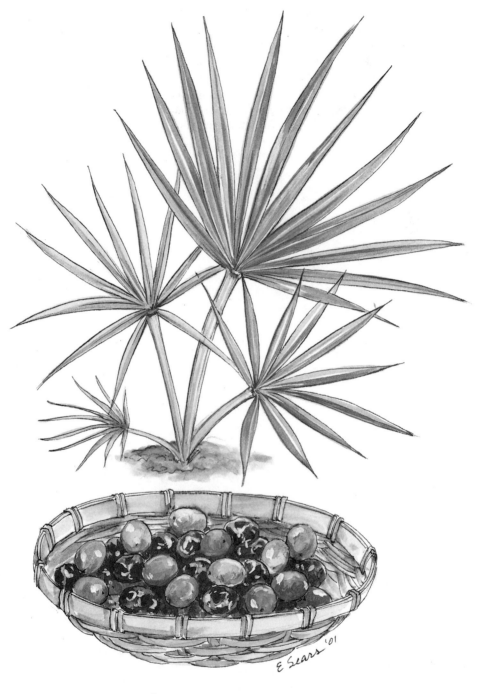

Serenoa repens

SAW PALMETTO

🌿 **LATIN NAMES:** *Serenoa repens, Sabal serrulata*

🌿 **FAMILY:** Arecaceae

🌿 **COMMON NAMES:** Saw palmetto, sabal, sawtooth palm, windmill palm, fan palm, scrub-palmetto

🌿 **HEALTH PATTERN:** Elimination

🌿 **PLANT DESCRIPTION:**

Saw palmetto is a small, low-growing palm tree that is native to Southeastern North America, particularly Florida and South Carolina. The stems that support the leaves have spiny teeth. The leaves, which are from 2 to 4 feet (approximately 1 meter) high, have a somewhat circular palm-shaped outline. They are bright green and composed of many slender lance-shaped divisions that fan out from a single point. The ripe fruit is olivelike, blackish-brown, about ½ to 1 inch (1.5 to 2.5 cm) long and half as wide, with a single seed inside. A single branch cluster may yield from 6 to 8 pounds (2700 to 3600 g) of the berries as they ripen from September through December (Felter & Lloyd, 1983; Leung & Foster, 1996). The berries, known as "drupes," are sheltered inside the thick foliage on small stems attached to the trunk. The hard saw teeth for which the plant is named run along the petiole, or leaf stalk, making collection of the protected berries very dangerous and difficult. The hardy, compact saw palmetto is very fire resistant, and it often grows in areas that are naturally prone to fire. Saw palmetto is considered a cash crop now in Florida. In 1998, the yield of dried berries was approximately 2000 tons, worth $50 million to the growers (Marks & Tyler, 1999).

🌿 **PLANT PART USED:** Ripe, dried, or fresh saw palmetto berry.

🌿 **TRADITIONAL EVIDENCE:**

Cultural Use

North American Indian. The Seminole Indians of the Southeastern United States use saw palmetto berries as a food source. They make baskets, brushes, and rope from the leaf stems. They also use the plant to make fish drags, fire fans, dolls, dance fans, rattles, and flint punk. The Choctaw use the stem in basketry (Moerman, 1998).

Hispanic. Saw palmetto attracts bees and makes a very good honey. The berry is sometimes mixed with Mexican damiana to make an aphrodisiac. Saw palmetto is considered when impotence is a concern, and it is widely used in Latin countries for the treatment of enlarged prostate (Grasso et al., 1995). The Mayans made an infusion of the leaves and roots and a decoction from the interior of the trunk of a species related to saw palmetto. This was given for dysentery and abdominal pain. A remedy for snake and insect bites and for skin ulcers was obtained from the interior of the trunk. The crushed root was applied to skin sores (Vogel, 1970).

European. The German Commission E has approved the internal use of saw palmetto berry for urination problems associated with benign prostatic hyperplasia (BPH) stages I and II (Blumenthal et al., 2000). Saw palmetto extracts are widely recommended by urologists in France, Germany, and Italy for the supportive treatment of BPH (Foster & Tyler, 1999). Ninety percent of prescriptions written for BPH in Europe are written for herbal medicines including saw palmetto (McPartland & Pruitt, 2000).

Culinary Use

North American Indians historically used saw palmetto berries as a food source, and early European settlers used them as a survival food (Leung & Foster, 1996). Because they have a rather disagreeable, soapy taste, the berries are not used currently as a commercial food item (Wren, 1988), but extracts of the berries are used as an aromatic ingredient in cognac (Duke, 1985).

Use in Herbalism

Saw palmetto has been used in many ways, such as in the making of thatched huts, mattresses, straw hats, and paper. Animals are said to enjoy the berries and to become fat when eating them. The berries have been used in herbalism as a nutritive tonic and expectorant. They also have been used to treat irritation of mucous membranes, coughing, bronchitis, whooping cough, laryngitis, asthma, and conditions associated with tuberculosis. Saw palmetto was recommended for use in conditions of wasting, or weight loss with fatigue, because it was believed to help weight gain and the improvement of strength. It was considered to be very nutritive (Duke, 1985).

The most pronounced effects of saw palmetto seem to occur with the reproductive tracts of both males and females and with the urinary tract symptoms that occur in men with BPH. Saw palmetto berries have diuretic, sedative, antiandrogenic, anti-inflammatory, antiexudative, and both antiestrogenic and estrogenic effects (Leung & Foster, 1996). Saw palmetto has been used to restore the sexual appetite and has been known to enlarge wasted organs such as the breasts, ovaries, and testicles with continued use (Felter & Lloyd, 1983) and to reduce pathologic enlargement of the prostate. Some find that the berries help relieve prostatic irritation and give tone to the gland rather than actually reducing hypertrophy. Saw palmetto relieves the aching, dull, throbbing pain in the prostate and reduces irritation associated with gonorrhea. Saw palmetto berries are used for the symptoms associated with BPH, such as hesitancy in initiation of the urinary stream, dribbling, urinary urgency, pressure over the bladder, and incomplete emptying of the bladder. Saw palmetto often is used in combination with other herbs such as stinging nettle for the relief of lower urinary tract discomfort.

Saw palmetto is also used in women with polycystic ovaries, pain related to ovarian cysts, and mittelschmerz. Master herbalist David Winston recommends using saw palmetto in combination with other herbs for polycystic ovary: chaste tree *(Vitex agnus-castus)*, dandelion root *(Taraxacum officinale)*, or Oregon grape root *(Berberis vulgaris)*; and for ovarian cysts and mittelschmerz he recommends using saw palmetto in combination with: chaste tree, corydalis *(Corydalis yanhusuo)*, and dan shen *(Salvia miltiorrhiza)* (Winston, 1999).

BIOMEDICAL EVIDENCE:

Most, if not all of the clinical trials on the use of saw palmetto are related to the effects of a standardized extract of the berries on the prostate and related urinary tract symptoms. Some literature states that saw palmetto has not had significant effects on prostate volume, while numerous other studies show that saw palmetto does decrease prostate volume. Some of these favorable studies do have limitations that need to be taken into consideration in clinical decision making.

Studies Related to Elimination

In a ninety-day open trial of 305 patients with mild-to-moderate symptoms of prostatic hyperplasia who fulfilled specific inclusion criteria, a 160 mg twice daily oral dose of saw palmetto extract, Prostaserene, improved symptoms such as urinary flow rates, residual urinary volumes, quality of life, and prostate size in 88% of patients. The prostate-specific antigen (PSA) was not altered by saw palmetto. Other medications, such as Proscar, which do reduce the PSA level, can run the risk of masking the development of prostate cancer during treatment (Braeckman, 1994).

Results of a multicenter, double-blind, placebo-controlled study of 44 men with BPH show that participants taking saw palmetto for six months (form and dose not reported), had a reduction in the size of epithelial tissue particularly in the transition zone from 17.8% to 10.7% as compared with controls that had no reduction (Overmyer, 1999).

In a study of 42 patients with BPH who received a saw palmetto extract called Strogen forte for twelve months, 68.4% experienced a decrease in night urination, 74.7% felt no residue, and 80% had no subjective complaints such as hesitancy or dribbling. Subjective complaints were 50% improved in the men after three months. Measurements of residual urine showed a decrease from an average of 62.8 ml to 35.1 ml after three months and 12.3 ml after twelve months. There were no adverse effects (Romics, Schmitz, & Frang, 1993).

In another placebo-controlled, double-blind trial of 94 outpatients with BPH given oral doses of 320 mg per day of a saw palmetto extract called Permixon, those who received the extract demonstrated significant improvement in objective and subjective lower urinary tract symptoms after thirty days of treatment. There were five reports of minor side effects such as headache from the standardized extract (Champault, Patel, & Bonnard, 1984).

A metanalysis of thirteen clinical trials on Permixon only demonstrated its highly significant effect over placebo in the treatment of symptoms related to BPH. "Despite limitations in the information provided by some clinical trials and the need for caution in interpreting their findings, there appears to be strong evidence that the use of Permixon increases the Qmax rate (peak urinary flow) in a consistent manner across studies" (Boyle, Robertson, Lowe, & Roehrborn, 2000, p. 538).

In a clinical trial that included 1098 participants with moderate BPH, saw palmetto extract (Permixon 320 mg) was comparable to 5 mg finasteride (Propecia) in decreasing lower urinary tract symptoms in men without affecting PSA levels or causing the untoward side effects, such as erectile dysfunction and altered libido, associated with the drug. Unlike, finasteride, the saw palmetto extract had little effect on prostate volume (Carraro et al., 1996).

In a prospective open-label six-month trial of 50 men with BPH who took saw palmetto, 160 mg capsules orally twice a day, there was a significant difference in subjective observation of symptoms as measured with the International Prostate Symptom Score but there was no significant difference with objective measures. These results need to be evaluated in light of the fact that the men knew they were receiving saw palmetto (Gerber, Zagaja, Bales, Chodak, & Contreras, 1998).

Saw palmetto 160 mg twice a day was compared with the selective alpha-blocker Alfuzosin, 2.5 mg three times per day, over the course of three weeks. Alfuzosin was found to be superior to saw palmetto in improving symptoms related to BPH (Grasso et al., 1995). Alfuzosin blocks alpha-receptors in the muscle of the prostate gland, which causes the muscle in the prostate to relax. This allows urine to flow freely past the prostate and relieves the urinary symptoms. Alfuzosin does not shrink the prostate. The study fails to mention the differences between potential side effects. Although no side effects were noticed in the three weeks of the study, alfuzosin has been known to cause headache; dry mouth; postural hypotension; drowsiness; diarrhea, constipation, nausea, vomiting, or abdominal pain; flushing; edema; chest pain; tachycardia; syncope; vertigo; and dizziness (www.netdoctor.co.uk/medicines/showpreparation.asp?id=4297, December 20, 2000). Aside from occasional gastrointestinal upset, side effects related to the oral intake of saw palmetto have not been reported (Marks & Tyler, 1999).

Studies Related to Other Health Patterns

Hormone Balance. See previously cited studies because the elimination studies in BPH patients also address the hormonal effects of saw palmetto on the prostate.

Mechanism of Action

The German Commission E states that saw palmetto only relieves the symptoms associated with an enlarged prostate; it does not reduce the enlargement (Blumenthal et al., 2000); however, some studies including one (open) study of 305 patients found that prostatic volume decreased significantly (by 10% as measured by transrectal echography, $p < .0001$) after ninety days on a treatment of saw palmetto extract (Prostaserene) 160 mg twice daily (Braeckman, 1994).

It has been suggested that saw palmetto's (and other extracts derived from saw palmetto such as Permixon) ability to reduce uncomfortable symptoms of the lower urinary tract related to BPH may be due to its ability to inhibit 5 alpha-reductase, an enzyme that converts testosterone to dihydrotestosterone, the compound that causes prostate cells to multiply excessively. However, this hypothesis is derived from in vitro data, and animal and human studies since have shown that there is no apparent effect on 5 alpha-reductase. New research has demonstrated alpha-1 adrenoceptor antagonism in vitro, but in vivo studies are necessary (Brinker, 1993/1994; Goepel, Hecker, Krege, Rubben, & Michel, 1999; Bayne, Donnelly, Ross, & Habib, 1999).

The antiestrogenic activity of saw palmetto in prostate tissue was demonstrated in a study of 35 patients with untreated BPH. It is hypothesized that one or more fractions of saw palmetto extract are able to "block by competition the translocation of estrogen receptors (cytosolic) to the nuclei" (DiSilverio, 1992, p. 313).

USE IN PREGNANCY OR LACTATION:

There are no known restrictions to the oral intake of saw palmetto during pregnancy and lactation (Blumenthal et al., 2000; McGuffin et al., 1997).

Herbal Caveat—Pregnancy or Lactation

Some herbs are contraindicated in pregnancy because of a risk of the herb or one of its constituents stimulating the uterus and therefore possibly promoting fetal loss. Many herbal practitioners do not recommend herbal remedies, in particular oral doses of herbs, during the first trimester of pregnancy and seek an alternative. However, herbs are successfully used during pregnancy, especially to prepare the body for the birth. Herbs are relatively unstudied in pregnancy and lactation, so patients need to be made aware through education of the potential benefits and risks of using herbs for health conditions that arise during pregnancy or lactation. The use of herbal remedies during pregnancy often warrants a referral to a knowledgeable herbal practitioner.

USE FOR CHILDREN:

Saw palmetto has been used traditionally for those who are poorly nourished and anorexic. Although there are no studies in teens, saw palmetto might be considered in those children with anorexia.

Herbal Caveat—Children

Children have special needs in regard to herbal therapies. They require lesser amounts of herbs and often respond well to mild teas and topical applications such as compresses and baths. The lowest dose of oral preparations should be tried first before increasing the amount given children. Caregivers should observe children closely for responses to herbal remedies. Younger children, particularly infants, have traditionally been given herbs either through their mother's breast milk or in the form of a homeopathic remedy because of their sensitivity to medicines and treatments and the immaturity of their liver. It is recommended that a person knowledgeable in the herbal treatment of children be consulted before the offering of any herb to a child for the first time.

CAUTIONS:

Side effects of stomach problems occur rarely with oral intake of saw palmetto (Blumenthal et al., 2000; McGuffin et al., 1997). Although finasteride (Propecia), which has similar results to saw palmetto in the relief of symptoms related to BPH, also is used in the medical treatment of hair loss, saw palmetto has not been shown to be beneficial for hair loss (Foster & Tyler, 1999).

Although some men notice relief of BPH-related symptoms after one month of taking saw palmetto, saw palmetto preparations must often be taken consistently for up to ninety days before improvement in the symptoms of enlarged prostate are noticed (McCaleb et al., 2000). There are no known contraindications or herb/drug interactions associated with saw palmetto (Blumenthal et al., 2000).

NURSING EVIDENCE:

Historical Nursing Use

No data are available at this time.

Potential Nursing Applications

Given the number of older men experiencing symptoms associated with enlarged prostate, nurses may want to explore the possibility of recommending the use of saw palmetto. Nurses also might want to explore the possibility of researching the prophylactic use of saw palmetto. Because its history demonstrates that saw palmetto has been eaten as a staple food, it might be interesting to look at the possibility of incorporating it into men's diets once a year for a certain period when it is in season to keep the size of the prostate gland in check. Perhaps saw palmetto supplements also could be added to the diet as is done with cranberry juice when the first symptoms of urinary discomfort arise. Tea can be used also, but it does not taste very good.

Nurses may also want to explore the use of Saw palmetto supplements in anorexic teens, women with ovarian pain, and polycystic ovaries.

Integrative Insight

Saw palmetto seems to have the ability to regulate the smooth flow of urine and increase comfort related to healthy urinary elimination. Regardless of its mechanism of action, saw palmetto has an extensive history, both traditionally and biomedically, of relieving discomfort associated with BPH. BPH is the most common urologic disorder affecting males over 40 years of age. It is present in more than 90% of men over the age of 65; however, only about 50% of men develop symptoms (Schulz et al., 1998). Stage I of BPH is associated with an increased frequency of urination, nocturia, delayed onset of urination stream, and weak urinary stream. Stage II BPH is associated with the beginning of the decompensation of the bladder function accompanied by formation of residual urine and urge to urinate. Saw palmetto relieves symptoms without interfering with the standard blood test for prostate cancer, the PSA test (McCaleb et al., 2000).

Saw palmetto has been shown to be an effective alternative to drug therapy for BPH, especially in those patients who are worried about serious adverse effects of drugs such as erectile dysfunction and hypotension. Saw palmetto standardized extracts usually cost about $15 to $45 per month compared with $45 to $85 for pharmaceutical therapy (Consumer Reports, 2000), and men often have symptomatic relief within three months of starting to take the herb. It would be interesting to study men with BPH who use saw palmetto that is not a standardized extract. The cost would be further reduced. Saw palmetto products have other ingredients in them such as pygeum or pumpkin seed, but single preparations are available.

When eaten, saw palmetto has been known to help those who exhibit wasting to put on weight and grow. If in future studies saw palmetto is found conclusively to shrink prostate tissue even though its signature is also to help promote growth, this would be another example of an herb with an adaptogen action, the ability to provide the body with whatever it needs for greater balance.

THERAPEUTIC APPLICATIONS:

Oral

Note: Saw palmetto is much less effective as a tea because the active ingredients are not water soluble; they are fat soluble (Foster & Tyler, 1999). They also do not taste very good.

Decoction: Use Approximately 0.5 to 1.0 g of dried berries three times daily (Newall et al., 1996).

Fluid extract 1:1 (g/ml): Take approximately 1 to 2 ml twice daily.

Fluid extract 1:2 (g/ml): Take 2 to 4 ml twice daily.

Soft native extract 10:1 to 14:1 (w/w) (contains about 85% to 95% fatty acids): Take 160 mg twice daily.

Dry normalized extract 4:1 (w/w) (contains about 25% fatty acids): Take 400 mg twice daily (Blumenthal et al., 2000).

Standardized extract: Take 160 mg twice daily, or 320 mg once daily (standardized to 85% to 95% fatty acids and sterols) (McCaleb et al., 2000).

Capsules/tablets: Take one 585 mg capsule or tablet up to three times daily (McCaleb et al., 2000).

Topical

The crushed root of saw palmetto can be applied to sores on the skin.

Environmental

This plant is very strong and has been used in the making of thatched huts, mattresses, and paper. Because of the increasing demand for the berry, major areas of production such as Florida in the United States have become cautious about the strain the demand places on plant populations and the balance within the ecosystem and have become protective of the crops.

Herbal Caveat—Therapeutic Applications

In traditional and conventional herbal medicine, amounts of herbs given to patients are based on individual needs. The amounts or "doses" recorded here are provided so that the health practitioner has a general idea of the amounts recommended for an adult patient. Dosing in herbalism not only refers to amount of plant used but also includes when, where, and how to take a plant medicine. These dosages should not be used as guidelines for indiscriminate intervention without proper assessment, critical thinking, and patient education on the part of the practitioner.

Note: Please see chapter 5 for detailed descriptions of how to prepare various applications.

PATIENT INTERACTION:

BPH is the most common urologic disorder affecting males over 40 years of age. It is present in more than 90% of men over the age of 65. However, only about 50% of men develop symptoms. Symptoms of BPH include increased frequency of urination, waking at night to urinate, delayed onset of urination stream, and weak urinary stream. A yearly digital prostate examination to check for enlargement of the prostate is recommended, especially if symptoms are noticed. If the prostate is enlarged, a blood test (PSA) is often performed as part of the examination.

BPH is often treated with surgery, but conservative treatment for this condition can be instituted with a change in daily habits. The bladder should be emptied as soon as the urge to void is noticed, to help reduce congestion and irritation. Overdistending the bladder should be avoided by not drinking large amounts of fluids very quickly. Excessive cold and prolonged sitting should be avoided also. Regular bowel habits and ample physical exercise are encouraged. Adrenomimetic drugs, such as ephedrine and phenylephrine in cold and flu preparations, and antihistamines and anticholinergics can exacerbate voiding difficulties, so these should be avoided.

Good prostate health can be threatened by the hormone dihydrotestosterone (DHT). DHT is converted from the male hormone testosterone in the prostate, particularly in men over 50. One of the effects of DHT is to cause prostate cells to multiply, which induces the prostate to become larger. It is thought that saw palmetto inhibits the conversion of testosterone into DHT in the prostate. Saw palmetto is often used by men for self-care when their prostate condition is not serious, when, for example, the physician says, "Let's watch and wait and see how it is in a few months." Saw palmetto can be taken as a standardized extract in capsules 160 mg twice a day. Most studies have shown that discomfort begins to subside within one to three months. Saw palmetto does not interfere with the results of a PSA test. If a patient's symptoms become worse or do not begin to resolve, be sure the patient considers speaking to his physician.

Although saw palmetto has been in the media for its effects on men's reproductive and urinary health, it also has a history of use in women. It is used to relieve pain related to ovarian conditions.

Herbal Caveat—Patient Interaction

Patients considering the use of an herb or formula of herbs in self-care benefit from education about the plant itself and the use of the plant in healing. This education can come through many sources, including local herbalists; plant specialists such as botanists; health practitioners such as nurses, nutritionists, naturopaths, and other physicians; and various written references including the scientific literature. Patients need to remember that their unique health care needs are not necessarily represented in any literature they may encounter. Therefore, it is recommended that a knowledgeable mentor be consulted before initiating self-care with any herb being used for the first time.

NURTURING THE NURSE-PLANT RELATIONSHIP:

Note: You may want to keep a journal of your experiences with the herb.

The berries of the saw palmetto plant produce a juice that is deemed by some "grazers" to be the worst tasting and worst smelling herb ever. Some people really like it. If you live in the southeastern United States and have access to someone who can give you some berries, you can try it for yourself. For this experiment, however, no tasting is involved. Shopping for saw palmetto is a good opportunity to experience what it is like to shop for herbs and herb products.

If you have access to the Internet, start by going to a website that has a search engine, such as www.frontierherbs.com. Type in "saw palmetto" and hit "enter." You will see a list of products and then a list of informational pieces on saw palmetto. Notice that saw palmetto may be sold in bulk as a whole herb, in capsules, in formula, and in potpourri. Take a few minutes and read the information entries about saw palmetto.

Next, go to a health food store or apothecary that carries herbal products. Ask the clerk or nutritionist to see all the saw palmetto products. Sometimes I have seen more than twenty different products that include saw palmetto in the ingredient list. Review the sections in chapters 4 and 5 on standardized extracts, and go to the store and read the labels of the saw palmetto products to determine which are standardized. Using the information on standardized herbal products from chapters 4 and 5 as a guide, see how many herbal product forms you can identify from the labels. What can you tell about the products from the labels? What questions, if any, do you have after this shopping experiment? Do you have enough information to choose a product without the help of an herbalist?

CHAPTER 13

Digestion

INTRODUCTION

CHEFS ARE SOME OF THE GREATEST SCIENTISTS and often are referred to as chemists of the kitchen. They are also great healers. Chefs know that the way food is prepared, the way it looks and smells, and the way it tastes are important to ensure the pleasure of the person eating it. Chefs also know that eating must be a healing experience. When people eat a meal, they want to feel good during and afterward. Because food is critical to survival, every culture throughout history has given a lot of attention to the preparation and presentation of food so that eating is energizing, healing, and pleasurable.

Spices are an important part of food preparation and presentation. Spices are defined as "various aromatic vegetable products used to season and flavor foods . . . something that gives zest or relish" (Merriam-Webster, 1999). In the vernacular, the words "herb" and "spice" are used interchangeably. Sometimes "herb" is used to refer to the medicinal use of plant material and "spice" is used to denote culinary use. Some use the term "spice" for ground plant material and the word "herb" for whole forms. The terms "spice" and "herb" are used here interchangeably to refer to the plant materials used in cooking to change the food in some way, to make it more palatable, pleasurable, or digestible.

Cooks have used small amounts of spices throughout history for therapeutic and culinary reasons. For example, rosemary was used to preserve meats before refrigeration was available, and lemons were used on board ships not only because they were refreshing to the palate but also because they were known to prevent scurvy. Good cooks know the science and the art of their craft and create appetizing and healing meals for their guests.

Because of this long tradition of using herbs and spices in food preparation, people often overlook the fact that the herbs are being used therapeutically in small amounts to aid digestion. They also have the potential for medicinal use. The herbs profiled in this chapter—lemon, ginger, and horseradish—are just three of the culinary herbs used to affect digestion in some way. Many other culinary herbs, such as dill, basil, and oregano, also have therapeutic value to promoting healthy digestion. Often these same herbs, which contain significant amounts of antimicrobial essential oils, helped prevent food spoilage before the era of refrigeration.

Healthy digestion begins in the mouth. Some digestive herbs help promote salivation. Some stimulate the appetite through the senses of smell and taste. Many digestive herbs are warm in nature. Warmth is necessary for healthy digestion. Many cultures note the importance of adding warmth to food either through the heat from the process of cooking or through the use of herbs and spices to promote digestive "fire," the secretion of digestive juices. The herbs profiled in this chapter may not only promote salivation or warmth but also may correct imbalances in digestion such as occur with nausea, anorexia, or vomiting.

The herbs profiled in this chapter, more than any other chapter, may be very familiar. They are almost always available in local markets and people often have them in their homes. These herbs are so common that they are often overlooked as healing agents. They are generally inexpensive and readily available herbs that nurses can easily add to their caring repertoire because most people, especially sick patients, need help in improving their digestion.

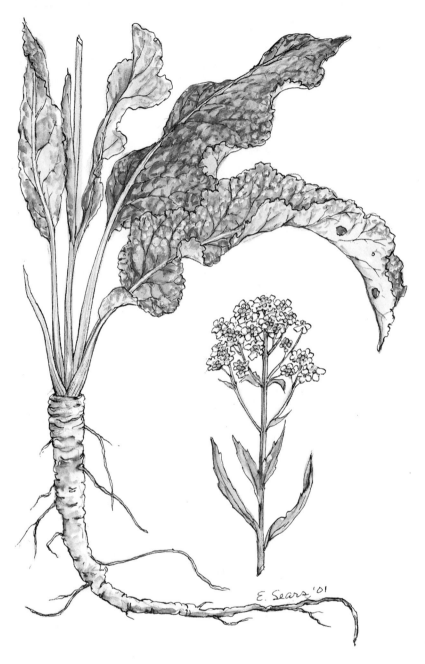

Armoracia rusticana

Horseradish

- **LATIN NAME:** *Armoracia rusticana*

- **FAMILY:** Brassicaceae

- **COMMON NAMES:** Horseradish, horseradish root, mountain radish, great raisefort, red cole

- **HEALTH PATTERN:** Digestion

- **PLANT DESCRIPTION:**

Horseradish is a vegetable in the same family as broccoli, cabbage, and cauliflower. It is a hardy, leafy, low-growing plant that can be planted early in the year and harvested before the heat of summer. The root is yellowish-white, cylindrical and fleshy, and about 1 inch (2 cm) thick. The roots, which contain mustard oil, can grow quite deep. When the root is crushed or grated, it releases a pungent, mustard-like odor and taste.

One of the volunteers on the herb farm where I worked learned just how large horseradish roots can be. I gave the strong man a spade, showed him the row of horseradish we had been growing for a few years, and asked him to harvest the roots. I told him to "just follow the roots" and left for a few hours. Upon returning, I could not find the man. There were signs of work having been done because I saw mounds of soil beside the area that had been the row of horseradish. I went over to take a look and found the man up to his shoulders in a very deep ditch! He said, "Well you told me to follow the roots!"

- **PLANT PARTS USED:** Root, leaf

- **TRADITIONAL EVIDENCE:**

Cultural Use

Asian. Horseradish is a warm and pungent herb that carries the energy of the metal element, related to the Five Element Theory used in Chinese medicine (Pitchford, 1993). It has a dispersing quality, meaning that it moves energy away from a central point. *Wasabi*, the green paste served as a condiment with sushi, is a Japanese horseradish.

North American Indian. Cherokee women use wild horseradish to promote menstrual flow. It also has been used for rheumatism, colds, and urinary stones; to increase the appetite and urinary output; and as a tonic. The roots are chewed for tongue and mouth diseases. It is used for asthma. An infusion was gargled for sore throat. The root is eaten as a condiment. The Iroquois drink an infusion of the roots for the blood and for diabetes. A poultice of the leaves is applied to the face for the treatment of toothache. The Delaware apply a poultice of the leaves for nerve pain (Moerman, 1998).

Hispanic. Hispanics in the southwestern United States use horseradish root in cooking and as medicine for bladder infections, gout, asthma, and colds. It is grated and put in vinegar and applied to sore limbs.

European. The German Commission E approved the internal use of horseradish for inflammation of the mucous membranes of the respiratory tract and as supportive treatment for infections of the urinary tract. It was approved for external use in the treatment of respiratory mucous membrane inflammation and to increase blood flow to areas of minor muscle aches (Blumenthal, Goldberg, & Brinckman, 2000). In Anthroposophical medicine, horseradish is used to stimulate and enliven metabolism, the nerve-sense system, and the head area (Husemann & Wolff, 1982).

Culinary Use

Horseradish root is added to various foods in small amounts as a flavoring. It is often served as a condiment with high protein foods, such as beef, to act as a digestive aid, although it was first used to mask the odor and taste of spoiled meat. Horseradish is a food source of chromium, magnesium, phosphorus, potassium, riboflavin, and vitamins A and C (Pedersen, 1998).

Use in Herbalism

Both the root and leaves of horseradish were used as medicine during the Middle Ages. It was a common condiment in Germany and Denmark. It is also reported to have been among the five bitter herbs, along with coriander, horehound, lettuce, and nettle, that the Jews ate during the Feast of Passover. The root was included in the *Materia Medica* of the London *Pharmacopoeias* of the eighteenth century. Horseradish was recommended for its stimulant action; its ability to increase circulation locally; and for its diuretic, mild laxative, and antiseptic actions. It was eaten with oily fish and rich meats to improve digestion. The root was eaten plain, steeped as a tea or in vinegar, or used in a sauce for its stimulant action on the digestive organs or to settle the stomach (Crellin & Philpott, 1990; Grieve, 1971). It also has been taken grated in water for pain in the stomach and bowels (Thomson, 1841).

Horseradish is used as a strong diuretic and is given to those with kidney stones and general edema. It is used internally for scurvy, rheumatism, and as an expectorant. Eating horseradish regularly throughout the day was said to stop coughs that occurred following influenza. The juice is mixed with glycerine, vinegar, and water and given to children for the relief of whooping cough. Horseradish also has been given to children for intestinal worms (Grieve, 1971).

Externally, horseradish, either tincture or the leaves soaked in vinegar, is applied as a counterirritant to areas affected by chronic rheumatism, sciatica, gout, joint pain, and swelling of the liver and spleen. Horseradish juice was applied to freckles to remove them (Grieve, 1971). Some herbalists use horseradish as an antioxidant to stimulate the body's immune system. When eaten, it clears the sinuses and therefore often is recommended to allergy sufferers. A tincture of horseradish also is used in wound healing (Vogel, 1991).

BIOMEDICAL EVIDENCE:

Although horseradish has been used medicinally for centuries, there has been little biomedical investigation of the use of the herb in healing.

Studies Related to Digestion

No published studies were found that support the traditional use of horseradish for medicinal purposes related to digestion.

Studies Related to Other Health Patterns

Immune Response. Some older German studies (Kienholz & Kemkes as reported in Blumenthal et al., 2000) have reported the antibacterial activity of horseradish in the treatment of urinary tract infections.

Mechanism of Action

One animal study of horseradish root (Sjaastad as reported in Blumenthal et al., 2000) found that the hypotensive effect of horseradish is related to its peroxidase enzymes, which trigger arachidonic acid metabolites.

USE IN PREGNANCY OR LACTATION:

In the 1800s, the American Eclectic physicians used horseradish to produce abortion (Crellin & Philpott, 1990), which may be why Blumenthal et al. (2000) state that the use of horseradish is not recommended during pregnancy and lactation. No differentiation is made between medicinal and culinary use by pregnant women.

Herbal Caveat—Pregnancy or Lactation

Some herbs are contraindicated in pregnancy because of a risk of the herb or one of its constituents stimulating the uterus and therefore possibly promoting fetal loss. Many herbal practitioners do not recommend herbal remedies, in particular oral doses of herbs, during the first trimester of pregnancy and seek an alternative. However, herbs are successfully used during pregnancy, especially to prepare the body for the birth. Herbs are relatively unstudied in pregnancy and lactation, so patients need to be made aware through education of the potential benefits and risks of using herbs for health conditions that arise during pregnancy or lactation. The use of herbal remedies during pregnancy often warrants a referral to a knowledgeable herbal practitioner.

USE FOR CHILDREN:

Horseradish root should not be administered to children under the age of four years (Blumenthal et al., 2000; Brinker, 1998; McGuffin, Hobbs, Upton, & Goldberg, 1997). No differentiation is made between medicinal and culinary use.

Herbal Caveat—Children

Children have special needs in regard to herbal therapies. They require lesser amounts of herbs and often respond well to mild teas and topical applications such as compresses and baths. The lowest dose of oral preparations should be tried first before increasing the amount given children. Caregivers should observe children closely for responses to herbal remedies. Younger children, particularly infants, have traditionally been given herbs either through their mother's breast milk or in the form of a homeopathic remedy because of their sensitivity to medicines and treatments and the immaturity of their liver. It is recommended that a person knowledgeable in the herbal treatment of children be consulted before the offering of any herb to a child for the first time.

CAUTIONS:

Although horseradish appears on the U.S. Food and Drug Administration's list of herbs as being generally recognized as safe (GRAS), it is a powerful condiment and medicament. It is very pungent and hot. The internal use of horseradish is contraindicated in conditions of stomach and intestinal disorders, and in kidney disorders. One person is reported to have experienced "vasomotor near collapse" after ingesting a small mound of wasabi (Japanese horseradish condiment) all in one bite because he did not know what it was (Spitzer, 1988). There is one other report of a Jewish man with hypertension collapsing with convulsive syncope at a Passover Seder after ingesting grated horseradish in an amount the size of a "large olive" (Rubin & Wu, 1988). Diners in Japanese restaurants should be aware that green wasabi horseradish paste is meant to be mixed with a small amount of *tamari* (soy sauce) and used as a condiment in very small amounts to facilitate the digestion. Those who attend Seders can take small amounts of horseradish or choose the bitter lettuce instead.

Side effects that have occurred with the internal use of horseradish are associated with discomfort of the gastrointestinal tract (Blumenthal et al., 2000). There are no known herb-drug interactions associated with eating horseradish (Blumenthal et al., 2000).

One source reports that some plant members of the cabbage and mustard family have been found to depress thyroid function and therefore proposes that horseradish not be used by those with hypothyroidism or those taking thyroxine (Newall, Anderson, & Phillipson, 1996); the source does not report whether this recommendation is based on animal or human data, and no research is cited to support the caution for horseradish.

For topical applications of horseradish, use preparations of horseradish root with a maximum of 2% mustard oil content. The leaf has been used traditionally after soaking it in vinegar. Be alert when applying horseradish topically so that blistering does not occur.

NURSING EVIDENCE:

Historical Nursing Use

Early nineteenth-century American nurses recommended horseradish root to promote appetite and digestion. It was also used internally and externally for chronic rheumatism. Horseradish syrup was used for hoarse colds and horseradish leaves were bound to patients' feet to relieve headache and colds (Child, 1997).

Anthroposophical nurses use horseradish root poultice in the care of patients with sinus discomfort (Bentheim, Bos, de la Houssaye, & Visser, 1980).

Potential Nursing Applications

Poor digestion causes food to move slowly through the gastrointestinal tract and thus to ferment. This is especially the case with protein foods, which can be harder for some to digest. Nurses may want to consider horseradish and its extensive traditional use as a digestive aid, especially when working with patients who have sluggish digestion. Horseradish is also an excellent addition to a regular, balanced diet when used as a condiment (i.e., in very small amounts mixed with other foods). Nurses may wish to consider researching not only the effects of ingesting small amounts of horseradish root as a digestive aid, but also the counterirritant effects of the topical use of horseradish for discomfort related to rheumatic complaints and sinus congestion and infection.

Integrative Insight

Horseradish has not really been explored from a biomedical perspective. Traditionally, it is so common that it is used in many cultures as a standard condiment to aid digestion. This herb is easy to grow and has such a strong history of use that nurses might find it a good herb to use clinically and to research. Horseradish seems to stimulate digestion through its warming action of the digestive tract. So many patients eat quickly and do not chew their food thoroughly. They often have discomfort related to indigestion or poor digestion. In addition to educating patients about the importance of chewing food, recommending condiments with food that strengthen digestive "fire" is a simple way to begin to address the issues related to nutrition and healthy digestion. A little horseradish goes a long way in helping those who need the benefits of protein-rich foods, such as meat and fish, but who often have trouble digesting them.

THERAPEUTIC APPLICATIONS:

Oral

Fresh Root. ½ to 1 teaspoon (2 to 4 g) before meals

Infusion. Steep ½ teaspoon (2 g) in 5 ounces (150 ml) of boiled water for five minutes. Drink several times daily.

Syrup. Steep ½ teaspoon (2 g) of root in 5 ounces (150 ml) boiled water in a covered container for two hours. Strain and add an equal amount of sugar ⅔ cup (150 g) to liquid 5 ounces (150 ml) to thicken.

Succus. You can obtain fresh pressed juice from about 1 ounce (20 g) of the root (Blumenthal et al., 2000).

Topical

Poultice. Grate the fresh root and spread it onto a linen cloth or thin gauze. Apply it locally with the cloth's surface against the skin until a warming sensation is felt (Blumenthal et al., 2000). For sinus, use ½ teaspoon of freshly grated root on tender sinus points. Cover the eyes with small pieces of cloth so that they are not exposed to the odor of the horseradish.

Environmental

The aroma of horseradish can be helpful in opening the sinuses.

Herbal Caveat—Therapeutic Applications

In traditional and conventional herbal medicine, amounts of herbs given to patients are based on individual needs. The amounts or "doses" recorded here are provided so that the health practitioner has a general idea of the amounts recommended for an adult patient. Dosing in herbalism not only refers to amount of plant used but also includes when, where, and how to take a plant medicine. These dosages should not be used as guidelines for indiscriminate intervention without proper assessment, critical thinking, and patient education on the part of the practitioner.

Note: Please see chapter 5 for detailed descriptions of how to prepare various applications.

PATIENT INTERACTION:

Horseradish root has many medicinal benefits in addition to its noted culinary uses. Horseradish aids in the digestion of foods; in particular, meat and fish. It also has antimicrobial properties and can be used externally for clearing the sinuses. A tincture of horseradish has been used traditionally for joint pain. It is a very pungent, hot herb and should be used in small amounts as a condiment and under the guidance of a knowledgeable health practitioner when being used internally or externally for medicinal purposes for the first time.

Herbal Caveat—Patient Interaction

Patients considering the use of an herb or formula of herbs in self-care benefit from education about the plant itself and the use of the plant in healing. This education can come through many sources, including local herbalists; plant specialists such as botanists; health practitioners such as nurses, nutritionists, naturopaths, and other physicians; and various written references including the scientific literature. Patients need to remember that their unique health care needs are not necessarily represented in any literature they may encounter. Therefore, it is recommended that a knowledgeable mentor be consulted before initiating self-care with any herb being used for the first time.

NURTURING THE NURSE-PLANT RELATIONSHIP:

Note: You may want to keep a journal of your experiences with the herb.

Try getting to know the strength of this plant through both a culinary and a therapeutic experience.

Culinary. Try eating some finely chopped horseradish root with fish or meat. For example, mix some pulverized horseradish root with some lemon juice, a little Worcestershire sauce, and tomato ketchup or sauce. Dip some shrimp in the cocktail sauce and feel your sinuses open and your mouth water as you chew.

Therapeutic. Obtain some fresh horseradish root, making sure to have someone help you identify it if you have never seen it or tasted it before. Powdered root can be used if fresh is not available. Peel and grate 1 teaspoon of the root. Take a small piece of natural fiber cloth and fold with the root inside. Test the compress on the inner aspect of your forearm. The compress should be removed as soon as a burning sensation begins to be felt. After learning how strong the root is, the compress can be placed on the sore sinus points on the face. The compresses should not be secured because they need to be able to be removed quickly if burning begins. When the heat builds, remove the compress for a moment and give the skin a brief rest. Reapply and remove until the root in the compress no longer causes an effect on the skin. The compress should be used no more than once per day. Use 1 to 2 teaspoons of powder and moisten the compress before applying. Horseradish powder often does not seem to heat the skin as much as the fresh root.

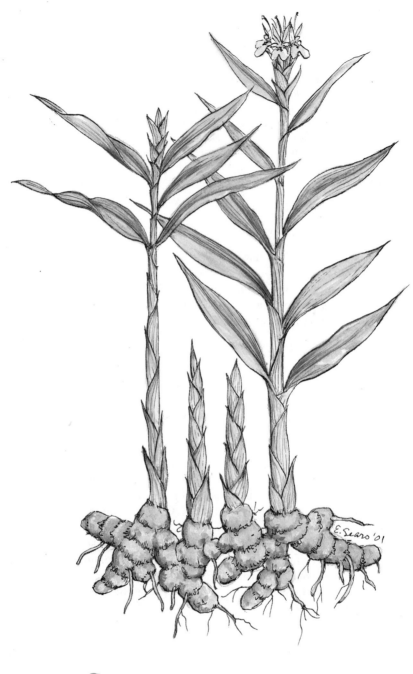

Zingiber officinale

Ginger

- LATIN NAME: *Zingiber officinale*

- FAMILY: Zingiberaceae

- COMMON NAMES: Ginger, common ginger

- HEALTH PATTERN: Digestion

- PLANT DESCRIPTION:
Ginger is thought to have originated in the tropical regions of Asia. It is cultivated in Jamaica, the West Indies, Africa, China, India, Vietnam, Sri Lanka, and Australia (DeSmet, 1997). Ginger is a perennial root that sends up a green shoot in the spring. This stalk reaches approximately 2 feet (0.7 meter) and develops several lanceolate-shaped leaves that die down annually. The flowering stalk grows directly from the root and develops an oblong scalloped spike from which a white or yellow blossom grows. Ginger flowers have an aromatic fragrance. Ginger roots must be allowed to grow for at least one year before harvest. They have an aromatic, spicy, and hot taste.

- PLANT PARTS USED: Root and rhizome

- TRADITIONAL EVIDENCE:
Cultural Use
Asian. Ginger has been used in China for at least 2500 years. It is currently an ingredient in almost half of all Chinese patent herbal medicines (DeSmet, 1997). Marco Polo reported seeing ginger in China between 1280 and 1290 A.D. Both fresh and dry ginger are included in the Chinese *Materia Medica*. Practitioners of Asian medicine make a distinction between the medicinal properties of fresh and dried ginger. Fresh ginger is known as "sheng jiang" and is classified as an herb that relieves wind chill; dry ginger is called "gan jiang" and is classified as an herb that warms the interior (Bensky & Gamble, 1993). Clinicians in China also use injectable forms of ginger in the treatment of rheumatism and low back pain (Wren, 1988).

Dried ginger root is used in traditional Chinese medicine (TCM) to warm the stomach and spleen energy systems in cases when either deficiency or excess are present. It also is used with symptoms such as epigastric pain, vomiting, dysentery, and abdominal pain with feelings of gnawing hunger. It also is used for lung-cold conditions such as thin, watery sputum; coughing; and congestion. Dried ginger also is used for (deficiency cold only) hemorrhage, which often manifests as uterine bleeding in women, and is contraindicated in TCM if the patient has a condition known as yin deficiency with heat. The skin of the ginger root is used to promote urination and decrease edema. Fresh ginger root is used to release the exterior of the body and disperse cold and for symptoms of cold in the stomach and may be used in cases of vomiting, coughing, and excess sweating (Bensky & Gamble, 1993).

Ginger has been reported in China to be very effective in the clinical treatment of rheumatism, acute bacterial dysentery, inflammation of the testicles, and malaria (Leung & Foster, 1996). Ginger also is applied externally to painful joints to decrease inflammation (Pedersen, 1998). The Japanese macrobiotic community uses fresh ginger extensively in topical ginger compresses for increasing circulation of blood and body fluids in an area of the body when stagnation exists such as during joint pain, toothache, backache, menstrual cramps, and passing kidney stones (Kushi, 1993).

Hispanic. Ginger is called "ajenjibre" in Spanish and is used to settle the stomach, break a fever, stimulate circulation, and in cooking.

Pacific Islander. Hawaiian natives have used wild ginger root for many years. The roots are pounded with salt to extract the juice that is used as a scalp wash for headaches and itching of the skin. Ginger juice is used as a hair dressing. Hawaiian dancers wear ginger flowers and other fragrant blossoms in their leis. The ashes from burned leaves are used for cuts and skin sores. The roots are pounded with salt then mixed with urine, and used for ringworm and white skin blotches. The flowers and roots are pounded and mixed with water and rubbed on the body during massages and as a bath for bruises and sprains. Ginger roots are cooked and placed in the tooth cavity for the relief of toothaches (Moerman, 1998).

African. A variety of ginger similar to that grown in the West Indies has been developed in Nigeria at the Root Crop Research Institute. In African folk medicine, ginger has been used to dispel intestinal gas, promote urinary output, and relieve nausea and vomiting (Iwu, 1993).

East Indian. Ginger has been cultivated in India since before recorded history. Ginger root, called in Sanskrit, "srangavera," has been classified in Ayurvedic medicine as having heating and drying properties. It has been widely used to promote digestive function, as an aphrodisiac, to dispel flatulence, strengthen memory, and "remove obstructions in the vessels." It is used in nervous conditions and incontinence of urine. Dry ginger is combined with black pepper and long pepper to make a carminative called "trikatu."

Ginger is used for colic, vomiting, coughs, colds, and painful spasms of the bowel. Fresh ginger root is chewed to relieve sore throats and hoarseness. Dried ginger infusion is taken for rheumatism and colds. Ginger is used in external applications for the treatment of symptoms of toothache, headache, cholera, cramps, and fainting. Wild ginger that is native to India, *Zingiber zerumbet,* has been used in many of the same ways as *Z. officinalis*, with the added uses for asthma, intestinal parasites, leprosy, and other skin diseases (Nadkarni, 1976).

European. Ginger was imported from China to Europe as a popular spice from the eleventh to the twelfth centuries. It was used during the Middle Ages to counter the plague (Lawless, 1998). Spaniards introduced ginger into the West Indies where it later became widely cultivated (Pedersen, 1998). The German Commission E approves the internal use of ginger for treatment of symptoms of digestive disturbance and for motion sickness. The British Herbal Compendium recommends the internal use of ginger for digestive disturbances, gastrointestinal colic, and the prevention of motion sickness and vomiting during pregnancy (Blumenthal et al., 2000).

Culinary Use

Ginger root is commonly used fresh and dried as a culinary spice, especially in Asian cooking. It is used commercially in many foods, such as beverages, baked goods, gelatins, puddings, meats, relishes, and condiments. Ginger oil is also used in soft drinks such as ginger ale and cola. It is used in liqueurs, bitters, and other alcoholic drinks. Ginger oil and extracts also are used to flavor candies and frozen dairy desserts (Leung & Foster, 1996). The various uses of ginger in cooking are quite extensive and include pickled ginger eaten as a condiment with Japanese sushi and crystallized ginger pieces found in English scones.

Use in Herbalism

Historical uses of ginger include aiding digestion, warming the stomach, clearing the vision, warming joints, and expelling flatulence. It has been used for gout, especially in older men (Culpeper, 1990). American Eclectic physicians recommended ginger as a stimulant, as an agent that could increase local circulation, and for its ability to increase nasal discharge and the flow of saliva. Chewing ginger was known to promote salivation. Swallowing it was known to stimulate digestion, increase the secretion of gastric juice, and dispel flatulence. Ginger was used to disguise the taste of drugs and to prevent nausea. It was given with other preparations in the treatment of dysentery, diarrhea, cholera, and vomiting. It was very useful in older individuals who had chronic digestive weakness with flatulence and gout. Ginger often was used to relieve gastrointestinal cramping, fevers, colds, and menstrual pain. It was used as a poultice for skin ulcers and headaches (Felter & Lloyd, 1983).

Ginger is widely used in current herbalism, too. It is used as an ingredient in medicinal preparations for digestion, constipation, flatulence, nausea, gastric acidity, and colds. It is recommended in tea form to promote the onset of menstruation, to increase energy, and aid mental focus (Weed, 1986). Ginger may be effective in the treatment of the nausea related to inner ear dysfunction. Some use fresh ginger juice in the treatment of thermal burns. Ginger's medicinal actions include the ability to lower cholesterol; provide relief from allergies, asthma, colds, and nausea; and to protect the body against parasites (Rister, 1999). It is used to reduce the inflammation associated with arthritis, rheumatism, and migraine and is used to stimulate blood circulation.

Health food stores sell ginger in the form of capsules, tablets, teas, extracts, and drinks. Fresh ginger root is available in many grocery stores. In aromatherapy, ginger essential oil is regarded as a powerful nerve tonic that is good for exhaustion and mental fatigue. It is best used in combination with other essential oils. It has an uplifting, comforting, and warming effect on the emotions and a stimulating effect on the mind (Lawless, 1998).

Cosmetic Use. Ginger oil is used as a fragrance in various cosmetics, soaps, lotions, detergents, creams, and perfumes, especially Asian and men's fragrances (Leung & Foster, 1996).

BIOMEDICAL EVIDENCE:

This is one herb that has been studied as a whole herb for its anti-nausea and anti-emetic effects. The results are conflicting. The majority of the research on the actions of ginger in relation to digestion has been performed using ginger powder in capsules, where the taste of the plant material is disguised. Many traditional forms of healing indicate that if ginger, or any plant medicine, is not tasted, the healing benefit cannot be fully achieved. Researchers want to protect the double-blind status of their studies but from an ethical standpoint some might be concerned that people are being given lesser treatment if not allowed to taste their medicine.

Another question still remains of whether or not fresh ginger tea, for example, might not have a completely different effect than powdered ginger. The effect of different forms of plant medicine is recognized in traditional practice. Animal studies have found that the effects of ginger were reversed (induced or inhibited contraction in veins of mice) depending upon whether the whole fresh rhizome was used or a processed ginger extract was used (Pancho, Kimura, Unno, Kurono, & Kimura, 1989).

Studies Related to Digestion

Powdered ginger rhizome, 1 g, given orally in a capsule, has been shown, after four hours, to significantly reduce vomiting and cold sweat associated with seasickness in a double-blind, randomized trial involving 80 healthy navy cadets, age 16 to19 years, who were unaccustomed to the high seas ($p < .05$). The protection index in regard to vomiting was found to be 72%. The ginger did not affect nausea and vertigo (Grontved, Brask, Kambskard, & Hentzer, 1988).

One study of 36 men and women with high susceptibility to motion sickness, who received 940 mg of powdered capsulated ginger, showed that the ginger was superior to dimenhydrinate (Dramamine) in relieving the symptoms of gastrointestinal distress (Mowrey & Clayson, 1982).

Another study of 28 volunteers in which 500 or 1000 mg powdered ginger, 1000 mg fresh ginger, and scopolamine were compared to placebo, showed that both powdered and fresh ginger partially inhibited tachygastria, but they did not protect against motion sickness under other various test conditions. Powdered ginger had no effect on gastric emptying (Stewart, Wood, Wood, & Mims, 1991).

Powdered ginger, given orally 250 mg four times a day, has been shown in a randomized, double-blind, crossover study to be significantly more effective than placebo (in 19 of 27 patients) in reducing or eliminating symptoms related to hyperemesis gravidarum as measured by a Likert scale using both subjective and objective data (Fischer-Rasmussen, Kjaer, Dahl, & Asping, 1990).

In a randomized, placebo-controlled trial in which 60 women, ages 16 to 65, before undergoing gynecologic surgery, were given 1 g of powdered ginger root, 10 mg metoclopramide, or placebo, the incidence of postoperative nausea during the first twenty-four hours was 28%, 30%, and 51%, respectively, a significance favoring the potential use of ginger preoperatively ($p < .05$) (Bone, Wilkinson, Young, McNeil, & Charlton, 1990). In a study of 120 gynecological patients more than 16 years old undergoing laparoscopic surgery, who received either 10 mg metoclopramide (Reglan), an oral dose of 1 g powdered ginger root, or placebo and no other premedication, there was a significant difference between the placebo and ginger groups as to the number of antiemetics required after surgery: 15% of the ginger group, 32% of the metoclopramide group, and 38% of the placebo group needed antiemetics. Ginger given orally one hour before anesthesia was as effective as metoclopramide 10 mg in reducing the incidence of post-operative nausea and vomiting (Phillips, Ruggier, & Hutchinson, 1993b).

In another trial of 108 female patients, age 17 to 75 years, undergoing laparoscopic surgery, it was concluded that not only was ginger powder in capsules, given in oral doses of 500 or 1000 mg, ineffective in reducing the incidence of postoperative nausea or vomiting, but there was a tendency for nausea and vomiting to increase in patients with the higher doses. The patients in this study received diazepam with the study capsules one hour before anesthesia and intravenous morphine was given post-operatively (Arfeen et al., 1995). A subsequent study supports the findings of the Arfeen et al study (Visalyaputra, Petchpaisit, Somcharaen, & Choavaratana, 1998). The investigators discuss the subjectivity of the findings in regard to nausea. They also write that vomiting was not thoroughly addressed in some of the studies, such as Philips et al., 1993, where it was found that there was no significant difference between placebo and ginger powder in regard to frequency of vomiting.

Ginger powder, 3 capsules of 530 mg each given thirty minutes before treatment, in 11 patients undergoing monthly photophoresis (ingestion of 8-MOP–psoralen), demonstrated one third the incidence of nausea after taking the ginger as measured on a subjective rating scale of 0 to 4 (Meyer, Schwartz, Crater, & Keyes, 1995).

Because ginger has an effect on the digestive tract, some practitioners have speculated that ingestion of ginger might have an effect on the absorption rate of pharmaceutical drugs. Studies have been conducted to measure gastric motility and/or emptying rate after ingestion of ginger. Although animal studies have shown that ginger may increase the bioavailability of certain drugs (Atal, Zutshi, & Rao, 1981), the data in humans is inconclusive. One gram of powdered dried ginger per day in capsules did not exert any effect on gastric motility or gastric emptying rate in 16 healthy volunteers as measured using a paracetamol absorption technique in a randomized, double-blind, crossover trial; however, the investigators acknowledge that further studies in pregnant women and people with gastrointestinal disease (situations in which gastric emptying can be altered) should be done (Phillips, Hutchinson, & Ruggier, 1993a). In another randomized, double-blind, crossover study of 12 males, a ginger product, identified as an "extract," 200 mg corresponding to 1 g of ginger rhizome, the ginger was shown to significantly improve gastroduodenal motility (Micklefield et al., 1999).

Studies Related to Other Health Patterns

Mobility. In a pilot study of seven patients with rheumatoid arthritis or arthritis deformalis, the consumption of 5 g fresh ginger or 0.5 to 1 g powdered ginger orally per day was shown to significantly reduce pain, increase joint mobility and decrease swelling and morning stiffness (Srivastava & Mustafa, 1989).

Comfort and Pain Relief. In a follow-up of the histories of 56 patients, 28 with rheumatoid arthritis, 18 with osteoarthritis, and 10 with muscular discomfort, who used powdered ginger every day, "three quarters" of the patients with arthritis were said to have experienced significant relief of pain and swelling and all of the patients with muscular discomfort were relived of pain after starting to take ginger. Patients sometimes took three to four times (and in some cases more) the test dose of 0.5 to 1.0 g powdered ginger per day, and they reported quicker and better relief than those who took the recommended levels. There were no reported adverse effects (Srivastava & Mustafa, 1992).

One case study shows the healing effect of powdered ginger, 500 to 600 mg in plain water, at the onset of migraine and the overall reduction of incidence of migraine over the course of a year when the patient increased their daily consumption of uncooked fresh ginger (Mustafa & Srivastava, 1990).

Elimination. In a study of 24 male subjects, 6 to 10 fresh ginger slices, 0.2 mm thick, placed over the affected testis was noted to instigate a subjective and objective cure from orchitis within 3 days as compared with the control group of 4 subjects for whom healing time was 8.5 days (Bensky & Gamble, 1993).

Restoration. In vitro studies examining various species of ginger, including *Z. officinale,* found that ginger contains nontoxic compounds that inhibit Epstein-Barr virus activation, which could contribute to the development of cancer prevention methods (Vimala, Norhanom, & Yadav, 1999).

Mechanism of Action

Dried ginger has been the subject of several clinical trials to determine whether or not it is useful in motion sickness. Dried ginger does not work like pharmaceutical drugs for motion sickness. The positive antiemetic activity has been attributed to an effect on gastric activity rather than on central nervous system mechanisms, specifically oculomotor and vestibular systems, that are characteristic of pharmaceutical antimotion sickness drugs (Holtmann, Clarke, Scherer, & Hohn, 1989).

It is hypothesized that the relief experienced by patients with arthritis when they take ginger is due to ginger's ability to interfere with cyclooxygenase and lipoxygenase enzymes of the prostaglandin and leukotriene biosynthetic pathways (Srivastava & Mustafa, 1989).

Powdered ginger, 2 g orally per day, has not been shown in a study of 8 healthy males to have any significant effect on bleeding time, platelet count, thromboelastography, and whole blood platelet aggregometry when compared with placebo, as measured before the ginger was given, and at three and twenty-four hours after the ginger was given (Lumb, 1994). In a small study of 7 females who consumed 5 g of *fresh* ginger daily, serum thromboxane B_2 levels decreased by 37% (each woman served as her own control) $(p < .1)$ (Srivastava, 1989).

Ginger and its extracts have been found to have strong antioxidant properties. It also contains high levels of protease and could possibly have applications similar to those of papain, bromelain, and other plant proteases (Leung & Foster, 1996) (e.g., help in digesting foods, protein foods in particular).

USE IN PREGNANCY OR LACTATION:

The use of ginger during pregnancy has been controversial and much research has been done on this issue. Experts have decided that there is no evidence that the therapeutic dosage of 1 g of dried root, the therapeutic dose required for antinausea activity, produces harm to the fetus or the mother (Blumenthal et al., 2000). However, some do not recommend ginger in large amounts during pregnancy, because of its potential to promote uterine bleeding (Brinker, 1998). "Large amounts" refers to doses greater than what would be found in foods each day (Leung & Foster, 1996). The Chinese *Materia Medica* recommends caution in using dry ginger during pregnancy, but not fresh ginger (Bensky & Gamble, 1993).

One midwife recommends tablespoonful doses of ginger root tea anytime nausea occurs during pregnancy. The small, frequent doses are especially effective for motion sickness and early morning nausea (Weed, 1986).

Chinese researchers have found that applying ginger paste to a specific acupuncture point on the mother can result in a 77% correction of breech-positioned babies (Rister, 1999).

The World Health Organization (WHO) monographs (1999) report that no information is available on the effect of ginger on the baby during lactation.

Herbal Caveat—Pregnancy or Lactation

Some herbs are contraindicated in pregnancy because of a risk of the herb or one of its constituents stimulating the uterus and therefore possibly promoting fetal loss. Many herbal practitioners do not recommend herbal remedies, in particular oral doses of herbs, during the first trimester of pregnancy and seek an alternative. However, herbs are successfully used during pregnancy, especially to prepare the body for the birth. Herbs are relatively unstudied in pregnancy and lactation, so patients need to be made aware through education of the potential benefits and risks of using herbs for health conditions that arise during pregnancy or lactation. The use of herbal remedies during pregnancy often warrants a referral to a knowledgeable herbal practitioner.

USE FOR CHILDREN:

The use of ginger is not recommended for children under six years (WHO, 1999). It is not clear whether this refers to culinary use or therapeutic use or both. Schilcher (1992) suggests using ginger with children for digestive concerns and travel sickness. Ginger can be used with children in small amounts in foods, teas, and compresses. Children often like sips of ginger ale when nauseated. With some experimentation to moderate the bite of the ginger, it is possible to make a homemade ginger ale for children by using fresh ginger root decoction, honey, and sparkling water.

Herbal Caveat—Children

Children have special needs in regard to herbal therapies. They require lesser amounts of herbs and often respond well to mild teas and topical applications such as compresses and baths. The lowest dose of oral preparations should be tried first before increasing the amount given children. Caregivers should observe children closely for responses to herbal remedies. Younger children, particularly infants, have traditionally been given herbs either through their mother's breast milk or in the form of a homeopathic remedy because of their sensitivity to medicines and treatments and the immaturity of their liver. It is recommended that a person knowledgeable in the herbal treatment of children be consulted before the offering of any herb to a child for the first time.

CAUTIONS:

Although some sources report no known side effects associated with the use of ginger (Blumenthal et al., 2000), TCM sources report that chewing fresh ginger has been shown to raise systolic blood pressure by 11.2 mm Hg and diastolic blood pressure by 14 mm Hg. Dry ginger also can raise blood pressure (Bensky & Gamble, 1993). Chinese medicine also cautions that ginger not be used in cases of interior heat. However, several case histories of patients who have taken up to 6 g of ginger powder for six months to three years without any adverse effects have been reported (Srivastava & Mustafa, 1989).

Those who have gallstones should consult a knowledgeable plant medicine practitioner before taking therapeutic amounts of ginger because of its ability to stimulate the flow of bile from the gallbladder (McGuffin et al., 1997).

One source suggests that "Ginger has been reported to possess both cardiotonic and antiplatelet activity in vitro and hypoglycemic activity in in vivo studies. Therefore, excessive doses may interfere with existing cardiac, antidiabetic, or anticoagulant therapy" (Newall et al., 1996, p. 136). Ginger may increase the bioavailability of certain pharmaceutical drugs (Atal et al., 1981).

NURSING EVIDENCE:

Historical Nursing Use

Nurses often provide ginger ale soft drink to nauseated patients. Ginger is one of the ingredients in the spice poultices nurses historically used as a counterirritant (Weeks-Shaw, 1914).

Potential Nursing Applications

Nurses may want to consider exploring the extensive traditional medicinal uses of ginger in caring for people with nausea, chronic joint pain, pain due to kidney stones, poor digestion, toothache, cold, and sore throat. Because ginger is so readily available, its use can be integrated into home care and self-care procedures. Nurses may want to do their own research into the use of ginger for easing nausea experienced during pregnancy or for patients who complain of poor digestion and flatulence. Nurses also might consider researching the use of ginger compresses to the kidney area to ease the pain associated with the passing of kidney stones.

Integrative Insight

There is much more biomedical data on ginger than most herbs. Questions then arise regarding interpretation of the data so that the information can be applied clinically. Some of the major issues regarding application of the data on ginger concern the form of the herb. Most of the studies used powdered ginger in capsules and it is unclear about the use of fresh ginger or ginger tea, for example. Traditional evidence and animal studies have shown that there are potentially significant differences, even opposite effects, that occur between the different forms of the herb.

In herbalism, people's different responses to various forms of herbs are taken into account. When people self-treat, they may not be unaware of these differences. Several years ago, I received a call from a pregnant woman who had been having severe first trimester nausea and occasional vomiting. She was taking ginger in capsules that she bought from a health food store and had been experiencing almost complete relief until she went to see her health care practitioner. The practitioner agreed with her choice of using ginger to ease the nausea, but suggested that she did not need to pay a higher price for a supplement when she could use fresh ginger instead.

Thinking the suggestion reasonable, the woman bought fresh ginger, made a tea, drank some, and promptly vomited. The fresh ginger did not help her at all. She went back to the capsules. This is an example of how perplexing working with medicinal plants can be. Did this woman feel better taking a capsule because she did not taste the ginger, even though, according to the data, fresh ginger might be more appropriate for use during pregnancy? If she could not take fresh ginger, would the dry ginger be okay if used with caution? These are the type of questions nurses need to ask if they use herbs or advise patients about the use of herbs. After an herb is studied from a biomedical perspective, the clinical work begins. Nurses can integrate the traditional data, the new biomedical data, and their own research and observation skills to further the clinical knowledge of the use of ginger.

THERAPEUTIC APPLICATIONS:

Oral

Powdered Rhizome. Take 0.25 to 1.0 g three times daily (Blumenthal et al., 2000).

Infusion or Decoction. Use 0.25 to 1.0 g in 5 ounces (150 ml) boiled water three times daily (Blumenthal et al., 2000).

Fluid Extract. 1:1 (g/ml): 0.25 to 1.0 ml three times daily (Blumenthal et al., 2000).

Tincture. 1:5 (g/ml): Up to 1 teaspoon (1.25 to 5.0 ml) three times daily (Blumenthal et al., 2000).

Standardized Extract. Take two 250 mg capsules thirty minutes before expected onset of symptoms, then two capsules every four hours (Blumenthal et al., 2000).

Topical

Massage. Blend 1 drop of ginger essential oil with a few drops of jasmine and sandalwood in 1 tablespoon (15 ml) of sweet almond oil and use for massage (Lawless, 1998).

Ginger Compress. Using 4 to 5 ounces (113 to 150 g) of freshly grated ginger root or 1 to 1½ ounces (28 to 42 g) of ginger powder, put the ginger into a small cloth bag and add it to 1 gallon (3.8 liters) of water that is simmering on the stove. Allow the mixture to gently steep, not boil, for five minutes. Holding both ends of a small towel, dip the middle into the ginger water. Wring it out and fold it to the desired size. You can also completely submerge the compress material and use a small hand towel to wring out the compress. Take care in applying the hot compress to the area of the body to be treated, making sure that the skin does not burn because of the heat. Replace the compress every three to four minutes for twenty minutes. The ginger compress will create increased circulation of blood and body fluids in areas of stagnation. Stagnation usually manifests as pain, inflammation, swelling, or stiffness. According to macrobiotic principles, ginger compresses are not used on the brain area, on the abdomen in pregnancy, for infants or the very old, when fever is present, or on the body area experiencing infection (e.g., pneumonia) or heat (Kushi, 1993).

Environmental

Bath. Put 2 to 3 tablespoons (28 to 42 g) of powdered ginger root into a small cloth bag or tea bag. Steep it in hot bath water to help relax muscles and relieve body pain (Pedersen, 1998).

Essential Oil Bath. Add 3 drops of ginger essential oil to the bath for nervous exhaustion, mental debility, frigidity, poor memory, impotence, or migraine.

Ginger essential oil can be added to other favorite essential oils for scenting the home environment through the use of an essential oil diffuser (Lawless, 1998), or just chop up some root and cook with it. The oils are strong enough to put out a stimulating fragrance.

Herbal Caveat—Therapeutic Applications
In traditional and conventional herbal medicine, amounts of herbs given to patients are based on individual needs. The amounts or "doses" recorded here are provided so that the health practitioner has a general idea of the amounts recommended for an adult patient. Dosing in herbalism not only refers to amount of plant used but also includes when, where, and how to take a plant medicine. These dosages should not be used as guidelines for indiscriminate intervention without proper assessment, critical thinking, and patient education on the part of the practitioner.

Note: Please see chapter 5 for detailed descriptions of how to prepare various applications.

PATIENT INTERACTION:

Ginger has been used for centuries not only as a culinary herb that improves digestion but also medicinally for discomfort associated with colds, poor digestion, nausea and vomiting, pain, and motion sickness. Some research supports these uses. The research on ginger has been done primarily on ginger in powdered capsulated form, even though ginger has been used traditionally either in its fresh form or as a tea made from dried whole herb. When using ginger internally for medicinal purposes, be careful because ginger is a very warm herb. It is best to consult with a knowledgeable plant medicine practitioner if planning to use medicinal amounts of ginger internally for more than a few days. Do not use ginger in medicinal amounts when high fever is present.

Herbal Caveat—Patient Interaction

Patients considering the use of an herb or formula of herbs in self-care benefit from education about the plant itself and the use of the plant in healing. This education can come through many sources, including local herbalists; plant specialists such as botanists; health practitioners such as nurses, nutritionists, naturopaths, and other physicians; and various written references including the scientific literature. Patients need to remember that their unique health care needs are not necessarily represented in any literature they may encounter. Therefore, it is recommended that a knowledgeable mentor be consulted before initiating self-care with any herb being used for the first time.

NURTURING THE NURSE-PLANT RELATIONSHIP:

Note: You may want to keep a journal of your experiences with the herb.

Experiencing the warmth of ginger both on the inside and the outside of the body is a good way to get to know ginger's personality. Buy a large plump piece of fresh ginger to make a tea and a kidney compress. One of the best preventive self-care practices is to gently warm the digestive fire and the kidneys. Asian medical theory states that when the kidney energy system is supported, the source of "qi" (life force) is supported. It is important to warm the kidney area, especially in the winter months or when fatigued.

To make a simple ginger tea, peel a portion of the ginger root and take five thin slices of the root and steep for fifteen minutes and strain. Try sipping the tea when your stomach is empty. As you drink the tea, you may actually feel the warming energy of the herb in your stomach.

To make a kidney compress, prepare the compress as directed in the topical applications section. Wring out the compress and fold it to a size that will lie comfortably on your back over both kidneys. Take care in applying the hot compress to the kidney area. Although the skin on the back is not as sensitive as other areas of the body, be careful not to burn your skin. Lie down with the ginger decoction nearby and place the compress over the kidneys. Cover up with a blanket and be sure to keep your feet warm. Replace the kidney compress every three to four minutes for twenty minutes. The ginger compress will create increased circulation and warmth to the kidneys area. After the twenty minutes of compress application, get into a warm bed (use hot water bottles to warm the bed), and rest for one hour.

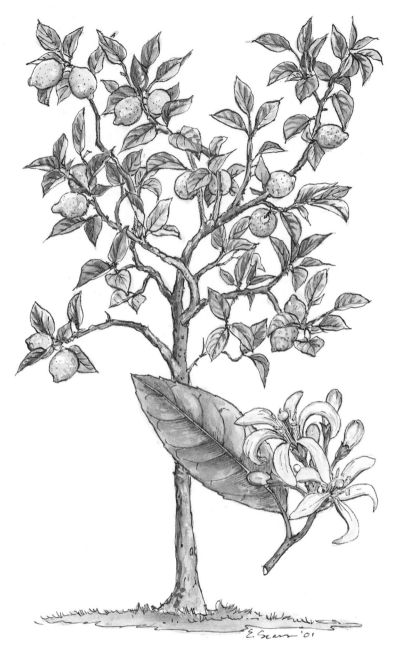

Citrus limon

Lemon

🌿 **LATIN NAME:** *Citrus limon*

🌿 **FAMILY:** Rutaceae

🌿 **COMMON NAME:** Lemon

🌿 **HEALTH PATTERN:** Digestion

🌿 **PLANT DESCRIPTION:**

The lemon tree is an evergreen that reaches 15 to 20 feet (5 to 7 meters) tall. The oval leaves are glossy, green, and smooth and approximately 2 inches (5 cm) long. The fragrant flowers are white on the inside and purple or pink on the outside. The fruit, known commonly as a lemon, is oblong with a bright yellow bitter rind and a juicy, very sour pulp. The lemon tree is native to Asia.

🌿 **PLANT PARTS USED:** Rind, juice, pulp, and volatile oil

🌿 **TRADITIONAL EVIDENCE:**

Cultural Use

Asian. The topical application of lemon juice is recommended for treating dandruff, hair loss, and seborrhea (Kushi, 1993). Although tangerine peel *(Citrus reticulata)* is the citrus most often used in TCM, lemon has similar qualities of being sour and bitter and moving "qi" in the middle burner (gastrointestinal tract area). Lemon is quite sour and somewhat astringent and can disturb the function of the liver if taken in excess.

North American Indian. The Seminole tribe of the southeast United States uses various citrus species for food. The branches from the trees have been used to make bows (Moerman, 1998).

Hispanic. Lemon is used in cases of congestion of bronchioles and asthma, sore throat, warts, and corns. A conserve of lemon rind is recommended for headaches. The Mayans have used blossoms of any citrus fruit for despair and for the nerves. Mexican Americans make a hot tea of lemon juice with honey for colds. Lemon tea with whiskey and cinnamon is used for fever. Dry lemon powder is used to stop excessive bleeding. One drop of lemon juice in the eye is used to treat a foreign body, although it is painful. Traditional Mexican American midwives drop lemon juice into the eyes of newborns to prevent disease (Kay, 1996).

East Indian. In Ayurvedic medicine, the sour taste associated with lemon among other foods and medicinal plants is said to "improve the taste of food, enkindle the digestive fire, add bulk to the body, invigorate, awaken the mind, give firmness to the senses, increase strength, dispel intestinal gas and flatus, give contentment to the heart, promote salivation, aid swallowing, moistening and digestion of food and give nourishment" (Lad & Frawley, 1986, p. 29).

Indian traditional medicine practitioners recommend putting a few drops of fresh lemon juice into the eye each morning when cataracts are forming to gradually break up the cataract and make the eyesight clearer day by day. A drink made of fresh lemon juice also has been used to treat smallpox, measles, and other forms of fevers. It is used during hemorrhage from the lungs, stomach, bowels, uterus, kidneys, and other internal organs and is used to treat rheumatism, gout, low back pain, and nerve pain. Hot lemon juice is used for colds, influenza, and pneumonia. A glass of lemon juice in water is taken by mouth before breakfast and at bedtime for a laxative effect. This preparation also is used for nausea and to relieve the thirst of diabetics. Lemon juice is recommended for vomiting and headaches. Lemon also is used in the treatment of leprosy.

External applications of lemon juice are used for nerve pain, backache, dandruff, acne, skin infections, sunburn, and scabies. Lemon oil is used topically for hip pain, rheumatism, and low back pain and also may be used for postpartum hemorrhage. Natives of India used lemons to make a pickle of the fruit in its own juice with salt. This pickle is a popular remedy for indigestion (Nadkarni, 1976).

European. Anthroposophical health practitioners recommend the use of lemon compress when a patient is in danger of losing consciousness as a result of fever and/or delirium. The heat of the head is drawn toward the feet by the lemon compress (Bentheim et al., 1980). Lemon inhalations also are used in caring for patients with asthma and croup.

Culinary Use

Lemon oil is used extensively to flavor many food products such as bitters, vermouths, sweet liqueurs, soft drinks, drink mixes, frozen dairy desserts, candy, baked goods, gelatins, puddings, breakfast cereals, and fats and oil, among others (Leung & Foster, 1996). Lemon is an alchemical ingredient in many culinary creations. My family has a secret recipe for lemon bread that has the qualities of a pound cake. The recipe is not a pound cake recipe however, and when the lemon zest and juice are added to the other ingredients that have been mixed together, the dough takes on a completely different consistency. Many chefs add lemon to their creations because it brings out the flavors in the food.

Use in Herbalism

Lemon increases salivary flow, an important first part of the digestive process (Christensen & Navazesh, 1984). Because of this, lemon has been used extensively in cooking. It also has an extensive history of use in medical herbalism. American Eclectic physicians recommended the use of lemon to reduce fevers; as a tonic; and to treat scurvy, a debilitating disease caused by a deficiency of vitamin C in the diet. English ships planning to make long voyages were required by law to carry an ample supply of lemon syrup and oil of lemon in an attempt to prevent scurvy among the sailors (Felter & Lloyd, 1983). The ships were required to carry enough lemon juice for every seaman to have one ounce daily after being at sea for ten days (Grieve, 1971).

The popularity of lemon as plant medicine declined in the United States in the nineteenth century. Before that time, lemon had been used for rheumatism and liver and gall bladder problems in addition to those conditions previously mentioned (Crellin & Philpott, 1990). In the early 1900s in the United States, people used a natural lithiated lemon-lime soda to make the blood more alkaline, thereby increasing protection against disease, energy level, enthusiasm, and clear complexion (Aita, Aita, & Aita, 1990). One physician claimed to have cured cases of obstinate hiccoughs with lemon. Lemon juice has been applied with a thin paint brush to enlarged tonsils to reduce the swelling. It was applied locally in cases of sunburn, uterine hemorrhage, and scrotal pruritus with beneficial effects. Lemon was used to treat hoarseness, cholera, rheumatism, and malaria (Felter & Lloyd, 1983). It also was used to promote perspiration and urine output. Lemon was sometimes given to counteract narcotic poisons, especially opium, and was beneficial in jaundice and heart palpitations (Grieve, 1971). Lemon juice also can be applied to hemorrhoids to reduce swelling and bleeding (Weed, 1986).

Lemon essential oil is used as a sedative and an antifungal and antiparasitic agent and to reduce the frequency of bouts of chronic bronchitis in institutionalized patients. Lemon floral water has been used to irrigate wounds (Buckle, 1997). Lemon essential oil has been used to relieve mental fatigue, listlessness, and emotional confusion. The scent is believed to stimulate the mind, increase memory, and improve intellectual performance. The oil is increasingly being used in hospitals to neutralize unpleasant odors, as a disinfectant, and to disperse stale air. It has been found to have a psychologically strengthening effect on patients, especially those with terminal illness (Lawless, 1998). A thousand lemons yield between 1 and 2 pounds of oil (Grieve, 1971).

Cosmetic Use. Lemon is excellent for improving the skin. The oil is used as a fragrance component in soaps, detergents, creams, lotions, and perfumes (Leung & Foster, 1996).

BIOMEDICAL EVIDENCE:

Few studies have directly addressed the therapeutic effects of lemon on digestion or any other health pattern. The studies presented here have to do with the salivation response (a critical part of digestion) and the use of lemon in oral care.

Studies Related to Digestion

One review article regarding the use of lemon-glycerine swabs for oral care of patients (a practice done in the United States at least since the 1930s) concluded that although the swabs are one of the five most commonly used materials for oral care, the glycerine dries the oral tissues and lemon is too irritating for most patients, such as those receiving chemotherapy, and those who have stomatitis or oral lesions. One study found that the pH of the oral cavity after the use of lemon-glycerine swabs was 2.6 to 3.9 instead of the normal 6.2 to 7.6, causing a chemically induced decalcification of the teeth. In addition, the lemon-glycerine inactivated salivary amylase in the saliva of the 15 participants in the study. It also was found that the lemon-glycerine solution had little or no effect on bacteria in the mouth and therefore had no antiseptic activity (Wiley, 1969).

Lemon has the ability to cause humans to salivate, an important part of digestion. So often, people eat in such a hurry that they do not thoroughly chew their food. Chewing and mixing food with saliva is a key to healthy digestion and to overall good health and longevity. Nurses also have known of the traditional understanding of the moistening properties of lemon on the mouth, where digestion begins. One study found that it is possible to overstimulate the salivation reflex associated with lemon. Although lemon stimulates salivation, excessive, frequent stimulation may cause "reflex exhaustion" (Warner, 1986). In a controlled study, it was found that human salivation increases when noise is present, and the weight of saliva produced correlates with the level of noise chosen (Corcoran & Houston, 1977). It might be hypothesized that the high level of noise in health care facilities has the potential to cause "reflex exhaustion" in patients, just as too much exposure to lemon can. These studies seem to suggest that patients who are having difficulty with salivation or digestion perhaps could benefit from a balanced amount of noise and exposure to the taste of lemon before eating.

Studies Related to Other Health Patterns

Immune Response. Lemon compresses have been used to significantly reduce fever as compared with plain water compresses alone. Lemon compresses used with Paracetamol were even more effective in gently lowering fever (Faschingbauer, 1995).

Mechanism of Action

Lemon's ability to stimulate digestion (i.e., salivation) seems to be related to its physical and chemical properties (Christensen & Navazesh, 1984). Lemon peel contains citroflavonoids, sometimes referred to as vitamin P, that are beneficial in vascular disorders where venous insufficiency results in hemorrhoids and varicose veins. The flavonoids are reported to be able to increase capillary resistance (Crellin & Philpott, 1990). Lemon contains a component in the essential oil, cymene, that is known to have analgesic properties. The essential oil also has antibacterial actions against methicillin-resistant *Staphylococcus aureus* (Buckle, 1997). Research into the effects of fragrance has found that lemon oil activates the hippocampus, an area of the limbic system in the brain related to emotions and feelings (Lawless, 1998).

USE IN PREGNANCY OR LACTATION:

Use of lemon during pregnancy or lactation has no known contraindications.

Herbal Caveat—Pregnancy or Lactation

Some herbs are contraindicated in pregnancy because of a risk of the herb or one of its constituents stimulating the uterus and therefore possibly promoting fetal loss. Many herbal practitioners do not recommend herbal remedies, in particular oral doses of herbs, during the first trimester of pregnancy and seek an alternative. However, herbs are successfully used during pregnancy, especially to prepare the body for the birth. Herbs are relatively unstudied in pregnancy and lactation, so patients need to be made aware through education of the potential benefits and risks of using herbs for health conditions that arise during pregnancy or lactation. The use of herbal remedies during pregnancy often warrants a referral to a knowledgeable herbal practitioner.

USE FOR CHILDREN:

Lemon compresses around the lower legs can be used for reducing high fevers in infants and children.

Herbal Caveat—Children

Children have special needs in regard to herbal therapies. They require lesser amounts of herbs and often respond well to mild teas and topical applications such as compresses and baths. The lowest dose of oral preparations should be tried first before increasing the amount given children. Caregivers should observe children closely for responses to herbal remedies. Younger children, particularly infants, have traditionally been given herbs either through their mother's breast milk or in the form of a homeopathic remedy because of their sensitivity to medicines and treatments and the immaturity of their liver. It is recommended that a person knowledgeable in the herbal treatment of children be consulted before the offering of any herb to a child for the first time.

CAUTIONS:

The topical use of lemon essential oil can cause phototoxicity. This condition is caused by a reaction between the essential oil, the skin, and ultraviolet light. Exposure to either radiation from a tanning bed or natural sunlight can produce a skin reaction. Reactions can vary from pigmentation of the skin to severe full-thickness burns. Components in lemon essential oil called furanocoumarins (oxypeucedanin and bergapten) are thought to be responsible for these reactions (Naganuma, Hirose, Nakayama, Nakajima, & Someya, 1985). It is recommended to avoid sunlight and tanning beds while wearing lotions or oils that contain lemon essential oil. Although it has been thought that lemon juice rubbed into a tattoo would cause the tattoo to fade after being exposed to ultraviolet light, animal studies have not confirmed this (Chapel, Leonard, & Millikan, 1983).

Although disputed by The Society of Plastics Industry, there is some evidence to suspect that lemon may act as a corrosive agent when drunk in polystyrene cups and that it is best to drink lemon out of a china cup instead (Cembrowski, 1980; Phillips, 1979). Lemons used in excess also can cause decalcification and erosion of the teeth (Wiley, 1969).

NURSING EVIDENCE:

Historical Nursing Use

Nurses have often recommended tea with honey and lemon for soothing sore throats and the cough associated with the common cold. In Germany in particular, lemon compresses also have been used successfully to reduce fever gently in patients seen for general medical care and in postoperative care (Faschingbauer, 1995; von Samson, 1995). The compresses are placed on the lower leg (see topical application). Nurses also offer 7-Up or other lemon-lime soft drinks to comfort those who are nauseated.

Potential Nursing Applications

Nurses may want to consider researching the benefit of including lemon in the diet of those who are having trouble eating or digesting food. Nurses may want to research the effects of lemon essential oil on the mind and the effect of the inhalation of a small amount of the oil on salivation and therefore digestion. Lemon compresses can be considered for comforting those with fever and their use can be taught as a self-care technique.

Integrative Insight

Lemon is so common that its therapeutic applications are often forgotten. Although little biomedical evidence supports the use of lemon for health concerns such as improving digestion, lowering fever, and wound healing, it is clear from traditional evidence that lemon is worthy of further consideration in nursing care. Lemon elicits from the body its signature for use as an herbal remedy, increasing salivation, and causing the puckering or astringing of tissues.

THERAPEUTIC APPLICATIONS:

Oral

Lemon juice can be taken liberally as a tea or juice.

Topical

Lemon Compress for the Chest. The room temperature should be regulated so that the patient is not chilled by drafts or by the room temperature itself. The patient is covered for warmth. A woolen cloth with safety pins attached is placed on the bed in preparation for being placed around the chest area. Place another piece of soft material on top of the wool that will fit around the chest. Then the dipping cloth is prepared. A bandage-type material that will go around the chest is folded to fit the chest and then rolled on both sides up to the middle. Place the bandage on another cloth that can be used to wring out the hot bandage. This cloth should have both ends rolled too. Place boiling water in a bowl and using a fork to hold the lemon submerged in the water, use a knife to cut the lemon in half into a star shape. Use the base of a glass to press the lemon halves. The lemon is cut under water so that the volatile oil does not escape. Then put the cloth with the bandage on it in the lemon water, holding onto the rolled ends so that they do not get wet. After fully soaking the cloth, lift it out of the water and wring it out quickly using the outer cloth to retain the heat but expressing as much water as possible. If the bandage is too wet it will cool down too quickly. With the patient sitting up, tap their back with the hot compress to get them used to the heat. Take the bandage out of the cloth and roll it out around the chest. As soon as the bandage is rolled around the chest of the patient, wrap the soft cloth and the woolen cloth around the chest and secure them with safety pins. The patient puts on a shirt over the whole compress or pack and then is tucked into bed. Leave the pack on for twenty to thirty minutes unless it gets cool or the patient becomes uncomfortable. The pack is removed and the patient dresses immediately to avoid getting chilled. If the patient falls asleep, the pack can be left on until the patient wakes up because the body may produce enough heat to keep the pack from cooling down.

Compress for Fever Reduction. The lemon water is prepared as described in the previous section, except the water temperature must be approximately 37.6°C. The compresses can be wrung out in the same fashion or by hand and are wrapped around the lower leg from the top of the metatarsals to below the kneecap while the patient is reclining. The lemon compresses are left in place for 60 to 120 minutes. Blood pressure, temperature, and perspiration are observed to be sure that the patient's temperature is lowered gently (Faschingbauer, 1995).

Massage. Add 2 drops of lemon essential oil to 1 tablespoon (15 ml) of sweet almond oil and use for massage (Lawless, 1998).

Environmental

Bath. Add up to 3 drops of lemon essential oil to a morning bath to overcome tiredness. Do not exceed 3 drops because the lemon oil may burn the skin.

Lemon Inhalation. Prepare the lemon in hot water the same way as preparing for a compress (see topical section). Place a towel over the patient's head and tell him or her to breathe slowly and deeply.

Vaporizer. Add a few drops of lemon essential oil to a vaporizer or air diffuser in the study or the sick room to create a clean, fresh, uplifting atmosphere, especially for depressed and fearful patients (Lawless, 1998).

Lemons used in air fresheners and cleaning agents make excellent disinfectants. "It is being employed increasingly in hospitals today, not only as a disinfectant but also because it neutralizes unpleasant odors and disperses stale air . . ." (Lawless, 1998, p.172). One study demonstrated that lemon juice (approximately 2 tablespoons, or 30 ml per liter [quart] of water) can significantly disinfect drinking water by killing *V. cholerae*. Not all ground water is disinfected by the same amount of lemon juice, however (D'Aquino & Teves, 1994).

Herbal Caveat—Therapeutic Applications

In traditional and conventional herbal medicine, amounts of herbs given to patients are based on individual needs. The amounts or "doses" recorded here are provided so that the health practitioner has a general idea of the amounts recommended for an adult patient. Dosing in herbalism not only refers to amount of plant used but also includes when, where, and how to take a plant medicine. These dosages should not be used as guidelines for indiscriminate intervention without proper assessment, critical thinking, and patient education on the part of the practitioner.

Note: Please see chapter 5 for detailed descriptions of how to prepare various applications.

PATIENT INTERACTION:

Fever is one of the best natural remedies for infection. The problems that usually occur with fever happen because the heat generated during the fever rises to the head, causing discomfort and delirium. Many people have forgotten the use of lemon compresses to draw the heat of fever from the head to the lower limbs. Lemon had been a fever remedy until just a few decades ago. Lemon compresses have been shown to lower fever by degrees and can be considered for use in self-care practices. Lemon is safe for internal use, but in excess can cause erosion and decalcification of the teeth. Lemon is an excellent digestive stimulant in that it stimulates salivation. Chewing food thoroughly and mixing it with saliva is important to maintaining healthy digestion. Lemon with a little water makes an excellent gargle for sore throat and colds. It is best to drink lemon water or tea out of a ceramic, glass or china cup, not plastic or Styrofoam.

Herbal Caveat—Patient Interaction

Patients considering the use of an herb or formula of herbs in self-care benefit from education about the plant itself and the use of the plant in healing. This education can come through many sources, including local herbalists; plant specialists such as botanists; health practitioners such as nurses, nutritionists, naturopaths, and other physicians; and various written references including the scientific literature. Patients need to remember that their unique health care needs are not necessarily represented in any literature they may encounter. Therefore, it is recommended that a knowledgeable mentor be consulted before initiating self-care with any herb being used for the first time.

Note: You may want to keep a journal of your experiences with the herb.

Lemons are so readily available that it is easy to forget how important they are to the diet and traditional medicine of many countries. Because lemons are common, it is easy sometimes to overlook their special healing qualities. Being *mindful* of the foods and herbs we ingest means recognizing these special qualities. How often have you eaten a lemon or any food mindfully? Mindfulness is a state of awareness that is similar to what in nursing is called "being present." Being completely and purposefully mindful of one's actions and focusing thought for a period of time can rest the mind from the stress of excessive thought. Eating something mindfully can be like eating it for the first time. Plants that cause a strong human sensory experience can be used when practicing mindfulness. Citrus fruits are such plants.

Mindfulness and Lemon. Find thirty minutes when you will not be disturbed (Bring a timer if you need to so that you don't have to watch the clock). Pick a quiet location and bring a lemon that has been washed, a paring knife, and a towel. Lay the towel out in front of you and place the lemon and knife on the towel. Sitting in a comfortable position, close your eyes and breathe deeply, in and out, eight times. First look at the lemon, examining the color and shape of the peel. If your thoughts wander, bring them back to the lemon. Smell and touch the lemon and then use the knife to cut open the lemon. Listen to your thoughts about the lemon and about this experiment in mindfulness. Then, using all of your senses again, explore the inside of the lemon, saving tasting the lemon for last! Taste the *zest* (the yellow outer peel), the *rind* (the inner white part of the peel), and the *pulp*. While tasting the different parts of the lemon be observant how and where you feel the essence of the plant affect your body. After experiencing the lemon through taste, sit and smell the lemon. Does the smell make you salivate? Does just thinking of your mindful experience of the lemon make you salivate? Record your experience.

CHAPTER 14

Energy

INTRODUCTION

WHEN NURSES LOOK INSIDE THE CHEST CAVITY at the heart of a patient undergoing open heart surgery, they see and sense the life force or energy that beats in the hearts of men and women. Where that energy comes from may be unknown, but there is no doubt that the heart is the primary generator for the life force in the human body (Pearsall, 1998). The heart sets the rhythm for the person's life, a rhythm of pulses—contraction and release—energizing moments of action and moments of rest. Energy is the ability to do work, to move, and to exert power. How energy is manifested is unique to each personality, but inside each person, stored in the heart and conveyed to each cell of the body through the blood, is pure energy or the life force.

People are aware of their energy level. They know when they feel energized, empowered, and active. People also know that, when their energy level is low, they feel fatigued and perhaps unable to face their work or the world. Positive or high energy levels are typically associated with health, and low energy levels are associated with diminished health and vitality. People seek medical help for fatigue and low energy. Fatigue was the third most common reason people in the United States sought help from their doctor and a complementary therapies practitioner in 1997 (Eisenberg et al., 1998).

Most people like to be active and usually feel better about themselves when they can be active. Very active people, such as athletes, are acutely aware of their energy levels and know when they are at the top of their game. People with healthy energy levels do not just have high levels of energy or power. They also have energy that flows smoothly throughout the body and is exhibited in a controlled manner. A professional runner may have healthy energy levels, for example, whereas a child with attention deficit hyperactivity disorder may have lots of energy but is not able to harness the energy and be effective in activities of daily life.

In Chinese medicine, the smooth flow of energy or "qi" in the body is said to be governed by the liver. Some herbs help balance the energy in the liver and facilitate the smooth flow of "qi" in the liver and other organs. In addition to "qi," the Chinese believe that the person is born with a certain quotient of energy called "jing," or essence. The amount of "jing" a person has determines vitality, resistance to disease, and longevity. "Jing" is determined by the health of the parents. It is stored in the kidneys, the brain, the semen and ova, and in the bone marrow. "Jing" is considered precious because it cannot be replaced. Once native or congenital "jing" is used, it is gone and the person dies. One of the "goals" of Chinese medicine is to use lifestyle and dietary and herbal interventions to support the person energetically so that they build up their store of acquired "jing" and do not have to use their native "jing."

"Jing" can be depleted through stress, insecurity, and overwork; men losing too much semen; women bearing more children than they can constitutionally support; environmental pollutants; use of alcohol, tobacco, and other intoxicants; and by eating too much protein or sweet foods (Pitchford, 1993). Ways to nourish the "jing" include lifestyle practices such as yoga and meditation and eating cooked, well-chewed foods.

Nurses often hear people talk about feeling low in energy or fatigued. Many people are not aware of how their lifestyle choices can affect their energy balance. For example, children may not realize that eating lots of candy, although it may give them an initial burst of energy, can ultimately cause them to feel fatigued. People who dislike their work and yet choose to stay on the job can become mentally and emotionally drained because their heart's desires are unfulfilled. These types of energy drains can ultimately affect physical health.

All herbs affect the energy systems of the body in some way and can be used to restore and balance energy. The herbs profiled in this chapter—ginseng, coffee, tea, and ephedra—affect the energy of the body as a whole, such as its ability to do work or increase mental awareness. These plants affect the energy system of the body in different ways and if used excessively by some, or even at all by others, can potentially have unhealthy consequences. People learn throughout life how to garner energy and use it wisely to fulfill their desires. It also is possible to learn how the appropriate use of herbs such as those included in this chapter can help restore and support the body's vital energy.

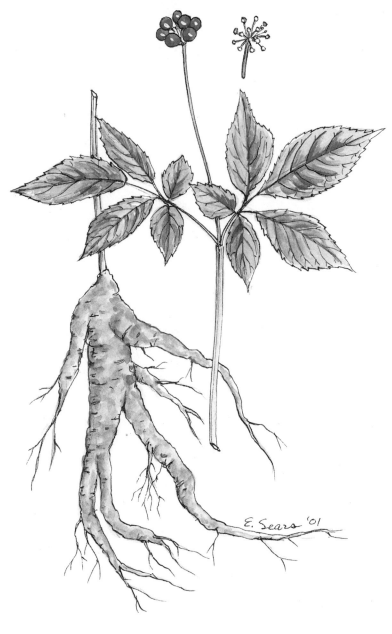

Panax ginseng

Ginseng

🍃 **LATIN NAMES:** *Panax ginseng, Panax schinseng Nees*

🍃 **FAMILY:** Araliaceae

Note: Do not confuse with Siberian ginseng *(Eleutherococcus sen-ticosus)* or American ginseng *(Panax quinquefolium)* an endangered, or legally protected species.

🍃 **COMMON NAMES:** Ginseng, white ginseng, Asian ginseng, true ginseng, Korean ginseng, red ginseng, Chinese ginseng

🍃 **HEALTH PATTERN:** Energy

🍃 **PLANT DESCRIPTION:**

Panax ginseng is a small perennial with a single stem with a few leaves, depending on the age of the plant. The first year of growth, ginseng has one leaf and three leaflets; the number of leaves change as it ages. Ginseng usually flowers the fourth year. The flowers are white and the berries are red. *Panax,* from the Greek, means "cure-all" and "ginseng" means "man essence or root." The shape of the branched root looks like the body of a man. Ginseng has a warm, slightly bitter and sweet taste. Cultivated plants are harvested in September or October after six to seven years of growth (Bensky & Gamble, 1993). American ginseng is sold in large quantities to China, whose own Chinese ginseng supply (of which there are five grades) has dwindled at times. Chinese ginseng is often adulterated (Felter & Lloyd, 1983). Good quality ginseng is not easy to differentiate from poor quality, especially for someone unfamiliar with the herb. In general, good quality ginseng root is thick, long, and intact with a thin cortex or bark. White ginseng should be pale yellow, and red ginseng should be reddish-brown and translucent. Freeze-drying ginseng has been found to prevent the decomposition of the saponins and increase the potency of the herb (Bensky & Gamble, 1993).

🍃 **PLANT PART USED:** Root

🍃 **TRADITIONAL EVIDENCE:**

Cultural Use

Asian. Ginseng is so revered in Asia that countries like Japan demonstrate their regard for the plant by housing a 1200-year-old specimen in the Imperial Treasure House in Nara, Japan (Bradley, 1992). Ginseng is known as a "fountain of youth" and is called "ren shen" (Chinese), "ninjin" (Japanese), and "insam" (Korean). Ginseng is classified as an herb that strongly tonifies the "qi" and enters the lung and spleen energy systems. There are numerous varieties of ginseng in China. The wild variety grown in the Jilin province is considered the best quality and therefore is very expensive. The ginseng that is culti-vated is either cured in rock candy and is used for treating "qi" and yin deficiency, or fresh dried root that also is known to tonify yin.

Fresh dried root is sometimes substituted for American ginseng, which is classified primarily as a yin tonic and is more cooling than Chinese ginseng, which is classified energetically as warm. Red gin-seng is steam cured, which causes its thermal or energetic quality to become even warmer. Korean ginseng is usually red ginseng and is stronger than Chinese ginseng. In China, ginseng is used primarily for severe collapse of "qi," which in the West would occur with conditions such as severe blood loss, impending collapse and shock, prolapse of organs, after high fever with lots of perspiration, and shortness of breath or labored breathing with sweating and weak pulse. It may be given to older people who need to feel more energetic or to people recovering from illness, depending on their symptom/sign pattern (Bensky & Gamble, 1993). Because Chinese ginseng is so warming, it cannot always be used. American ginseng, which is cooler, and Codonopsis root, "dang shen," which is more thermally neutral, are often substituted. Cooking ginseng with rice is thought to bring out its tonifying quality and decrease its stimulating qualities. Ginseng rice may be used by children, for example.

Japanese Kampo medicine employs ginseng in much the same way as Chinese medicine, as a warming "qi" tonic (Rister, 1999).

North American Indian. North American Indian use of ginseng centers around the use of American ginseng, not the *P. ginseng* re-ferred to in this profile.

Russian/Baltic. In Russia, ginseng is used to stimulate and re-store the immune system in diseases such as cancer and acquired im-munodeficiency syndrome (AIDS) (Zevin, 1997).

European. Ginseng, powdered root or tea, is approved by the Ger-man Commission E for use in geriatric and tonic preparations for in-vigoration during times of fatigue, convalescence, debility, and declin-ing capacity for mental and physical work (Blumenthal, Goldberg, & Brinckman, 2000).

Culinary Use

Ginseng is used in soft drinks, chewing gum, instant tea, premixed juices, and various functional foods.

Use in Herbalism

Historically, ginseng has been used in many Eastern countries to pro-mote health, sexual potency, and longevity, rather than to heal dis-ease per se. It also is used as a whole body tonic and is an adaptogen (Brekhman & Dardymov, 1969) used to support the healthy balance of the immune and stress response systems and to increase physical and mental performance. It is used traditionally to help those recov-ering from disease. Traditional uses of the "cure-all" ginseng include anemia, asthma, diabetes, cancer, dysentery, fatigue, gastritis, insomnia, and many more. Ginseng leaf is more cooling than the root and is used more in the summer months.

Cosmetic Use. Ginseng is used in numerous cosmetic products.

BIOMEDICAL EVIDENCE:

Both human and animal research support the traditional use of ginseng for improving energy (i.e., physical and mental performance). There are some studies that do not support the traditional use of ginseng for increasing energy. Most of the studies involve the use of capsulated and/or ginseng standardized extract.

Studies Related to Energy

Ginseng was shown to significantly reduce the fatigue in 12 student nurses working night shift who were given 1200 mg of capsulated ginseng in a double-blind, placebo-controlled, crossover clinical trial. Mood, performance, and competence were improved at night in comparison with daytime behavior (Hallstrom, Fulder, & Carruthers, 1982).

A daily dose of 200 mg of standardized ginseng extract was shown to significantly increase athletic performance in twenty-eight 20- to 30-year-old males in a placebo-controlled, double-blind, twenty-week German study (Forgo & Schimert, 1985, as reported in McCaleb, Leigh, & Morien, 2000).

Supplement capsules containing vitamins, minerals, and standardized ginseng extract were shown in one multicenter, double-blind clinical trial to significantly decrease fatigue after six weeks in people suffering long-term fatigue (at least 15 years) as reported by both patients and physicians (LeGal, Cathebras, & Struby, 1996).

In a study of Korean ginseng, given 100 mg twice a day for twelve weeks to 16 healthy males, the ginseng was found to be superior to placebo in improving attention, mental processing, sensory motor function, and auditory reaction time (D'Angelo et al., 1986).

One double-blind, placebo-controlled, three-week study of people in their early twenties, found no significant ergogenic effect on peak aerobic performance (measuring exercise time, heart rate, workload, and so on), after supplementation with one 200 mg tablet of standardized 7% ginseng daily (Allen, McLung, Nelson, & Welsch, 1998).

In a randomized, double-blind, placebo-controlled trial of 36 healthy men, no significant ergogenic improvement (e.g., no physical or psychologic impact) was shown after participants took an oral standardized extract of ginseng in 200 or 400 mg doses per day for eight weeks as compared with placebo (Engels & Wirth, 1997).

Studies Related to Other Health Patterns

Lifestyle Choices. Ginseng has been known to be able to help the body stabilize after excessive intake of alcohol. *P. ginseng,* in oral doses of 3 g per 65 kg of body weight, increased blood alcohol clearance from 32% to 51% in 10 of 14 healthy male volunteers, 14% to 18% in 3 volunteers, and 0% in one subject, forty minutes after their last drink in a study in which each subject served as their own control (each subject's blood alcohol level was 0.18%) (Lee, Ko, Park, & Lee, 1987).

Hormone Balance. In a study of 66 men, those who received 4 g of ginseng extract orally each day for three months showed a significant increase in testosterone levels and in the number and motility of sperm (Salvati et al., 1996).

Red ginseng, 6 g given orally for thirty days, significantly reduced cortisol/dehydroepiandrosterone (DHEA-S) ratio and Cornell Medical Index and State-Trait Anxiety Inventory scores in 12 postmenopausal women with symptoms of fatigue, insomnia, and depression, demonstrating the positive effect of ginseng on stress-related hormones (Tode et al., 1999).

Comfort and Pain Relief. In animal studies, ginseng has been shown to relieve pain and increase the effectiveness of other pain medications such as Talwin and aspirin, without causing drowsiness. Ginseng exhibits both central and peripheral analgesia (Mitra, Chakraborti, & Bhattacharya, 1996).

Immune Response. In a comparison between wild (higher priced) and cultivated ginseng, wild ginseng was shown to have a total ginsenoside content of 45% and cultivated ginseng 37%. Oral doses of wild ginseng had a significantly greater effect on stimulation of cytotoxic T-cells in mice, whereas cultivated ginseng did not (Mizuno et al., 1994).

Restoration. A prospective study of 4634 people greater than 40 years old living in areas where ginseng is produced, from August 1987 to December 1992, demonstrated that those people taking ginseng extract had a significantly lower risk of gastric cancer. It is hypothesized that ginseng has a nonorgan-specific preventive effect against some cancers (Yun & Choi, 1998 as reported in Blumenthal et al., 2000).

Mechanism of Action

One of the challenges in researching ginseng is its complex chemical nature. Ginseng has been used traditionally for generations, and thousands of papers and books have been written on ginseng. There is an extensive knowledge base on the botany and chemistry of ginseng, but experienced researchers still do not claim to understand if and how ginseng works based on objective biomedical evidence. The active constituents in ginseng are the eighteen different triterpenoid saponins, some of which are known as "ginsenosides" by Japanese researchers and "panaxosides" by Russians. Some ginseng saponins produce effects directly opposed to other ginseng saponins (Foster & Tyler, 1999). "For example, ginsenoside R b1 exhibits CNS-depressant, hypotensive and tranquilizing actions whilst ginsenoside R g1 exhibits CNS-stimulant, hypertensive, and anti-fatigue actions" (Newall, Anderson, & Phillipson, 1996, p. 148). This was apparent with callers on the Natural Healthcare Hotline service at the Herb Research Foundation, where some people with hypertension who were taking ginseng would call in and report lower blood pressure even though the literature reports that ginseng should not be used if the person has high blood pressure.

The stimulant effects of ginseng are quite different from other substances such as coffee, which stimulate the body under any circumstance. Ginseng only stimulates the body when it is needed such as when the body is under stress. Ginseng has been shown to support and strengthen the adrenal gland (Shibata et al., 1985 as reported in McCaleb et al., 2000). Although ginseng is often used to increase virility and animal studies have demonstrated an increase in sexual response in both male and female animals related to ginsenosides, some state that the ginsenosides did not exhibit sex hormonal effects (Wong, 1984 as reported in Leung & Foster, 1996). The ginseng roots studied by Youn did not contain estradiol or estriol (DeSmet, 1992).

Animal studies have shown that the same dose of ginseng "may induce a physiological response which varies in degree and/or direction depending on the biological timing" (i.e., the time of day that the ginseng is given) as measured by changes in circadian rhythm (Cai, Hui, & Yu, 1990, p. 142).

USE IN PREGNANCY OR LACTATION:

Although Ginseng has not been shown to be teratogenic (World Health Organization [WHO], 1999), some sources (Bradley, 1992; Weed, 1986) suggest not using ginseng during pregnancy. The German Commission E and traditional Chinese medicine (TCM) do not have a contraindication for ginseng in pregnancy (Bensky & Gamble, 1993; Blumenthal et al., 2000). During labor, ginseng root can be chewed to lend energy for sustaining labor, especially difficult labor. Extracts of ginseng can be used for those who cannot chew the root. Some midwives and herbalists also recommend ginseng during the postpartum period for helping the stabilization of hormones, especially when the woman experiences depression (Weed, 1986).

Herbal Caveat—Pregnancy or Lactation

Some herbs are contraindicated in pregnancy because of a risk of the herb or one of its constituents stimulating the uterus and therefore possibly promoting fetal loss. Many herbal practitioners do not recommend herbal remedies, in particular oral doses of herbs, during the first trimester of pregnancy and seek an alternative. However, herbs are successfully used during pregnancy, especially to prepare the body for the birth. Herbs are relatively unstudied in pregnancy and lactation, so patients need to be made aware through education of the potential benefits and risks of using herbs for health conditions that arise during pregnancy or lactation. The use of herbal remedies during pregnancy often warrants a referral to a knowledgeable herbal practitioner.

Ginseng is not usually indicated for use in children. A child's life force is usually quite strong and dietary interventions are recommended first for children recuperating from minor illness.

Herbal Caveat—Children

Children have special needs in regard to herbal therapies. They require lesser amounts of herbs and often respond well to mild teas and topical applications such as compresses and baths. The lowest dose of oral preparations should be tried first before increasing the amount given children. Caregivers should observe children closely for responses to herbal remedies. Younger children, particularly infants, have traditionally been given herbs either through their mother's breast milk or in the form of a homeopathic remedy because of their sensitivity to medicines and treatments and the immaturity of their liver. It is recommended that a person knowledgeable in the herbal treatment of children be consulted before the offering of any herb to a child for the first time.

CAUTIONS:

No significant drug interactions or side effects have been reported, but ginseng should not be taken with other stimulants including caffeine. Ginseng is contraindicated in people with hypertension and acute illness (Bradley, 1992). Ginseng is contraindicated in TCM during acute illness such as colds and flu because of its strongly tonifying and warming qualities. Prolonged or excessive use has been associated with low risk (Chandler, 1988), but some still recommend that ginseng not be taken for more than three months at a time and preferably one month on two months off (Baldwin, Anderson, & Phillipson, 1986).

The documented side effects of ginseng are diarrhea, insomnia, and skin eruptions. An oft-quoted study by Siegel from 1979 about "ginseng abuse syndrome" has been discredited by reputable researchers, stating that the study had significant faults in its methodology including that the subjects were given excessive doses of ginseng (Foster & Tyler, 1999; WHO, 1999).

Insulin dosages may need to be adjusted in those diabetic patients who take ginseng (Brinker, 1998). Seven cases of mastitis and one case of postmenopausal bleeding have been reported related to ingestion of unspecified ginseng products (WHO, 1999).

Energetically, ginseng is very warming and is contraindicated in TCM for conditions known as "yin deficiency with heat" (e.g., thirsty, warm or hot feeling). The neck of the ginseng root, usually found near the wider top, is broken off and not used when the patient seeks the "qi" tonic action (e.g., to increase energy). This part of the root has mild emetic effects.

One source suggests not taking ginseng with vitamin C, its natural antagonist (Weed, 1986). Take care when purchasing ginseng. Some expensive ginsengs cost as much as $20 (U.S.) per ounce (Foster &

Tyler, 1999). There can be considerable variation in the panaxoside (various saponins) content of ginseng root and ginseng products. In one study in which 24 samples of ginseng *(P. ginseng* and *P. quinquifolium)* roots or products were analyzed, 8 were reported as containing no panaxosides at all. However, 1 of the 8 samples was a 60-year-old herbarium sample that had been attacked by insects. The roots in the study yielded higher panaxoside content than did the products (Liberti & Der Marderosian, 1978).

NURSING EVIDENCE:

Historical Nursing Use

No data are available at this time.

Potential Nursing Applications

Although there are many fields of acute care nursing, many nurses continue to work with the chronically ill and those who are rehabilitating from serious illness. Nurses may wish to collaborate with other practitioners such as TCM practitioners and physical therapists in studying the effects of ginseng in patients recuperating from debilitating illness. Nurses may want to consider researching the clinical potential of using ginseng to help manage patients' pain and lower insulin need in diabetic patients. Nurses also may want to consider the possibility of using ginseng themselves when working night shifts and long hours during nursing shortages.

Integrative Insight

Ginseng is a good example of why nurses cannot just rely on research to provide a definitive answer as to when, why, and how they should consider supporting the clinical use of an herb. Biomedical research provides valuable information that can be added to the bank of knowledge on a particular herb. But even though ginseng has had at least 30 years of scientific research—clinical trials, animal studies, and thousands of years of traditional use—biomedical scientists still are perplexed and do not completely understand how and why it works. Part of the reason ginseng is not understood from a biomedical paradigm is that it has constituents that have completely opposite actions; for example, one ginsenoside is tranquilizing and another is antifatiguing. Ginseng is an adaptogen that promotes energy and increases human and animal performance only when necessary. Ginseng does not just stimulate the body regardless of the need, the way that other plants like coffee do. Research cannot explain the ability of ginseng to "know" what to do in the body to bring greater harmony, energy, balance, and health to the patient. Observation of caregivers such as nurses is important to furthering the understanding of the use of medicinal plants such as ginseng and how the relationship between plant and patient affects health and well-being.

Oral

Dried Root as Decoction. Use 0.6 to 2 g as a daily dose in the morning for up to three months (Blumenthal et al., 2000; Bradley, 1992). Use 0.6 to 3 g one to three times daily eaten or prepared as tea (McGuffin, Hobbs, Upton, & Goldberg, 1997). If using as a single herb, simmer the sliced whole root in water for forty-five minutes, or if the root is expensive, use a special ginseng cooker available at Asian markets or herb stores.

Fluid Extract. (1:1 g/ml): 1 to 2 ml daily

Tincture. (1:5 g/ml): 1 to 2 teaspoons (5 to 10 ml) daily

Standardized Extract (4% Total Ginsenosides). 100 mg twice daily

Topical

No data are available at this time.

Environmental

No data are available at this time.

Herbal Caveat—Therapeutic Applications

In traditional and conventional herbal medicine, amounts of herbs given to patients are based on individual needs. The amounts or "doses" recorded here are provided so that the health practitioner has a general idea of the amounts recommended for an adult patient. Dosing in herbalism not only refers to amount of plant used but also includes when, where, and how to take a plant medicine. These dosages should not be used as guidelines for indiscriminate intervention without proper assessment, critical thinking, and patient education on the part of the practitioner.

Note: Please see chapter 5 for detailed descriptions of how to prepare various applications.

PATIENT INTERACTION:

Ginseng has been revered in China as a "cure-all" and as an adaptogen herb, meaning that it helps bring greater overall balance to the body, mind, and spirit rather than treating specific disease. It has been researched and used for many years. *P. ginseng,* the herb many westerners know as the "fountain of youth" herb is very warming, and the Chinese know very well that it is contraindicated in many conditions, especially as people age, because often there is excess heat in the body. This is one of the reasons why the Chinese buy large amounts of American ginseng each year, even though they have access to Chinese ginseng. American ginseng is thermally a cooler herb. Also it may not be appropriate for some people to take *P. ginseng.* For example, many Westerners have fatigue and weakness that is not related to a deficiency condition such as is found in people recuperating from blood loss or illness. Many Westerners are fatigued and weak because of the opposite condition, excess. They may be overweight as one example. In general, taking ginseng in cases of excess is generally contraindicated in traditional Chinese herbal medicine unless used in formulation by a knowledgeable practitioner for a specific reason. Other herbs can be used to help decrease the excess condition, thereby increasing energy in the body. Check with a practitioner before using ginseng for more than an occasional cup of tea.

Herbal Caveat—Patient Interaction

Patients considering the use of an herb or formula of herbs in self-care benefit from education about the plant itself and the use of the plant in healing. This education can come through many sources, including local herbalists; plant specialists such as botanists; health practitioners such as nurses, nutritionists, naturopaths, and other physicians; and various written references including the scientific literature. Patients need to remember that their unique health care needs are not necessarily represented in any literature they may encounter. Therefore, it is recommended that a knowledgeable mentor be consulted before initiating self-care with any herb being used for the first time.

NURTURING THE NURSE-PLANT RELATIONSHIP:

Note: You may want to keep a journal of your experiences with the herb.

Go to your nearest Chinese herb shop and ask to look at the different grades of ginseng whole root. Be sure to ask the prices on each one. Don't forget, you probably won't be able to tell the difference in grades with the naked eye! Then purchase a piece of "ren shen." For this tasting, you will need only a piece that weighs 1 to 2 *qian* (pronounced chen), or 3 to 6 g (about ¼ ounce). Slice it and put it in a small pot with 1½ cups (360 ml) water. Raise the water just to the boiling point and take it off the heat. Cover and let it steep for 4 hours. After the steeping, raise the temperature again until steam is rising from the water and gently simmer for 3 hours. The water level should be two thirds of the original level after cooking. After the tea cools down, sip the tea paying attention to what you experience in your body with this root that for many has represented the fountain of youth. The root is edible and can be eaten as well. The taste is sweet and slightly bitter. Record your energy levels before and after the herb tasting.

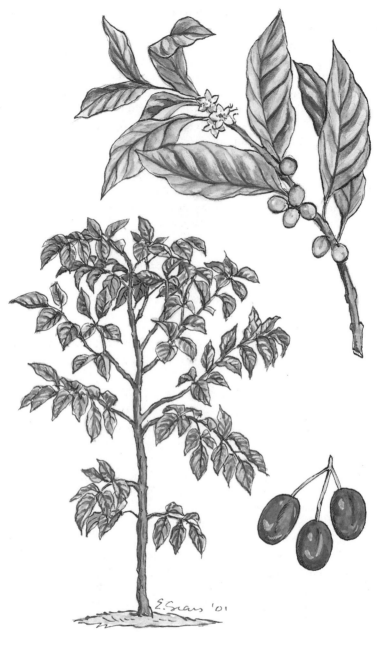

Coffea arabica

Coffee

LATIN NAME: *Coffea arabica L.*

FAMILY: Rubiaceae
Note: Do not confuse coffee with coffeeberry *(Karwinskia humboldtiana)*

COMMON NAMES: Coffee, Arabian coffee, caffea, arabica, espresso, café, mocha

HEALTH PATTERN: Energy

PLANT DESCRIPTION:

Coffee is a tree that is native to Arabia and which in the wild grows to 30 feet (10 meters). The cultivated tree is kept shorter to expedite harvesting of the berries. The leaves are evergreen, smooth and shiny, and approximately 6 inches (15 cm) long. The flowers are white and grow in clusters. The berries, also called "cherries," take three years to appear after starting the plant. They are red with two seeds that are green and flat on one side with a line running lengthwise down the middle of the seed. After the outer pulp of the berry is removed either by a dry or wet process, the seeds are roasted to develop the volatile oil so that the aroma is enhanced. The coffee season lasts from September to December. Robusta coffee comes primarily from African countries, and Arabica coffee comes from Central and South America.

Good coffee is said to be firm and solid and able to immediately sink when placed in water. Roasted coffee is lighter and more aromatic than green coffee (Felter & Lloyd, 1983; Leung & Foster, 1996). Decaffeinated coffee is produced by extracting the caffeine with a solvent before roasting. Instant coffee is made by extracting the roasted and ground coffee with water while under pressure. The extract is then freeze-dried or spray-dried (Leung & Foster, 1996).

PLANT PARTS USED: Seed (bean) and leaf (contains more caffeine)

TRADITIONAL EVIDENCE:

Cultural Use

Asian. In TCM, it is believed that while coffee may tonify the yang somewhat, it readily drains kidney (energy system) yang and can aggravate the liver energy system.

East Indian. Coffee is referred to in Sanskrit as "mlechca-phala" and in Hindi as "kafi." It is thought to hasten old age and decrease longevity because it disturbs the normal metabolism. It has been used for asthma, delirium tremens, whooping cough, heart palpitations, cholera infantum, chronic diarrhea, gout, early stages of typhoid fever, malaria, opium, and alcohol poisoning. It is given in spoonfuls after surgery to patients as an antiemetic.

Middle Eastern. The Arabs serve coffee, as do the Turks, in a little cup with the grounds. They roast and grind the coffee immediately before serving, add the coffee to a pot with sugar and water, and boil it. The coffee is served with the grounds in the cup. It is believed that the grounds neutralize any excessively stimulating qualities associated with the caffeine in the coffee (Vogel, 1991).

European. Coffee was introduced to Europe in the sixteenth century (Grieve, 1976).

Culinary Use

Coffee is best used right after roasting. The roasted seeds are ground and infused into a very popular beverage known by the common name for the seed of the plant, "coffee," also referred to as a cup of "java" or "Joe." Coffee is widely used as a flavoring agent in alcoholic and non-alcoholic beverages, ice cream, candy, baked goods, and sauces (Leung & Foster, 1996). Used coffee grounds are helpful in composting.

Use in Herbalism

An infusion of roasted coffee has been used as a stimulant and an antiemetic. It mildly stimulates digestion and increases biliary flow and intestinal peristalsis. Coffee is used to decrease a feeling of fullness after a large meal and to regulate the bowels. It also has a diuretic action. It increases circulation and, if drunk too much, can overstimulate the nervous and digestive systems. Those who are drowsy or intoxicated have used strong, black coffee to increase mental alertness and "sober up." Coffee also is drunk by hard laborers during cold winter months.

Infusion of coffee is given along with a gentle purgative and warm footbath for fullness in the head (congestive headache) and pain in the back. Coffee and coffee syrup have been used successfully in whooping cough, rheumatism, gout, gravel, malaria, dropsies of the heart, postpartum hemorrhage, and asthma. Coffee and tea produce therapeutic results that caffeine alone does not (Felter & Lloyd, 1983). Coffee enemas are sometimes recommended as part of nonconventional cancer programs to stimulate and assist the liver in detoxification, while taking large quantities of recommended nutritional supplements. Coffee is given generally recognized as safe (GRAS) status, but caffeine is being reevaluated (Leung & Foster, 1996).

Coffee charcoal, the ground outer part of the green dried coffee seed that is roasted and carbonized, is used for relieving symptoms of acute diarrhea and also is applied topically for mild inflammation of the oral mucosa (Schilcher, 1992).

BIOMEDICAL EVIDENCE:

In the United States, approximately 80% of adults regularly drink coffee (La Croix, Mead, Liang, Thomas, & Pearson, 1986). The percentages may be just as high or higher in other countries. Coffee and the lifestyle rituals surrounding coffee are a huge part of many cultures. Nurses who are observant of cultural traditions can identify how these rituals are demonstrated patient by patient. Numerous studies have been conducted on the physiologic effects of caffeine, a constituent in coffee, in relation to energy levels; however, fewer studies, some of which are included here, have been conducted on coffee as a whole herb. Several epidemiologic studies have been conducted on coffee consumption and its relationship with health.

Oftentimes these studies are not specific regarding the way the coffee is prepared, or in the case when coffee as a beverage is being studied, the number of cups of coffee consumed. As with all botanical studies, it is best to specifically identify the form of plant used. The way coffee is prepared is important to various health-related risk factors. Not all of the studies presented here are specific enough in regard to botanical preparation.

Studies Related to Energy

Coffee was shown in a randomized, crossover study of 32 participants, to produce mild autonomic nervous system stimulation, increased alertness, and elevation in mood. Although different beverage strengths were used (coffee beverage with 75 and 150 mg of caffeine), and caffeine did show some dose-dependent effects on some of the autonomic responses, caffeine level was shown not to be an important factor (Quinlan et al., 2000).

Coffee has traditionally been used to relieve symptoms of the common cold. In a study of 100 subjects, 53 of whom were healthy and 47 of whom had colds who reported changes in mood and/or performance, 35 people were assigned to drink coffee, 32 to drink decaffeinated coffee, and 33 to drink juice. A significant increase in alertness and psychomotor speed, alleviating the cold symptoms, was demonstrated in the coffee group and, to a certain extent, in the decaffeinated coffee group as well (Smith, Thomas, Perry, & Whitney, 1997).

Studies Related to Other Health Patterns

Lifestyle Choices. In a recent case study by a home health care nurse, the care plan for a man with diabetes and chronic obstructive pulmonary disease was a complete failure until the nurse offered to bring a cup of coffee to the patient and have their meeting over coffee. The patient responded so favorably that all of the team members started seeing the patient earlier in the day with a shared cup of coffee. The patient was much more active and amenable to participating in his rehabilitation. He told the nurse his story, a pleasant memory, that as a police officer, he had always started the day with his fellow officers over a cup of coffee (Lesley, 1998).

In a study of 2638 people, 90% of whom drank coffee regularly, approximately one-third stopped drinking caffeinated coffee because they thought it was not healthy for them. Only 10% of those who stopped drinking caffeinated coffee did so at the suggestion of a physician. Two-thirds of the sample continued drinking caffeinated coffee. In a survey of 700 physicians, 75% recommended changes in caffeine consumption to patients with insomnia and other symptoms evaluated in the study that are often related to excessive coffee/caffeine intake. Only 68% of physicians recommended lifestyle changes in relation to caffeine consumption to pregnant women (Soroko, Chang, & Barrett-Connor, 1996).

Mobility. In one large study of the relationship between coffee or tea drinking and cardiovascular health in over 5000 men and 5000 women, it was found that despite the similarities between coffee and tea (i.e., the caffeine content), coffee consumption was associated somewhat with a beneficial effect on coronary risk factors and mortality, whereas tea was not (Woodward & Tunstall-Pedoe, 1999). Habitual coffee drinking has been shown to be related to lower blood pressure with and without adjustment for alcohol use, cigarette smoking, body mass index, glucose tolerance, and green tea consumption (Wakabayashi et al., 1998). It also has been linked to hypertension in numerous other studies of coffee consumption during the workday (Lane, Phillips-Bute, Pieper, 1998).

Hormone Balance. One nine-week study of coffee randomly assigned 107 volunteers to one of three groups: Group A drank 4 to 6 cups of coffee each day that had been prepared by boiling, known pharmaceutically as a filtered decoction. Group B drank the exact same amount of coffee, but the coffee was percolated. Group C drank no coffee. Group A demonstrated a significant rise in serum cholesterol and low-density lipoprotein (LDL) levels after nine weeks, whereas Groups B and C showed no changes. The change in Group A was thought to be due to boiling the coffee (Bak & Grobbee, 1989). Instant coffee also is associated with increased serum LDL and lower triglyceride levels in Japanese men (Miyake et al., 1999).

Digestion. A large prospective study conducted over ten years has shown that coffee drinking has been shown to be linked with decreased risk of gallstone disease in 46,008 men (Leitzman et al., 1999).

Emotions and Adaptation. A review article reported that caffeine not only increases anxiety in psychiatric patients but also that patients drinking coffee are prescribed significantly higher doses of phenothiazines than those who drink decaffeinated coffee. It was suggested that the prescribing physicians may have detected greater agitation in the coffee drinkers and prescribed more of the drug. It also has been shown that caffeine lengthens the seizures associated with electroconvulsive therapy. It is well known that patients with diagnosed anxiety or panic disorders fare better when reducing or abstaining from coffee (Kruger, 1996).

Elimination. Caffeinated coffee was found to stimulate colon motor activity 23% more than decaffeinated coffee, 60% stronger than plain water, and equaled the elimination effect of a 1000 kcal meal in a small sample of 12 healthy participants (Rao, Welcher, Zimmerman, & Stumbo, 1998).

Mechanism of Action

Coffee is classified as a narcotic stimulant (Duke, 1985). One major constituent known to be at least partially responsible for the stimulant activity of coffee is the caffeine content. The caffeine content of green coffee can be between 0.06% to 0.32%, less after roasting. One cup of coffee usually contains approximately 100 mg of caffeine. Caffeine is addicting. It acts by blocking the normal action of adenosine, resulting in an overactive adenosine system, abnormal sedation, and therefore a subsequent craving for caffeine whenever the effect wears off (Duke, 1985). Adenosine is known to inhibit dopamine release, so if its action is blocked, excess dopamine in the body results. It is speculated that caffeine could aggravate those psychiatric conditions, such as schizophrenia, which are thought to be linked to increased dopamine levels. Coffee and many psychiatric medications form an insoluble flaky precipitate in vitro and if this were found to be so in vivo, it is hypothesized that there could be exacerbation of psychotic symptoms. Caffeine may be a drug of abuse (Kruger, 1996). Roasted coffee contains much less of other constituents such as tannins and trigonelline that are found in green coffee. Coffee also contains chlorogenic acid, which also has significant diuretic, stimulant, and cholorectic properties. Roasted coffee contains high levels of niacin (Leung & Foster, 1996). It is used in many analgesic preparations because it potentiates the effect of aspirin and paracetamol (Wren, 1988). Experiments in animals and three human volunteers confirmed that enzymes from green coffee seed can convert type O to type B blood (Duke, 1985).

Coffee is effective in relieving symptoms associated with asthma because it contains xanthines, such as theobromine and theophylline, which help stop bronchospasm (Duke, 1997). The following list shows the caffeine content of some common coffee beverages (Duke, 1985) (180 ml is equivalent to approximately 6 ounces):

6 ounces (180 ml) espresso coffee = 310 mg
180 ml boiled coffee = 100 mg
180 ml instant coffee = 65 mg

The method of preparation is more important than the original plant's caffeine content in determining how much caffeine is in the final product (Foster & Tyler, 1999). Some studies have shown that coffee that is filtered through paper traps cholesterol-raising constituents such as cafestol and kahweol (Miyake et al., 1999; Urgert & Katan, 1997).

USE IN PREGNANCY OR LACTATION:

Some sources say that coffee should not be used by people trying to conceive or during pregnancy because of the caffeine (McGuffin et al., 1997; Weed, 1986). Another source reports that caffeine consumption was not associated with infertility in a study of 1818 women who drank up to 2 cups of coffee per day (Joesoef, Berel, Rolfs, Aral, & Cramer, 1990). Another source also reports no correlation between coffee and infertility in 210 women (Caan, Quesenberry, & Coates, 1998). Caffeine has been shown to reduce iron levels in breast milk and therefore is contraindicated during lactation (Brinker, 1998).

Herbal Caveat—Pregnancy or Lactation

Some herbs are contraindicated in pregnancy because of a risk of the herb or one of its constituents stimulating the uterus and therefore possibly promoting fetal loss. Many herbal practitioners do not recommend herbal remedies, in particular oral doses of herbs, during the first trimester of pregnancy and seek an alternative. However, herbs are successfully used during pregnancy, especially to prepare the body for the birth. Herbs are relatively unstudied in pregnancy and lactation, so patients need to be made aware through education of the potential benefits and risks of using herbs for health conditions that arise during pregnancy or lactation. The use of herbal remedies during pregnancy often warrants a referral to a knowledgeable herbal practitioner.

USE FOR CHILDREN:

Although in some cultures coffee is given to children to drink, coffee is said by some to be contraindicated in children because it produces sleeplessness and therefore can inhibit growth (Nadkarni, 1976).

Herbal Caveat—Children

Children have special needs in regard to herbal therapies. They require lesser amounts of herbs and often respond well to mild teas and topical applications such as compresses and baths. The lowest dose of oral preparations should be tried first before increasing the amount given children. Caregivers should observe children closely for responses to herbal remedies. Younger children, particularly infants, have traditionally been given herbs either through their mother's breast milk or in the form of a homeopathic remedy because of their sensitivity to medicines and treatments and the immaturity of their liver. It is recommended that a person knowledgeable in the herbal treatment of children be consulted before the offering of any herb to a child for the first time.

CAUTIONS:

A fatal dose of caffeine in humans is 10 g (Leung & Foster, 1996). A dose of caffeine, 1 g or more, or coffee drunk to excess leads to nervousness, irritability, dejected spirits, mental confusion, trembling, headache, and ringing in the ears. Some overusers can suffer from chronic coffee poisoning with symptoms such as emaciation, dusky skin, expressionless features, dilated pupils, trembling lips and tongue, sleep disturbance, poor appetite, diarrhea or constipation, neuralgic pain, dizziness and headache, and impotence (Felter & Lloyd, 1983).

Coffee should not be consumed by those with anxiety or panic disorders and there is some question about the advisability of using caffeine by people with any psychiatric disorder, especially those disorders affected by increased dopamine levels or in patients taking psychiatric medications or sedative hypnotics (Brinker, 1998; Kruger, 1996). There is some conflicting evidence that coffee is linked to myocardial infarction and different types of cancer and is mutagenic. The mutagenicity of coffee can be inactivated by sodium sulfite, sodium bisulfite, and metabisulfite. Some have suggested adding these chemicals to coffee to reduce potential mutagenicity (Leung & Foster, 1996).

Coffee should not be used long-term or excessively. Because coffee stimulates gastric secretion, people with gastric ulcer should not drink it. People with glaucoma should not drink coffee because it has been shown to increase intraocular pressure, at least temporarily (McGuffin et al., 1997). Coffee that is not filtered through filter paper has been shown to increase serum concentrations of total cholesterol and LDL (Miyake et al., 1999; Urgert & Katan, 1997). According to one source, coffee is contraindicated in kidney inflammation and high-grade inflammation (Brinker, 1998).

Coffee may interact with iron, ephedrine, monoamine oxidase (MAO) inhibitors, adenosine, clozapine, benzodiazepines, beta-blockers, phenylpropanolamine, lithium, aspirin, phenytoin, oral contraceptives, cimetidine, furafylline, verapamil, disulfiram, fluconazole, mexiletine, and quinolone antibiotics (Brinker, 1998). Coffee charcoal is very absorbent and may limit absorption of medications given at the same time (Schilcher, 1992).

Coffee is commonly adulterated with cereals, sawdust, bark, acorns, figs, lupine, beans, peas, and baked liver (Nadkarni, 1976). Coloring agents are used to improve the appearance of lesser quality beans.

NURSING EVIDENCE:

Historical Nursing Use

Nurses routinely offer coffee as a part of a clear liquid or regular diet to patients.

Potential Nursing Applications

One major nursing application regarding coffee is to educate people about the medicinal values of the plant and how to use it judiciously. For example, nurses may want to tell people with asthma that if for any reason they were to forget their medication/inhaler, and were to begin wheezing, they could drink a few cups of coffee while they arrange to get their medication. Asthma can be life threatening and coffee has been reported to be successfully used in potential emergencies. Public health nurses and those who work with wellness programs can teach the benefits and risks of the use of coffee and how coffee can become a substance of abuse for some people. Nurses working with psychiatric patients need to be aware of the potential for skewed behavioral observations in those patients reacting to coffee intake. Nurses also need to consider creating clearer guidelines for providing coffee to ill and postoperative patients.

Integrative Insight

Research on coffee supports its common traditional use in many countries as an energy booster. Coffee is so readily available that most people do not even consider that when they prepare their morning cup of coffee they are self-medicating. People rarely consider that they may be overmedicating themselves when they drink it every day. Coffee is a powerful stimulant. Some cultures believe that although it may boost energy, it does so in a way that depletes the life force, therefore hastening the aging process.

Using coffee as an example is a terrific way to teach people about the safe and effective use of herbs in general. Coffee is a good example because people are familiar with it. When people are taught herbal principles such as that the preparation of a plant remedy has a lot to do with its therapeutic action, they understand because people who consider themselves coffee lovers know first hand that there are differences in "therapeutic action" of coffee products, depending on how the coffee is prepared. People also know that the same coffee preparation can affect people differently.

People might benefit from being more mindful about their use of coffee because overconsumption and abuse can lead to major imbalances of body, mind, and spirit. Coffee is actually strong medicine. The herb is used extensively in hospital care. Many of the medicinal plants used in clinical herbalism are not nearly as toxic, considering median lethal doses, as a cup of coffee (Duke, 1985), yet coffee is provided with other medications after surgery and other biomedical procedures often without question. Nurses have a wealth of biomedical and traditional evidence on coffee and may want to reevaluate their practices of providing coffee liberally without providing the patient education and information about the potential benefits and risks of its use.

THERAPEUTIC APPLICATIONS:

Oral

One 6 ounce (180 ml) cup of coffee contains about 100 mg of caffeine.

Coffee Charcoal. The daily dose is 9 g (Schilcher, 1992).

Topical

Health practitioners sometimes recommend coffee enemas for conditions such as cancer and asthma. The purpose of the coffee enema is to assist in the detoxification of the body, specifically by stimulating the liver. This is strong medicine and should be conducted under the guidance of a knowledgeable health practitioner.

Coffee charcoal is used topically for gangrenous ulcers and inflammation of the mouth (Felter & Lloyd, 1983).

Environmental

The aroma of roasted coffee is a powerful deodorizer and mild antibacterial.

Herbal Caveat—Therapeutic Applications

In traditional and conventional herbal medicine, amounts of herbs given to patients are based on individual needs. The amounts or "doses" recorded here are provided so that the health practitioner has a general idea of the amounts recommended for an adult patient. Dosing in herbalism not only refers to amount of plant used but also includes when, where, and how to take a plant medicine. These dosages should not be used as guidelines for indiscriminate intervention without proper assessment, critical thinking, and patient education on the part of the practitioner.

Note: Please see chapter 5 for detailed descriptions of how to prepare various applications.

PATIENT INTERACTION:

Coffee is used extensively as a beverage in many countries. It also has some strong medicinal actions and has historically been used for such discomforts as trouble breathing, headache, colds, and flu. As with any plant remedy, using coffee is associated with risks and benefits. Coffee contains the constituent caffeine. This is a very stimulating substance and used to excess can be addicting and debilitating. Coffee and caffeine also have been known to be lifesaving, as in the case of an asthmatic person who has an attack and does not have their medicine with them. This is not to say that a person can manage their asthma illness with a cup of coffee.

For those who are concerned about their excessive coffee use, examples of alternatives are roasted dandelion root beverage or chicory root. For those who take prescription medications, especially drugs for mental illnesses, check with a knowledgeable health practitioner about other beverages that will not pose a risk of changing the effect of the drugs. Coffee and/or caffeine have been shown to interact with several medications.

Herbal Caveat—Patient Interaction

Patients considering the use of an herb or formula of herbs in self-care benefit from education about the plant itself and the use of the plant in healing. This education can come through many sources, including local herbalists; plant specialists such as botanists; health practitioners such as nurses, nutritionists, naturopaths, and other physicians; and various written references including the scientific literature. Patients need to remember that their unique health care needs are not necessarily represented in any literature they may encounter. Therefore, it is recommended that a knowledgeable mentor be consulted before initiating self-care with any herb being used for the first time.

Note: You may want to keep a journal of your experiences with the herb.

Most nurses are very familiar with coffee. Some may have a very intimate relationship with this plant in regard to its use. Some nurses may even suspect that they cannot get through a day without at least one cup of coffee. It is addicting, more so to some than others. Because of this, I offer the following two options for nurturing the relationship with this plant:

1. If you are somewhat familiar with coffee as a beverage and want to use it medicinally, try this old remedy when you may feel fullness in the head (congestive headache) and pain in the back. Prepare a wine glass full of an infusion of coffee and sip it as you soak your feet in a warm footbath for twenty minutes. The footbath is an old nursing remedy for taking excessive energy (stuffiness) from the head and the coffee is a stimulant that moves the process along and helps with the headache.

2. If you have been drinking coffee in an amount you deem excessive, and you believe your relationship with coffee to be unhealthy, your nurturing experiment includes refraining from coffee and taking back your power. If you can't live without a cup of coffee, you may have turned over your power to the coffee plant! This is an unhealthy relationship. Refraining from coffee is not easy for most people because coffee is everywhere, but there are some things you can do.

Try looking for a coffee substitute. Serious coffee drinkers know that they can never replace the actual cup of coffee. So keep the ritual as much the same as possible and use a different herb. Some people do not realize that they are stimulated not only by the caffeine in coffee but also by drinking a hot beverage and the ritual of preparing the drink. Coffee substitutes provide the stimulation of a hot beverage. Try a roasted chicory or grain beverage for instance. There are products, often found in health food stores, that have to be percolated just like coffee. And if your daily coffee ritual includes instant coffee, then use an instant grain beverage substitute. You can still have your ritual of preparing an aromatic hot beverage. Dandelion root beverages are better for some people because the dandelion helps regulate blood sugar, often an underlying concern in people who need a coffee pick-me-up. Dandelion root beverages come in instant form, too.

There is still the issue of energy to deal with because the body gets addicted to the rapid energy "buzz" from the coffee. For the first few days coming off coffee, you may experience headache and flulike symptoms. Drink plenty of water and take walks, preferably in the woods where you can breathe in some new stimulating aromas like juniper, pine, fir, and spruce, which can be invigorating yet soothing to the mind and emotions. Take a sauna or hot bath and then calm your nervous system with a massage with warm oil. Roasted coffee has a good amount of niacin in it (Leung & Foster, 1996), which also can add to the "boost" that people feel when drinking it. You may want to consider taking a vitamin B supplement that includes niacin when stopping daily coffee intake. Healing a coffee addiction does not happen overnight. It can take months to heal. Meditation or centering can be very helpful during this time to tune into what the body needs to make the adjustment and adapt. Coffee is a powerful adrenal stimulant. "Ask" your adrenal glands what they need to heal. Record your experiences.

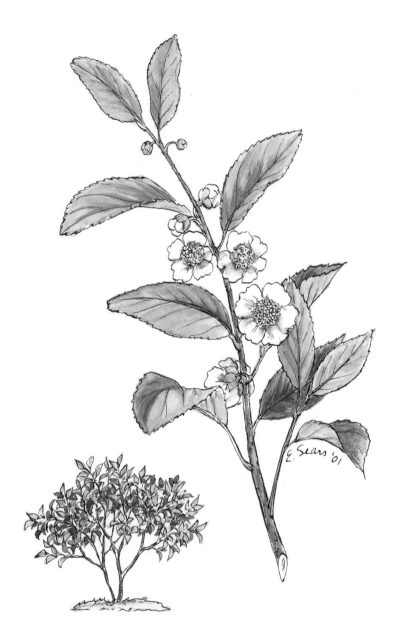

Camellia sinensis

Tea

🍃 **LATIN NAME:** *Camellia sinensis L. Kuntze*

🍃 **FAMILY:** Theaceae

🍃 **COMMON NAMES:** Tea, black tea, green tea, Chinese tea, oolong tea, thea

🍃 **HEALTH PATTERN:** Energy

🍃 **PLANT DESCRIPTION:**

Tea is a small evergreen shrub that in the wild can grow to a height of 30 feet (10 meters) but cultivated grows to approximately 7 feet (3½ meters). It is native to Asia. The leaves are alternate, dark green, and lanceolate or elliptical. There is either a single white flower or two or three bunched together. Each flower has five to nine petals. The fruit is the size of a small nut. Green tea is the leaf that is steamed and dried, and black tea is made from leaves that are rolled, fermented, and dried (Duke, 1985). Oolong tea is slightly fermented and considered an intermediary between black and green tea. In China, tea that has been harvested is not used until it is one year old because of the "intoxicating" effects of new tea (Felter & Lloyd, 1983).

🍃 **PLANT PARTS USED:**

The leaf buds and young leaves are used and together are known as a "tea flush" (Leung & Foster, 1996). The first buds and new leaves picked are the first flush, and the second growth that is harvested is known as the "second flush." The first flush is considered the best quality tea leaf.

🍃 **TRADITIONAL EVIDENCE:**

Cultural Use

Asian. Tea or "ch'a" has been used in China for thousands of years. In Japan, green tea is called "ocha." It is a cold and bitter herb that clears heat from the eyes and refreshes the spirit. Green tea is used among Kampo practitioners topically for burns and as an infusion to ward off colds and flu (Rister, 1999). Green tea is a recognized cancer preventive in Japan (Fujiki et al., 1999). The tea ceremony in Japan is a reknowned ritual of beauty and grace. It has social, esthetic, and religious aspects and takes practitioners much time to learn and perfect, just as with any other art form. The tea ceremony has a tension-reducing effect both on practitioners and guests (Keenan, 1996). Many religious sects drink tea to stay alert during meditation.

North American Indian. Native Americans have used tea as a beverage, and the Makah tribe use a poultice of the leaves to stop bleeding (Moerman, 1998).

East Indian. Tea is called "chai" in India. Both green and black teas are used in India. The green is considered to be more of a stimulant. Tea is used medicinally as a stimulant and occasionally as a gargle or injection. It is used for headache, neuralgia, and nervous depression.

European. Tea is a common beverage among Europeans, especially the British. Afternoon tea is a large part of the culture in Britain and "high tea" has become a popular event in many countries fashioned after Victorian tradition.

Culinary Use

Green tea is the most common beverage used by humans after water (Graham as reported in McGuffin et al., 1997). It is used as a flavoring agent and is used in baked goods, alcoholic beverages, candy, and puddings (Leung & Foster, 1996). Green tea, in particular, is growing in popularity and is being used in several functional foods. Many black teas are adulterated with other herbs, fragrant oils, and so on. For instance, Earl Gray tea is a black tea with bergamot oil, making it a popular tea to aid digestion after a meal. Tea is also a source of food coloring.

Use in Herbalism

Tea has been used as a cancer cure, an astringent, and a stimulant. It has been used to relieve headache, nervous and digestive complaints, amebic and bacterial dysentery, gastroenteritis, and hepatitis. Tea has been used for wounds, malaria, epilepsy, fever, smallpox, and much more. Tea bags are applied to sunburned areas, swollen eyelids, and tired eyes and used as a compress for headache (Duke, 1985).

BIOMEDICAL EVIDENCE:

Few clinical trials have been conducted on the energy effects of tea in humans. Green tea is thought to have the greatest potential for further development among natural products being reviewed for their cancer preventive properties. The studies on tea include the use of whole infused leaf.

Studies Related to Energy

Green tea has significant thermogenic and fat-oxidizing properties. In a small study of 10 healthy men, green tea extract in capsule form (50 mg caffeine and 90 mg epigallocatechin) was shown to significantly increase twenty-four-hour energy expenditure, significantly reduce twenty-four-hour respiratory quotient, and increase urinary excretion of norepinephrine as compared with placebo and caffeine (Dulloo et al., 1999).

Tea has been shown to promote significant increases in alertness and information processing capacity, which did not decline throughout the day, as compared with water in a study of 19 healthy participants who received 400 ml of hot black tea three times a day (Hindmarch, Quinlan, Moore, & Parkin, 1998). Another study of 30 participants demonstrated that black tea, 1 to 2 cups per day containing approximately 75 mg total caffeine, produced similar alerting effects to coffee despite lower caffeine levels and was less likely to disrupt sleep (Hindmarch et al., 2000).

Studies Related to Other Health Patterns

Lifestyle Choices. The mortality rate in 2665 practitioners of the Japanese tea ceremony, "chajin," was lower as compared with all Japanese women. It is hypothesized that this may be due to the regular ingestion of green tea but also is thought to be due to other factors such as the unique lifestyle of the *chajin*. Another study is being conducted to control for the lifestyle of the *chajin* (Sadakata, Fukao, & Hisamichi 1992).

Restoration. In a phase I/II study of 14 participants, green tea was shown to inhibit prostaglandin E_2 levels (used as colorectal carcinogenesis markers) in the rectal mucosa of 71% of the subjects who received a single dose of standardized green tea powder mixed in warm water. Further study is planned to explore the potential of green tea as a chemoprotective agent in colorectal cancer (August et al., 1999).

A prospective study of 8552 Japanese people has shown that those who were diagnosed with cancer and who consumed more than 10 Japanese cups of green tea per day received their diagnosis 7.3 years later for females and 3.2 years later for males than those who drank less than 3 Japanese cups of green tea per day. In a study of 472 participants, the women with stage I and II breast cancers who consumed more than 5 cups of green tea per day had a lower recurrence rate, 16.7 %, and longer disease-free period of 3.6 years than those consuming less green tea. Because stage III cancer patients did not show significant associations with green tea consumption, it was concluded that green tea may be more effective in early stages of breast cancer (Suganuma et al., 1999).

Both black and green teas are rich sources of flavonoids (antioxidants), known as "catechins," "thearubigins," and "theaflavins." In a crossover study of 21 healthy volunteers who received a single dose of tea (2 g black or green tea solids in 300 ml of water, with or without milk), there was a significant increase in plasma antioxidants, and the addition of milk to the tea did not change the increase in antioxidants (Leenen, Roodenburg, Tijburg, & Wiseman, 2000).

Skin Care. Green tea oral extract and topical applications (0.2 mg), given pretreatment and posttreatment, were shown in one study that included in vitro, animal, and human investigations, to significantly protect skin against the psoralen plus ultraviolet A–induced phototoxicity often occurring in patients with psoriasis by inhibiting deoxyribonucleic acid (DNA) damage. The topical application almost completely abolished the erythema caused by treatment (Zhao et al., 1999).

Digestion. Drinking plain black Ceylon tea (1.5 g per 250 ml boiled water) with each of three meals significantly reduced the frequency of phlebotomies needed in 18 patients with diagnosed hemochromatosis because intestinal iron absorption was reduced 70% by the addition of the tea. The type of Ceylon tea used in the study was chosen because of its high tannin content (Kaltwasser et al., 1998).

Mobility. In a study of 20 normotensive men, black and green tea were not found to significantly affect blood pressure when consumed regularly over a period of seven days (Hodgson, Puddey, Burke, Beilin, & Jordan, 1999).

Immune Response. Green tea ethylacetate extract demonstrated significant inhibitory effects against microorganisms known to cause dental caries in vitro, but black tea showed no antibacterial activity (Rasheed & Haider, 1998).

Elimination. In a ten-week, randomized, crossover study of 65 participants during which the subjects drank six cups of black tea per day following a standardized protocol for preparation for four weeks, the tea was shown to soften stool more effectively than placebo as measured by self-report (Bingham et al., 1997).

Mechanism of Action

Although tea leaves contain up to 4% caffeine, a cup of tea contains between 10 and 50 mg of caffeine because it is prepared as an infusion (Foster & Tyler, 1999). In a study of 19 healthy adults, which showed that tea significantly improved cognition and psychomotor performance, the investigators compared the response to caffeine and concluded that the energy effect of tea is not solely due to the caffeine, but also is due to the presence of other biologically active substances, expectancy of the subject, or sensory attributes such as the temperature of the beverage (Hindmarch et al., 1998).

In most studies, black and green teas have similar effects. In one review article, four of the effects of tea are summarized as follows: (1) Effects that are related to the polyphenolic antioxidants that lower oxidation of LDL cholesterol and therefore may be associated with decreased heart disease and cancer risk. (2) Tea and its antioxidants induce metabolic enzymes (primarily cytochrome P450, 1 A1, 2 B1 and glucuronyl transferase) that increase the formation and excretion of detoxified metabolites of carcinogens. (3) Tea lowers the growth rate of tumors. (4) Tea changes the flora of the intestines, increasing beneficial bacteria *(Lactobacilli* and *Bifidobacteria)* and reducing harmful bacteria (Weisburger, 1999).

In vitro studies have shown that during the fermentation process of making black tea from green tea, conversion of antioxidant catechins in green tea to partially polymerized theaflavin or thearubigin has no effect on its antioxidant scavenging abilities (Halder & Bhaduri, 1998). Milk does not impair the bioavailability of the catechins in black or green tea (van Het Hof, Kivits, Weststrate, & Tijburg, 1998). The antioxidants in green tea, mainly epigallocatechin-3-gallate (EGCG), are thought to be responsible for the chemopreventive properties of green tea (Mukhtar & Ahmad, 1999). EGCG also has been shown to inhibit tumor promotion in mouse skin through a reduction of specific binding of 12-O-tetradecanoylphorbol-13-acetate (TPA) and okadaic acid to their receptors, called a "sealing effect" (Fujiki et al., 1999). The polyphenols in black tea have been shown to convert dietary non-heme iron into a form that makes it unavailable for absorption (Kaltwasser et al., 1998).

USE IN PREGNANCY OR LACTATION:

Because of the caffeine, some sources report that black tea should be avoided by those women wishing to conceive and those who are pregnant (Brinker, 1998; Weed, 1986). One study of 210 women found that women who drank more than ½ cup of tea per day had a significant increase in fertility (Caan, Quesenberry, & Coates, 1998).

Herbal Caveat—Pregnancy or Lactation

Some herbs are contraindicated in pregnancy because of a risk of the herb or one of its constituents stimulating the uterus and therefore possibly promoting fetal loss. Many herbal practitioners do not recommend herbal remedies, in particular oral doses of herbs, during the first trimester of pregnancy and seek an alternative. However, herbs are successfully used during pregnancy, especially to prepare the body for the birth. Herbs are relatively unstudied in pregnancy and lactation, so patients need to be made aware through education of the potential benefits and risks of using herbs for health conditions that arise during pregnancy or lactation. The use of herbal remedies during pregnancy often warrants a referral to a knowledgeable herbal practitioner.

USE FOR CHILDREN:

Green tea is more effective than black tea for relieving discomfort associated with diarrhea in children. One heaping teaspoon of tea is decocted in a cup of boiled water for fifteen minutes. Some children just won't drink it because of the taste (Schilcher, 1992). One source (Brinker, 1998) does not recommend the use of tea in children because of its ability to decrease the body's absorption of iron necessary for proper growth and development in children.

Herbal Caveat—Children

Children have special needs in regard to herbal therapies. They require lesser amounts of herbs and often respond well to mild teas and topical applications such as compresses and baths. The lowest dose of oral preparations should be tried first before increasing the amount given children. Caregivers should observe children closely for responses to herbal remedies. Younger children, particularly infants, have traditionally been given herbs either through their mother's breast milk or in the form of a homeo-pathic remedy because of their sensitivity to medicines and treatments and the immaturity of their liver. It is recommended that a person knowledge-able in the herbal treatment of children be consulted before the offering of any herb to a child for the first time.

CAUTIONS:

Tea has been considered relatively harmless in healthy individuals who take the tea in moderation, but those who use tea to excess, thereby increasing their dose of caffeine and tannins, may experi-ence nervous and dyspeptic symptoms, with green tea being more injurious (Grieve, 1971). Tea is more likely to produce nervous sys-tem complaints and insomnia as compared with coffee (Felter & Lloyd, 1983).

Green tea is a significant source of vitamin K. One case reports the possible inhibition of warfarin by green tea consumption (Taylor & Wilt, 1999).

The tannins in tea are thought to be carcinogenic; however, adding milk has been found to bind the tannins to a protein in the milk, thereby preventing any harmful effects (Duke, 1985; Foster & Tyler, 1999). Fermented or black tea is not recommended for long-term use (McGuffin et al., 1997). Tea should not be taken in excess, in particular by those with liver disease (Shulz et al., 1998).

Brinker (1998) lists several speculative contraindications related to the intake of a caffeinated beverage, not tea as a whole. They in-clude kidney disorders, duodenal ulcer, heart disorders, psychologic disorders, and pregnancy. Brinker reports the following potential and actual drug interactions, primarily related to the caffeine content in tea: MAO inhibitors, ephedrine, chlorpromazine, adenosine, clozapine, benzodiazepines, beta-blockers, lithium, aspirin, phenytoin, quinolone antibiotics, and oral contraceptives.

NURSING EVIDENCE:

Historical Nursing Use

Nurses have been known to recommend black tea and prune juice as a laxative. Some lactation nurses recommend topical applications of tea bags to sore nipples in the early stages of breastfeeding.

Potential Nursing Applications

Nurses may want to consider the addition of green tea to clear liq-uid diets as an option. Oncology nurses may want to research the addition of information regarding tea to their dietary recommen-dations. Nurses may want to consider researching the long-term benefits and risks to health promotion related to tea con-sumption. The topical application of tea in wound healing also might be studied.

Integrative Insight

Biomedical evidence has identified the caffeine content in tea as being one of the primary reasons for its energy effects. Tea needs further study regarding its other potential health benefits. As with coffee, patients could benefit from more education about the benefits and risks of tea drinking. People who drink lemon with their black tea might choose to use a "spot" of milk instead, if they knew about the risks of excessive intake of tannins. The other important aspect of tea drinking, which has begun to be researched, is the health benefits of the ritual that occurs with black and green tea drinking, such as the health benefits of an afternoon tea break or the calming effects of participating in the Japanese tea ceremony. The effects of tea drinking may go far beyond the antioxidants and caffeine. Nurses know the importance of maintaining patients' daily activities or rituals. Familiarity supports stress reduction and psychologic orientation, which can lead to improved healing. Encouraging tea rituals might be very helpful in this way for some patients.

THERAPEUTIC APPLICATIONS:

Oral

Each 6 ounce (180 ml) cup of tea can contain between 10 and 50 mg of caffeine according to one source (Foster & Tyler, 1999) and 100 mg according to another (Leung & Foster, 1996).

Green Tea. Use 1 teaspoon (2.5 g) of green tea per cup. Commercial tea bags hold as little as 0.5 g. Steep in slightly cooled boiled water for about three minutes. Two to three cups a day is considered an average dose of tea (McCaleb et al., 2000). One study showed that green tea, in bags or loose, has less caffeine than black tea. The amounts of caffeine per cup were from 19 to 36 mg (Bunker & McWilliams, 1979).

Black or Oolong Tea. Steep tea in boiled water for three to five minutes. One source recommends steeping tea for at least fifteen to twenty minutes to get the fullest benefit of the tannin properties and a more bitter taste (Schulz et al., 1998).

Standardized Extract. Use 250 to 400 mg per day of extract standardized to 90% polyphenols (McCaleb et al., 2000).

Topical

Tea bags are applied to sunburned areas, swollen eyelids, and tired eyes and used as a compress for headache. They are also very soothing when applied to nipples during the early stages of lactation. Tea bags can be applied to sore, even fissured nipples, after nursing in addition to having a lactation specialist evaluate the baby's suck.

Environmental

The essential oil of tea is very stimulating and intoxicating and is rarely used (Felter & Lloyd, 1983).

PATIENT INTERACTION:

Tea drinking is a favorite pastime in many nations. Just recently, scientists have begun to understand more about the potential and historical health benefits associated with drinking both black and green teas. Black and green teas come from the same plant, they are just prepared differently; black tea leaves are steamed and fermented. Green tea is considered stronger medicinally because it has a higher content of tannins. Tannins, a plant constituent, have an affinity for protein and because excessive amounts of tannins can be harmful, tea is best drunk with milk to bind the tannins. Most people who drink green tea know that it does not taste very good with milk and most people drink it plain, the way it is drunk in Asia. Black tea can easily be taken with milk as the British do.

NURTURING THE NURSE-PLANT RELATIONSHIP:

Note: You may want to keep a journal of your experiences with the herb.

Both Asians and the British have a highly developed social ritual around the drinking of tea. To get to know tea, try planning tea time for an afternoon with some close friends. Plan to make a plate of finger sandwiches with the crust of the bread removed and the sandwiches cut into triangular quarters with some small amounts of your favorite fillings. Make some scones or biscuits if you have the time and serve them with your favorite jam, and have some delicate sweets as well. Prepare some pots of black and green tea you have purchased at your favorite gourmet beverage shop and have cream and a sweetener available for the black tea.

Serve your guests their choice of tea and then serve yourself. Breathe deeply of the aroma of your cup of tea and rest easily in your chair. Focus on enjoying the moment with your guests and let your troubles melt away for the time being. Sip your tea, noticing how you feel in your body, without drinking so much tea as to become too energized. The tea should only gently refreshen and enliven the mind and body. Perhaps you will want to have two teacups available for each guest so that both green and black teas can be tried for a real East–West experience!

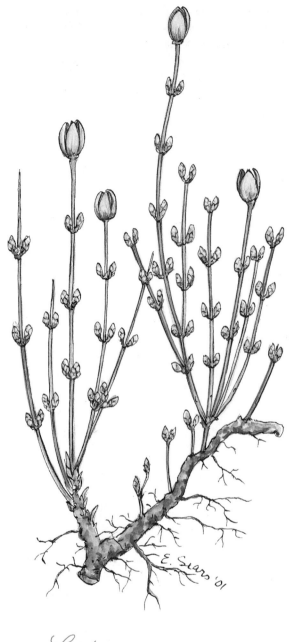

Ephedra sinica

Ephedra

🌿 **LATIN NAMES:** *Ephedra sinica S., Ephedra equisetina, Ephedra vulgaris*

Note: *Ephedra nevadensis S.,* known as "Mormon tea," and other ephedra species that do not contain the alkaloid ephedrine are discussed in the North American Indian and Hispanic sections only.

🌿 **FAMILY:** Ephedraceae

🌿 **COMMON NAMES:** Ephedra, amsania, budshur, chewa, huma, shrubby, soma, khama

Note: Although the Latin word *ephedra* can be translated as "horse tail," the herb known commonly as horsetail is from a different plant, *Equisetum arvense.*

🌿 **HEALTH PATTERN:** Energy

🌿 **PLANT DESCRIPTION:**

Ephedra is one of the oldest medicinal herbs on the planet. It was one of seven herbs identified from fossil pollen on the skeletal remains of Neanderthals from 60,000 years ago in Iraq. Ephedra is an erect, perennial shrub with short green branches and small triangular leaves that are scalelike and joined into the base into a sheath (Grieve, 1971). It is a flowering plant. The small white flowers turn into red fruit followed by two-seeded cones. Ephedra has a strong pinelike fragrance (McCaleb et al., 2000). There are over forty species of ephedra that grow in India, China, regions near the Mediterranean, Mongolia, Afghanistan, and North and Central America. East Indians have observed that rainfall has a tremendous impact on the quantity of alkaloid in the plant. Annual rainfall has an inverse relationship to the quantity of ephedrine, and an occasional heavy rain shower also affects the quantity (Nadkarni, 1976). It is slightly bitter and astringent in taste and causes a slight numbness of the tongue (WHO, 1999).

🌿 **PLANT PARTS USED:**

Green stems harvested in the fall before winter frost gives the most alkaloid (Nadkarni, 1976). The nodes joining the leaf segments are considered toxic in Chinese and Kampo medicine and should be removed before using (Rister, 1999). The dried branch, root, and berries contain very little alkaloid and usually are not used.

🌿 **TRADITIONAL EVIDENCE:**

Cultural Use

Asian. Ephedra, known as "ma huang," has been used for more than 5,000 years in TCM. Ephedra is classified as an herb that releases the exterior (opens the pores so that the illness or pathogen can escape), disperses cold, and enters the lung and bladder energy systems. By opening the pores, it supports the movement of lung "qi" and helps relieve wheezing. It promotes urination and reduces edema as well. Ephedra is almost always used in combination with other herbs. It is not used for prolonged periods of time because it induces sweating that weakens the body over a period of time. The herb is decocted by itself first, so that the foam that forms on the surface of the water can be removed before the other herbs are added to the formula. The same cautions are followed with use in the East as are recommended in Western herbalism (Bensky & Gamble, 1993). In Chinese herbal medicine, the herb is also honey-cured and stir-fried. This type of *ma huang* contains a higher concentration of antiasthmatic, antitussive, antibacterial, and antiviral components (Leung & Foster, 1996) and also reduces the tendency of the herb when used for longer periods of time to cause excessive perspiration (Bensky & Gamble, 1993).

Ephedra, "mao," is used in Kampo medicine in much the same way as in TCM.

North American Indian. The species of ephedra used by North American Indians are *E. nevadensis, E. torreyana, E. trifurca,* and *E. viridis. E. nevadensis* (Mormon tea) is alkaloid free, which means that ephedrine and its derivatives are not present in these plants (Foster & Tyler, 1999). The Apache and many other tribes traditionally have used the plant as a beverage tea and as a medicinal tea for venereal diseases. The Navajo use ephedra for kidney disease and the Shoshoni use a poultice of the powdered twig for sores on the skin. Others use the stem of the plant for gastrointestinal discomfort and itching of the skin. The stems also are used during the sweat bath and as a tea for cough, constipation, diarrhea, backache, menstrual discomfort, and anemia (Moerman, 1998).

Hispanic. Mexicans smoke tobacco and ephedra (Mormon tea) leaves, known as "canutillo del campo," for discomfort associated with headache and for urinary tract complaints. "Canutillo" meaning "little tube" is also a name given to horsetail, *Equisetum arvense* (Duke, 1985; Kay, 1996).

East Indian. In India, the ephedra "Khanda" or "Kharna," plant used for its ephedrine content is *E. nebrodensis.* Ephedra may be the plant source from which the famous drink of *Rishis* (ascetics) has been made. Ephedra is used to treat symptoms related to bronchial asthma; however, it is not recommended for prolonged use. The paroxysms associated with asthma may be controlled temporarily by ephedra, but the ephedra does not affect the "cause" of the paroxysms. A juice of the berries is used for respiratory conditions, and a tea is used for discomfort associated with rheumatism, asthma, syphilis, and poor digestion. Many Indians use ephedra because it is cheaper and is thought to have fewer side effects than the drug ephedrine (Nadkarni, 1976).

European. The German Commission E approves the use of ephedra internally for respiratory conditions with mild bronchospasms in adults and children over six years of age (Blumenthal et al., 2000).

Culinary Use

Ephedra is not used in cooking.

Use in Herbalism

Ephedra has been used in herbalism to reduce swelling of the mucous membranes and as an antispasmodic, reducing the discomfort of those with rheumatism, asthma, or allergies. It has been used prophylactically in hypotension associated with pneumonia and influenza (Grieve, 1971). Ephedra has been used for conditions such as urticaria, enuresis, incontinence, narcolepsy, myasthenia gravis, and chronic postural hypotension (WHO, 1999). Ephedra has been used for many years for treating the discomfort associated with asthma, allergic conditions, and nasal congestion. It also is used as a stimulant in many herbal diet and athletic performance enhancing formulae for which there is no supporting research (Foster & Tyler, 1999). Traditionally, ephedra has not been used for weight loss or performance enhancement. Ephedra herb has been used as a diaphoretic and the root has been used as an antiperspirant, two opposite actions (Leung & Foster, 1996).

BIOMEDICAL EVIDENCE:

Ephedra's effect on energy levels has not been studied. Much of the biomedical evidence addresses the effects of ephedrine, not ephedra as a whole herb. Ephedra is being included more and more in "natural" diet drugs because of the ephedrine research. Although the focus of this chapter is on the herb, the ephedrine studies have been included.

Studies Related to Energy

In a Danish study of 180 obese participants, in which participants ate a low-calorie diet and took either 20 mg ephedrine, 200 mg caffeine, an ephedrine-caffeine combination of the same doses, or placebo, there was a slight improvement in weight loss in the ephedrine-only group; the most significant changes occurred in the ephedrine-caffeine group. Forty-four of those receiving ephedrine or caffeine reported side effects, such as headache and fatigue, as compared with 3 patients in the placebo group (Toubro, Astrup, Breum, & Quaade, 1993).

Ephedrine has been shown in a double-blind, placebo-controlled study with a small sample of 6 normal weight people to significantly increase energy expenditure as compared with placebo with an increase of 22 kcal per 3 hours for 10 mg, for example. However, ephedrine in oral dose combination with caffeine (20 mg/200 mg) was shown to increase thermogenesis even more in normal weight people, 30 kcal per 3 hours. Given the limitation of a small sample, it is clearly demonstrated that there is a synergistic effect between ephedrine and caffeine not only related to thermogenesis but also in relation to changes in heart rate and systolic and diastolic blood pressures (Astrup, Toubro, Cannon, Hein, & Madsen, 1991). A study of 5 healthy females showed that chronic ephedrine treatment, 20 mg three times a day for three months, led to a sustained 10% elevation in metabolic rate compared with controls (Astrup, Madsen, Holst, & Christensen, 1986).

At least one small human clinical trial has supported what herbalists have observed over time, that the effects on the body of the use of whole herb ephedra are quite different from the use of ephedrine. A study on the pharmacokinetics of whole herb ephedra use in 12 normotensive subjects who took four capsules of powdered ephedra, 375 mg each, with breakfast and then dinner, demonstrated no significant changes in blood pressure (two participants actually had a decrease in diastolic blood pressure), and a significant increase in heart rate in 50% of the participants from 78 ± 6 bpm to 86 ± 9 bpm, without clinical symptoms such as palpitations (White et al., 1997).

Studies Related to Other Health Patterns
No data are available at this time.

Mechanism of Action
Ephedrine and pseudoephedrine are the alkaloid constituents said to be responsible for the action of ephedra. The pharmaceutical drug, ephedrine, is no longer extracted from ephedra but is chemically synthesized in a laboratory because it is difficult to extract the very small quantity of ephedrine found in the leaf of the ephedra plant (Foster & Tyler, 1999). Ephedrine is known to stimulate the central nervous system (CNS), dilate the bronchioles and constrict blood vessels. Ephedrine raises both diastolic and systolic blood pressures and pulse pressure (WHO, 1999). Ephedrine increases metabolic rate by stimulating the release of noradrenaline from sympathetic nerve channels (Liu, Toubro, Astrup, & Stock, 1995).

The ephedrine in ephedra is not absorbed as quickly as pharmaceutical ephedrine even though it is thoroughly excreted in the same amount of time (White et al., 1997). Ephedrine and pseudoephedrine stimulate alpha- and beta-adrenoceptors. Giving repeated doses of ephedrine is less effective because of depletion of norepinephrine stores (tachyphylaxis) (Bruneton, 1999). Because it stimulates alpha-adrenoceptors of the muscle cells in the bladder, ephedrine increases resistance to urination, thereby explaining ephedra's use in urinary incontinence and bedwetting (WHO, 1999). The pseudoephedrine in ephedra has been shown to be the main anti-inflammatory constituent (Hikino, Konno, Takata, & Tamada, 1980).

USE IN PREGNANCY OR LACTATION:

Ephedra is contraindicated when trying to conceive and during pregnancy and lactation (McGuffin et al., 1997; Weed, 1986). Ephedra is not abortifacient in rats (Lee, 1982 as reported in WHO, 1999).

Herbal Caveat—Pregnancy or Lactation

Some herbs are contraindicated in pregnancy because of a risk of the herb or one of its constituents stimulating the uterus and therefore possibly promoting fetal loss. Many herbal practitioners do not recommend herbal remedies, in particular oral doses of herbs, during the first trimester of pregnancy and seek an alternative. However, herbs are successfully used during pregnancy, especially to prepare the body for the birth. Herbs are relatively unstudied in pregnancy and lactation, so patients need to be made aware through education of the potential benefits and risks of using herbs for health conditions that arise during pregnancy or lactation. The use of herbal remedies during pregnancy often warrants a referral to a knowledgeable herbal practitioner.

USE FOR CHILDREN:

Some sources report that ephedra is not to be used with children under six years of age (WHO, 1999). There are no contraindications for using this herb in the Chinese *Materia Medica,* but dosages of whole herb are modified for children. With so many more children being diagnosed with asthma at younger ages, practitioners may want to consider an ephedra formula as a first approach, rather than starting a small child on steroid inhalers and bronchodilators, which have not necessarily been clinically tested in children either. The risk-benefit might show that ephedra should be considered. Maximum daily dose of ephedrine from ephedra is 2 mg/kg body weight (Schulz et al., 1998).

Because of the abuse of ephedra (alkaloid-containing) products by some young people seeking a "natural high" and because of the report of toxic overdoses, the American Herbal Products Association recommends that manufacturers include a warning statement on the label of their ephedra products that says that the product is not to be used by persons under 18 years of age (McGuffin et al., 1997).

Herbal Caveat—Children

Children have special needs in regard to herbal therapies. They require lesser amounts of herbs and often respond well to mild teas and topical applications such as compresses and baths. The lowest dose of oral preparations should be tried first before increasing the amount given children. Caregivers should observe children closely for responses to herbal remedies. Younger children, particularly infants, have traditionally been given herbs either through their mother's breast milk or in the form of a homeopathic remedy because of their sensitivity to medicines and treatments and the immaturity of their liver. It is recommended that a person knowledgeable in the herbal treatment of children be consulted before the offering of any herb to a child for the first time.

Alkaloid-containing species of ephedra have been shown to cause contraction of the uterus and elevated blood pressure in animals. Frequent use may result in nervousness, and those with hypertension, heart disease, diabetes, or thyroid conditions should use ephedra only under the guidance of their health practitioner (Foster & Tyler, 1999). Ephedra herb has been shown to have less of a hypertensive action than pure ephedrine (British Herbal Pharmacopoeia, 1983 as reported in Schulz et al., 1998). In addition, ephedra should not be used by those with glaucoma, enlarged prostate, suicidal ideation, stomach ulcers, anorexia, bulimia, or for prolonged periods (Bruneton, 1999; Brinker, 1998; McGuffin et al., 1997).

Ephedra is not to be used at the same time as an MAO inhibitor because it could cause fatal hypertension. It should not be used at the same time with ergot derivatives or oxytocin, cardiac glycosides, halothane, or guanethidine (WHO, 1999). Although several drug interactions with *ephedrine* are cited here, it is speculative that ephedra has the same effect. The drug interactions are listed here because the amount of ephedrine in ephedra plant is 2400 to 22,500 ppm (Duke, www.ars-grin.gov/cgi-bin/duke/farmacy2.pl). In addition to MAO inhibitors and the drugs previously listed, the following drugs have known interactions with ephedrine: theophylline, caffeine, dexamethasone, ammonium chloride, sodium bicarbonate, reserpine, and amitriptyline (Brinker, 1998).

Potential side effects of ephedra include insomnia, acute pain in the cardiac region, hypertension, palpitations, flushing, tingling and numbness of the extremities, persistent constipation, psychosis, and loss of appetite. After prolonged use, insomnia and dermatitis may occur (Nadkarni, 1976).

Some people now use ephedra for weight loss and athletic performance enhancement. It has become a plant of misuse and abuse. It is bought and sold in recreational formulas for the sole purpose of achieving a euphoric state. In the United States, one report states that the Food and Drug Administration had a record of more than 600 adverse reactions to ephedra products including 22 deaths as of 1996 (Dickinson, 1996). A more recent report of the Council for Responsible Nutrition states that there were 1173 suspected cases of adverse reactions to ephedra and only 121 of those cases had actual detailed information available for investigation. Of the 121 cases, 8 deaths were investigated as *possibly* being caused by ephedra. "This value represents 6.7% of the 121 adverse event reports [AERs] that were considered to contain sufficient quantity of information for scientific analysis of trends. Despite this, there is not enough information to do a detailed analysis of each of these individuals (i.e., complete hospital records), and therefore, specific conclusions cannot be drawn as to the role of ephedra in these reactions" (Council for Responsible Nutrition, www.crnusa.org/crncantoxreportindex.html).

There is a potential public health issue whenever people choose to misuse a medicinal plant or formulation on the market. The sale of ephedra may be regulated in some areas because its constituent, ephedrine, can serve as a precursor for the creation of methamphetamine, "speed"; however, controlling the sale of ephedra in order to control the potential access to ephedrine, which is cumbersome to extract and very little can be extracted from the plant, is viewed as excessive by some (Foster & Tyler, 1999).

It is estimated that approximately 12 million people may have used supplements containing ephedra in the United States in 1999 alone (Haller & Benowitz, 2000). Although a ban on recreational products may be welcomed by some, controls on whole herb use by responsible practitioners is not. Some people who died using recreational herbal products not only ingested ephedra but also other stimulants. Many of the ephedra products sold for recreational and weight loss purposes contain significant amounts of caffeine. The caffeine is included in the products either as straight caffeine or in the herbs guarana or kola nut, which both contain caffeine. Caffeine augments the release of catecholamines, an effect that, when combined with that of ephedrine, could lead to increased stimulation of the CNS and cardiovascular systems. Herbs containing caffeine in formulation with ephedra have been shown to increase the rate of ephedrine absorption from ephedra (Gurley, Gardner, White, & Wang, 1998). It is also important to remember that numerous over-the-counter drugs, at least in the United States, contain the drugs ephedrine and pseudoephedrine. They do not typically have warning labels about the risks of simultaneous use of caffeine with the drugs even though there is potential for a consumer to use both.

Recent studies of supplements containing ephedra in formulation show that significantly lower amounts of ephedrine (alkaloid) are reported than are present when analyzed. In an evaluation of 20 products, variations between label claim and actual total alkaloid content were found to be as much as 154% (Gurley, Gardner, & Hubbard, 2000). Nurses need to be aware of the potential for inaccurate reporting on both sides of the issue around herbs such as ephedra, which often are herbs that have a connection to a common drug like ephedrine. Nurses need to help patients critically evaluate the data presented in the biomedical literature and the media. How ephedra is used or misused is key to understanding the importance of the data as well as how the details of the issue are reported.

NURSING EVIDENCE:

Historical Nursing Use

No data are available at this time.

Potential Nursing Applications

Nurses' ethnographic and historical studies might provide greater insight into the therapeutic benefits and risks of the use of ephedra as a whole herb. Nurses who help patients make health decisions for chronic conditions may want to watch for research about the use of ephedra herb in the treatment of asthma. Researchers need to do more comparison studies between the traditional use of the whole herb and the use of pharmaceutical ephedrine products not only in the acute treatment of an attack but also in the length of time without an attack following the treatment with the herb or drug. Nurses can help clarify the data for patients on the differences between ephedra whole plant and ephedrine. They also can help patients identify safe use practices for the whole herb and ephedra products.

Integrative Insight

There is much to be learned from this herb about health and balance. After all, the plant itself is one of the oldest living plants on the planet. It has survived and adapted to huge changes in its environment. One might wonder if ephedra has survived so long because of the antiaging properties of the ephedrine constituent. The ephedrine in ephedra is very stable and is not decomposed by light, air, or heat. Age does not seem to affect its activity. Studies have shown that if kept in a dry place, the ephedrine content in ephedra does not decrease (Nadkarni, 1976).

The use of this herb is being threatened even though the tradition behind the use of ephedra is extensive. It is a special herb to many. One of the traditional uses of ephedra was the drink known as "soma," an ephedra juice also known as the drink of "perpetual youth" and used by hunters to enhance their skill (Rister, 1999). Ephedra can boost the energy levels in the body, but it has never been used until recently to speed up the body so that it will lose weight. Nor has the herb been used to "get high," unlike plants such as opium poppy. The use of this plant has changed drastically from being a restorative drink of *rishis* in India and a long-time healing agent for asthma in China to being used to lose weight and get high.

Many practitioners and their patients may be kept from ever experiencing the benefits of ephedra because of the choices of a few to misuse and abuse the herb. Ephedra could become illegal for public use in some countries. Nurses must be aware of the sociopolitical processes that affect the regulation of herbs. It is also important to understand the historical benefits of an herb, especially when its safety is being called into question after centuries of safe use. The key is knowledge. Nurses can support and promote the public's responsible use of ephedra.

THERAPEUTIC APPLICATIONS:

Oral

Whole Herb. 1.2 to 2.3 g for adults and 40 mg/kg for children (Blumenthal et al., 2000)

Fluid Extract. (1:1) 1.2 to 2.3 ml single dose

Standardized Extract. 12 to 25 mg total ephedrine two to three times per day (McCaleb et al., 2000)

Capsules/Tablets Whole Herb. 500 to 1000 mg two to three times per day (McCaleb et al., 2000)

Tincture. Take 15 to 30 drops up to three times per day (McCaleb et al., 2000) or 5.75 to 11.5 ml (1:5 [g/ml]) as a single dose (Blumenthal et al., 2000).

Topical

Ephedra root powder is used for excessive perspiration and has potential to be used in antiperspirant preparations (Leung & Foster, 1996).

Environmental

No data are available at this time.

Herbal Caveat—Therapeutic Applications

In traditional and conventional herbal medicine, amounts of herbs given to patients are based on individual needs. The amounts or "doses" recorded here are provided so that the health practitioner has a general idea of the amounts recommended for an adult patient. Dosing in herbalism not only refers to amount of plant used but also includes when, where, and how to take a plant medicine. These dosages should not be used as guidelines for indiscriminate intervention without proper assessment, critical thinking, and patient education on the part of the practitioner.

Note: Please see chapter 5 for detailed descriptions of how to prepare various applications.

PATIENT INTERACTION:

Many safety issues surround the use of ephedra at this time. This herb should only be used in self-care after significant research and study to be sure that it is appropriate for you. Check with a knowledgeable health practitioner to learn how to use this herb wisely.

Herbal Caveat—Patient Interaction

Patients considering the use of an herb or formula of herbs in self-care benefit from education about the plant itself and the use of the plant in healing. This education can come through many sources, including local herbalists; plant specialists such as botanists; health practitioners such as nurses, nutritionists, naturopaths, and other physicians; and various written references including the scientific literature. Patients need to remember that their unique health care needs are not necessarily represented in any literature they may encounter. Therefore, it is recommended that a knowledgeable mentor be consulted before initiating self-care with any herb being used for the first time.

NURTURING THE NURSE-PLANT RELATIONSHIP:

Note: You may want to keep a journal of your experiences with the herb.

If you have never experienced ephedra, you are about to join those who have used this herb for health, healing, and longevity for approximately 5000 years or more. Begin by purchasing some dried herb, preferably *Ephedra sinica,* also known as Chinese *ma huang.* Although this herb is traditionally used in combination with other herbs, for the purpose of this sensory experience, you can use it singly. Take approximately 1 teaspoon of the herb and steep it in 1 cup of boiled water for five to ten minutes. If you have high blood pressure, perspire excessively, or are on cardiac or asthma medications, do not drink the tea, just smell the aroma of the tea as it cools down. If you are able to do the tasting, as you take a sip, focus your attention on your body and where you feel the effects of your tea. How does the tea affect your energy levels? Take a moment to think about how this one herb is able to sustain such a lengthy history of use, how it can have a reputation as a "fountain of youth" tea in some cultures, and how it can cause such controversy in modern times. Record your response.

CHAPTER 15
Emotions and Adaptation

INTRODUCTION

Joy, anger, sadness, elation, and numerous other feelings called emotion (e-energy in motion) come and go like the waves on the sea during the course of life. They become part of illness when the emotion no longer flows through a person with the gentle strength and predictability of the tide coming in and going out. People who are emotionally ill often are stuck in a feeling, such as the depressed person who feels sadness but is unable to feel any joy in life. The ability to experience this rhythmic flow of emotions is part of the adaptation response to stressors in life.

Herbs have been used throughout history to facilitate the adaptation response and to provide support for a healthy emotional life. In Ayurveda, for example, emotions are considered both in the assessment of the patient and as part of intervention. Foods and herbs are known for their potential to support healing of body, mind, and spirit. "The unified body-mind science of Ayurveda allows us to use herbs to help counteract mental states and emotional problems" (Lad & Frawley, 1986, p. 35). In Ayurveda, certain tastes not only are associated with particular foods and herbs but also with certain emotional states. For example, envy is a "sour" emotion and anger is a "pungent" emotion. In traditional Chinese medicine, herbal healers also are knowledgeable of the effects of emotions on the health or illness of a person and the effects of foods and herbs on emotional well-being and balance. In the Five Element theory, each element—wood, fire, earth, metal, and water—is associated with an organ and an emotion. For example, the liver and gall bladder are associated with anger and irritability, the spleen and stomach with worry and anxiety, and the heart and small intestine with joy or mania (Wicke, 1992). The Chinese have treated mental and emotional illness with traditional healing methods such as diet and herb therapy for centuries. A very specific science and logic are applied to the selection of the appropriate herbs or foods for balancing the emotions.

The plants presented in this chapter—St. John's wort, kava, passion flower, and Siberian ginseng—are just a few examples of medicinal herbs that have an effect on emotions and the adaptation response. How certain plants cause emotional changes in people when ingested, inhaled, or absorbed is still virtually unknown. Some theories are described here, and herbs and their adaptogen actions are discussed in more detail in chapter 20.

Emotions are still not clearly understood scientifically. "For a long time, neuroscientists have agreed that emotions are controlled by certain parts of the brain. This is a big 'neurocentric' assumption–and I now think it is a wrong (or at least incomplete) one" (Pert, 1997, p. 132). It is now known that emotion is related to neuropeptides and their receptors found in cells throughout the body. As scientists continue the exploration of what emotion is to begin with and how herbs create the responses they do in some people, perhaps there will be a meeting of the minds. Until that time, it may be premature to expect that we can fully understand how herbs affect emotions. It may even be the case that how herbs affect human emotions is unique to the individual user. But one thing is abundantly clear—herbs do influence emotional balance and the ability to adapt. Just take a walk through a garden to smell the roses, cut open a lemon, or drink a cup of kava tea to experience it yourself!

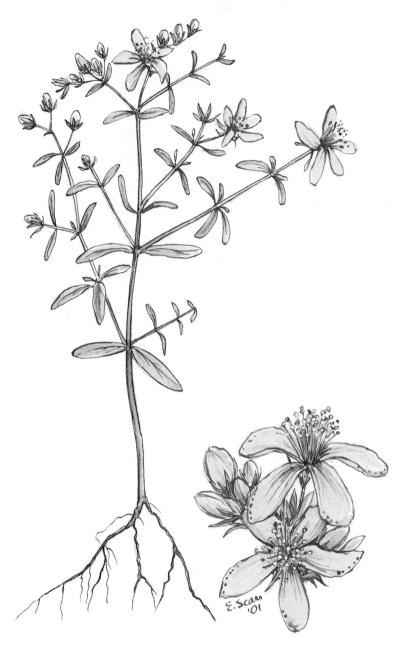

Hypericum perforatum

St. John's Wort

- **LATIN NAME:** *Hypericum perforatum*

- **FAMILY:** Clusiaceae

- **COMMON NAMES:** St. John's wort, Saint-John's-wort, Saint-Joan's-wort, klamath weed, hypericum, amber, goatweed, Johnswort, tipton weed, hardhay

- **HEALTH PATTERN:** Emotions and adaptation

- **PLANT DESCRIPTION:**

The Latin name for St. John's wort, *Hypericum,* is from the Greek meaning "over an apparition," referring to the plant's long historical use as a means of warding away evil spirits. St. John's wort is an herbaceous perennial that grows wild along uncultivated ground, roadsides, and woods. It prefers sunny and dry locations. Although native to Europe, the plant was imported into North America where it grows freely. It is considered a noxious weed among farmers and ranchers. The plant grows to a height of 1 to 3 feet (1 meter), has a two-edged stem, and numerous yellow flowers. The flowers and the body of the small, oval leaves have many tiny dots visible when held up to light, making the leaves appear perforated, which gives the plant its species name, *perforatum.* Mythologically, the dots have been said to be symbolic of the battle between St. John and the devil's pitchfork. The flower has five sepals and five petals. Rubbing the St. John's wort bud or flower between the fingers produces a purple-red stain, caused by hypericin and other active compounds. Good quality tinctures and oil infusions have a deep red color. The herb has been described as having a balsamic, astringent taste (Felter & Lloyd, 1983). St. John's wort is harvested when it blooms. The flowers typically bloom in midsummer, near the time of the Feast of St. John the Baptist (June 24), which is thought to partially explain its name.

- **PLANT PARTS USED:**

The above-ground parts of the plant—the leaves, unopened buds, and flowers—are used. The flowers and buds found in the top 3 inches (6 cm) of the plant are the preferred parts. The seeds also can be used medicinally.

- **TRADITIONAL EVIDENCE:**

Cultural Use

North American Indian. Various North American tribes have used several different species of St. John's wort for medicinal purposes. The Cherokee use the plant as an antidiarrheal, a topical ointment for sores, a snakebite remedy, a gastrointestinal aid, an abortifacient, and as a treatment for venereal disease (Moerman, 1998). The Iroquois use the plant for fever and to prevent sterility. The Montagnois use the plant as a cough medicine (Moerman, 1998).

Hispanic. St. John's wort is known among some Hispanics as *yerba de san juan.* The aerial plant parts are used to support the nerves, for nerve injury, and in the healing of those with mood swings and depression.

East Indian. In India, St. John's wort is known as *bassant, balsunt,* or *dendlu.* The leaves are used as a vermifuge, for diarrhea, and for prolapse of the anus and uterus. The herb is used as a purgative, astringent, diuretic, and emmenagogue (Nadkarni, 1976).

Russian/Baltic. St. John's wort is mentioned in an old Russian Proverb: "It is as impossible to make bread without flour as it is to heal people without St. John's Wort" (Zevin, 1997, p. 137). The Russian people use St. John's wort for pulmonary (bronchial asthma) and gastrointestinal complaints, to promote the flow and filtration of urine from the kidneys, and to promote the flow of bile. It is used for headache and nervousness. The oil is applied topically for the healing of wounds and burns. A tincture is often gargled for healing sores of the throat and mouth.

European. St. John's wort is known in Germany as *Johanniskraut,* in France as *millepertuis,* and in Spain as *corazoncillo* (Brinker, 1998). It has been used in Europe since antiquity. Medical herbalists such as Hippocrates, Pliny, and Galen have written of the medicinal uses of St. John's wort. There are numerous folk beliefs and superstitions about the power of St. John's wort. The most common belief is that the herb has the ability to protect a person from evil spirits. A European custom developed in which sprays of St. John's wort were hung over the doors of houses and churches on the eve of St. John's Day (the summer solstice) to ward off evil spirits (Lawless, 1998). The primary European uses of the herb are as a wound-healing agent; diuretic; and as a treatment for neuralgia, sciatica, and various psychological disorders.

Culinary Use

St. John's wort is listed by the Council of Europe as a natural source of food flavoring which can be added to foods as long as the hypericin content does not exceed 0.1 mg/kg in the finished product (Newall, Anderson, & Phillipson, 1996). It is regulated in the United States as a flavoring agent in alcoholic beverages. Only hypericin-free alcohol distillate form is allowed (McGuffin, Hobbs, Upton, & Goldberg, 1997). St. John's wort is patented as a possible food preservative (Duke, 1985).

Use in Herbalism

St. John's wort is best known for its use in promoting the healing of wounds, bruises, and sprains and treating nervous and psychiatric disorders. It is used in times of stress and is also an effective sleep aid and antiviral. American Eclectic physicians gave St. John's wort for hysteria, nervous affections with depression, urinary tract complaints, diarrhea, and jaundice. Older people who feel lonely and sad can drink tea made with St. John's wort. It also can be taken by those who experience difficulty concentrating. St. John's wort is used for its anti-inflammatory properties when used externally. It is used topically in the form of oil or tincture for wounds, bruises, and tumors (Felter & Lloyd, 1983). Historically, St. John's wort has been drunk in a boiled wine for healing "inward hurts and bruises . . . vomiting and spitting of blood and it is good for those that are bitten or stung by any venomous creature, and for those that cannot make water" (Culpepper, 1990, p. 99).

St. John's wort has been used extensively to repair nerve damage. I have used it internally and/or externally with stroke and brain-injured patients. St. John's wort has been used in the treatment of spinal cord injury, shock, and concussion (Felter & Lloyd, 1983). Some herbalists also use it with patients who have pain related to shingles.

Cosmetic Use. St. John's wort is an excellent red dye for wool and violet-red dye for silk.

BIOMEDICAL EVIDENCE:

Several clinical trials on St. John's wort have been conducted and published. The studies primarily used standardized extracts, not whole herb, in tea, tincture, or liquid extract forms. Much of the current research on St. John's wort looks at the use of the plant medicine for depression. Although St. John's wort has been traditionally used for mild to moderate depression, several clinical studies have focused on the use of the herb for major depression.

Studies Related to Emotions and Adaptation

A metanalysis of human trials on the effect of St. John's wort extract (standardized to hypericin) for patients experiencing depression includes twenty-three randomized trials (fifteen placebo-controlled and eight comparison trials to other pharmaceutical drugs). Most of the studies included in the analysis are short-term studies of approximately eight weeks. The total sample of the metanalysis includes over 1757 outpatients, most of whom had mild-to-moderate symptoms of depression. St. John's wort standardized extract was found to be significantly superior to placebo and was as effective as other pharmaceutical antidepressants when used singly or in combination. Overall, the metanalysis demonstrates that there are fewer short term side effects with St. John's wort (19.8%) as compared with pharmaceutical antidepressants (52.8%). The specifics about the nature of these side effects are presented in the following text (Linde et al., 1996).

St. John's wort standardized extract LI 160, 300 mg three times per day has been shown to be comparably effective as maprotiline (Ludiomil) (Harrer, Hubner, & Podzuweit, 1994), and imipramine (Tofranil), pharmaceutical antidepressants (Vorbach, Hubner, &

Arnoldt, 1994), and significantly more effective than placebo (Hansgen, Vesper, and Ploch, 1994; Hubner, Lande, & Podzuweit, 1994; Sommer & Harrer, 1994) in alleviating symptoms of depression (as determined by comparison with the *Diagnostic and Statistical Manual* [DSM] III-R or *International Classification of Diseases* [ICD]-09 codes). Fewer side effects were observed in those taking the St. John's wort extract than those taking the pharmaceutical antidepressants. Side effects primarily included mild gastrointestinal complaints, dry mouth, and dizziness. In one drug monitoring study by Woelk, Burkard, and Grunwald (1994), the most common side effects noted in a sample of 3250 patients who received *Hypericum* extract LI 160, were gastrointestinal (0.6%), allergic reactions (0.5%), and fatigue (0.4%).

Questions are still being raised about the significance of the data generated from these human trials. Vitiello (1999) wrote of the following concerns: (1) many of the studies enrolled patients that did not meet the diagnostic criteria for major depression as found in the DSM III, III-R, or IV; (2) the studies are short-term; (3) many have small samples; and (4) the doses of pharmaceutical comparators used in some of the studies were much lower than is commonly considered therapeutic for depression. Studies are being funded by centers such as the National Center for Complementary and Alternative Medicine in the United States that address some of the limitations of previous clinical trials. A new study in progress is the first large-scale controlled clinical trial in the United States to assess whether the herb has a significant therapeutic effect in patients with clinical depression. The $4.3 million study involves 336 patients with major depression. The Duke University Medical Center in Durham, North Carolina, is coordinating the 3-year study, which has 13 clinical sites around the country. Three different treatment groups are in the trial. One group will receive an initial dose of 900 mg per day of St. John's wort (form not stated); a second will receive a placebo; and the third will receive Zoloft (a commonly used antidepressant). Patients who respond positively to their randomly assigned treatment will be continued on it for another 4 months. (http:// nccam.nih.gov/nccam/fcp/factsheets/stjohnswort/stjohnswort.htm, April, 2001).

St. John's wort standardized oral extract, 900 mg/d given for four weeks followed by 1200 mg/d for four weeks, in a study of 200 adults diagnosed with major depression and a baseline Hamilton rating scale of 20, was not significantly effective (26.5%) as compared with placebo (18.6%) in relieving symptoms associated with the illness (Shelton, Keller, Gelenberg, Dunner, Hirschfeld, Thase, Russell, Lydiard, Crits-Cristoph, Gallup, Todd, Hellerstein, Goodnick, Keitner, Stahl, & Halbreich, 2001).

Standardized extract of St. John's wort, 300 mg three times a day for four weeks in combination with daily light treatment for 2 hours was found effective during a randomized study in relieving 20 subjects' symptoms of seasonal affective disorder (SAD), a subgroup of major depression (Martinez, Kasper, Ruhrmann, & Moller, 1994).

One descriptive study of 20 participants identified the following four decision-making themes for the reasons people (in this case the participants were all women) choose St. John's wort for self-treatment of symptoms of depression:

- Personal health care values: Participants shared a belief in having control over their treatment.
- Mood: Participants used St. John's wort because they felt sadness and hopelessness and experienced suicidal ideation and lack of energy.
- Perceptions of seriousness of disease and risks of treatment: Participants did not believe that they were seriously depressed and that pharmaceutical drugs have major side effects.
- Accessibility: St. John's wort is easily accessible and many of the participants had already experienced no relief from therapy and/or did not believe that their physician had knowledge of how to help them with their depressed feelings (Wagner et al., 1999).

Studies Related to Other Health Patterns

Immune Response. Plant constituents of St. John's wort, hypericin and pseudohypericin, have been shown to inhibit encapsulated viruses such as *Herpes simplex* I and II and human immunodeficiency virus (HIV) (Lavie et al., 1989). In one study, 14 of 16 patients with acquired immunodeficiency syndrome (AIDS) were clinically stable (per Karnovsky index) for 40 months (stable or increasing counts of absolute CD4 values and improvements in CD4/CD8 ratios in the majority of patients) when given an intravenous St. John's wort preparation called Hyperforat, 2 ml two times per week (Steinbeck & Wernet, 1993).

Mechanism of Action

The exact mechanism related to St. John's wort's antidepressant activity is still unclear. Three of the major constituents found in the plant, hypericin, pseudohypericin, and hyperforin, have been, and continue to be, investigated. Although in vitro studies demonstrate that hypericin from St. John's wort inhibits monoamine oxidase (MAO) (Suzuki, Katsumata, Oya, Bladt, & Wagner, 1984), this has not been shown to be true in humans. There are some theories that St. John's wort affects neurotransmitters such as serotonin, dopamine, or gamma-aminobutyric acid (GABA), but there are no definitive answers. "Most recent investigations definitely suggest that other constituents in the whole extract, rather than hypericin and related compounds, are responsible for the efficacy in mild to moderate forms of depression" (Foster & Tyler, 1999, p. 332). It could be that several mechanisms are responsible for St. John's wort's antidepressant action, explaining its few side effects. "The advantage of this combined action is fewer side effects, because the total response is not due to a single strong action (Duke, 1997, p. 159).

Two constituents of St. John's wort, hypericin and pseudohypericin, have been shown to be antiretroviral in vitro and in vivo. Synthetic hypericin is currently being investigated as an antiretroviral agent to be used with the blood transfusion supply (Leung & Foster, 1996).

Hypericin is absorbed in the intestines and concentrates near the skin (Leung & Foster, 1996), which is why taking St. John's wort may lead to susceptibility to phototoxicity. The elimination half-life of the St. John's wort constituents hypericin and hyperforin are 24 and 9 hours, respectively (studies by Staffeldt et al. and Biber et al. as reported in Vitiello, 1999). Livestock that have consumed St. John's wort have become phototoxic.

St. John's wort's wound healing action is most likely explained by the plant's tannin. The tannin (10%) is thought to exert wound healing "through its astringent and protein-precipitating actions" (Foster & Tyler, 1999, p. 331). St. John's wort also contains a number of flavonoids (Leung & Foster, 1996) that are known to exert an anti-inflammatory action.

A human study conducted by Ereshefsky and colleagues of 16 healthy subjects divided into extensive and poor metabolizers found that "[St. John's wort] does not interact with CYP2D6 or CYP3A4. SJW is a significantly weaker inhibitor of CYP3A4 than grapefruit juice" (as reported in Treasure, 2000). While St. John's wort may, under certain circumstances, modulate cytochrome P450 isoforms, in particular 3A4, potentially inducing detoxification of drugs, it also contains quercetin, which is a 3A4 inhibitor (Treasure, 2000).

USE IN PREGNANCY OR LACTATION:

Brinker (1998) suggests that St. John's wort is contraindicated in pregnancy because of the possibility of its acting as an abortifacient and exerting uterine stimulant effects (based on in vitro and animal studies). There are naturopaths and herbalists who have extensive experience in recommending St. John's wort during pregnancy without any side effects to mom or baby. As a psychiatric clinical specialist, I have had women and therapists ask about the use of St. John's wort for depression that occurs in pregnancy. It is important that the woman be carefully assessed and that the benefits and risks of the use of *any* antidepressant substance, synthetic or herbal, be discussed. The potential side effects of St. John's wort are significantly fewer than the synthetic antidepressants, and it may be more comforting to a woman needing medication to choose a substance that will offer the possibility of fewer side effects.

St. John's wort is also used during labor. Susan Weed suggests St. John's wort tincture made from fresh herb as a remedy to "control spasms of the back, sides and uterus" during labor (1986, p. 68). Some midwives, including one trained in England that I used to work with, often use St. John's wort oil to gently massage the perineum during labor in preparation for delivery and to promote healing of the perineum.

Herbal Caveat—Pregnancy or Lactation

Some herbs are contraindicated in pregnancy because of a risk of the herb or one of its constituents stimulating the uterus and therefore possibly promoting fetal loss. Many herbal practitioners do not recommend herbal remedies, in particular oral doses of herbs, during the first trimester of pregnancy and seek an alternative. However, herbs are successfully used during pregnancy, especially to prepare the body for the birth. Herbs are relatively unstudied in pregnancy and lactation, so patients need to be made aware through education of the potential benefits and risks of using herbs for health conditions that arise during pregnancy or lactation. The use of herbal remedies during pregnancy often warrants a referral to a knowledgeable herbal practitioner.

USE FOR CHILDREN:

St. John's wort oil can be the treatment of choice in children who have first-degree burns, such as sunburn, after the burn is cooled. A gauze dressing soaked in St. John's wort oil is applied for about ten hours to help in healing the burn and preventing formation of scar tissue. St. John's wort tea also can be given as a sedative to children (1 teaspoon [3 to 5 g] of cut herb to $6\frac{1}{2}$ oz [200 ml] water, 2 to 3 cups per day for children over 3 years; children [age 1 to 3] 1 cup per day) (Schilcher, 1992). St. John's wort tea also has been given at bedtime for bed-wetting (Duke, 1985) and as an antidepressant.

Fluid Extract. A school age child should receive 10 drops (extract dilution not defined) up to three times per day; a small child should receive 5 drops two times per day (Schilcher, 1992).

Herbal Caveat—Children

Children have special needs in regard to herbal therapies. They require lesser amounts of herbs and often respond well to mild teas and topical applications such as compresses and baths. The lowest dose of oral preparations should be tried first before increasing the amount given children. Caregivers should observe children closely for responses to herbal remedies. Younger children, particularly infants, have traditionally been given herbs through their mother's breast milk or in the form of a homeopathic remedy because of their sensitivity to medicines and treatments and the immaturity of their liver. It is recommended that a person knowledgeable in the herbal treatment of children be consulted before the offering of any herb to a child for the first time.

CAUTIONS:

St. John's wort is recommended for mild-to-moderate depression. Patients with severe depression should check with a health practitioner knowledgeable about the use of St. John's wort in the treatment of symptoms related to depression and their mental health practitioner, before using it in self-treatment so that the risks and benefits can be discussed. When considering the use of St. John's wort to treat symptoms related to depressed mood, patients and nurses must also consider the known benefits of noninvasive psychotherapies such as cognitive-behavioral therapy. Two studies by Kovacs et al. (1981) and Weissman et al. (1981) (as reported in Bergin and Garfield, 1994, p. 761) found that at one year follow-up, acutely depressed patients who received psychotherapy without medication functioned better than those who received pharmacotherapy. Four controlled studies reported in Bergin and Garfield (1994) also demonstrated that over a long-term period, antidepressant medications were more efficacious in symptom reduction and relapse prevention than placebo or psychotherapy. Psychotherapy, however, was more effective in helping patients deal with problems in living, social functioning, and interpersonal relationships.

Although some texts including the German Commission E monographs have warned against phototoxic reactions with simple use of St. John's wort, human studies have demonstrated that photosensitivity does not occur when St. John's wort is used at the recommended doses of standardized extract (900 mg) (Blumenthal, Goldberg, & Brinckman, 2000). Severe cutaneous phototoxicity was observed in 48% of 23 HIV-infected adult patients enrolled in a clinical trial of the use of high doses of hypericin, a constituent of St. John's wort (Gulick et al., 1999). If high doses of hypericin are consumed, such as 600 mg standardized extract of hypericin three times a day or a single dose of 3600 mg, then the consumer may experience a slight increase in photosensitivity (Brinker, 1998).

Although no significant data have suggested that St. John's wort *(Hypericum)* causes phototoxicity in humans, especially at normal doses, it is still recommended that people with fair skin avoid excessive exposure to sunlight or ultraviolet (UV) light when using St. John's wort (McGuffin et al., 1997). UV light is best avoided immediately following topical applications of St. John's wort oil or cream. Aqueous or water extracts of St. John's wort contain only a small amount of hypericin (Schilcher, 1992). The hyperforin in freshly macerated St. John's wort oil is unstable and can break down within thirty to ninety days, decreasing the potential medicinal benefit of the oil. It is therefore recommended that the oil be preserved in a bottle where no air can get into it (Leung & Foster, 1996).

There had been no reported drug-herb interactions with St. John's wort (Blumenthal et al., 2000); however, one recent small open-label study of 8 healthy subjects demonstrated that St. John's wort standardized extract taken 300 mg three times a day for fourteen days reduced the plasma concentration of HIV-1 protease inhibitor, indinavir, by a mean of 57%. Because HIV-1 protease inhibitors are part of the 3A4 cytochrome P450 system, which St. John's wort induces, questions are being raised about the interaction of the plant remedy with other drugs (Piscitelli, Burstein, Chaitt, Alfaro, & Fallooon, 2000). For further information on herb-drug interactions and the cytochrome P-450 issue, please see the Mechanism of Action section.

There are some *potential* interactions of St. John's wort with foods or pharmaceuticals. The speculation that St. John's wort not be used with other MAO inhibitors is based on earlier in vitro data that the antidepressant action of St. John's wort might be related to its ability as an MAO inhibitor. More recent data have not necessarily supported this concern. Patients taking therapeutic amounts of St. John's wort may still want to stay away from tyramine-containing foods such as cheeses, beer, and wine. Animal studies have shown that St. John's wort enhances sleeping time of the narcotic effect of alcohol and antagonizes the effects of reserpine (Brinker, 1998). Because it is speculated that St. John's wort's antidepressive effect may be related to its action on neurotransmitters, it is possible that it may interact with selective serotonin reuptake inhibitors (SSRIs) such as Prozac. Patients may be best advised to make a choice between the herbal or pharmaceutical remedy and that a three-week wash-out period should occur before switching between St. John's wort and pharmaceutical antidepressant medications.

St. John's wort is not genotoxic or mutagenic in animals and the median lethal dose (LD_{50}) was found in one animal study to be greater than 5000 mg/kg (study by Leuschner as reported in Schulz, Hansel, & Tyler, 1998).

St. John's wort may be labeled a noxious weed where you live. Check with local authorities before attempting to grow this plant in an herb garden. One medicinal garden I worked with had plenty of St. John's wort when I became the caretaker. Despite the herb's reputation for being weedy, it always stayed right where it was originally planted, unlike some other plants like celandine and mugwort. Nevertheless, take care to know how the plant acts in your area.

NURSING EVIDENCE:

Historical Nursing Use

No data are available at this time.

Potential Nursing Applications

St. John's wort not only has been used for mild to moderate depression but also has been used extensively for the occasional blues or down-in-the-dumps emotions that people experience from time to time throughout life. Nurses may want to consider using and researching St. John's wort as an antidepressant for patients with mild-to-moderate symptoms, such as those who are experiencing normal grief and loss, and for those with symptoms of seasonal depression.

Most of the scientific research regarding St. John's wort has looked at the standardized extract. Nurses might consider the use and research of St. John's wort tea, tincture, and oil. For example, St. John's wort oil is unsurpassed in its versatility as an intervention for wound healing in patients with the inflammation, bruising, and/or skin breakdown associated with first-degree burns, decubitus ulcers, and perineal tears from labor. I also have had excellent results using St. John's wort oil in patients with fibromyalgia. The oil can be applied to trigger points to help with the pain associated with the illness and to help calm and soothe the nervous system. Nurses may also want to explore the use of St. John's wort in patients with nerve damage or pain related to such conditions as stroke, spinal cord injury, and shingles.

Integrative Insight

St. John's wort is a plant remedy that not only has many years of safe traditional use but also has undergone significant scientific investigation, at least of the standardized extract. Recently, as exemplified in this herb profile, there has been conflicting data about the risks and benefits of St. John's wort in terms of the biomedical evidence. It is important for nurses to use the principles in chapter 19, "Reasonable Research," when evaluating the data as it emerges in the media. There are numerous reports that can be confusing to the public and professionals alike when plant information or research data is not clearly defined. For example, when the public reads reports that state that St. John's wort is ineffective against depression, they may be inclined to not consider the herb as an option. What this kind of report leaves out is the therapeutic application studied (e.g., standardized extract, tea, liquid extract) and that the research was conducted with patients diagnosed with major depression and that there is evidence that St. John's wort is effective in mild to moderate depression. An analogy for this omission might be press reports that over-the-counter lozenges are not effective for sore throat when there is only research that lozenges are not effective in cases of strep throat, not the minor throat irritation that occurs with the common cold. Inadequate reporting and misinformation about herbs can potentially have a negative effect on the role herbs play in achieving the goal of health care for all people. Nurses are responsible for presenting herb information in context. Because of its prominence in the media and in the research arena, St. John's wort may be the first of many opportunities nurses have for collecting seemingly conflicting data about the therapeutic use of a plant remedy with decades of traditional use in healing, and helping patients decide if the herb is something that might be helpful for their unique health concern.

The following clinical example is provided to demonstrate how considering the option of using St. John's wort might change the clinical picture of a patient with symptoms related to depression.

Clinical Example. A 40-year-old breastfeeding mother is experiencing moderate postpartum depression. She is not suicidal. She has gained more than 25 kg with this, her second pregnancy. Her self-esteem is poor and her relationship with her husband is very strained. She lives day-to-day and is still able to keep a job, although she has little energy. It takes months before she decides to speak to her primary care practitioner about her health concerns. She is diagnosed with depression and given a pharmaceutical antidepressant. She is told that it would be best to stop breastfeeding because the drug is excreted in breast milk. She does and the grief she experiences accentuates her depression. She experiences significant adverse effects related to the use of the drug, such as severe fatigue. Her biggest concern with the medication is her loss of libido. The rift with her husband grows because of their prolonged sexual distance related to postpartum recovery, then depression, and then loss of libido related to the medication.

What might have happened to this mother and her family had she been presented with St. John's wort as an option, based on the significant traditional evidence of its positive effect in postpartum depression? Some practitioners might be concerned with using St. John's wort when a mother is lactating, or that no significant clinical trials of its benefit in postpartum depression have been conducted. If the mother had been offered the option of taking St. John's wort or a pharmaceutical, told of the clinical data that exist regarding the herb's efficacy both traditionally and biomedically, and that there are rare accounts of side effects, might she have chosen the St. John's wort instead of medication? In addition, what might have happened if she had also been given the option of psychotherapy in combination with an antidepressant or St. John's wort? The woman was desperate and ill when she saw the health practitioner the first time and was not in the best position to think through her options. Unfortunately, in this scenario the patient's options were limited by the knowledge of the practitioner. Her subsequent choice to follow her practitioner's advice to take the drug led to her feeling more fatigued and to a loss of libido, thereby intensifying her life stressors and making her ability to heal the baseline depression even more difficult.

Nurses often assist patients to weigh the benefits and the risks of one treatment plan over another. The integrative nurses may work alone with the patient, such as in the case of the advanced practice nurse, or they may work with the patient and their health care team to evaluate and choose the best course of action. Although St. John's wort may offer less risk of adverse effects, the person may not want to take an herb, tea, or tincture. In this case, choosing the pharmaceutical and/or the psychotherapy might be better. In the clinical example described here, this is not the case and the new mother might have been better off with an herbal remedy and/or psychotherapy.

Nurses need to be informed and provide patients with options, as depicted in this clinical example. The benefits and risks of a number of options should be explored with the patient and/or their family. The herbal option, in the case of St. John's wort, may be appropriate for some patients. Nurses should consider the effects of treatments such as pharmaceutical antidepressants that may have significant side effects and seek out potential alternatives, herbal and otherwise.

Psychotherapy for example has been shown to be as beneficial as psychopharmacotherapy in treating depression. Although this mother may have wanted an oral medicine, plant or synthetic, to help her postpartum depression, psychotherapy itself might have been a much better choice. Unfortunately, the treatment used resulted in the patient adding to her troubles rather than spending some time finding the best holistic solution. Nurses can help patients weigh all of the evidence about their health choices, including St. John's wort, so that they can make a holistic, educated, and informed decision that takes into account the short- and the long-term effects.

THERAPEUTIC APPLICATIONS:

Oral

Standardized Extract. Although hypericin continues to appear on the labels of some St. John's wort products in some countries as the substance to be calibrated to in the standardization process, Germany no longer allows the labeling of standardized products based on hypericin content (Foster & Tyler, 1999) because research has shown that a single constituent, such as hypericin, is not solely responsible for the health-promoting effects of the herb.

Tea. Take 1 to 2 teaspoons fresh or dry herb per cup water one to two times per day (Duke, 1997). Tea is not registered in Germany because of lack of evidence of efficacy (Blumenthal et al., 2000).

Liquid Extract. (1:1 g/ml) ½ teaspoon (2 ml) twice daily (Blumenthal et al., 2000)

Dry Extract. 5–7:1 (w/w) 300 mg three times daily (Blumenthal et al., 2000)

Oil. Oily preparations can be taken internally for dyspepsia (Blumenthal et al., 2000; Leung & Foster, 1996).

Topical

Oil. St. John's wort infused oil, (fresh mashed flowers in olive oil), can be applied topically for the healing of wounds and first-degree burns. It also makes an excellent massage oil for sore joints and muscles, such as occurs in gout, fibromyalgia, and rheumatism.

Tincture. Tincture is often gargled for healing sores of the throat and mouth.

Environmental

Hanging St. John's wort above the front door in the home has been used to ward off evil spirits. The odor of St. John's wort was thought to be the reason the spirits stayed away. "The possessed or insane were also obliged to inhale the odour of the crushed leaves and flowers, or drink a potion of it, in an effort to rid them of their madness" (le Strange as quoted in Lawless, 1998, p. 6).

Bath. St. John's wort infusion can be added to footbaths.

Herbal Caveat—Therapeutic Applications

In traditional and conventional herbal medicine, amounts of herbs given to patients are based on individual needs. The amounts or "doses" recorded here are provided so that the health practitioner has a general idea of the amounts recommended for an adult patient. Dosing in herbalism not only refers to amount of plant used but also includes when, where, and how to take a plant medicine. These dosages should not be used as guidelines for indiscriminate intervention without proper assessment, critical thinking, and patient education on the part of the practitioner.

Note: Please see chapter 5 for detailed descriptions of how to prepare various applications.

🍃 PATIENT INTERACTION:

St. John's wort has a long history of safe use in the relief of symptoms such as depressed mood, stress, insomnia, and wounds. This herb can be taken orally as a tea, tincture, liquid extract, or standardized extract and used topically as an infused oil. Much of the research on the effects of St. John's wort has been on the standardized extract, while the extensive traditional evidence has been on the whole herb forms. When using St. John's wort, do not exceed recommended amounts because of the possibility of your skin becoming more sensitive to light as a result of a constituent in the herb called hypericin. Animals have been known to have problems with phototoxicity when ingesting too much St. John's wort. Do not expose yourself to sunlight or any source of ultraviolet light immediately after using St. John's wort oil topically.

Do not combine this plant medicine with antidepressant medications, such as the drug indinavir. When deciding how to treat symptoms related to depression, you will need to choose a therapy that is right for you. Ask your health practitioner about the benefits and risks of trying St. John's wort, drug therapies, and/or psychotherapy. People who take therapeutic amounts (as opposed to an occasional cup) of St. John's wort should not eat cheese or drink alcohol.

Herbal Caveat—Patient Interaction

Patients considering the use of an herb or formula of herbs in self-care benefit from education about the plant itself and the use of the plant in healing. This education can come through many sources, including local herbalists; plant specialists such as botanists; health practitioners such as nurses, nutritionists, naturopaths, and other physicians; and various written references including the scientific literature. Patients need to remember that their unique health care needs are not necessarily represented in any literature they may encounter. Therefore, it is recommended that a knowledgeable mentor be consulted before initiating self-care with any herb being used for the first time.

🍃 NURTURING THE NURSE-PLANT RELATIONSHIP:

Note: You may want to keep a journal of your experiences with the herb.

The summer is the best time to get to know St. John's wort. Try finding a place where it grows, identify the plant, and take a look at the little holes on the petals. Gently roll a petal between your fingers and see if the flower leaves the confirmation of a reddish-purple stain. Make an herbal infused oil from fresh St. John's wort flowers and buds, following the instructions in chapter 5, and after a long day, massage the oil into tired joints and muscles as you sip a cup of St. John's wort tea made from the dried delicate yellow flowers and buds. Record how you feel, both physically and emotionally, before and after using St. John's wort.

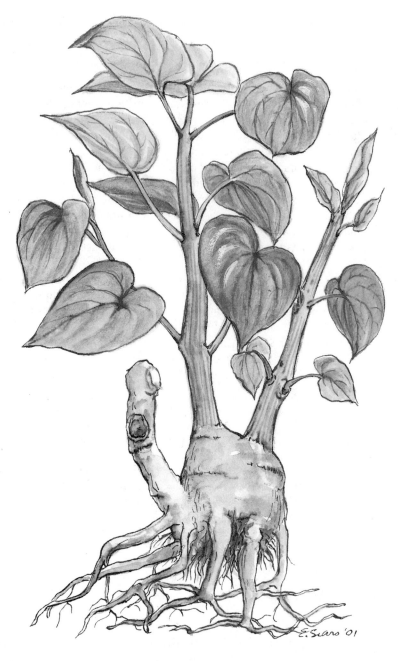

Piper methysticum

Kava

🍃 **LATIN NAME:** *Piper methysticum Forst.*

🍃 **FAMILY:** Piperaceae

🍃 **COMMON NAMES:** Kava, kava kava, intoxicating pepper, awa, ava, ava pepper

    Note: Kava is known by numerous vernacular names in the various Polynesian, Micronesian, and Melanesian countries.

🍃 **HEALTH PATTERN:** Emotions and adaptation

🍃 **PLANT DESCRIPTION:**

The name *Piper methysticum* means "intoxicating pepper." Kava, a member of the pepper family, is a plant of unclear origin, but is presently cultivated extensively by a number of Pacific Island countries. Vanuatu is considered the center of the cultivation of kava because 80 of the known 118 cultivars occur there (Foster & Tyler, 1999). Kava is a perennial, deciduous shrub that often grows to more than 9 feet (3 meters) in height. The leaves are large and heart shaped with short spikes of flowers. The root is large, thick, and sometimes tuberous and is referred to as the "stump" (Lebot, Merlin, & Lindstrom, 1997). At ten months, the roots can weigh up to 2 pounds (1 kg) (Leung & Foster, 1996). The root is a black-grey color on the outside and white on the inside. The taste is pungent, bitter, and astringent (Felter & Lloyd, 1983) and causes numbness of the mouth. The odor is similar to lilacs (Wren, 1988). The psychoactive components of the plant are mostly concentrated in the lower stem and upper root (Norton, 1998).

🍃 **PLANT PARTS USED:** Root, leaf

🍃 **TRADITIONAL EVIDENCE:**

Cultural Use

    Pacific Islander. In Hawaii, kava is known as *awa* and as *sakau* in Micronesia. Kava refers to the herb and to a beverage made from the plant. The importance of kava in many Pacific island communities, especially Micronesia, can be compared to that of wine in Europe. Kava is used as a sacred drink and a cash crop. It is not used for medicinal purposes as it once was. Kava continues to be used for religious, political, and social reasons today. Religiously, kava is believed to act as a transporter to the realm of the gods (Lebot et al., 1997). Politically, kava (either the drink or the root itself) is thought to promote good will and peace. For example, Pope John Paul II drank kava with the prime minister of Fiji during his visit to the island in 1986. The

Kava cup is depicted on the flag of the state of Pohnpei in Micronesia (Norton, 1998).

Traditionally, some island cultures have viewed kava use by women as a "shameful homosexual act" because of the association of the drink with women, in particular the female genitalia. It is believed that the smell of kava drink is similar to the smell of female genitalia. Some Pacific Islanders, including Hawaiians, have used kava leaf inserted in the vagina as an abortifacient. Animal studies on rats have not supported the traditional claim that kava affects fertility (Lebot et al., 1997).

Australian. The Aborigines of Australia learned of kava from missionaries from Fiji and Polynesia in the 1980s. Aboriginal leaders supported the integration of kava into their own culture as a substitute for alcohol. Kava is now reported to be an abused substance among Aboriginals, especially in Northern Australia, where some are said to be using fifty times the amount used by Pacific Islanders (Singh & Blumenthal, 1997). It is thought that kava may be misused in Australia because the people using the herb do not have the historical connection with the plant that often includes certain traditional and ceremonial restraints and guidelines for appropriate use.

European. In current German phytomedicine practice, kava extract is approved for anxiety, stress, and restlessness (Blumenthal et al., 2000).

Culinary Use

Kava is made from the upper portion of the root and drunk as a ceremonial beverage (Duke, 1985). The root, although traditionally chewed by a male community member, is now more often ground, pounded, or grated, and then soaked and macerated in cold water to bring out its active constituents. It is numbing to the tongue. Felter and Lloyd (1983) report that the taste resembles soapsuds and tannin.

Use in Herbalism

Kava is used for its sedative, antispasmodic, anticonvulsant, diuretic, stimulant, analgesic, and antiseptic properties. Its psychoactive properties are considered comparable or superior to valium, alcohol, nicotine, and cocaine (Lebot et al., 1997) without the addictive qualities. Kava is used for enhancing feelings of "interpersonal universalism and goodwill" (Lebot et al., p. 210) and has been used in Pacific Island countries when attempting to solve disputes peacefully.

The sleep that kava induces is said to be restful and deep. Kava has been used traditionally for conditions such as migraine, backache, menstrual problems, ureter pain, and spasm associated with chronic cystitis, respiratory infections, and tuberculosis. It has been combined with pumpkin seed oil to treat irritable bladder (Leung & Foster, 1996). Gonorrhea has been treated internally with a 20% oil of kava resin in sandalwood oil (Grieve, 1971).

Because of the muscle relaxant action of kava, it can be recommended before a visit to the chiropractor's office. The herb relaxes the muscles so that the chiropractic adjustments and work on the body are much easier to perform.

In small doses, kava is tonic and stimulating, while in larger doses it produces a type of drowsy intoxication. It is used as a bitter stimulant for the stomach and for bed-wetting in children and incontinence in the elderly, especially when the incontinence is due to muscular weakness. Kava also has been known to be helpful in symptoms related to neuralgia (especially due to the fifth cranial nerve such as in dental neuralgia), dysuria, renal colic, and hemorrhoids (Felter & Lloyd, 1983).

BIOMEDICAL EVIDENCE:

Very few human trials supporting the traditional use of kava have yet to be conducted. The human trials that have been published have been conducted using standardized extracts of kava. One animal study is cited here because it does compare natural kava extract with isolated kavalactones.

Studies Related to Emotions and Adaptation

Two capsules of a standardized extract of kava called Kavatrol (60 mg kavalactones in each capsule), given twice daily for four weeks, was found to significantly reduce daily stress and state anxiety (nonpsychopathologic stress and anxiety) without adverse effects when compared with placebo in a double-blind, controlled trial of sixty subjects (Singh, Ellis, & Singh, 1998).

In a study of 101 patients diagnosed with anxiety disorder of nonpsychotic origin, those patients given one capsule of WS 1490, a lipophilic extract of kava root containing 90 to 110 mg dry extract (70 mg kavalactones) per capsule, three times a day for 24 weeks, demonstrated a significant reduction of scores on the Hamilton Anxiety Scale as compared to those who received placebo. Although both groups showed a decrease in anxiety, the kava group decreased from a mean score of 30.7 at week 0 to a score of 9.7 at week 24, and the placebo group went from 31.4 to 15.2. A possible limitation of this study is that the investigator's inclusion criteria consisted of four different anxiety disorders (Volz & Kieser, 1997).

The strength of *natural* kava extracts was demonstrated when concentrations of kavalactones were found to be significantly lower in animals that were injected with isolated kavalactones than those animals that were injected with natural extracts containing several kavalactones (study by Keledjian et al. as reported in Lebot et al., 1997). This data may point to the potential benefit of human use of natural kava extracts as opposed to individual kavalactones.

Studies Related to Other Health Patterns

Hormone Balance. One eight-week German study of a kava extract (Laitan) has been found to reduce symptoms such as hot flashes and irritability attributed to menopause in women after one week of treatment (Warnecke study as reported in Blumenthal et al., 2000).

Mechanism of Action

Kava root contains starch (> 60%), fiber, water, sugars, proteins, minerals, and 3% to 20% kavalactones, depending on age and cultivation (Leung & Foster, 1996). One way to recognize kava is that the fresh root has a local anesthetic action in the mouth, an action thought to be caused by kavain, a kavalactone. "The superficial effects of kavain are equivalent to and last as long as those of cocaine . . . the kavalactones are particularly interesting as superficial anesthetics because they manifest no toxicity in the tissues" (Lebot et al., 1997, p. 71). One researcher found that an alcoholic solution of kavain given by subcutaneous injection induced a local anesthesia that lasted for hours or even days. Because higher doses caused peripheral nerve paralysis, the researcher concluded that kavain was unsuitable as a local anesthetic (study by Baldi as reported in Lebot et al., 1997).

Kava is known for more than its local anesthetic properties. The first comprehensive studies done on kava in Germany beginning in the 1950s found that kava also has muscle relaxant properties, antimycotic activity, analgesic effects, and can potentiate barbituric narcosis. There are six major kavalactones in kava, all of which are physiologically active. The kavalactones have varying effects: some are short acting while others are long acting and vary in induction periods. This finding helps explain the observed differences in physiologic effects of crude extracts of kava on humans (Lebot et al., 1997). The muscle relaxant activity of kava is related to kavalactones known as dihydrokavain and dihydromethysticin, which directly affect muscular contractility (Leung & Foster, 1996). Kava contains two constituents, dihydrokavain and dihydromethysticin, that have known analgesic qualities similar to aspirin that may be helpful as pain-relieving agents.

Although kava has psychoactive properties, it is neither hallucinogenic nor stupefacient. Animal studies suggest that kava may promote relaxation by binding to GABA receptors in the brain, but that the action is not as direct as the binding of barbiturates (study by Jussofie et al. as reported in McCaleb, Leigh, & Morien, 2000). Animal studies also suggest that kavalactones, kawains, and methysticins reduce excitability of the limbic system in rabbits, an effect similar to benzodiazepines (Schulz et al, 1998). Kava consumption, unlike alcohol, does not impair the ability to think clearly before falling asleep, and kava is not addictive (Lebot et al., 1997).

The sedative effect of kava may be related to its dopamine antagonistic properties. This hypothesis was formed after observation of four patients who took standardized extracts of kava and developed clinical symptoms suggestive of central dopaminergic antagonism and from the fact that kava has been helpful in the relief of schizophrenic symptoms in some Aborigines in Australia (Schelosky, Raffauf, Jendroska, & Poewe, 1995).

Because reversible scaly skin eruptions can occur as a result of excessive kava intake, it has been hypothesized that kava may interfere with cholesterol metabolism necessary for normal keratinocyte formation (Norton, 1998).

☘ USE IN PREGNANCY OR LACTATION:

Although some sources report that kava is not recommended during pregnancy and lactation (Blumenthal et al., 2000; McGuffin et al., 1997), another states that contraindication is speculative related to kava's ability to relax the body and uterine tone (Brinker, 1998). Some herbalists have been known to give kava in the case of threatened miscarriage due to its antispasmodic action. According to Duke (1997), no data support contraindication at this time.

Herbal Caveat—Pregnancy or Lactation
Some herbs are contraindicated in pregnancy because of a risk of the herb or one of its constituents stimulating the uterus and therefore possibly promoting fetal loss. Many herbal practitioners do not recommend herbal remedies, in particular oral doses of herbs, during the first trimester of pregnancy and seek an alternative. However, herbs are successfully used during pregnancy, especially to prepare the body for the birth. Herbs are relatively unstudied in pregnancy and lactation, so patients need to be made aware through education of the potential benefits and risks of using herbs for health conditions that arise during pregnancy or lactation. The use of herbal remedies during pregnancy often warrants a referral to a knowledgeable herbal practitioner.

☘ USE FOR CHILDREN:

The German Commission E and the American Herbal Products Association have issued the warning that kava not be used by children under the age of 18 (Blumenthal et al., 2000). However, Hawaiian herbal healers use kava extensively for "general debility in children . . . and with those children having a disorderly stomach and . . . thick, white coating of the tongue. . . . Tannese women drink kava medicinally and give it to their children (a one-teaspoon dose is considered to cure whooping cough)" (Singh & Blumenthal, 2000, p. 50).

Herbal Caveat—Children
Children have special needs in regard to herbal therapies. They require lesser amounts of herbs and often respond well to mild teas and topical applications such as compresses and baths. The lowest dose of oral preparations should be tried first before increasing the amount given children. Caregivers should observe children closely for responses to herbal remedies. Younger children, particularly infants, have traditionally been given herbs either through their mother's breast milk or in the form of a homeopathic remedy because of their sensitivity to medicines and treatments and the immaturity of their liver. It is recommended that a person knowledgeable in the herbal treatment of children be consulted before the offering of any herb to a child for the first time.

Adhering to the recommended dosage and proper use of kava is very important. Kava is best taken at bedtime and should not be taken before operating machinery or vehicles. "Temporal limitations from 4 weeks to 3 months are recommended in Australia and required in Germany" (McGuffin et al., 1997, p. 87). The effects of kava may be influenced by its preparation (i.e., whether it is chewed or not) and whether or not it is taken with food. Eating immediately before ingestion of kava may render it ineffective (Singh & Blumenthal, 1997).

Although kava acts as a soporific drug, putting the drinker to sleep within thirty minutes, no aftereffects such as are experienced by alcohol drinkers are experienced if kava is consumed in reasonable quantities (Lebot et al., 1997). Some kava drinkers have reported experiencing photophobia related to pupil dilation, diplopia, and disturbances in oculomotor balance (Lebot et al., 1997).

Although animal studies have shown that alcohol, barbiturates, and psychopharmacologic agents may potentiate the effect of kava on the concentration of kavalactones in the brain (Blumenthal et al., 2000; Lebot et al., 1997), a recent German study by Herberg (1993) demonstrated no negative synergistic effect of alcohol and kava extract (WS 1490) in humans with a 0.05% blood alcohol level (as reported in Blumenthal et al., 2000). Other German observational studies with large human samples of 4049 patients taking 105 mg per day of a kava standardized extract (70% kavapyrones), and 3029 patients taking 800 mg per day of a kava extract standardized to 30% kavapyrones, resulted in minimal side effects in both studies, 1.5% and 2.3%, respectively. The reversible side effects were gastrointestinal complaints, allergic skin reactions, headache, or dizziness (studies by Hansel and Hofmann & Winter as reported in Schulz et al, 1998). Allergic skin reactions do occur in rare cases (Jappe, Franke, Reinhol, & Gollnick, 1998).

A kavalactone extract (dihydromethysticin) may cause exfoliative dermatitis. Ongoing use may cause inflammation of the body and the eyes and subsequent ulcers and peeling of the skin (Duke, 1985). Excessive use of kava (as demonstrated among Aboriginal heavy drinkers), 310 to 440 g of kava per week as a beverage (Mathews et al., 1988), can lead to general ill health, skin rash, skin yellowing (kava dermopathy), shortness of breath, malnutrition, liver damage, and changes in red and white blood cells and platelets (Lebot et al., 1997, p. 200). The symptoms are relieved when kava consumption is discontinued (Foster & Tyler, 1999). The symptom pattern associated with kava dermopathy may indicate that it interferes with cholesterol metabolism necessary for normal keratinocyte formation (Norton, 1998).

One report published in the United States notes a possible drugherb interaction between kava and the benzodiazepine, alprazolam (Xanax), in which the reporting physicians suggest a dangerous additive effect of kava with the alprazolam based on in vitro studies showing that the two substances act on the same GABA receptors. The patient discussed in the report experienced lethargy and disorientation even though he claims that he was taking appropriate amounts of kava and alprazolam. He also was taking other medications including cimetidine (Reglan). No results of an investigation were reported (Almeida & Grimsley, 1996). Although there have been safety concerns about chronic, excessive kava consumption, no deaths have resulted (Lebot et al., 1997).

Four patient case histories have demonstrated that pharmaceutical preparations of kava, such as Laitan and Kavasporal, seemingly antagonize dopamine and therefore may be contraindicated in the treatment of Parkinson's disease (Brinker, 1998; Schelosky et al, 1995).

NURSING EVIDENCE:

Historical Nursing Use

No data are available at this time.

Potential Nursing Applications

So many diseases are being linked to increasing stress conditions. Nurses work not only with patients who deal with the physical, mental, and spiritual effects of *daily* stress but also those who have psychopathology resulting from significant stress and anxiety. Nurses may want to consider using and researching the effects of kava on psychiatric patients, such as those recuperating from posttraumatic stress disorder. Kava also might be considered very useful with patients being treated at pain management clinics with nonpharmacologic methods because of the chronic nature of their health concerns. For instance, adult patients with chronic back pain and muscle spasms might find kava extremely helpful not only with their physical symptoms but also for those family members who want to be more tolerant of the chronic illness in their loved one.

Integrative Insight

Kava has been used primarily in one part of the world where it has been part of cultural ritual and traditions. Although kava has been shown to clearly reduce anxiety and tension and promote goodwill in Micronesian and Polynesian cultures, one might wonder if the plant medicine would have the same effect in people who do not use it in the same cultural framework. Scientifically, kava has been shown to reduce anxiety and stress in humans and may offer those living in a high tech world some respite where so many acute and chronic illnesses are influenced or induced by unmanageable stress. However, as has already been seen with the introduction of kava in Australia, this herb may best be used with some special attention to the cultural ways in which it has been used historically. The use of kava in the West may provide significant information about the relationship between the action of a medicinal plant and its cultural/traditional use. Just as it takes years to prepare and perfect a pharmaceutical drug or therapeutic medical or nursing procedure, it may take some time to understand and perfect the best way to receive the benefits of using kava outside of the Pacific Island cultures. Nurses can facilitate this learning process by including a thorough sociocultural assessment of how patients prepare and use kava.

THERAPEUTIC APPLICATIONS:

Oral

The methods of preparing kava on Fiji and Tonga include the "chewing and pounding" method. Another method used to ensure the intoxication of the drinker, is to use hot water to extract dry or green root stock and then allow the beverage to cool before drinking. The hot water extraction method increases the strength of the drink (Singh & Blumenthal, 1997). Chewing and pounding traditionally are performed by healthy young girls or boys. They rinse their mouths and then chew the root without mixing saliva into it. After the chewing, the root is dry and has increased significantly in weight (Singh & Blumenthal, 1997). In Fiji, kava root also may be pounded or grated before chewing.

German pharmacopeial grade kava must contain not less than 3.5% total kavalactones calculated as kavain (Blumenthal et al., 2000). The traditional kava drink contains approximately 250 mg of kavalactones.

Powdered Root in Capsules. 400 to 500 mg capsules up to six times per day (McCaleb et al., 2000)

Liquid Extract. 1:2 (g/ml) ½ to 1 teaspoon (3 to 6 ml) per day in divided doses (as reported in Blumenthal et al., 2000) or 15 to 30 drops in a small amount of water up to three times per day (McCaleb et al., 2000)

Standardized Extract. 70 mg of kavalactones 2 to 3 times per day (McCaleb et al., 2000)

Whole Root, Cut. 1.7 to 3.4 g per day (equivalent to 60 to 120 mg kavapyrones) (Blumenthal et al., 2000)

Dry Normalized Extract Containing 30% (300 mg/g) Kavapyrones. 0.2 to 0.4 g (200 to 400 mg)

Topical

The juice from kava has been used externally for skin diseases, including leprosy.

Poultice. Fresh leaf or juice used for intestinal complaints, abcesses, or earache

Douche. Used for vaginitis (Duke, 1985)

Environmental

No data are available at this time.

PATIENT INTERACTION:

The history of kava use includes certain cultural rituals of preparation and use. You may want to familiarize yourself with the traditional use of kava before taking it for the first time. Kava root and drink have been used in Pacific Island cultures to promote peace and good will and there are strict guidelines regarding its use so that its sedative properties are not abused. Kava root is not addicting but has occasionally been misused when not taken within the context of ritual and traditional use.

Medicinally, kava is a sedative, topical anesthetic, and muscle relaxant. Kava root may be helpful with muscle spasms, anxiety, stress, restlessness, and pain. When taking kava root drink or liquid extract, a mild numbing sensation will occur in the mouth. While eating certain foods has been part of the ritual use of kava, some report that eating should not occur at the same time as taking kava because the kava may then be ineffective. Do not take kava at the exact same time as other pharmaceutical drugs or supplements. Consider checking with a knowledgeable practitioner before taking kava if you are taking any medications or supplements routinely. Kava can be taken 30 minutes before bed to assist restful sleep. Kava in appropriate dosages can cause drowsiness, so do not operate vehicles or heavy equipment after taking kava. Drinking alcoholic beverages at the same time as taking kava may significantly increase the sedative action of kava and is not recommended.

NURTURING THE NURSE-PLANT RELATIONSHIP:

Note: You may want to keep a journal of your experiences with the herb.

Achieving the desired sedative and mind-relaxing benefits of drinking kava root beverage is not the only goal of the kava ceremony. The ceremony itself is as important as achieving the desired effects of the plant. The Japanese tea ceremony is much like the Pacific Island kava ceremony. These ceremonies are national treasures and are used in promoting peace and good will. Both ceremonies are choreographed for the health benefit to server and guest. There is a known stress reduction effect from tea ceremonies. A tea ceremony is conducted as a nonverbal way of saying, "welcome . . . be at peace." Try preparing a kava drink and serving it to a guest with full awareness that your act of preparation can be a potent stress reducer for you, the giver, as well as the receiver. Prepare a relaxing kava root drink for yourself after a stressful day with just a few drops of extract in a small amount of water to start. Record your experience with kava.

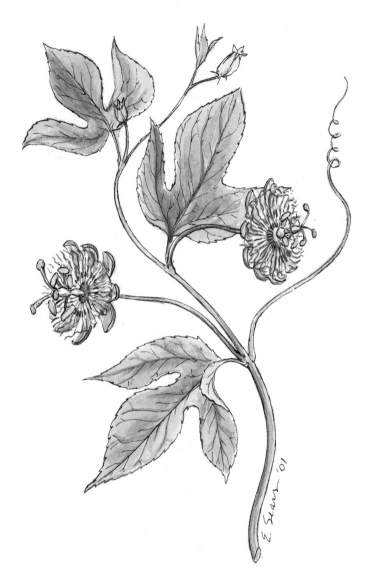

Passiflora incarnata

Passion Flower

🌿 **LATIN NAME:** *Passiflora incarnata L.*

🌿 **FAMILY:** Passifloraceae

🌿 **COMMON NAMES:** Passion flower, apricot vine, grenadille, maypop, passiflora, passion vine, wild passion flower, purple passion flower

🌿 **HEALTH PATTERN:** Emotions and adaptation

🌿 **PLANT DESCRIPTION:**

Passion flower is a perennial vine that can climb to a height of 27 feet (9 meters). The plant has three to five lobed, finely serrated leaves and large, sweet-smelling flowers that are flesh colored or yellow and tinged with purple. The ripe berry is orange and approximately the size of an apple. It has a yellow pulp and is sweet and edible. (Be sure to clearly identify the plant species because some *Passiflora* berries are not edible.) The plant was named for the resemblance of the blossom to the crown of thorns used in the passion and crucifixion of Christ (Grieve, 1971). The plant is native to the United States, particularly the southern states (Leung & Foster, 1996).

🌿 **PLANT PARTS USED:** Leaves, dried aerial parts, and the whole plant

🌿 **TRADITIONAL EVIDENCE:**

Cultural Use

North American Indian. Passion flower grows in America but only in the warmer climates such as in the southeastern states where it is known as *maypops*. Indian tribes use passion flower both medicinally and as food. The Cherokee use the root for boils, as an anti-inflammatory for brier and locust wounds, as an aid in weaning babies, and as a liver aid. It was also used topically for earache (Moerman, 1998). The Cherokee also use the plant juice as a beverage. The fruit is eaten raw, the young shoots and leaves are boiled or fried and eaten as greens, and the leaves are cooked in grease as a potherb (Moerman, 1998). The Houmas tribe uses the roots of the plant as a blood tonic (Moerman, 1998).

Hispanic. Passion flower was first used medicinally by the Aztecs as a sedative for insomnia and nervousness and taken back to Europe by the Spanish explorers (Blumenthal, Goldberg, & Brinckman, 2000). The Maya used the crushed whole plant as a poultice for swelling and internally for ringworm (Vogel, 1970). In Mexican culture, the herb, known as *granada china* or *passiflora* is often used as a tea for *nervios* or nervous conditions. Passion flower is used for heart conditions as well because "the heart is believed to be the source of *nervios*" (Kay, 1996, p. 61).

East Indian. The Indian *Materia Medica* lists only *P. foetida,* known in Sanskrit as *mukkopeera.* A decoction is used in the treatment of asthma and the leaf is applied to the head for headache (Nadkarni, 1997).

Russian/Baltic. In Russian herbalism, passion flower is often used in combination with valerian for symptoms of insomnia (Zevin, 1997).

European. Passion flower is used extensively in Europe. Euphytose (EUP), a combination of six herbal extracts including passion flower, is an herbal product that has been marketed and widely used in France since 1927 for its anxiolytic effect (Bourin, Bougerol, Guitton, & Broutin, 1997). The German Commission E has approved passion flower for use in nervous restlessness. It is also used for mild sleeplessness, tenseness, restlessness, and anxiety (Blumenthal et al., 2000). The herb is found in several sleep aides marketed in Britain. It is also sold as a sedative chewing gum.

Culinary Use

The Council of Europe lists passion flower as a natural source of flavoring (Newall et al., 1996). The plant also is used for flavoring alcoholic and nonalcoholic beverages and frozen dairy desserts (Leung & Foster, 1996).

Use in Herbalism

Passion flower is used in herbalism as a sedative, hypnotic, antispasmodic, and analgesic. It has been used in the past specifically for neuralgia, generalized seizures, hysteria, tachycardia, headaches, asthma, insomnia, and dysmenorrhea. Some herbalists use passion flower for treating the symptoms of Parkinson's disease. Passion flower often is used in combination with other herbs such as valerian, chamomile, and hops for promoting relaxation, rest, and sleep. Passion flower/ephedra combinations have been used for rhinitis, nasal congestion, sinus drainage, respiratory allergies, headaches, sinus headaches, and colds (Pedersen, 1998). Passion flower/chamomile combinations have been used for anxiety, muscle tension, insomnia, and nervous headaches (Pedersen, 1998).

✿ BIOMEDICAL EVIDENCE:

No published studies are available on the use of passion flower as a single herb in humans in regard to the herb's effect on emotions and adaptation.

Studies Related to Emotions and Adaptation

As previously described, EUP, a French herbal product containing six herbal extracts including 40 mg of passion flower, significantly improved Hamilton anxiety scores in those participants given two tablets three times a day for twenty-eight days as compared with placebo in a double-blind trial of 182 patients with adjustment disorder with anxious mood (Bourin et al., 1997).

Animal studies have shown that passion flower can act as a sedative at high doses and an anxiolytic at low doses (Leung & Foster, 1996). There is also evidence that a fluid extract of Passion flower can prolong sleep time and affect locomotor activity in rats and can protect rats from the convulsive effect of pentylenetetrazole (Speroni & Minghetti, 1988).

Studies Related to Other Health Patterns

Sleep and Rest. In vivo (animal) studies have shown that a passion flower extract increased sleeping time induced by hexobarbital in mice and potentiates pentobarbital; however, the doses of passion flower given far exceeded those typically given in human doses (Brinker, 1998; Schilcher, 1992).

Comfort and Pain Relief. The analgesic effect of passion flower has been shown in animal studies. One study demonstrated an increase in the nociceptive threshold in response to pain as measured by tail flick (Speroni & Minghetti, 1988).

Mechanism of Action

The effectiveness of passion flower (particularly related to alleviating Parkinson's disease symptoms) may be explained by two compounds found in the plant known as harmine and harmaline alkaloids (Duke, 1997). Although some sources say that passion flower contains cyanogenic glycosides, *P. incarnata* does not. Other *Passiflora* species may contain cyanogenic glycosides (Newall et al., 1996).

USE IN PREGNANCY OR LACTATION:

There are no known contraindications for the use of passion flower during pregnancy (Blumenthal et al., 2000; McGuffin et al., 1997). The *Eclectic Medical Journal,* 1896, reported the successful use of two drachms of injectable passion flower given for postpartum puerperal eclampsia with convulsions (Felter & Lloyd, 1983). Susan Weed (1986) suggests using passion flower during pregnancy to control hypertension. The dosage she recommends is 2 to 4 capsules or 15 drops of tincture three times a day for several weeks. Some sources report that the harman and harmaline alkaloids in passion flower have been shown to increase uterine stimulant activity in animals (Newall et al., 1996; Brinker, 1998) and suggest that passion flower may be contraindicated in pregnancy.

On occasion, I have used passion flower in a tea formulation to help women who have been unsuccessful in conceiving a child. So often women become very anxious when they are unsuccessful in conceiving easily. Passion flower can prove helpful (and successful) in preparing a woman for pregnancy. When using herbs with a woman trying to conceive, always confirm that she is not undergoing medical infertility treatment. Also take a full menstrual cycle history and monitor her cycle closely.

Herbal Caveat—Pregnancy or Lactation
Some herbs are contraindicated in pregnancy because of a risk of the herb or one of its constituents stimulating the uterus and therefore possibly promoting fetal loss. Many herbal practitioners do not recommend herbal remedies, in particular oral doses of herbs, during the first trimester of pregnancy and seek an alternative. However, herbs are successfully used during pregnancy, especially to prepare the body for the birth. Herbs are relatively unstudied in pregnancy and lactation, so patients need to be made aware through education of the potential benefits and risks of using herbs for health conditions that arise during pregnancy or lactation. The use of herbal remedies during pregnancy often warrants a referral to a knowledgeable herbal practitioner.

USE FOR CHILDREN:

Passion flower is used for children in Germany as part of a sedative tea containing lemon balm, lavender, and St. John's wort (Blumenthal et al., 2000; Schilcher, 1992). Early American Eclectic physicians used passion flower for nervous conditions and insomnia in infants and children. It also was used in cases of whooping cough with convulsions (Felter & Lloyd, 1983).

Herbal Caveat—Children
Children have special needs in regard to herbal therapies. They require lesser amounts of herbs and often respond well to mild teas and topical applications such as compresses and baths. The lowest dose of oral preparations should be tried first before increasing the amount given children. Caregivers should observe children closely for responses to herbal remedies. Younger children, particularly infants, have traditionally been given herbs either through their mother's breast milk or in the form of a homeopathic remedy because of their sensitivity to medicines and treatments and the immaturity of their liver. It is recommended that a person knowledgeable in the herbal treatment of children be consulted before the offering of any herb to a child for the first time.

CAUTIONS:

One case of hypersensitivity vasculitis may have been attributed to passion flower. The 77-year-old man involved in the reported case was taking diclofenac and cyclopenthiazide, and the rash may have been due to an herb-drug interaction (Fugh-Berman & Cott, 1999). No side effects or other toxic effects have been reported with passion flower. Acute toxicity values of *P. incarnata* are greater than 900 mg/kg in mice (Speroni & Minghetti, 1988).

In the United States, passion flower may be entwined with a very toxic plant, *Abrus precatorius L.*, so care must be taken when harvesting from the wild.

Historical Nursing Use

No data are available at this time.

Potential Nursing Applications

Nurses work with patients who are anxious and irritable because they are not feeling well and are having to undergo painful tests, uncomfortable procedures, and sometimes hospitalization. Entering the health care system can be an extremely anxiety-producing experience for people, and nurses are often the ones who must find ways to diffuse the anxiety and tension patients experience. Passion flower may present nurses with a clinical way of helping patients adapt to the health care environment and their illness. Nurses may want to consider the potential clinical benefits of passion flower tea, liquid extract, and even gum for the symptoms patients experience related to anxiety, insomnia, and stress. Nurses may want to research the potential benefit of passion flower in pain management, mental illness, and the management of a stressful hospital milieu. Nurses also may want to consider setting up n-of-1 or case studies, regarding the use of passion flower in women trying to conceive.

Integrative Insight

Passion can be likened to intense emotion. It also can be defined as suffering. Numerous triggers cause the tension, stress, and suffering that people sometimes feel on a daily basis as they go through life. Nurses observe certain patterns among these internal and external triggers, and they may observe patterns in how patients react and respond to those triggers. Nurses also may find, as they seek to individualize care for the stressed and emotionally suffering patient, that each person's experience of anxiety or stress that can lead to illness or imbalance is also slightly different in its expression. How is it then, that an herb like passion flower can be used so effectively in so many people for calming the nerves, promoting restful sleep, and relieving anxiety?

Passion flowers are intriguing and beautiful and are considered unique by some. Somehow, this unique flower seems to understand the passion, suffering, or strong emotion a person feels and is able to make it better. The way passion flower works may have something to do with its phytochemical constituents, but the mechanism of action is not really known. What is known from years of use of this herb is that there is always hope for relief from suffering and passion or intense emotions. Nurses in many countries are observing the effects of a fast-paced, technologically advanced world on peoples' well-being. Some of those effects are not healthy at all and lead to serious, often chronic illness. Herbs such as passion flower offer patients and nurses alike an opportunity for physical and psychologic support in times of passion when feelings are just too intense and the body and mind do not seem to adapt to the stressors that have challenged them.

THERAPEUTIC APPLICATIONS:

German pharmaceutical grade passion flower must contain not less than 0.4% flavonoids (Blumenthal et al., 2000). Other European monographs state that the crude plant formula should contain not less than 0.8% total flavonoids and that harmala alkaloids should not exceed 0.01% (Leung & Foster, 1996). As with many plants, no clear data exist regarding one specific active component of the plant, so standardization information is not available.

Oral

Tea. To 6½ ounces (200 ml) of boiling water add 1 tablespoon of crude herb (Schilcher, 1992). One to four cups (240 to 960 ml) of tea per day are recommended (Schilcher, 1992; Blumenthal et al., 2000).

Fluid Extract. 1:1 (g/ml) ½ teaspoon (2 ml), three to four times per day (Blumenthal et al., 2000; Pedersen, 1998).

Tincture. 1:5 (g/ml) 2 teaspoons (10 ml), three to four times per day (Blumenthal et al., 2000)

Dried Herb. 2 g three to four times per day (Blumenthal et al., 2000)

Topical

Compress. Use cotton saturated with *Passiflora* and place it on a carious tooth for toothache (Felter & Lloyd, 1983, p. 1441). The Maya used the crushed whole plant as a poultice for swelling (Vogel, 1970).

Environmental

No data are available at this time.

Herbal Caveat—Therapeutic Applications

In traditional and conventional herbal medicine, amounts of herbs given to patients are based on individual needs. The amounts or "doses" recorded here are provided so that the health practitioner has a general idea of the amounts recommended for an adult patient. Dosing in herbalism not only refers to amount of plant used but also includes when, where, and how to take a plant medicine. These dosages should not be used as guidelines for indiscriminate intervention without proper assessment, critical thinking, and patient education on the part of the practitioner.

Note: Please see chapter 5 for detailed descriptions of how to prepare various applications.

PATIENT INTERACTION:

Passion flower has been used extensively for insomnia and anxiety related to stress. In animal studies, higher doses have been found to have sedative effects while lower doses relieve anxiety. When purchasing a passion flower product, read the label carefully to ensure the product contains *P. incarnata*. This herb is most often used in combination with other herbs such as valerian and hops. Talk to a health practitioner if your anxiety or stress is not relieved by self-care such as taking herbs or if you are having thoughts of harming yourself or others.

Herbal Caveat—Patient Interaction

Patients considering the use of an herb or formula of herbs in self-care benefit from education about the plant itself and the use of the plant in healing. This education can come through many sources, including local herbalists; plant specialists such as botanists; health practitioners such as nurses, nutritionists, naturopaths, and other physicians; and various written references including the scientific literature. Patients need to remember that their unique health care needs are not necessarily represented in any literature they may encounter. Therefore, it is recommended that a knowledgeable mentor be consulted before initiating self-care with any herb being used for the first time.

NURTURING THE NURSE-PLANT RELATIONSHIP:

Note: You may want to keep a journal of your experiences with the herb.

This flower has a very unique design. To get to know passion flower, find a place where it is growing or obtain some photos of it. Describe the plant. To experience the healing properties of this beautiful herb, consider making a tea and drinking it before bed. This is a good plant remedy to try when you may be having the insomnia that often accompanies rotating shift work. While drinking the tea, take a moment to consider those things you are passionate about. Record your experiences.

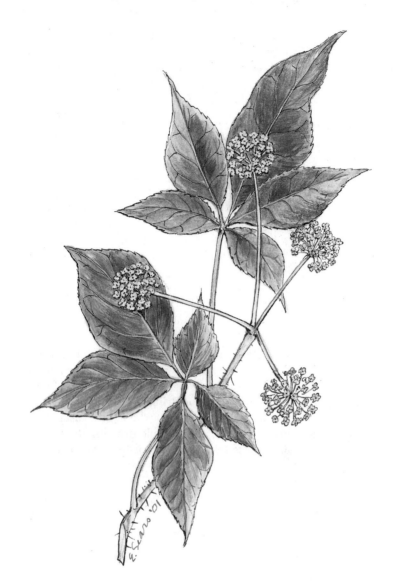

Eleutherococcus senticosus

Siberian Ginseng

🍃 **LATIN NAME:** *Eleutherococcus senticosus*
(Chinese reports refer to the plant as *Acanthopanax senticosus* [Farnsworth, Kinghorn, Soejarto, & Waller, 1985].)

🍃 **FAMILY:** Araliaceae

🍃 **COMMON NAMES:** Siberian ginseng, eleutherococc, eleuthero, eleuthero ginseng, Ussurian thorny pepperbush, wujiaseng, devil's shrub, wild pepper, touch-me-not, spiny eleutherococc

🍃 **HEALTH PATTERN:** Emotions and adaptation

🍃 **PLANT DESCRIPTION:**
Siberian ginseng is not a true ginseng, nor is it grown in Siberia. Siberian ginseng grows abundantly in the Khabarovsk and Primorsk districts in the Soviet Union (Farnsworth et al., 1985). Siberian ginseng has been developed in the Soviet Union as an alternative to *Panax ginseng*. It is often confused with *Panax ginseng* but is not the same plant (see chapter 14), nor does it contain plant constituents called ginsenosides that are characteristic of the *Panax* species (Farnsworth et al., 1985). The plant is a thorny shrub that grows to heights of eight to ten feet (2½ to 3 meters). It grows in the harsh climate of Manchuria and is therefore very hardy. It has several prickly stems with light gray or brownish bark (McCaleb et al., 2000). The plant has three to seven serrated leaflets on each stem. The taste of the root is characterized as sharp, aromatic, and slightly sweet (Schulz et al., 1998, p. 273). Roots with the highest concentration of plant constituents known as eleutherosides occur just before the leaves fall in the autumn (McCaleb, Leigh, & Morien, 2000).

🍃 **PLANT PARTS USED:** Root and root bark

🍃 **TRADITIONAL EVIDENCE:**
Cultural Use

Asian. Siberian ginseng is called *ciwujia* in Chinese medicine. The Chinese have been using Siberian ginseng for 2000 years. The root is a remedy for bronchitis and other respiratory infections, heart ailments, insomnia, and is used as a general tonic to restore vigor and memory and improve general health and longevity (Blumenthal et al., 2000; Duke, 1985). It also is used in rheumatoid arthritis, diabetes, heart disease, and certain cancers (Foster & Chongxi, 1992).

Russian/Baltic. The Pharmacological Committee of the U.S.S.R. Ministry of Health approved a 33% extract of Siberian ginseng for human use in 1962. Numerous studies on extracts of Siberian ginseng have been done in the Soviet Union since the 1950s and are published in the Russian language. The plant is used as an adaptogen and tonic (Farnsworth et al., 1985).

Culinary Use

No data are available at this time.

Use in Herbalism

Siberian ginseng is used primarily in herbalism as an adaptogen in that it supports the body in its ability to adapt to changes in the environment and other stressors. Siberian ginseng came into worldwide use in the twentieth century when the Russians began looking for an alternative to red ginseng that was less expensive and would still help people cope with stress, stimulate the immune system, and prevent respiratory disorders (Rister, 1999). Through research, Russians know that people who take Siberian ginseng 12 weeks before cold and flu season can experience a significant decrease in the incidence of respiratory illness (Kalashnikov, 1977 as reported in Rister, 1999). The plant also has been used as a stimulant of mental and physical performance and is a "legal stimulant" used in athletic training. It also is used to help those with cancer or depression and is reported to be effective in treating insomnia (Duke, 1985). It has also been used in treating high altitude sickness.

BIOMEDICAL EVIDENCE:

Numerous human (totaling over 6000 subjects), animal, and in vitro studies have been conducted, primarily in the Soviet Union, on the effect of Siberian ginseng extract. Many of the human studies have investigated Siberian ginseng's adaptogen action as human subject performance related to physical exertion, visual acuity, hearing, color discrimination, motion sickness, and mental alertness. "There are numerous reports of the ability of *E. senticosus* (ES) extracts to inhibit or modulate a disease process, including atherosclerosis, pyelonephritis, hypertension, diabetes, rheumatic heart lesions, pneumoconiosis, hypotension, neurosis and arrhythmias. . . . Evidence to support the adaptogenic nature of ES extracts in both animal models and humans is extensive" (Farnsworth et al., 1985, p. 207). These studies are published in Russian. No studies were found regarding the use of Siberian ginseng as tea or for applications for which a form of the herb other than as an extract was used.

Studies Related to Emotions and Adaptation

One study compared physical work capacity in 6 male athletes taking Siberian ginseng extract, 33% ethanol, or placebo. The subjects had significantly higher physical work capacity with Siberian ginseng (23.3%) as compared to placebo (7.5%). It is thought that the increase may be due to higher oxygen metabolism (Asano et al., 1986). Generalizability of the results of this study is limited because of the small sample size.

Russian studies report a doubling of the lifetime (survival) and improved state of blood in mice treated with Siberian ginseng during chronic irradiation with a total of up to 7000 rads. Other adaptogenic effects observed in human or animal studies include increase in mental and physical efficiency, a reduction of the symptoms related to alarm states, antioxidant actions, immune system stimulation, and the restoration of blood albumin after massive bleeding (Brekhman & Dardymov, 1969, p. 423).

Studies Related to Other Health Patterns

Sleep and Rest. In vivo animal studies have been conducted with Siberian ginseng. One study found that Siberian ginseng caused a dose-dependent decreased sleep latency and increased sleep duration. In vitro controlled studies demonstrated a decrease in hexobarbital metabolism (Medon, Ferguson, & Watson, 1984).

Restoration. In a randomized, placebo-controlled, double-blind, crossover study of 24 patients, Siberian ginseng root (a preparation called ACTION) given in oral daily doses of 1250 mg, was shown to significantly improve selective memory ($p < .02$) and subjective feeling of being more active ($p < .02$) in middle-aged participants (Winther, Ranlov, Rein, & Mehlsen, 1997).

Siberian ginseng has been shown in animal studies to delay tumor intake, delay or prevent metastasis, and delay the induction of chemically induced or spontaneous tumors in mice. Animal studies also have demonstrated that Siberian ginseng significantly increases the ability to tolerate toxic medications and improve the antitumor effect of medications used in the treatment of various cancers (Farnsworth et al., 1985).

Mechanism of Action

As is common with numerous plant medicines, despite the numerous human, animal, and in vitro studies that have been conducted, pharmacologic explanations for the mechanism of action are not well defined (Farnsworth et al., 1985). The primary use for Siberian ginseng is as an adaptogen (Brekhman & Dardymov, 1969), a substance that "must be innocuous, must have a nonspecific action, and has a normalizing action irrespective of the direction of the pathologic state" (Farnsworth et al., 1985, p. 157). Data obtained through animal studies support an inhibitory effect of Siberian ginseng on hepatic enzymes rather than induction as the mechanism of action (Medon et al., 1984). In vitro studies have shown that Siberian ginseng binds with both estrogen and progestin receptors (Farnsworth et al., 1985). It also acts as a monoamine oxidase (MAO) inhibitor (Duke, 1997). Key compounds identified in Siberian ginseng root are eleutherosides A–G (Brekhman & Dardymov, 1969).

USE IN PREGNANCY OR LACTATION:

Siberian ginseng is not contraindicated in pregnancy (McGuffin et al., 1997). Numerous animal studies have not shown any harmful effects of the use of Siberian ginseng in pregnancy and lactation (Judin studies as reported in Farnsworth et al., 1985). There has been one report of androgenicity in an infant whose mother was taking Siberian ginseng in pregnancy. Further analysis of the capsules the mother took revealed that the capsules sold as Siberian ginseng actually contained silk vine not *E. senticossus*. Follow-up pharmacologic studies with animals did not show any androgenicity with Siberian ginseng (Leung & Foster, 1996).

Herbal Caveat—Pregnancy or Lactation

Some herbs are contraindicated in pregnancy because of a risk of the herb or one of its constituents stimulating the uterus and therefore possibly promoting fetal loss. Many herbal practitioners do not recommend herbal remedies, in particular oral doses of herbs, during the first trimester of pregnancy and seek an alternative. However, herbs are successfully used during pregnancy, especially to prepare the body for the birth. Herbs are relatively unstudied in pregnancy and lactation, so patients need to be made aware through education of the potential benefits and risks of using herbs for health conditions that arise during pregnancy or lactation. The use of herbal remedies during pregnancy often warrants a referral to a knowledgeable herbal practitioner.

USE FOR CHILDREN:

One study of children ages 9 to 15 given Siberian ginseng extract 1 drop for each year of age per day for 6 weeks followed by a 2-week break and then $3\frac{1}{2}$ more months of treatment, showed significant improvement in symptoms related to pulmonary tuberculosis (e.g. physical exercise tolerance) without side effects (Sobkovich study as reported in Farnsworth et al., 1985).

Herbal Caveat—Children

Children have special needs in regard to herbal therapies. They require lesser amounts of herbs and often respond well to mild teas and topical applications such as compresses and baths. The lowest dose of oral preparations should be tried first before increasing the amount given children. Caregivers should observe children closely for responses to herbal remedies. Younger children, particularly infants, have traditionally been given herbs either through their mother's breast milk or in the form of a homeopathic remedy because of their sensitivity to medicines and treatments and the immaturity of their liver. It is recommended that a person knowledgeable in the herbal treatment of children be consulted before the offering of any herb to a child for the first time.

CAUTIONS:

No toxicity has been found in the numerous human studies involving more than 6000 subjects or in the animal studies exposing rats, mice, rabbits, dogs, minks, deer, lambs and piglets to Siberian ginseng extract. In one study, the LD_{50} for powdered Siberian ginseng root in mice was more than 30 g/kg (Farnsworth et al., 1985, p. 207). There has been one report of a possible herb-drug interaction between Siberian ginseng and digoxin, in which serum digoxin levels increased to toxic levels, although the patient did not experience symptoms of toxicity (McRae, 1996). McRae reports that the capsules the patient was taking were analyzed and found to have "no digoxin or digitoxin contamination" (McRae, 1996, p. 294); however, no analysis was carried out to determine whether the herb capsules did in fact contain Siberian ginseng either. The patient's serum digoxin levels remained high when the digoxin was discontinued (the patient was still taking the herb). Once the herb was discontinued, the digoxin level decreased from 4.0 nmol/L to 2.2 nmol/L in five days. When the Siberian ginseng was introduced again, the patient's digoxin levels rose steadily once again until the herb product was discontinued (McRae, 1996). Because the capsules were never analyzed and found to actually contain Siberian ginseng, no final conclusions were drawn to support the hypothesis that there may be a drug-herb interaction between digoxin and Siberian ginseng.

In addition to silk vine, there is a report of adulteration of Siberian ginseng with caffeine. An investigation of powdered Siberian ginseng imported into the United States showed that Siberian ginseng can be misidentified with some so-called Siberian ginseng products containing more than six plants other than Siberian ginseng (Tyler, 1993). Siberian ginseng has been shown to have hypoglycemic effects and should be used with caution in diabetes. The herb also has been shown to increase the efficacy of antibiotics (monomycin and kanamycin) in humans (Brinker, 1998). Siberian ginseng is contraindicated in high blood pressure (in excess of 180/90 mm Hg) because of the potential for increased production of adrenaline (Farnsworth et al., 1985); however, the normalizing, adaptogenic effect of Siberian ginseng on the human body has demonstrated that because of the glycosides found in the plant, Siberian ginseng also can actually lower blood pressure (McGuffin et al., 1997). Some recommend that the plant only be used for extended periods of time if periodic breaks are taken every one to three months (Brinker, 1998).

NURSING EVIDENCE:

Historical Nursing Use

No data are available at this time.

Potential Nursing Applications

The nursing literature includes the concept of adaptation mostly noted in the work of nursing's systems theorists such as Roy and Newman. Much can be learned about the body's ability to adapt and the adaptogenic characteristics of Siberian ginseng by using the herb in caring for patients with stress-related conditions. A potentially useful nursing study might be to provide Siberian ginseng tea or liquid extract to caregivers of chronically ill patients and then study whether or not this is useful in reducing perceived stress and caregiver burden. Nurses also may want to consider the clinical use of Siberian ginseng with patients with stress-related conditions, immune deficiency symptoms, generalized weakness, and rheumatism. Siberian ginseng might also be explored for use in preparing cancer patients who elect to undergo chemotherapy and radiation treatments.

Integrative Insight

Siberian ginseng has been shown to be a very effective herb for helping improve the body's ability to adapt to change and environmental and physical stressors. It has been studied and used extensively in Russia and China. The importance of the herb is now being recognized more and more in other countries. Its exact mechanism of action as an adaptogen is not fully understood. (See chapter 20 for further information on adaptogen action.) Siberian ginseng is one herb that may be helpful in furthering an understanding of the herb-body relationship. Siberian ginseng seems to be able to help the body's self-regulatory mechanisms, but how it does what it does is still unknown.

In China, herbs are classified by their influence on certain symptom patterns. Siberian ginseng influences the *qi*, or energy of the body, as a tonic. Perhaps herbs that tonify *qi* or raise energy as does Siberian ginseng will need to be studied by new techniques to fully grasp how they influence the energy systems of the body that supply the vital organs. Nurses too are skilled at pattern recognition. They may want to consider how their observational skills and ability in health pattern recognition may add to the knowledge of adaptogen herbs such as Siberian ginseng.

THERAPEUTIC APPLICATIONS:

Oral

Oral dosage forms are available in liquid, tincture, tablet, crude herb, and tea. There are no clear standardization criteria available for Siberian ginseng.

Powdered Root. 2 to 8 g per day (McCaleb et al., 2000)

Fluid Extract. (1:1 g/ml) ½ teaspoon (2 to 3 ml); ½ to 2 teaspoons (2 to 12 ml) per day of 33% ethanol extract (McCaleb et al., 2000); ½ to 3 teaspoons (2 to 16 ml) 33% ethanol extract one to three times a day for up to sixty consecutive days (Farnsworth et al., 1985)

Tincture. (1:5 g/ml) 2 to 3 teaspoons (10 to 15 ml)

Tea. Add 1 teaspoon powdered herb to 1 cup (240 ml) of hot water; steep for 5 to 10 minutes.

Topical

Siberian ginseng is best known for its internal use.

Environmental

No data are available at this time.

Herbal Caveat—Therapeutic Applications

In traditional and conventional herbal medicine, amounts of herbs given to patients are based on individual needs. The amounts or "doses" recorded here are provided so that the health practitioner has a general idea of the amounts recommended for an adult patient. Dosing in herbalism not only refers to amount of plant used but also includes when, where, and how to take a plant medicine. These dosages should not be used as guidelines for indiscriminate intervention without proper assessment, critical thinking, and patient education on the part of the practitioner.

Note: Please see chapter 5 for detailed descriptions of how to prepare various applications.

PATIENT INTERACTION:

Siberian ginseng, an herb known as an "adaptogen," may be particularly helpful in supporting the body to adapt to changes, such as can occur in the interaction between a person and his or her environment or when experiencing many kinds of stress. It has been used extensively to increase physical and mental performance and stamina. When purchasing a Siberian ginseng product, be sure to read the label carefully to ensure the product contains *E. senticosus*. There are other ginsengs that are not the same plant (genus or species) as Siberian ginseng. If you are diabetic and taking insulin, notify your health care provider that you are taking Siberian ginseng because your insulin dosage may need to be adjusted.

Siberian ginseng should be taken for no more than two months without a break because of its stimulation of the immune system.

Herbal Caveat—Patient Interaction

Patients considering the use of an herb or formula of herbs in self-care benefit from education about the plant itself and the use of the plant in healing. This education can come through many sources, including local herbalists; plant specialists such as botanists; health practitioners such as nurses, nutritionists, naturopaths, and other physicians; and various written references including the scientific literature. Patients need to remember that their unique health care needs are not necessarily represented in any literature they may encounter. Therefore, it is recommended that a knowledgeable mentor be consulted before initiating self-care with any herb being used for the first time.

NURTURING THE NURSE-PLANT RELATIONSHIP:

Note: You may want to keep a journal of your experiences with the herb.

Nurses are hardworking people who often find that the work of caring for others is physically, mentally, and emotionally stressful. Using Siberian ginseng extract may be helpful for increasing the ability to adapt to changes in the environment and for handling the physical and emotional challenges of providing nursing care. Siberian ginseng is thought to increase resistance to illness, potentially making it beneficial for those working in health care environments loaded with infectious and often resistant organisms.

Record in a notebook or day planner your rating of the following statements. Then purchase a liquid extract of Siberian ginseng, take as directed, and rate the statements again after each week of taking the herb. Make note of any changes.

Using a scale of 0 to 10, with 10 being "definitely agree" and 0 being "no agreement," rate the following statements:

1. I feel full of energy when I wake up.
2. I have a great appetite.
3. I have lots of energy at work.
4. I feel physically strong.
5. I feel strong emotionally.
6. I sleep well.
7. I handle environmental stress with ease.
8. When I exercise I feel like I have more stamina and endurance.

CHAPTER 16

Mobility

INTRODUCTION

MOBILITY IS MORE THAN THE CONCEPT RELATED to the total body process of moving through space known as ambulation. Mobility, as a health pattern, incorporates a much broader meaning. In this chapter, the term "mobility" refers to the movement and flow that occurs either as an activity of a total being or the activity within an organ, the mind, or a bodily system such as the circulatory or respiratory system. Mobility or activity at the level of the whole body "reveals the intimate association of the vital processes of the body, as well as the structural interrelationships and coordination . . . there is a functional interrelationship between body parts" (Todd, 1937, p. 17). This can be seen when a person starts to ambulate quickly and heart rate and respiratory rate increase as a result of the increased mobility.

Traditional herbalists recognize the broad concept of mobility in caring for people. Herbs may be given to reduce stiffness, move the blood, or stimulate circulation of blood or body fluids. Traditional medicine systems, such as in China, also recognize the importance of the movement of energy in the body. Fluids in the body are thought to follow the movement of energy. Stagnation of fluids and energy in the body is considered the cause of illness. In herbalism, both mobility within the body, body fluids, and systems and the smooth and harmonious rhythm of that mobility pattern are important to health.

Movement or mobility is equated with life. "Everything moves, and in the pattern of movement, Life is objectified" (Todd, 1937, p. 3). The connection between mobility and life can be observed in the pregnant woman who finds it difficult to believe that she is carrying a child until she feels the baby *move* within her body for the first time. Life is often understood in terms of movement or mobility. Those who care for people who have lost a certain aspect of mobility, whether through loss of limb, such as in the paraplegic, or loss of system function, such as in the diabetic, can observe the significant changes and coping strategies that occur in the life of the person. The loss of mobility can lead to major lifestyle shifts and even significant emotional distress. Psychiatric nurses also observe the effects of stagnation or immobility when they care for the mentally ill. These patients' thoughts and emotions are often stuck or immobile.

Health is not a fixed state; it is a process. Mobility as a pattern of health implies a constant movement or flow that allows for adaptation to new events and environmental stimuli. When mobility is strong and flow is optimal within an organ, a system, or the whole body, life goes on. Activity occurs and is productive. When the body and its organs and systems are mobile, a person often is unaware of the body's experiences throughout the day. The body just carries out the will of the individual almost effortlessly. Consider, for example, young children when they are learning to walk. Standing takes tremendous effort at first. They hold on to a fixed object and sway and rock until they find their balance. Then when they take their first step on their own without support, they experience their world in a new way because they are now vertically mobile. Within a short period of time, if the child is healthy, walking becomes effortless, rhythmic, and unconscious. The child is able to "flow" through space. Mihaly Csikszentmihalyi, a researcher of flow, describes it as effortless movement. He writes, "In flow there is no need to reflect, because the action carries us forward as if by magic" (1990, p. 54). It is often when flow or mobility is disturbed that attention or reflection is given to its importance in health and life because a disturbance in flow or mobility manifests as illness or disease.

Underlying all disease, illness, and pain or discomfort is a change in mobility and flow. Pain, for example, can be a manifestation of the impairment or blockage of mobility or flow in the body. The herbs selected for this chapter—cayenne, rosemary, arnica, cinnamon, and wintergreen—were chosen because they have a strong connection with enhancing mobility and flow in some way. These herbs may have an effect on circulation of energy or body fluids such as blood. They may improve the flow of thoughts and memory, or they may help the whole body be more mobile, as is necessary when the body stiffens in conditions such as rheumatism and arthritis.

Comfort and mobility are interrelated health patterns. The herbs chosen for this chapter may improve comfort levels and provide pain relief or have connections with other health patterns such as energy. They are included in this chapter on mobility because in working with them as a nurse, I have found that the essence or underlying signature of their action in the body is significantly related to the pattern of influencing mobility.

Just as a person becomes unconscious of mobility when there is no problem, a practitioner's knowledge of these herbs' influence on mobility becomes remote and is even forgotten at times. Maintaining mobility is key to healthy living and should be included in any preventive health program. Nurses are in key positions within health care systems to promote mobility—active lifestyle, attention to the flow and health within internal organs, and healthy circulation of blood and energy. Adding herbs to the care plan when attending to the health pattern of mobility has the potential to enhance optimal flow and life satisfaction.

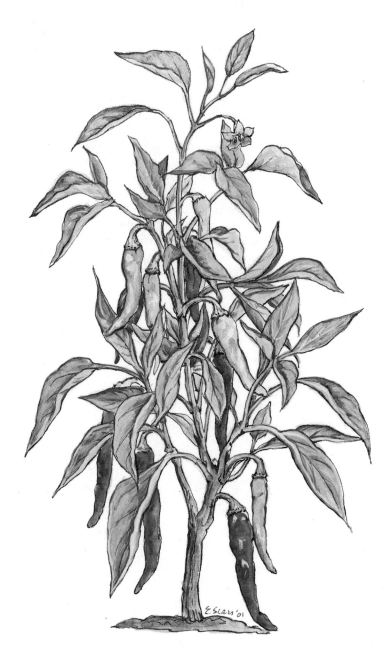

Capsicum frutescens

Cayenne

🍃 **LATIN NAMES:** *Capsicum frutescens*, *Capsicum annuum*, *Capsicum chinense*

🍃 **FAMILY:** Solanaceae

🍃 **COMMON NAMES:** Cayenne, cayenne pepper, chili pepper, red pepper, Mexican chili, Louisiana long pepper, Tabasco pepper, African capsicum, African chili, hot pepper

🍃 **HEALTH PATTERN:** Mobility

🍃 **PLANT DESCRIPTION:**

The word *cayenne* is from the Greek meaning "to bite," alluding to the pungent properties contained in the pepper and the seeds. There are several species of capsicum, all varying in their degrees of pungency. *C. annuum* includes the mild varieties known as paprika, bell pepper, and sweet pepper. A green pepper is an unripe red pepper. These mild peppers contain similar constituents to the hot varieties but with little or no pungent principles. Varieties of *C. frutescens* and *C. chinense* produce the hot, pungent, spicy types. A resin with a highly active principle called capsaicin is extracted from the hot varieties of capsicum (Leung & Foster, 1996).

The fruit, or pepper pod, of the *C. chinense* and *C. frutescens* varieties matures in the autumn. The pod takes various forms. Some are large, small, oblong, round, or pointed and are smooth and shiny. The pod may be green, yellow, or scarlet in color and contains numerous flat seeds. All varieties of capsicum have a faint, characteristic odor and an extremely hot, pungent taste. Some varieties are so intense that chewing even the smallest fragment causes an intolerable burning sensation in the mouth. Good quality powdered cayenne pepper is a bright red or yellow color. Several varieties are cultivated in the United States, especially in the areas that have a hot climate. Some of the hottest peppers are grown in Africa.

🍃 **PLANT PARTS USED:** The fruit pod, known as the pepper, leaf, and oil from the seeds

🍃 **TRADITIONAL EVIDENCE:**

Cultural Use

Asian. The Chinese use cayenne topically in ointments to treat myalgia and frostbite (Blumenthal et al., 2000).

North American Indian. Cayenne powder has been used by the Navajo as a means of weaning children from the breast (Willard, 1991). The Cherokee use cayenne as a stimulant (Willard, 1991), for colds, to reduce fevers, for colic, and for the treatment of gangrene (Moerman, 1998). Since cayenne grows easily in the southwest area of the United States, many of the indigenous Indian tribes used it in stews, soups, and as a condiment (Moerman, 1998).

Hispanic. The Maya have been said to use the cayenne leaf liniment for rheumatism. Mayan inhabitants of Mesoamerica had at least thirty-two known therapeutic plant remedies for conditions such as respiratory problems; earaches; and sores, infected wounds, and fresh burns that included cayenne as an ingredient (Cichewicz & Thorpe, 1996). Mexican Amerindians dip a cotton swab in cayenne and apply it to painful tonsils for relief. They treat earache by putting ground chili into the ear (Kay, 1996). Hispanic Americans drink a mild tea made from red chili (the Aztec name for cayenne pepper) to "warm the bones" during colder winter months. Chili caribe, a mild red chili, is used to increase circulation, and the chili powder is even put in shoes to warm the feet. Salves are made from cayenne to put on the chest to loosen mucus.

The Incas put cayenne peppers in the lakes where they caught fish so that the fish were spiced before being caught and cooked (Dasgupta & Fowler, 1997). The Tarahumara chew cayenne with other plants to treat headaches.

Pacific Islander. Cayenne preparations have historically been used in Hawaii for backache, rheumatism, and swollen feet.

African. Cayenne has been used in central Africa for its calming and analgesic properties (Duke, 1985).

East Indian. In Ayurvedic medicine, a plaster of cayenne, garlic, and liquid amber is used topically as a rubifacient and local stimulant. Mustard seeds also may be added as a counterirritant. (Blumenthal et al., 2000).

Cayenne paste is used externally as a local circulatory stimulant for the tonsils in tonsillitis and diphtheria. It is made into a lozenge with sugar and used for hoarseness. Cayenne is used in formulas with other herbs to treat gout, rheumatism, cholera, delirium tremens, and snake bite. Dried cayenne and/or tincture are used internally for flatulence, dyspepsia, and atony of the digestive organs (Nadkarni, 1976).

European. Standardized capsaicin-containing products have been approved in Germany for use in painful muscle spasms in the spine, shoulders, and arms (Leung & Foster, 1996).

Culinary Use

The earliest evidence of the use of chili peppers in the human diet is from excavations in Mexico that show that cayenne was in use as early as 7000 years ago (Blumenthal et al., 2000) and continues to be eaten today with most every meal. The pepper is eaten as a vegetable when either green or red, in the raw, dried, pickled, or cooked state.

It is used all over the world to add a pungent, spicy flavor to many foods. Varieties of chili provide a wide range of heat from the hot spicy types to the cool, sweet green of the bell pepper. Pungency is determined by a taste test and is usually expressed in Scoville (heat) units (Leung & Foster, 1996) or British thermal units (BTU).

Sweet peppers are used in pickles, salads, and meat and vegetable dishes, in curries, and in many Mexican foods. The yellow-orange color of paprika, derived from a variety of pepper pods, is used as a natural vegetable coloring agent in Morocco, Europe, and the United States. Hungarian paprika is hot and somewhat sweet like cayenne pepper. Cayenne is a source of vitamin C (Foster & Tyler, 1999), and paprika is higher in vitamin C than citrus fruits. Curry powder is made by grinding roasted dry chili with other spices such as coriander, turmeric, and cumin.

Cayenne peppers are steeped in hot vinegar that is used as a flavoring for meats and fish. Chilies are used in India as an ingredient in various curries, chutneys, and pickles (Nadkarni, 1976). A fresh condiment called mandram and made in the West Indies is used as a chutney. Made of thinly sliced cucumbers, shallots, chives, onions, lemon or lime juice, Madeira, and a few crushed pods of the cayenne pepper, it is eaten for weak digestion and loss of appetite (Grieve, 1971). Cayenne, ground and whole, is used as a spice in many food products, alcoholic and nonalcoholic beverages, frozen dairy desserts, candy, meats, baked goods, puddings, gelatin, and condiments and relishes (Leung & Foster, 1996).

Use in Herbalism

Cayenne is a warm, powerful stimulant, and is recognized as a substance that increases circulation. Cayenne has been used in folk remedies for asthma, dyspepsia, low back pain, sore throats, pneumonia, rheumatism, and skin sores. It has been used for treating cancer and tumors and is regarded as an aphrodisiac, a stimulant to the central nervous system, a digestive aide, and a tonic with the ability to induce sweating, dispel intestinal gas, and promote cessation of hemorrhage through astringent action.

In the early 1900s in the West, it was believed that cayenne was the best remedy for delerium tremens. People ate the hot peppers in soup to help relieve nausea and decrease the craving for alcohol. The hot peppers were believed to prevent vomiting, restore gastric tone, and promote the digestion of wholesome food in the chronic alcoholic (Felter & Lloyd, 1983).

Cayenne has a history of use in reducing chronic renal congestion by increasing capillary activity and reducing irritation. It is believed to affect the bladder and rectum similarly in cases of bladder spasms, diarrhea, constipation, and hemorrhoids. Capsicum has been used to treat low-grade fevers where there is dryness and constriction of the tissues with dry tongue and diminished salivary secretion. Cayenne also has been used internally for angina pectoris. Early Western physicians used it to treat the elderly who were experiencing low body heat, depressed vitality, and sluggish reactions, with tired and painful muscles (Felter & Lloyd, 1983).

Externally, cayenne was used in the early 1900s as a gargle for various kinds of sore throats. It was applied to skin ulcers, toothache, and frostbite. Cayenne powder was sprinkled into socks as a remedy for cold feet (Felter & Lloyd, 1983).

Cayenne is used as a powerful local stimulant with no narcotic effect. It is applied topically as a liniment or a poultice to cause a counterirritant effect, the reddening of the skin by increasing the local circulation. It causes dilation of the vessels, which, in turn, increases the supply of blood to the treated area of the body. Cayenne tincture and the extract of capsaicin, a plant constituent, are used in topical counterirritant preparations to treat arthritis, rheumatism, neuralgia, low back pain, and mild frostbite. Cayenne continues to be used internally to treat diarrhea, colic, cramps, and toothache. American herbalist John Christopher used cayenne in the care of patients with ulcers.

Cayenne is used as a synergist, a remedy that acts to enhance the action of others, in many herbal preparations, such as general tonics, laxatives, sedatives, and hay fever remedies (Leung & Foster, 1996). Cayenne is also used for arthritic pain in the form of various creams, ointments, liniments and other topical applications. It also has been used to treat herpes zoster outbreaks; backache, sprains, and strains; diabetic neuropathy, especially in the feet; postmastectomy pain; psoriasis; and cluster headaches (Ottariano, 1999). Cayenne also is used by the military, police forces, and private citizens as a spray for personal defense.

BIOMEDICAL EVIDENCE:

The evidence presented in the next section reports cayenne's effect in patients with illness and discomfort affecting their mobility and flow. Much of the research that has been done on cayenne in patients with mobility issues has been focused on the pain associated with immobility. Although the studies presented here may focus on pain relief, the study is included under mobility because of the underlying nature of the discomfort (e.g., the stiffening and hardening associated with arthritis or rheumatism). Preference has been given to those studies in which the investigators describe changes in mobility related to pain relief. Please take special note that many of the following studies discuss capsaicin, a constituent in cayenne, not cayenne as a whole herb.

Studies Related to Mobility

Capsaicin cream, 0.075% applied four times a day, has been shown to be significantly effective in increasing mobility and reducing pain in patients with diabetic neuropathy in an 8-week double-blind, vehicle-controlled study of 219 patients with diabetes types I and II (Capsaicin Study Group, 1992).

Capsaicin cream, 0.025% applied topically four times a day for four weeks, was found to significantly reduce trigger-point pain and increase grip strength in a study of 45 patients with fibromyalgia (McCarty, Csuka, McCarthy, & Trotter, 1994).

Topical capsaicin reduced joint pain experienced by 70 rheumatoid and osteoarthritis patients by 57% and 33%, respectively, in a double-blind, placebo-controlled trial in which the patients applied 0.025% capsaicin cream to their sore knees four times a day for four weeks (Deal et al., 1991).

A 0.075% capsaicin cream, applied four times a day, was found to significantly reduce pain by 40% in 14 patients with osteoarthritis of the hands as compared with placebo. The pain relief in the 7 patients with rheumatoid arthritis was not significant (McCarthy & McCarty, 1992).

Studies Related to Other Health Patterns

Pain Relief and Comfort. In a nonrandomized, unblinded study, 12 of 14 patients with postmastectomy pain syndrome experienced significant improvement in pain levels and sensory loss after using capsaicin cream 0.025% topically for four weeks. Fifty percent were still experiencing pain relief 6 months after initial treatment with capsaicin (Watson, Evans, & Watt, 1989).

Seventy-eight percent of patients with postherpetic neuralgia who participated in a nonrandomized trial in which they used topical capsaicin cream 0.025% four times a day for four weeks experienced improvement in symptoms (Watson, Evans, Watt, & Birkett, 1988).

Skin Care. Although cayenne applied topically can cause burning and pain, in a study at the Yale Pain Management Center, 11 patients with painful mucositis related to their cancer therapy had decreased or no mouth pain after eating capsaicin-laced taffy (Nelson, 1994).

A case study of a 30-year-old patient with apocrine chromhidrosis showed that the patient was successfully treated with capsaicin cream 1 to 2 times daily suggesting a possible relationship between substance P (see later discussion) and apocrine sweat production (Marks, 1989).

Elimination. Instillation of a capsaicin solution (1 mM) into the bladders of 16 patients with either spinal hyperreflexia, bladder instability, or hypersensibility resulted in the reduction in frequency in 14 participants and achievement of continence in 10 of those 14 with incontinence. There was a significant increase in cystometric capacity and the effects of the treatment lasted 6 to 12 months (Cruz, Guimaraes, Silva, Rio, Coimbra, & Reis, 1997). "Capsaicin should therefore be regarded as a useful medical treatment in patients with detrusor hyper-reflexia before surgical options are considered" (Dasgupta & Fowler, 1997, pp. 849, 851).

Digestion. Although many practitioners advise patients not to consume cayenne peppers when they have ulcers or dyspepsia, descriptive studies have found that the differences between 190 Chinese ulcer patients or controls with and without dyspepsia in the frequency of chili pepper use and the amount of chili used is not significant (Kang et al., 1995). Results of the study seem to support previous data that cayenne has a protective effect against gastroduodenal mucosal injury in humans (Yeoh et al., 1995).

Energy. Metabolic and carbohydrate oxidation rates were shown to increase when cayenne is added to a meal. The increase in energy expenditure only occurs right after a meal. It is thought that this activity of cayenne may be related to beta-adrenergic stimulation (Yoshioka et al., 1995). Cayenne has been shown in a small study of 12 young adults to significantly increase metabolic rate with a mean increase of 25% (Henry & Emery, 1986, p. 167).

Immunity. Cayenne has been found to have as much as four to six times as much vitamin C as oranges, and it inhibits bacteria, *Bacillus cereus* and *B. subtilis,* in vitro, which are both known to be present in food poisoning. Some species of cayenne also have been found to inhibit *Streptococcus pyogenes* and *Clostridium* species in vitro. The significant antimicrobial activity of cayenne in vitro may help explain cayenne's extensive use among a number of cultures such as the Mayan (Cichewicz & Thorpe, 1996).

Mechanism of Action

Capsaicin is a pungent constituent extracted from capsicum pods and seeds. It stimulates sweating and salivation (Duke, 1985). People develop a tolerance to the burning sensation of cayenne peppers in the mouth, but this is due to an affective shift rather than physiologic desensitization (Tominack, 1987). Capsaicin has been studied for topical use. It is known that a single application of capsaicin will produce local pain, inflammation, and hypersensitivity, but longterm and/or repeated application leads to desensitization, analgesia, and anti-inflammatory activity. Capsaicin-induced analgesia and desensitization has been explained according to neuropeptide release and depletion, but the specific mechanism of action has yet to be determined (Leung & Foster, 1996). It is believed that capsaicin works by decreasing the amount of the neurotransmitter called substance P. Substance P found in capsaicin has been shown to deplete serotonin and may play an important role in the pathogenesis of chronic pain (McCarty et al., 1994). Substance P is an undecapeptide distributed in afferent sensory fibers, and it acts as a neurotransmitter for the communication of pain and itch sensations along the peripheral nerves to the spinal column. Substance P also is a mediator of inflammation in the skin and other bodily tissues (Bernstein, 1991). Depletion of this neurotransmitter prevents the brain from perceiving peripheral pain. The initial depletion of substance P takes several days, so the ointment must be applied regularly during that time. One source suggests that when using capsaicin treatments in clinical situations, the treatment should be used for at least one week before significant effects can be expected (Bjerring & Arendt-Nielsen, 1990).

In a study of 220 participants, 30-minute applications of capsaicin cream(1 g/L in 70% alcohol) created an erythematous reaction to the skin that occurred more often proximally in the body and in younger subjects. The flare resulting from the cream reached its maximum size between the concentrations of 0.5 and 10 g/L. The initial sensation from the capsaicin application was heat (Helme & McKernan, 1985). In a small study of 10 participants, a 1% capsaicin ointment was applied to both forearms daily and found to reduce immediate inflammatory skin response, depending on the number of capsaicin applications. Capsaicin may have a stabilizing effect on mast cells (Bjerring & Arendt-Nielsen, 1990).

The traditional use of cayenne for improving circulation has been supported in a correlational study that showed that cayenne consumption enhances a fibrinolytic effect in humans, which is thought to be a possible explanation of why Thais, who eat cayenne regularly, have a very low incidence of thromboembolism (Visudhiphan, Poolsuppasit, Piboonnukarintr, & Tumliang, 1982).

USE IN PREGNANCY OR LACTATION:

In the past, some herbalists have used cayenne in controlling postpartum hemorrhage, but herbalists and midwives now believe that other herbs are more appropriate. Cayenne can slow down the hemorrhage, but it also stimulates circulation so that the uterine bleeding may return with renewed vigor after a short time. Additionally, capsicum does not act to contract the uterus, which is necessary if the bleeding is to be stopped (Weed, 1986). American herbalist Dr. John Christopher said that capsicum's hemostatic effect dissipates quickly and causes more bleeding later on. From the standpoint of traditional Chinese medicine (TCM) understanding, cayenne would not be the most likely choice for excessive postpartum bleeding. Often women who have just given birth are yin and blood deficient, both TCM symptom sign patterns that manifest as interior heat. Using a hot, blood moving herb in a patient with an interior heat condition and excessive bleeding would not be the first choice of herb in the Chinese system and would most likely be contraindicated because of its extremely hot nature.

There are no known contraindications to the oral intake of cayenne during pregnancy, although it may cause some gastrointestinal irritation. It is not known if the pungent components of cayenne are secreted into breast milk (Newall, Anderson, & Phillipson, 1996).

Herbal Caveat—Pregnancy or Lactation

Some herbs are contraindicated in pregnancy because of a risk of the herb or one of its constituents stimulating the uterus and therefore possibly promoting fetal loss. Many herbal practitioners do not recommend herbal remedies, in particular oral doses of herbs, during the first trimester of pregnancy and seek an alternative. However, herbs are successfully used during pregnancy, especially to prepare the body for the birth. Herbs are relatively unstudied in pregnancy and lactation, so patients need to be made aware through education of the potential benefits and risks of using herbs for health conditions that arise during pregnancy or lactation. The use of herbal remedies during pregnancy often warrants a referral to a knowledgeable herbal practitioner.

USE FOR CHILDREN:

Because of the extreme thermal (hot) nature of cayenne, the herb is not often recommended for therapeutic use in children. Children can learn about the flavor and health benefits of cayenne by including it in their food in small to moderate amounts. Health practitioners have reported that cayenne peppers have been used inappropriately for punishment and physical abuse in children (Tominack, 1987). Cayenne has also been used topically as a deterrent to nail biting in children; however, this is not recommended because children may get the preparation in their eyes or other sensitive mucous membranes, which can cause considerable pain.

Herbal Caveat—Children

Children have special needs in regard to herbal therapies. They require lesser amounts of herbs and often respond well to mild teas and topical applications such as compresses and baths. The lowest dose of oral preparations should be tried first before increasing the amount given children. Caregivers should observe children closely for responses to herbal remedies. Younger children, particularly infants, have traditionally been given herbs either through their mother's breast milk or in the form of a homeopathic remedy because of their sensitivity to medicines and treatments and the immaturity of their liver. It is recommended that a person knowledgeable in the herbal treatment of children be consulted before the offering of any herb to a child for the first time.

CAUTIONS:

Cayenne is a very hot herb! If using this herb orally, it is best not to take it in capsules. Tasting an herb can help a person regulate the amount of herb they take; the sensory mechanism of taste provides helpful feedback in making the decision about how much herb is appropriate for the individual. Excessive doses of cayenne have been reported to cause severe irritation of mucous membranes, nausea, vomiting, and diarrhea and can cause a strong burning sensation.

Cayenne applied externally has been known to produce dermatitis. Its use is contraindicated on injured skin or near the eyes. In places like India, where there is a high incidence of cayenne intake, submucous fibrosis of the palate has been observed. Although some authors have reported that red peppers are carcinogenic, the low incidence of gastric cancer in Latin America suggests that cayenne may actually help prevent cancer (Duke, 1985).

The German Commission E recommends that cayenne not be used externally for more than two days, with a fourteen-day time period between applications. It has been suggested that continued external use on the same area may cause damage to nerves in the skin. However, other experts state that capsaicin-containing preparations must be used daily for up to several weeks in order to be effective (McGuffin, Hobbs, Upton & Goldberg, 1997). It is highly recommended that capsaicin creams and ointments be applied with disposable gloves and that eye and facial contact be avoided. Capsaicin is practically insoluble in cold water and only slightly soluble in hot water, so it is difficult to completely wash it off the skin. Traces that may remain on the hands or other areas can easily be transferred to sensitive mucous membranes up to several hours after contact. Capsaicin may be removed from the affected part by bathing in vinegar (Foster & Tyler, 1999).

Oral ingestion of cayenne may cause gastrointestinal irritation; however, researchers have stated that it does not influence the healing of ulcers and does not have to be avoided by those with this condition. Ingestion of cayenne may interfere with monoamine oxidase inhibitors and antihypertensive drugs and may increase the hepatic metabolism of drugs (Newall et al., 1996). "Acute use of cayenne increases the hexobarbital hypnotic effects and plasma concentration, but chronic use actually decreases its effects and concentration" (Brinker, 1998).

NURSING EVIDENCE:

Historical Nursing Use

Nurses have a long history of the use of cayenne as a counterirritant (Harmer & Henderson, 1955). Cayenne also has been used in spice plasters and poultices. The spice plaster is made with a teaspoon each of cayenne, ginger, cinnamon, and clove mixed with one-half ounce of flour and enough brandy to make a paste. The poultice is made by sewing the spices into a cloth bag and dipping the bag into brandy or whiskey before applying the bag to the body part to be treated (Weeks-Shaw, 1914).

Potential Nursing Applications

Nurses might consider recommending the addition of an occasional serving of cayenne pepper to the adult diet. Cayenne makes an excellent condiment and has numerous health benefits. Capsaicin creams have been included in numerous clinical trials. Nurses may want to consider researching the use of capsaicin cream or cayenne compresses for pain relief and increasing mobility in patients with arthritis, rheumatism, or fibromyalgia.

Integrative Insight

Because of the extreme thermal (hot) nature of cayenne, special care must be taken in using it therapeutically and recommending it for use in patient self-care. With education and experience, cayenne can be a very helpful herb to use in topical and internal applications when there is blood and/or *qi* stagnation, especially of a "cold" nature. There are systems of assessment, such as in Chinese medicine, that help determine the thermal nature of a condition, especially as it may manifest in the joints and muscles of the body. If these assessment systems are unknown, one can also try an external application such as a poultice and, through observation of an initial trial, determine if the patient benefits from the heat and counterirritant action to a particular body part. Nurses are generally familiar with recommending hot and cold applications for structural injury. There are times during the healing process when heat or cold feels better to the patient. In general, cold is applied immediately after an injury to decrease inflammation, and heat is applied later to relax the muscles that have been protecting the injury. The heat in topical herb applications is not only used to stimulate joints and muscles but also is used to stimulate internal organs such as the lungs where thick stringy mucus may be lodged. Using a basic understanding of when applying heat might be helpful is foundational to the use of cayenne.

From a traditional Chinese medicine (TCM) viewpoint, the use of cayenne internally needs even more consideration because of its extremely hot nature. Cayenne would most likely be contraindicated in patients such as the elderly, who often have yin deficiency (interior heat) conditions. Although taking cayenne internally has many beneficial joint-pain relieving and gastrointestinal-protecting phytochemical activities that may be helpful for elderly patients, it also may aggravate other symptoms related to heat in the interior of the body, which can cause a dissipation of fluid, potentially leading to such symptoms as stiffness and stagnation.

Therapy must always be individualized with traditional, biomedical, and nursing evidence brought into the decision-making process. Because of the extreme thermal nature of this herb, a clinical Western or Chinese herbalist may need to be consulted, especially when considering using the herb for long-term use.

THERAPEUTIC APPLICATIONS:

Oral

> **Cayenne or Capsicum Powder.** 30 to 120 mg
>
> **Tincture of Capsicum.** 0.3 to 1 ml (Wren, 1988); frequency was not given.

Topical

It is recommended that to get the full benefit of creams containing cayenne or capsaicin, they should be applied at least four to five times daily until relief is obtained. This process could take three to four weeks to achieve maximum pain relief. After relief is noticed, capsaicin can be applied less often (Ottariano, 1999). It is recommended that the capsaicin preparation be applied with disposable gloves and that eye and facial contact be avoided because a burning sensation may occur.

> **Liniment.** Use a hot oil or alcohol preparation that contains dried cayenne powder. Apply topically by friction.
>
> **Ointment or Salve.** Use a semiliquid preparation containing 0.02% to 0.05% capsaicinoids in an emulsion base. Apply to the affected area. It is available as an over-the-counter preparation in the pharmacy.
>
> **Plaster.** Use a semisolid paste or plaster containing 10 to 40 g capsaicinoids per cm^2. Apply locally.
>
> **Tincture.** (1:10 g/ml), 90% ethanol, applied locally (Blumenthal et al., 2000)

Environmental

Chile peppers are traditionally dried by hanging them in the kitchen either on a string or as a wreath. They are very ornamental and serve as a good reminder to consider using cayenne in cooking or for healing.

Herbal Caveat—Therapeutic Applications

In traditional and conventional herbal medicine, amounts of herbs given to patients are based on individual needs. The amounts or "doses" recorded here are provided so that the health practitioner has a general idea of the amounts recommended for an adult patient. Dosing in herbalism not only refers to amount of plant used but also includes when, where, and how to take a plant medicine. These dosages should not be used as guidelines for indiscriminate intervention without proper assessment, critical thinking, and patient education on the part of the practitioner.

Note: Please see chapter 5 for detailed descriptions of how to prepare various applications.

PATIENT INTERACTION:

This herb is hot and whether used in cooking or therapeutically needs the same care as if handling a pot of boiling water. Cayenne peppers used internally can help digestion and metabolism of food and have traditionally been used for their effect on circulation and flow in the body. Cayenne also has been used topically as a counterirritant or as a stimulant of blood flow to a body part or internal organ. Capsaicin (a constituent in cayenne pepper) cream can be used externally for pain, but when applied to the skin, it should not be used on or near any open sores. The cream is best applied with plastic gloves because the cream does not come off the hands easily with water. Vinegar can be used to remove cream that gets on the skin. When applied, capsaicin cream may cause a burning or tingling sensation at first. This is the normal action of the plant therapy. It is not normal for the skin to blister or cause excruciating pain during a topical application of cayenne. Studies have shown that significant pain relief may not occur for two to four weeks.

Herbal Caveat—Patient Interaction
Patients considering the use of an herb or formula of herbs in self-care benefit from education about the plant itself and the use of the plant in healing. This education can come through many sources, including local herbalists; plant specialists such as botanists; health practitioners such as nurses, nutritionists, naturopaths, and other physicians; and various written references including the scientific literature. Patients need to remember that their unique health care needs are not necessarily represented in any literature they may encounter. Therefore, it is recommended that a knowledgeable mentor be consulted before initiating self-care with any herb being used for the first time.

NURTURING THE NURSE-PLANT RELATIONSHIP:

Note: You may want to keep a journal of your experiences with the herb.

There are two ways to really experience the healing properties and personality of cayenne. One is by tasting it in spicy Indian, Thai, Mexican, African, or Chinese food. Cayenne can clear the sinuses and bring beads of perspiration to anyone's forehead! The second way is to try a topical application such as a cayenne compress or capsaicin cream to a sore joint. Cayenne can provide an opportunity to learn about counterirritant effects on the skin. Applying cayenne to the skin can truly be a warm and memorable experience.

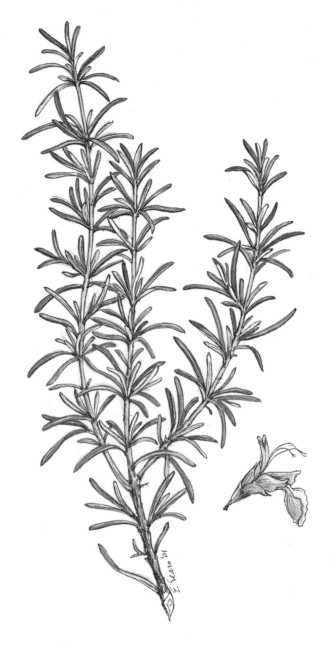

Rosmarinus officinalis

Rosemary

@ **LATIN NAME:** *Rosmarinus officinalis*

@ **FAMILY:** Lamiaceae

@ **COMMON NAMES:** Rosemary, garden rosemary, polar plant, compass-weed, compass plant, incensier (Old French according to Grieve, 1971)

@ **HEALTH PATTERN:** Mobility

@ **PLANT DESCRIPTION:**

The name rosemary is derived from the Latin meaning "dew of the sea." Rosemary is a many branched, bushy evergreen perennial shrub native to the Mediterranean area and Portugal. It is now cultivated in the United States, France, Spain, Morocco, South Africa, China, Australia, and the United Kingdom. Its branches grow 1.5 to 3 feet (0.6 to 1.3 meters) tall and bear aromatic, linear leaves that are dark green above and white below. The leaves are about 1 inch (2.5 cm) long with smooth edges. Miniature pale blue orchidlike flowers appear from April to May. The plant has a highly aromatic odor similar to camphor that is wakening rather than dulling (Husemann & Wolff, 1982). Rosemary has a bitter taste.

Rosemary is frequently cultivated in kitchen gardens and as a houseplant. There is an old English belief that rosemary will only truly thrive in the home where the mistress is really the master of the house! In early England, some women considered their husbands to be so touchy about this point that they suspected the men of injuring healthy rosemary plants that grew about the home (Grieve, 1971).

@ **PLANT PARTS USED:** Leaf, twig, and root

@ **TRADITIONAL EVIDENCE:**

Cultural Use

Asian. In China, rosemary leaves and branches have been used for hundreds of years for the treatment of headaches. Baldness was treated by mixing an infusion of rosemary herb with borax and applying it topically to the scalp (Leung & Foster, 1996). The essential oil of rosemary is bitter and pungent with a warm, drying property. Its secondary quality is stimulating, restoring, astringent, and dissolving. It is believed to have stimulant actions on the heart and arterial, liver, and adrenal systems. In Chinese medicine, rosemary oil is used for its action of stimulating the neuroendocrine pathways, causing a release of noradrenaline. This results in a general stimulating and restorative effect, which is useful for fatigue, depression, low motivation, and decreased endurance as a result of Yang deficiency. It enters the lung, spleen, heart, and liver (Holmes, 1998/1999).

Hispanic. The Spanish revere rosemary as one of the bushes that gave shelter to the Virgin Mary in the flight into Egypt. They call it *Romero,* the Pilgrim's Flower. In Spain it has been considered a protector from evil influences. It was believed that young fairies who took the shape of snakes would lie among the branches (Grieve, 1971). Hispanics use this herb as a tea for improving circulation and in bathing for sore muscles. Midwives place the steeped leaves of rosemary on the umbilical stump of newborns to keep it from getting infected. Menopausal women also drink the tea to help relieve feeling depressed. Rosemary also is used for numerous conditions including epilepsy, paralysis, blindness, cataracts, vaginitis, promoting menstruation, liver and digestive complaints (Kay, 1996).

European. Rosemary has been used in Europe since ancient times as a general tonic, a stimulant, and a carminative for dyspepsia. In French hospitals, it was the custom to burn rosemary sprigs with Juniper berries in sick rooms to purify the air and prevent the spread of infections (Grieve, 1971). Rosemary was used in old England as a tonic, astringent, diaphoretic, and stimulant. Oil of rosemary was used to treat headaches, calm nervousness, and decrease intestinal gas. It was used frequently as an external preparation in hair lotions because it was believed that rosemary stimulated the hair follicles to become active and thus prevent baldness (Grieve, 1971).

Small quantities of rosemary wine were taken to quiet a weak heart that was subject to palpitations. It also was used to decrease edema of the lower extremities through its action on the kidneys. Because of its stimulant action on the brain and nervous system, it was used as an effective remedy for headaches and poor circulation (Grieve, 1971). A warm tea made of young rosemary tops, leaves, and flowers was used as a remedy for relieving headaches, colic, colds, and nervous conditions, including depression. A jam made by mixing the freshly gathered tops with three times their weight in sugar was said to have the same effect (Grieve, 1971).

German health care practitioners use rosemary internally for indigestion and as a support for rheumatic conditions. Externally it is used for the treatment of circulatory disturbances (Foster & Tyler, 1999). It is licensed in Germany as a standard medicinal tea for internal and external use. Rosemary is used internally as a carminative for gastrointestinal problems. The oil is used externally on areas to increase circulation and is also added to liniments as a fragrant stimulant. It is used externally as an aqueous infusion and essential oil in baths, liniments, ointments, and other topical applications for rheumatic diseases and circulatory problems (Blumenthal et al., 2000). Rosemary and coltsfoot leaves are rubbed together in the palms to mix them and then smoked for asthma and other afflictions of the throat and lungs (Grieve, 1971). In many parts of Wales, it is still a custom to cast rosemary sprigs onto the coffin after it has been lowered into the grave, presumably to strengthen one's remembrance of the departed (Grieve, 1971).

Rosemary is used whenever intense warmth is needed in a person's metabolism and circulation, digestion, menstruation, or the circulatory processes in the limbs. Injectable rosemary is the approach used to address symptoms related to diabetes. Rosemary is thought to act as a stimulant for increased consciousness of internal organs, especially the pancreas. Injectable rosemary is also given for certain symptom patterns of psychosis. It is used as aroma therapy with the pure etheric oil and adjunctively during massage, embrocation, or bath therapy. Rosemary also is compounded and given as potentized oral drops and pilules.

Culinary Use

Rosemary is extensively used as a cooking herb to flavor a variety of meats, baked goods, vegetables, and other foods. Rosemary oil is used in small amounts to flavor alcoholic beverages, frozen desserts, candy, puddings, and other similar products. Extracts of rosemary oil have been found to have antioxidant (food preserving) properties similar to butylated hydroxyanisole (BHA) and butylated hydroxytoluene (BHT), two preservatives commonly used in the food industry. However, the large amounts of the oil that would be necessary to preserve foods are not safe when taken internally because of causing irritation of the stomach, intestines, and kidneys. The highest maximum use level considered safe for use in food is about 0.41% (4098 ppm) (Leung & Foster, 1996).

Use in Herbalism

People in ancient times were well acquainted with rosemary, believing that it had the power to strengthen the memory (Grieve, 1971). Shakespeare even wrote about it in *Hamlet* when Ophelia says, "There's rosemary, that's for remembrance" (Lawless, 1998). Because of its reputation for promoting memory, rosemary became a symbol of fidelity for lovers. It is used at weddings entwined in the bride's wreath. A branch of rosemary tied with beautiful ribbons is given to the wedding guests as a symbol of love and loyalty. It also is used at funerals, festivals, as incense during religious ceremonies, and in magical spells (Grieve, 1971).

Rosemary has been used as a stimulant, antispasmodic, and emmenagogue (Felter & Lloyd, 1983) and as a mouth rinse for gum disease and bad breath. It was used in the late 1800s to help strengthen eyesight (Culpeper, 1990).

In aromatherapy, rosemary essential oil is used for osteoarthritis and rheumatoid arthritis (Buckle, 1997) and as a tonic for the nerves, heart, and circulation. It is an effective nerve stimulant, helpful for memory loss, lethargy and general dullness, and improving alertness.

The scent is refreshing and invigorating, has an uplifting effect on the spirit, seems to dispel confusion, and promotes mental clarity. Rosemary oil is used for fainting, migraine and other headaches, and to decrease dizziness (Lawless, 1998). Rosemary oil is used to help decrease elevated cholesterol; decrease rheumatism and muscular pain; and relieve lung congestion, sore throat, and canker sores (Keville & Green, 1995).

Cosmetic Use. Rosemary oil is used extensively in the cosmetics industry as a fragrance or as a masking agent. It is used in soaps, perfumes, detergents, creams, lotions, colognes, and toilet waters.

BIOMEDICAL EVIDENCE:

A thorough search of the literature revealed no published human studies supporting the traditional use of rosemary for health concerns related to mobility. However, animal and in vitro studies have been conducted.

Studies Related to Mobility

The oral ingestion and inhalation of rosemary oil significantly stimulates motor activity in mice. It is not known if a single constituent is responsible for the increase in motor activity in animals or if the activity is due to a synergistic action among plant constituents within rosemary oil (Kovar, Gropper, Friess, & Ammon, 1987).

Studies Related to Other Health Patterns

Restoration. Animal and in vitro studies support that rosmanol, a constituent in rosemary, has antioxidant properties (Inatani, Nakatani, & Fuwa, 1983). In one study, those animals injected intraperitoneally for five days with 200 mg/kg rosemary extract and carnosol had a significant decrease in mammary tumor growth as compared with controls, thereby demonstrating the possible use of rosemary as a breast cancer chemopreventive agent (Singletary, MacDonald, & Wallig, 1996).

A methanol extract of rosemary applied topically to laboratory-induced skin tumors and ear inflammation in mice significantly inhibited the growth of the skin tumors and inflammation. For example, in mice given 1.2 or 3.6 mg of rosemary extract 5 minutes before being given a tumor-promoting compound, the number of tumors that developed in the mice decreased by 54% or 64%, respectively (Huang et al., 1994).

Mechanism of Action

The German Commission E reports that in humans, rosemary is an irritant to the skin. However, it acts to increase local blood supply when used externally. It has been shown to exert an antispasmodic action on gall passages and on the small intestines and to increase blood flow through the coronary artery (Blumenthal et al., 2000). Rosemary oil stimulates the adrenal glands, the motor nerves, and the gallbladder (Keville & Green, 1995).

Rosemary is a source of natural antioxidants (Leung & Foster, 1996). The antioxidant found in rosemary, rosmanol, has a demonstrated antioxidant activity four times higher than BHA and BHT (Inatani et al., 1983). Antioxidants from rosemary are nonvolatile and more stable at high temperatures as compared with the synthetic antioxidants BHT and BHA (Huang et al., 1994). Ninety percent of the antioxidant activity in rosemary is attributed to carnosol and carnosic acid (Aruoma, Halliwell, Aeschback, & Loligers, 1992).

Rosemary's antioxidants and other compounds may work to prevent oxidation and the breakdown of acetylcholine in the brain, leading to a potential prevention and/or suppression of the symptoms of Alzheimer's disease (Duke, 1997).

Rosemary's flavonoid constituent, diosmin, is more effective in decreasing capillary fragility and permeability than rutin and is much less toxic (Leung & Foster, 1996). One plant constituent, camphor, is a known stimulant for the central nervous system, respiratory system, and circulation (study by Eichholz as reported in Kovar et al., 1987). Camphor and cineole (another plant constituent in rosemary) are epileptogenic compounds (Steinmetz as reported in Burkhard, Burkhardt, Haenggeli, & Landis, 1999). One of the rosmaricine derivatives has been proven to cause smooth muscle stimulant effects in vitro as well as some pain-relieving activity (Leung & Foster, 1996). In vitro data from one study of the effect of rosemary essential oil on rabbit vascular smooth muscle cells suggests that the oil of rosemary leaf interferes with both calcium ion influx and intracellular calcium ion release of vascular smooth muscle cells and has a direct relaxant effect (Aqel, 1992). "Rosmarinic acid has been suggested as a possible potential treatment for septic shock, since it suppresses the endotoxin-induced activation of complement, the formation of prostacyclin, both hypotensive phases, thrombocytopaenia and the concomitant release of thromboxane Az" (D. Tattje, as reported in Wren, 1988).

Another constituent of rosemary, thujone, is abortifacient (Duke, 1985) but is present in proportionally low amounts. Doses of rosemary extract traditionally used by women as an abortifacient have been shown in animal studies to interfere with embryo implantation but do not interfere with normal development after the implantation phase, even when the extract was given during the organogenic period (Lemonica, Damasceno, & Di-Stasi, 1996).

USE IN PREGNANCY OR LACTATION:

There are no known restrictions for the use of rosemary during lactation (Blumenthal et al., 2000), but it is not recommended during pregnancy (McGuffin et al., 1997). Large doses of rosemary have been used as an abortifacient. It is a uterine stimulant and so has been used for delayed menses. Rosemary tea has been used for fertility control and as an emmenagogue (deLaszlo & Henshaw, 1954). Pregnant women should avoid therapeutic doses of rosemary.

Susan Weed (1986) recommends rosemary with licorice root, raspberry leaf, and skullcap taken as a tea for postpartum depression, to help increase the flow of milk during lactation, add calcium to the diet, and tone the liver.

Herbal sitz baths can help speed the healing of the perineum after childbirth, helping to prevent infection and promote pain relief. Potential herbs that are used for this purpose include rosemary, goldenseal, oak bark, witch hazel, and myrrh. If a woman has perineal stitches the herbal sitz baths are limited to one per day (Weed, 1986).

Herbal Caveat—Pregnancy or Lactation

Some herbs are contraindicated in pregnancy because of a risk of the herb or one of its constituents stimulating the uterus and therefore possibly promoting fetal loss. Many herbal practitioners do not recommend herbal remedies, in particular oral doses of herbs, during the first trimester of pregnancy and seek an alternative. However, herbs are successfully used during pregnancy, especially to prepare the body for the birth. Herbs are relatively unstudied in pregnancy and lactation, so patients need to be made aware through education of the potential benefits and risks of using herbs for health conditions that arise during pregnancy or lactation. The use of herbal remedies during pregnancy often warrants a referral to a knowledgeable herbal practitioner.

USE FOR CHILDREN:

Diluted rosemary tincture or powdered rosemary can be applied directly to an infant's umbilical stump to promote healing and prevent infection. It can be used at every diaper change to help the stump dry and kill bacteria that may be present (Weed, 1986).

Herbal Caveat—Children

Children have special needs in regard to herbal therapies. They require lesser amounts of herbs and often respond well to mild teas and topical applications such as compresses and baths. The lowest dose of oral preparations should be tried first before increasing the amount given children. Caregivers should observe children closely for responses to herbal remedies. Younger children, particularly infants, have traditionally been given herbs either through their mother's breast milk or in the form of a homeopathic remedy because of their sensitivity to medicines and treatments and the immaturity of their liver. It is recommended that a person knowledgeable in the herbal treatment of children be consulted before the offering of any herb to a child for the first time.

CAUTIONS:

The use of rosemary essential oil can cause overstimulation of the body and may increase blood pressure (Keville & Green, 1995) and therefore is contraindicated in patients with hypertension (Buckle, 1997). Because in vitro data suggest that the oil of rosemary leaf interferes with both calcium ion influx and intracellular calcium ion release of vascular smooth muscle cells (Aqel, 1992), cardiac patients may be affected by the use of rosemary oil.

Because of its uterine stimulant effects that promote menstruation, rosemary should not be used by women who are experiencing excessive uterine bleeding (McGuffin et al., 1997). Also, bath preparations that contain rosemary oil have been known to cause erythema. Cosmetics and toiletries that contain the oil can cause dermatitis in individuals who are hypersensitive (Duke, 1985). There has been at least one report of diagnosed allergic contact dermatitis in a 56-year-old man who used rosemary leaf topically as a plaster for knee pain (Fernandez et al., 1997).

Rosemary oil should not be used internally by those who have epilepsy (Holmes, 1998/1999). Although the cases of seizures related to the use of essential oils reported in the literature occurred with sage, eucalyptus, pine, and thyme, rosemary does contain cineole and camphor, which are known to be epileptogenic compounds (Burkhard et al., 1999).

Rosemary oil (verbenone type) has some neurotoxicity because of the presence of the ketone verbenone. For this reason, it is contraindicated in pregnancy and nursing, in infants and children, and in those with liver problems. Rosemary verbenone is not used in patients with estrogen-dependent cancer (Holmes, 1998/1999).

NURSING EVIDENCE:

Historical Nursing Use

No data are available at this time.

Potential Nursing Applications

Nurses may want to consider the long history of traditional use of rosemary herb and essential oil for comforting patients by increasing circulation and warmth, relieving joint pain, and stimulating the mind. Elderly patients often experience a warm rosemary footbath as the best remedy for helping ease the discomfort related to the generalized aches and pain and cold extremities they experience, especially when they are in an unfamiliar place such as a hospital or nursing home. The essential oil of rosemary can be very helpful when used appropriately for massage and or aromatherapy. Nurses in the United Kingdom, Germany, and Switzerland use rosemary essential oil with patients who complain of headache, stress, pain, and burns (Buckle, 1997). Nurses may want to consider studying the effects of rosemary on patients whose memories are impaired, such as those with Alzheimer's disease or dementia, as long as the patient's blood pressure is within normal limits.

Nurses are experts in balneology, the science of bathing. Perhaps the next step for some practitioners and patients is to extend the science and add plants such as rosemary to the bath water when appropriate. Nurses working with the elderly might consider providing rosemary shampoos and baths to their patients. According to Duke (1997), rosemary shampoos, baths, and tea may have an effect "similar to tacrine or huperzine" in the patient with Alzheimer's disease because several of the plant constituents known to retard the breakdown of acetylcholine are readily absorbed through the skin and "some probably cross the blood-brain barrier" (p. 38).

Integrative Insight

Rosemary and its constituents have many potential uses in nursing practice, especially as topical applications. When deep, penetrating warmth is needed, think of rosemary. If a patient's digestive "fire" is low consider suggesting the use of rosemary in food. If the patient is always feeling cold and stiff, consider rosemary baths. Rosemary essential oil or prepared bath oil may be more convenient for patients, but taking the time to prepare a bath infusion of fresh or dry rosemary leaf can add to the healing experience. As previously noted, healing components in rosemary, such as those that retard acetylcholine breakdown, can be absorbed through the skin and scalp. Working with a plant such as rosemary by growing it, harvesting it, and preparing it for use in cooking or as a therapeutic application puts both the caregiver and the patient in position to receive the benefits of the plant. Rosemary is for remembrance. Using rosemary can *remind* nurses that they too receive the benefit of the healing plant remedies they prepare for others.

THERAPEUTIC APPLICATIONS:

Oral

Infusion. 2 g in 5 ounces (150 ml) water three times daily (Blumenthal et al., 2000)

Tincture. 2 tsp (10 ml) three times daily (Blumenthal et al., 2000)

Fluid Extract. $\frac{1}{2}$ teaspoon (2 ml) three times daily (Blumenthal et al., 2000)

Essential Oil. Not more than 2 drops orally per dose (Blumenthal et al., 2000)

Topical

Fomentation. Saturate a cloth with hot rosemary decoction with or without the addition of the essential oil. Fold the cloth and apply to the affected area (Blumenthal et al., 2000).

Ointment. Apply to the affected area the semisolid preparation of rosemary essential oil, 6% to 10% essential oil, in a base of lanolin or petroleum jelly. This may be spread on a clean cotton or linen cloth for local application (Blumenthal et al., 2000). Rosemary is used on sluggish, underactive skin, and on dry, mature skin. It is used for cellulite and skin parasites (Keville & Green, 1995).

Massage. Mix 6 drops of the oil into 1 tablespoon almond oil and massage clockwise into the solar plexus, chest, or temples. This treatment has been used for general exhaustion, headaches, palpitations, and other stress-related symptoms (Lawless, 1998).

Environmental

Bath. Decoct about 2 oz (50 g) of leaf in 1 quart (1 L) of water, then let stand covered for 15 to 30 minutes (Blumenthal et al., 2000). Strain and add to the bath water. The bath may be very stimulating, especially in cases of low blood pressure, and is best done early in the day so as to not interfere with sleep. Add 8 to 10 drops of essential oil to bath water after the tub is filled, as a restorative for lethargy and hangovers (Lawless, 1998).

Put a few drops of the essential oil into a handkerchief or in an oil burner and inhale to improve memory and relieve headaches, migraine, dizziness, and mental and physical fatigue. Putting a cotton ball with a few drops of rosemary oil in the car may help improve alertness while driving. This also can be helpful for respiratory complaints. Rosemary essential oil can be used in a diffuser or vaporizer to scent the air during meditation to promote clarity of mind. "It purifies the environment on a physical and psychic level" (Lawless, 1998, p. 205). A few sprigs of rosemary or a few drops of the essential oil can be put into drawers or linen closets to keep moths or other insects away.

Herbal Caveat—Therapeutic Applications

In traditional and conventional herbal medicine, amounts of herbs given to patients are based on individual needs. The amounts or "doses" recorded here are provided so that the health practitioner has a general idea of the amounts recommended for an adult patient. Dosing in herbalism not only refers to amount of plant used but also includes when, where, and how to take a plant medicine. These dosages should not be used as guidelines for indiscriminate intervention without proper assessment, critical thinking, and patient education on the part of the practitioner.

Note: Please see chapter 5 for detailed descriptions of how to prepare various applications.

PATIENT INTERACTION:

When you think of rosemary think "warmth." Rosemary leaf used internally and externally can improve the circulation in the extremities and deeply warm the interior of the body as well. Plant constituents in rosemary improve memory and also may prevent the breakdown of acetylcholine, a process that is thought to be related to the development of Alzheimer's disease. The health benefits of rosemary can be absorbed through the skin when taking a bath or using a rosemary shampoo. Rosemary baths can be stimulating to the mind and warming to the body and are best taken in the morning. Do not use rosemary oil if you are experiencing hypertension, epilepsy, or have liver problems without consulting a knowledgeable practitioner first. Rosemary may be irritating to the skin of some individuals.

Herbal Caveat—Patient Interaction

Patients considering the use of an herb or formula of herbs in self-care benefit from education about the plant itself and the use of the plant in healing. This education can come through many sources, including local herbalists; plant specialists such as botanists; health practitioners such as nurses, nutritionists, naturopaths, and other physicians; and various written references including the scientific literature. Patients need to remember that their unique health care needs are not necessarily represented in any literature they may encounter. Therefore, it is recommended that a knowledgeable mentor be consulted before initiating self-care with any herb being used for the first time.

NURTURING THE NURSE-PLANT RELATIONSHIP:

Note: You may want to keep a journal of your experiences with the herb.

If you have a time when you're feeling a bit tired and sluggish before going to work try taking a warm rosemary bath and breathing in the stimulating vapors. Don't make the water too hot or you may have to go back to bed after the bath. Use a loofah sponge or a natural bristle brush to scrub your skin during the bath. Always scrub towards the heart for increasing circulation and alertness. Don't forget to massage your scalp!

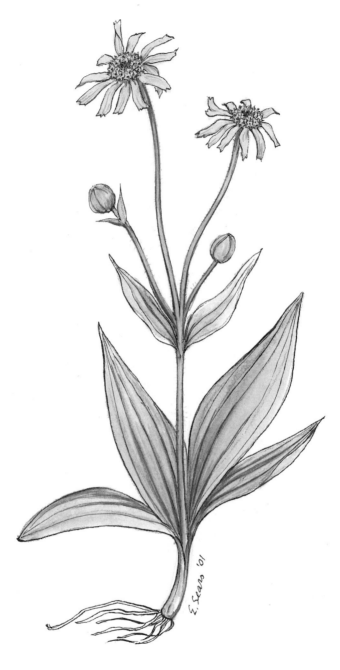

Arnica montana

Arnica

🍃 **LATIN NAME:** *Arnica montana*

🍃 **FAMILY:** Asteraceae

🍃 **COMMON NAMES:** Arnica, European arnica, mountain tobacco, leopard's bane, wolf's bane, mountain daisy, mountain snuff

Note: The focus of this herb guide is the use of herbs, not homeopathic medicines. Homeopathic forms of arnica are often used by patients accessing the health care system for the treatment of injuries and having surgeries; therefore, homeopathic arnica is included in this profile. Unless the word "homeopathic" is used, the form of arnica being referred to is the herbal form. Please refer to chapter 5 for more information about the science of homeopathy.

🍃 **HEALTH PATTERN:** Mobility

🍃 **PLANT DESCRIPTION:**

The name *arnica* is the ancient Greek name for the plant and is derived from *arnakis* meaning "lamb's skin." The name is used because the ovate leaves, which form a flat rosette on the ground, are very soft. From the leaves rise one or more central stalks about 1 to 2 feet (about ½ meter). The tip of each stalk bears a single yellow to orange flower from June to August. The flowers are collected whole and dried before use. The entire plant is rather hairy with a rough-textured or fuzzy feel to the leaves and stalk. The plant has an unpleasant odor. The leaves have smooth edges and are opposite each other on the stem. The rhizome found beneath the soil is brown and rough with a thick bark; internally it is whitish and spongy. Grieve (1971) recommends harvesting the rhizome in autumn after the leaves have turned brown. Felter and Lloyd (1983) harvest the rhizomes in the spring.

🍃 **PLANT PARTS USED:** Dried whole plant, flower, and rhizome.

🍃 **TRADITIONAL EVIDENCE:**

Cultural Use

North American Indian. North American Indians, in particular the Catawba tribe, use *Arnica acaulis* or leopard's bane as an infusion for back pain. The Okanagan tribe has used a poultice of mashed *Arnica cordifolia* for swelling related to rheumatism and as a love medicine. As a love potion, powdered plant is applied to the face while the person is in the water facing east and reciting certain words along with the name of the beloved (Moerman, 1998; Vogel, 1970).

Hispanic. The commonly used plant known as *arnica* in the Hispanic culture and used for rheumatism, poor circulation, and ulcers is false arnica, or *Heterotheca grandiflora*, and should not be confused with *A. montana* (Kay, 1996).

Russian/Baltic. The Russians have been cultivating arnica on a large scale since 1955. In Russian folk medicine, arnica boiled in water is recommended for poor digestion and stomach problems such as ulcers, spasms, and intestinal cramps. It also was used for epilepsy, colds, influenza, and bladder problems. External uses included the application of arnica lotions or a cold wash to promote the fast healing of minor wounds, bruises, scrapes, minor burns, and frostbite. It also was used to treat furuncles, carbuncles, abscesses, and cutaneous ulcers. Russians also have used the herb to treat inflammations of the genitals and to strengthen a weak heart (Duke, 1985).

A tea made of arnica is a common remedy for many health concerns. Small doses are used to tone the central nervous system, and larger doses are used to act as a sedative and to reduce stomach cramps. It is used as a vasodilator and to reduce serum cholesterol. Russian herbalists use arnica to reduce cardiac inflammation, increase bile flow, and control uterine hemorrhage during childbirth. Internal use is only recommended under the guidance of a knowledgeable practitioner (Zevin, 1997).

European. Arnica has a long history of use in Europe for bodily injuries that result in limitations to mobility. St. Hildegarde of Bingen is said to have used arnica during the twelfth century. German armed forces used arnica to treat shock during World War II (McIvor, 1973). Germany markets more than 100 drug preparations containing arnica extract (Duke, 1985).

Culinary Use

Arnica is rarely used internally because of toxicity concerns. In the United States, the Food and Drug Administration (FDA) lists arnica as an unsafe herb, and it is only approved for food use in small amounts in alcoholic beverages and homeopathic dilutions (Newall et al., 1996).

Use in Herbalism

Topical arnica applications in the form of oil, ointment, jelly, and tincture are quite common and currently are recognized by the German Commission E as antiphlogistic or anti-inflammatory for use in hematoma, sprains, bruises, contusions, rheumatic pain of muscles and joints, and for edema related to fracture (Blumenthal et al., 2000; Schulz, Hansel, & Tyler, 1998). It is used in the form of a tincture or salve externally for sprains and bruises because it stimulates the peripheral circulation of blood (Ottariano, 1999). For sprains and strains, arnica used topically usually results in the subsiding of swelling or congestion after twelve to twenty-four hours. I have observed topical arnica infused oil quickly reduce pain related to sprains and injuries and help swelling and bruising to disappear within two to four days.

Arnica is often used in antidandruff preparations (Leung & Foster, 1996) and in hair tonics because it is believed to make the hair grow (Duke, 1985). Arnica also has been used extensively in folk medicine for wounds. Arnica has antifungal properties, which may explain its use as a foot powder.

Arnica is not taken internally in whole herb form or preparations. Oral homeopathic preparations of arnica, because they are diluted to the point at which the molecules of arnica are chemically undetectable, are used for many conditions. These include abscesses, apoplexy (stroke), back pain, baldness, bed sores, black eye, bronchitis, bruises, chest ailments, cramps, diarrhea, exhaustion, fever, halitosis, paralysis, rheumatism, seasickness, sore feet, sore nipples, sprains, stings, trauma, and wounds. Arnica homeopathic preparations also are used for mental and physical shock, trauma, pain and swelling, dental extraction, bone fractures, headache, and concussion (Willard, 1991).

Even though internal use of arnica has been shown to cause adverse reactions, the Eclectics, early American botanical physicians, successfully used very small doses of the oral tincture to treat anemia with weak circulation, general debility, diarrhea, and edema of the lower extremities (Felter & Lloyd, 1983). Traditionally, arnica tincture also has been successful as a folk remedy for tumors and liver, stomach, and intestinal cancers (Duke, 1985).

Arnica tincture or infusion is used as a compress to treat acute inflammation of the joints, especially for chronic arthritis conditions (Duke, 1985). Herbalists also recommend arnica liniment for rheumatoid arthritis. Mixing two parts witch hazel with one part arnica tincture is sometimes recommended to be used topically in patients with rheumatoid arthritis to help lesson the potential for a skin reaction to the arnica tincture (Moore, 1993).

Breathing the vapors of the tincture of *A. montana* flowers from a suitable medium may reduce the desire to smoke tobacco products (Brinker & Alstat, 1995).

Cosmetic Use. Arnica contains an oil used in perfumery (Duke, 1985).

BIOMEDICAL EVIDENCE:

Few studies presently support the traditional use of arnica for improving mobility (e.g., reducing edema, bruising, and stiffness), especially during recuperation from injury or for reducing pain. No published studies on the topical use of arnica infusions, tincture, lotion, ointment, or oil were found. There have been a few published studies on the effects of the internal use of homeopathic arnica on postoperative swelling, pain, and bruising. A few of these studies, including one review of the literature, have been included here. The studies do not support the use of oral homeopathic arnica for its traditional use of improving mobility and pain. Arnica (herbal) topical remedies have not been studied, however.

Studies Related to Mobility

A review of studies done on the effects of homeopathic arnica on tissue trauma has demonstrated no significant data supporting its use (Ernst & Pittler, 1998). There were no significant effects of oral doses of homeopathic arnica (dilutions 30C and 10M) on laboratory-induced bruising as compared with placebo (Campbell, 1976). Limitations of these two studies include small sample sizes ($N = 11$ and $N = 15$), the use of homeopathic doses of the herb, and the fact that the bruises were experimentally induced and were expected by the subjects, which may affect the results of the use of an energy medicine such as a homeopathic remedy.

Another randomized, double-blind, placebo-controlled study of 400 long-distance runners who used oral doses of homeopathic arnica (dilution 30X), hoping to reduce muscle soreness after running, found no significant differences as measured by two-day visual analog scales, Likert scales, and race time (Vickers, Fisher, Smith, Wyllie, & Rees, 1998).

Studies Related to Other Health Patterns

Comfort and Pain Relief. A study published in a homeopathic journal (McIvor, 1973) discusses treating 200 patients with arnica three days before dental surgery for removal of impacted third molars or cyst removal from the mouth and then twice daily after surgery if swelling was noted. Although the investigator does not clearly report in what form the arnica was given or what dose or potency, it is written that the "pure tincture needs to be used in potency form" (p. 83) to avoid irritation to the mucous membranes. This means that arnica must be used in a highly diluted form. Ninety percent of the 200 arnica-treated patients are reported to have returned for suture removal in three days without noticeable edema or bruising, and very few complained of pain. The investigator reports less bleeding during surgery and no accounts of dry socket or infection in those patients treated with arnica. Although the lack of clarity of the methodology of this study raises concerns, the observations of this, most-likely, homeopathic study are intriguing; however, another double-blind trial of 118 participants undergoing wisdom teeth removal found that arnica seemed to increase pain and swelling as compared with placebo and was not as effective as metronidazole (Kaziro, 1984).

Mechanism of Action

Arnica contains sesquiterpene lactones called dihydrohelenalin and helenalin, which have been shown to be antibacterial and antifungal in vitro. Helenalin has been shown to be anti-inflammatory in animals (Leung & Foster, 1996). The presence of sesquiterpene lactones gives arnica an oxytoxic action, which may explain why some folk healers have used arnica as an abortifacient. Recent studies confirm that arnica preparations and its constituents have the following effects: antiseptic, anti-inflammatory, antifungal, antibiotic, antisclerotic, antitumorous, bacteriostatic, cytotoxic, and granulopoietic (DeSmet, 1992). Some plants in the Asteraceae family may cause sensitivity, resulting in contact dermatitis or other allergic effects. It is thought that the sensitivity may be caused by the sesquiterpene lactones of the helenalin type (Schulz et al., 1998).

USE IN PREGNANCY OR LACTATION:

Pregnant women have been known to have spontaneous abortions after the use of oral arnica preparations, and therefore arnica is contraindicated in pregnancy (Brinker, 1998; DeSmet, 1992; McGuffin et al., 1997). Homeopathic arnica is taken internally and used for shock (Weed, 1986) and after delivery when the mother is exhausted or has had delivery involving the use of instruments (McIvor, 1973).

Herbal Caveat—Pregnancy or Lactation

Some herbs are contraindicated in pregnancy because of a risk of the herb or one of its constituents stimulating the uterus and therefore possibly promoting fetal loss. Many herbal practitioners do not recommend herbal remedies, in particular oral doses of herbs, during the first trimester of pregnancy and seek an alternative. However, herbs are successfully used during pregnancy, especially to prepare the body for the birth. Herbs are relatively unstudied in pregnancy and lactation, so patients need to be made aware through education of the potential benefits and risks of using herbs for health conditions that arise during pregnancy or lactation. The use of herbal remedies during pregnancy often warrants a referral to a knowledgeable herbal practitioner.

USE FOR CHILDREN:

Arnica tincture or other topical applications should be used cautiously on the sensitive skin of children because the plant is a highly allergenic member of the Asteraceae family and has been known to cause dermatitis. As with the use of any topical cream, tincture, or lotion (such as sunscreen) for children, it is good practice to skin test a remedy on a small area of skin, such as the inner aspect of the arm of the child, before using the remedy on a larger area. Some advise against topical use of arnica in children (Schilcher, 1992).

Herbal Caveat—Children

Children have special needs in regard to herbal therapies. They require lesser amounts of herbs and often respond well to mild teas and topical applications such as compresses and baths. The lowest dose of oral preparations should be tried first before increasing the amount given children. Caregivers should observe children closely for responses to herbal reme-

---

dies. Younger children, particularly infants, have traditionally been given herbs either through their mother's breast milk or in the form of a homeopathic remedy because of their sensitivity to medicines and treatments and the immaturity of their liver. It is recommended that a person knowledgeable in the herbal treatment of children be consulted before the offering of any herb to a child for the first time.

CAUTIONS:

Note: These cautions relate to the use of the whole arnica plant, its flower, or root, not the homeopathic form.

Arnica has been known to cause contact dermatitis or other allergic reactions in some people. Arnica-sensitive individuals are known to cross-react to extracts of other Asteraceae species that contain the same or similar helenalin constituent. For this reason, these people should avoid contact with all plants and plant products that contain helenalin. In 1984, a patent was registered for a process that separates the allergens from arnica and other Asteraceae species. However, because these constituents are the pharmacologically active ones, the allergen-free preparations of arnica may actually be ineffective (DeSmet, 1992).

Extended use of arnica on damaged skin such as cutaneous ulcers or open injuries frequently causes edematous dermatitis with formation of vesicles. Eczema may develop with extended topical use (Blumenthal et al., 2000), especially if arnica is applied then covered with a bandage or tight clothing. Although arnica has been used traditionally for wound healing, it is no longer recommended for use on open wounds or broken skin (McGuffin et al., 1997; Moore, 1993).

Arnica whole plant remedies can seriously irritate mucous membranes. Ingestion may cause burning sensations in the stomach, vomiting, diarrhea, dizziness, muscular weakness, change in pulse rate (either a decrease or an increase), and collapse. Using the tea or tincture internally can result in exaggerated redness of the face, increased pulse rate, heart and respiratory dysfunction, cerebral symptoms, rigor, or bloody expectoration. One ounce (30 ml) of ingestion of the tincture has been reported to cause serious but not fatal symptoms (Leung & Foster, 1996). Two fluid ounces (60 ml) of the tincture taken orally has produced death (Felter & Lloyd, 1983). Because of these effects, arnica is rarely, if ever, taken internally *except* as a *homeopathic* dilution (McGuffin et al., 1997).

Even though internal use of arnica has been shown to cause many adverse reactions, the early American Eclectic physicians successfully used very small doses of the tincture for anemia with weak circulation, general debility, diarrhea, and edema of the ankles (Felter & Lloyd, 1983). The Eclectics understood the plant to cause heat in the throat, nausea, vomiting, diarrhea, spasms in the musculature of the limbs, inflammation of the alimentary canal, and coma when taken internally in large doses (Felter & Lloyd, 1983). In small internal doses, arnica has been known to cause accelerated pulse, increased perspiration, increased urine output, headache, and giddiness. It is a specific stimulant to the spinal nerves. Aqueous and alcohol extracts of arnica contain choline and two unidentified plant substances that can cause toxic gastroenteritis, nervous disturbances, intense muscular weakness, and death (Duke, 1985). For these reasons, the risk of using arnica internally has not supported its use, especially when other plant remedies can be used.

NURSING EVIDENCE:

Historical Nursing Use

Arnica appears in early nursing texts as one of the medicaments nurses studied. The applications are not discussed (Harmer & Henderson, 1955).

Potential Nursing Applications

Based on extensive traditional evidence, nurses may want to consider not only using arnica for patients with joint pain and injuries but also researching the objective and subjective effects of topical applications of arnica in patients with minor pain and injuries.

Integrative Insight

For many years, I have used and recommended topical arnica oil with lavender for patients with ankle and low back sprains, wrist and elbow pain, carpal tunnel syndrome, bruising, fractures, and joint pain. It is important to help the body stay mobile during these types of conditions because the tendency is for the body to tighten and protect the injury long after the initial insult warrants the protection. Herbal applications such as arnica oil massage encourage the stimulation of circulation and oxygen exchange in the injured area of the body. Arnica prevents stagnation and promotes healing. One integrative care protocol for healthy adults with ankle sprains includes icing and elevation, followed by gentle massage with arnica oil, and air cast. The air cast should be removed a few times a day so that icing and arnica oil can be repeated. Many patients are able to manage their pain with this protocol alone or with the addition of an occasional analgesic. Nurses in outpatient and school-based clinics may want to consider the addition of gentle arnica massage to their protocols for minor injuries, especially those related to sports. Arnica oil also can be used before warming up before athletic activity.

THERAPEUTIC APPLICATIONS:

Oral

Arnica is not currently recommended for oral use. However, arnica is a homeopathic remedy in which extremely small dilutions of the plant are used for a wide variety of complaints usually related to injury. In addition to its homeopathic use for injury, arnica (dilution of 6X) has historically been given to epileptics, and arnica (dilution of 3X) may prevent seasickness if taken before boarding ship and then every hour while on board (Grieve, 1971).

Topical

Compress. To make a compress, add 1 tablespoon (15 ml) of arnica tincture to $\frac{1}{2}$ quart ($\frac{1}{2}$ L) of water. The compress may be renewed every two hours (Duke, 1985).

Oil. Arnica oil is made with one part of the plant drug to five parts of vegetable oil. Ointments are used that contain 15% arnica oil (Blumenthal et al., 2000). Both oil and ointment are available commercially.

Mouthwash. For mouthwashes, dilute the tincture to ten times the volume with water (Blumenthal et al., 2000).

Salve. A salve can be made with 1 oz (28 g) of the dried flower and 1 oz (30 ml) of cold-pressed olive oil. The salve is used topically for chapped lips, inflamed nostrils, bruises, joint pain, skin rash, and acne (Willard, 1991).

Environmental

No data are available at this time.

Herbal Caveat—Therapeutic Applications

In traditional and conventional herbal medicine, amounts of herbs given to patients are based on individual needs. The amounts or "doses" recorded here are provided so that the health practitioner has a general idea of the amounts recommended for an adult patient. Dosing in herbalism not only refers to amount of plant used but also includes when, where, and how to take a plant medicine. These dosages should not be used as guidelines for indiscriminate intervention without proper assessment, critical thinking, and patient education on the part of the practitioner.

Note: Please see chapter 5 for detailed descriptions of how to prepare various applications.

PATIENT INTERACTION:

Whole herb arnica teas, tinctures, and extracts are no longer recommended for internal use. Homeopathic arnica, an extremely dilute form of the herb, is taken internally for certain conditions usually associated with injury. Arnica is most often used externally in the form of compresses, oils, or salves for the care of restricted mobility and pain related to injuries. Some people have had allergic reactions to the topical use of arnica preparations. Be sure to tell your health care provider if you may have an allergy to plants in the Asteraceae (daisy) family.

Herbal Caveat—Patient Interaction

Patients considering the use of an herb or formula of herbs in self-care benefit from education about the plant itself and the use of the plant in healing. This education can come through many sources, including local herbalists; plant specialists such as botanists; health practitioners such as nurses; nutritionists, naturopaths, and other physicians; and various written references including the scientific literature. Patients need to remember that their unique health care needs are not necessarily represented in any literature they may encounter. Therefore, it is recommended that a knowledgeable mentor be consulted before initiating self-care with any herb being used for the first time.

NURTURING THE NURSE-PLANT RELATIONSHIP:

Note: You may want to keep a journal of your experiences with the herb.

Nursing is a very active profession. Patient care is physically demanding and sometimes painful. Don't let those little aches and pains build up. When you get home from work, take a moment to turn your attention to your arms and legs and then your back, neck, and feet. Are you sore? You may have been so busy caring for others that you are not aware that you have stressed or strained a muscle or joint.

Get to know the healing effects of arnica by trying the herbal salve or oil when you come home from a physically strenuous day. Although both can be soothing to sore joints and muscles, arnica oil tends to be more warming and penetrating. Try massaging the herbal oil into those tender spots on your arms, legs, feet or back after a bath or shower when your skin is still warm and your pores are open. Better yet, you relax and have someone else help you with the oil massage!

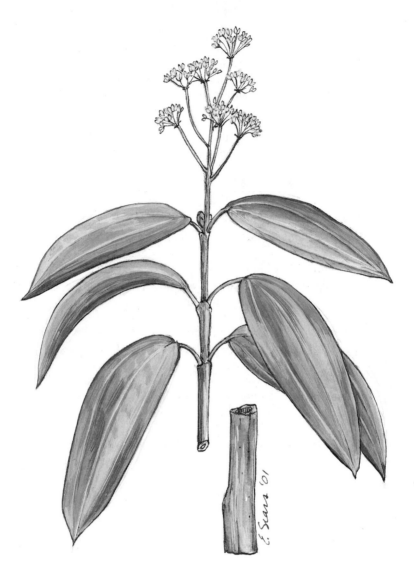

Cinnamomum zeylanicum

Cinnamon

🌿 **LATIN NAMES:** *Cinnamomum zeylanicum, Cinnamomum ceylanicum, Cinnamomum verum* (true cinnamon) (Ceylon), *Cinnamomum aromaticum, Cinnamomum cassia* (often the most common on the market) (China), *Cinnamomum burmanii* (Batavia), *Cinnamomum loureirii* (Saigon), *Cinnamomum laubatii* (Queensland)

🌿 **FAMILY:** Lauraceae

🌿 **COMMON NAMES:** Cinnamon, cassia, cinnamon bark, cinnamon oil, cassia oil, Chinese cinnamon; *Cinnamomum laubatii* also is known as camphorwood, pepperberry, pepperwood, and brown beech.

🌿 **HEALTH PATTERN:** Mobility

🌿 **PLANT DESCRIPTION:**

Cinnamon comes from the cinnamon tree, a medium-sized evergreen that grows from 10 to 35 feet (3 to 12 meters) tall. It is native to India, Sri Lanka, China, Indonesia, Vietnam, and is cultivated in parts of Africa, South America, and the West Indies (WHO, 1999). Cinnamon bark usually is harvested from trees that are at least seven years old (Bensky & Gamble, 1993). The bark has the warm, aromatic, and sweet odor that is characteristic of cinnamon. The leaves are similar in taste and odor. During harvesting, the bark is peeled from the shoots and branches. As it dries, it curls into quills, the long rolls from which commercial cinnamon sticks are later cut (Felter & Lloyd, 1983).

🌿 **PLANT PARTS USED:** Dried bark, leaves, and twigs.

🌿 **TRADITIONAL EVIDENCE:**

Cultural Use

Asian. Cinnamon, called *gui zhi,* has a long history of use in TCM. Its medicinal use has been recorded in Chinese texts as far back as 2700 B.C.E. (Blumenthal et al., 2000). It is classified as an herb that relieves wind chill and disperses cold in the muscles, meridians, and the exterior of the body. Cinnamon has been used to warm the kidney energy system and to tonify the yang in states of decreased physical vitality. Symptoms that may indicate a yang deficiency condition include aversion to cold, cold limbs, weak back, decreased libido, impotence, and frequent urination. Cinnamon also is used in TCM to treat decreased spleen and kidney yang symptoms of abdominal pain, decreased appetite, and diarrhea, and for wheezing due to the failure of the kidneys to grasp the *qi* (Bensky & Gamble, 1993). It is used to supplement the body's fire to warm and tone the spleen and kidney energy. These properties make it effective for certain types of pains in the chest and abdomen, diarrhea, and decreased function of the kidney. It also has been used with success in the treatment of asthma (Blumenthal et al., 2000). Cinnamon is contraindicated in conditions of deficiency of yin with heat, heat in the blood, and virulent heat.

In traditional Japanese herbal medicine, cinnamon, called *keishi,* is considered a warming herb used to prevent symptoms of misplaced *qi,* or energy, rising in the body. Cinnamon "leads fire back to its source," meaning that it corrects upward-floating energies that should be restrained by the internal organs. It acts to redirect excess energy in the upper half of the body and to revitalize deficient energy in the lower half of the body. Cinnamon does this by warming what is called *the gate of vitality* in the kidneys. It is used for fever, headaches, inflammation caused by sinusitis and colds, and to allay redness in the face caused by embarrassment or irritation. Cinnamon tea and tincture are used effectively for the relief of intestinal gas. Cinnamon oil has been used for many years as a remedy for wasp stings because it blocks the body's manufacture of inflammatory chemicals that create pain at the sting site (Rister, 1999). *C. cassia* bark has been used to treat Oketsu syndrome, a disease similar to disseminated intravascular coagulation (DIC), thought to be due to the advancement of inflammatory processes (Kubo, Shiping, Wu, & Matsuda, 1996).

Hispanic. A preparation of cinnamon has been used by the Mexican people to treat earaches (Kay, 1996). Hispanics also add milk to a cinnamon tea made from the boiled sticks for stomachache. Cinnamon tea with cloves is given for chest cold. Cinnamon also is used for headache, reducing fever, and as an antiviral agent.

East Indian. Cinnamon is known as *gudatvak* in Sanskrit. In India, the bark and leaves are used as a carminative, stimulant, galactagogue, and diaphoretic (Lassak, 1986). Cinnamon also was used as a popular aphrodisiac and antiseptic. Ayurvedic medicine includes the use of cinnamon as an infusion, decoction, powder, and distilled oil. These preparations may be used for bowel complaints such as dyspepsia, flatulence, diarrhea, and vomiting. Cinnamon is used as a stimulant to the uterine muscle fibers to control menorrhagia and to stimulate labor during childbirth. It is used for gastrointestinal cramps, toothache, and paralysis of the tongue. Chewing the bark is recommended to relieve nausea and vomiting. Cinnamon has been used in India to treat typhoid fever, gonorrhea, tuberculosis, lupus, and headaches (Nadkarni, 1976).

Middle Eastern. In Arabic, cinnamon is called *darasini* (Nadkarni, 1976). Arabs value cinnamon as a symbol of wealth. In Arabic medicine, the bark, branches, and root of cinnamon are used as an anticonvulsant or antihelminthic, to dispel intestinal gas, and as an insecticide. An extract of the root and bark is used as a sedative and applied externally to alleviate toothache pain (Ghazanfar, 1994).

European. Cinnamon bark is used for the treatment of appetite loss, dyspepsia, and mild gastrointestinal spasms. The German Standard License has listed cinnamon bark infusion as useful for flatulence, feelings of distention, mild cramping, and gastrointestinal disorders associated with decreased production of gastric juice (Blumenthal et al., 2000). The French use cinnamon bark to treat symptoms of digestive problems, functional asthenias, and to facilitate weight gain (Blumenthal et al., 2000).

Culinary Use

Cinnamon is used abundantly as a spice in curries and sweets. The cinnamon-like flavor in gum, candies, and toothpastes is usually derived from cassia, not cinnamon. Cinnamon, cassia, and their bark oils are used as flavorings in many foods, alcoholic and nonalcoholic beverages, frozen dairy desserts, candies, baked goods, gelatins and puddings, meat and meat products, condiments, relishes, soups, and gravies. Powdered cinnamon is used as an ingredient in home baking and cooking. The ground bark of cinnamon is widely used as a flavoring in herbal teas and tonics.

Use in Herbalism

Cinnamon bark has been used for thousands of years in both Eastern and Western cultures and has been valuable in the spice trade. Cinnamon was used in ancient Egypt as a medicine, food spice, and perfume. Cinnamon was one of the spices used in the mummification process. It was considered valuable enough to be offered in the temple during religious rites. Cinnamon is mentioned in the Bible several times and was one of the ingredients in the holy ointment of Moses (de Waal, 1980).

Cinnamon bark has been used as a stimulant, tonic, digestive aid, and astringent. It has been used both as an emmenagogue and for uterine hemorrhage and menorrhagia. Cinnamon used internally will control hemorrhage in the body, but it has a specific effect upon the uterus, acting to stop bleeding by causing contraction of the uterine musculature (Felter & Lloyd, 1983).

Cinnamon has been used for the treatment of diarrhea, rheumatism, colds, heart and abdominal pains, hypertension, kidney problems, disorders of the female reproductive tract, and cancer. In folk medicine, cinnamon has been used for impotence, frigidity, shortness of breath, vaginitis, rheumatism, neuralgia, wounds, and toothache. In aromatherapy, cinnamon essential oil is used as an inhalation in relieving tension, steadying the nerves, and invigorating the senses (Keville & Green, 1995). The oil also is used for its antibacterial, antiviral, and antifungal properties.

Cosmetic Use. Cinnamon is used in topical liniments, suntan lotions, nasal sprays, mouthwash, and toothpaste. It is used frequently as a fragrance for soaps, detergents, creams, lotions, and perfumes.

BIOMEDICAL EVIDENCE:

Cinnamon has traditionally been used for numerous symptoms related to the health pattern of mobility, including increasing circulation, moving the energy in meridians, warming and stimulating the body, and relieving symptoms related to conditions such as rheumatism. No human trials were found that support the traditional use of cinnamon for health concerns related to mobility. Some animal and in vitro data are presented here.

Studies Related to Mobility

In a controlled animal study, there was a significant reduction in laboratory-induced inflammation during the acute stage in mice given oral doses of cinnamon bark (70% methanolic extract 50–500 mg/kg), suggesting that there is an active constituent (or constituents) in cinnamon that has an inhibitory effect on inflammation (Kubo et al., 1996).

Studies Related to Other Health Patterns

Digestion. Animal studies have demonstrated that water extracts of *C. cassia* 100 mg/kg, given intraperitoneally to rats, significantly inhibited ulcerogenesis induced by cold stress or water immersion stress and that the cinnamon extract prevented serotonin-induced ulcer, possibly by increasing the blood flow of gastric mucosa. This activity was as high as cimetidine (Reglan) (Akira, Tanaka, & Tabata, 1986; Tanaka et al., 1987).

Hormone Balance. In vitro studies have shown that cinnamon and other spices such as cloves, bay leaf, and turmeric may have a role in glucose metabolism by potentiating insulin activity more than threefold (Khan, Bryden, Polansky, & Anderson, 1990). These elements are continuing to be researched for future use in studies of insulin resistant type II diabetics (Imparl-Radosevich et al., 1998).

Immune Response. Fluconazole-resistant strains of *Candida albicans* have been reported (Rex, Rinaldi, & Pfaller, 1995). One pilot study of 5 patients with HIV and oral candidiasis who received eight commercial cinnamon lozenges per day demonstrated significant improvement in the symptoms of 3 of the 5 participants. Investigators identify the concentration of cinnamon necessary for the anti-candidal effect and state that although effective levels are unlikely to be achieved systemically, therapeutic levels can be obtained locally in the oropharynx (Quale, Landman, Zaman, Burney, & Sathe, 1996). A study published in Chinese in the *Chinese Journal of Nursing* found that a 50% cinnamon bark mouth rinse also was effective against oral candidiasis (Cao, 1993 as reported in Quale et al., 1996).

Mechanism of Action

Cinnamaldehyde has been shown to have antipyretic and sedative activities in animals and is a constituent in cinnamon that can cause skin irritation in humans, especially among bakers and spice factory workers who handle cinnamon powder (Leung & Foster, 1996; Meding, 1993). Cinnamon has antifungal, antiviral, bacteriocidal, and larvicidal activity (DeSmet, 1992); in particular, a 0.1% extraction of cinnamon bark completely suppressed *Candida, E. coli,* and *Staphylococcus* growth (Duke, 1985). The leaf oil is antiseptic and anesthetic. Oil of cinnamon leaf is not interchangeable with oil of cinnamon bark because the two have different constituents (Wren, 1988).

USE IN PREGNANCY OR LACTATION:

Cinnamon is not recommended for therapeutic use in pregnancy (McGuffin et al., 1997). Cinnamon, as well as other herbs such as nutmeg, sassafras, and camphor, contains very small amounts of a chemical called safrole. Safrole has been shown to readily cross the placenta in mice, resulting in DNA damage to the developing fetus. It has been suggested that cinnamon does not present any special risk during pregnancy in humans provided that internal doses do not exceed the amounts used in foods, but that extended use of the oil should be restricted in pregnancy (DeSmet, 1992).

Cinnamon was used in the early 1900s to stop uterine hemorrhage occurring at any time, especially after childbirth (Felter & Lloyd, 1983). Cinnamon also has been reported as an abortifacient. However, current information reveals that in older reference books, cinnamon *(C. cassia)* was confused with *Cassia fistulosa,* which is known to contain substances called anthraquinones, compounds that cause stimulation of smooth muscle fibers in the gastrointestinal tract and uterus. Older records claiming that cinnamon is an abortifacient are most likely referring to *Cassia fistulosa* rather than *Cinnamomum.* There are no case reports that absolutely define *Cinnamomum* as an abortifacient (DeSmet, 1992).

Herbal Caveat—Pregnancy or Lactation

Some herbs are contraindicated in pregnancy because of a risk of the herb or one of its constituents stimulating the uterus and therefore possibly promoting fetal loss. Many herbal practitioners do not recommend herbal remedies, in particular oral doses of herbs, during the first trimester of pregnancy and seek an alternative. However, herbs are successfully used during pregnancy, especially to prepare the body for the birth. Herbs are relatively unstudied in pregnancy and lactation, so patients need to be made aware through education of the potential benefits and risks of using herbs for health conditions that arise during pregnancy or lactation. The use of herbal remedies during pregnancy often warrants a referral to a knowledgeable herbal practitioner.

Excessive use of cinnamon-flavored cosmetics and gum should be discouraged because of the potential damage to skin and sensitive mucosa. Pediatricians have reported that children have been found to repeatedly suck or sniff toothpicks dipped in cinnamon oil, primarily cassia oil, to get "high" (Schwartz, 1990).

Herbal Caveat—Children

Children have special needs in regard to herbal therapies. They require lesser amounts of herbs and often respond well to mild teas and topical applications such as compresses and baths. The lowest dose of oral preparations should be tried first before increasing the amount given children. Caregivers should observe children closely for responses to herbal remedies. Younger children, particularly infants, have traditionally been given herbs either through their mother's breast milk or in the form of a homeopathic remedy because of their sensitivity to medicines and treatments and the immaturity of their liver. It is recommended that a person knowledgeable in the herbal treatment of children be consulted before the offering of any herb to a child for the first time.

@ CAUTIONS:

Cinnamon bark and leaf oils can irritate skin and mucous membranes if applied topically. The bark oil is more irritating (Keville & Green, 1995). There is one report of a 7-year-old child demonstrating toxic symptoms after drinking about 2 ounces of cinnamon oil when challenged by a friend to do so. His symptoms included burning sensation in the mouth, chest, and stomach; double vision; dizziness; vomiting; and sleepiness (Pilapil, 1989). Ingestion of small amounts of undiluted cinnamon oil can cause tachycardia, shortness of breath, lightheadedness, and facial flushing (Schwartz, 1990).

Cinnamaldehyde has been identified as the leading substance responsible for allergic reactions caused by cosmetics or perfumes (DeSmet, 1992). Allergic symptoms may include urticaria, swelling of the lips and tongue, itching, burning, or blistering of the oral mucosa from the use of dental preparations containing cinnamon. The lowest concentration causing positive reactions in patch tests was 0.01%. Symptoms often resolve when the preparations containing cinnamon are withdrawn; however, it is suggested that persons with a disposition for skin reactions should not use products that contain cinnamon.

Some people who use toothpaste that contains cinnamonaldehyde develop oral lesions. The reaction may be due to a hypersensitivity reaction rather than an autoimmune response. Studies also have shown that repeated and prolonged exposure is needed to trigger the oral symptoms (Lamey, Rees, & Forsyth, 1990). One case study reports that cinnamon may have been related to the development of squamous cell carcinoma of the tongue in a 24-year-old woman who chewed five packs of cinnamon gum daily. The woman did not chew tobacco or consume alcohol (Westra, McMurray, Califano, Flint, & Corio, 1998).

Cinnamon should not be used internally with tetracycline. Cinnamon bark (2 g in 100 ml) markedly reduced the in vitro dissolution of tetracycline hydrochloride from gelatin capsules. In the presence of cassia bark about 20% of tetracycline hydrochloride was in solution after thirty minutes in contrast to 97% when only water was used (DeSmet, 1992).

The median lethal dose (LD_{50}) of cinnamon by intravenous injection in mice is 18.48 ± 1.8 g/kg of crude herb (Chang & But, 1986).

NURSING EVIDENCE:

Historical Nursing Use

Cinnamon has been used historically in nursing in spice poultices and plasters to produce a counterirritant effect at the site of treatment (Weeks-Shaw, 1914).

Potential Nursing Applications

Nurses may want to consider the use of cinnamon from the Chinese perspective, to create warmth in the body as it circulates throughout the meridians. Warmth in herbalism is considered one key to the health of the body and the internal organ systems. Cinnamon has been used traditionally to warm or stimulate digestion and circulation. Nurses often are aware of the chilled extremities of their patients as they lie in bed and recuperate from illness, but many people have cold extremities and poor circulation on a daily basis, not just when they are acutely ill. When extremities are cold, it is not as easy to move freely.

Athletes always warm up their bodies before working out. Nurses might want to experiment with the use of a cinnamon beverage tea when getting an elderly nursing home patient warmed up for a walk or for the recuperating patient who is healing after having a cast removed from a fractured extremity.

Cinnamon oil has established antibacterial, antiviral, and antifungal effects. Nurses may want to research the topical and internal use of cinnamon when caring for patients with conditions such as oral candidiasis when mouth care is uncomfortable for the patient.

Integrative Insight

Immobility is often painful. Bodies and organ systems need to move to maintain health, just as the water on the Earth needs to move or run to remain pure. Stagnant blood, organs, and bodies can be likened to a stagnant pool of water waiting for a splash to occur so that new oxygen can be infused into it. Cinnamon is an herbal catalyst. It is stimulating to the circulation and has an opening effect on the energy vessels, or meridians, of the body. Cinnamon has the ability to adapt to the need of the body. It is used to stimulate blood circulation and yet it can control hemorrhage when necessary—two seemingly opposite effects. Although cinnamon warms the body and can even be irritating (too warm) to the skin at times, it also can relieve inflammation, a condition often thought of as having too much heat. Cinnamon tastes good and is readily available. As a plant medicine, its warming and adapting healing qualities simply await further exploration.

THERAPEUTIC APPLICATIONS:

Oral

Tea. The recommended daily dose is not more than 2 to 4 g of the cut or ground bark. Prepare a cinnamon infusion with 3 to 5 g of ground cinnamon per 1 cup (240 ml) of water. To make a decoction, use 0.7 to 1.3 g in 5 oz (150 ml) of water, three times daily. It is best to use cinnamon in pieces as large as possible because it loses its potency quickly in storage.

Liquid Extract. The recommended use of cinnamon liquid extract (1:5 g/ml) for medicinal purposes is ½ to 1½ teaspoons (3.3 to 6.7 ml) three times daily (Blumenthal, Goldberg, & Brinckman, 2000).

Topical

For massage, add 2 drops each of the essential oils of cinnamon, frankincense, and orange into 1 tablespoon (15 ml) of almond oil.

Environmental

Up to 2 drops of essential oil of cinnamon can be used in the bath for nausea, depression, stress-related conditions, and exhaustion.

Cinnamon bark is used as incense and for fumigation, in potpourri, and to scent linens and clothes (Lawless, 1998). The Greeks used the bark as a spice with which to perfume their linens to keep the moths away.

A few drops of cinnamon essential oil can be used in a vaporizer to scent the air in the home. The fragrance is said to clear the head, get rid of unwanted smells, prevent the spread of infection, and act as a mood elevator to aid in meditation (Lawless, 1998).

Herbal Caveat—Therapeutic Applications

In traditional and conventional herbal medicine, amounts of herbs given to patients are based on individual needs. The amounts or "doses" recorded here are provided so that the health practitioner has a general idea of the amounts recommended for an adult patient. Dosing in herbalism not only refers to amount of plant used but also includes when, where, and how to take a plant medicine. These dosages should not be used as guidelines for indiscriminate intervention without proper assessment, critical thinking, and patient education on the part of the practitioner.

Note: Please see chapter 5 for detailed descriptions of how to prepare various applications.

Cinnamon has been used for centuries as a spice in food and beverages as well as cosmetics. Cinnamon also is used medicinally as a warming and stimulating herb that can help when a person is nauseated, feels cold, or is experiencing stiffness and pain due to rheumatism. Cinnamon bark can be made into a tea. Cinnamon oil also is used medicinally, but because the oil can be very irritating to skin and mucous membranes such as those in the mouth, it is best to use cinnamon oil in very small amounts and only occasionally. Even chewing too much cinnamon gum is a potential health hazard. Cinnamon oil should not be taken internally for medicinal purposes without the guidance of a knowledgeable practitioner. Cinnamon in any form should not be taken in medicinal amounts during pregnancy or by those who are taking the drug tetracycline.

Herbal Caveat—Patient Interaction

Patients considering the use of an herb or formula of herbs in self-care benefit from education about the plant itself and the use of the plant in healing. This education can come through many sources, including local herbalists; plant specialists such as botanists; health practitioners such as nurses, nutritionists, naturopaths, and other physicians; and various written references including the scientific literature. Patients need to remember that their unique health care needs are not necessarily represented in any literature they may encounter. Therefore, it is recommended that a knowledgeable mentor be consulted before initiating self-care with any herb being used for the first time.

🍃 NURTURING THE NURSE-PLANT RELATIONSHIP:

Note: You may want to keep a journal of your experiences with the herb.

Cinnamon is probably one herb you will have tried before. Take a moment to get reacquainted with cinnamon by sitting down and enjoying a piece of toast with butter and powdered cinnamon. Think of cinnamon's medicinal qualities and breathe in the fragrant aroma of the herb. How and what do you feel when you breathe in the scent of cinnamon?

Try making a decoction of cinnamon bark. You can use the cinnamon sticks in your pantry. When you have a moment, do a tea tasting. Sit quietly and sip a room temperature or slightly warm cinnamon decoction. Note the qualities of the herb, its tastes, smells, and where you feel its warming action in your body.

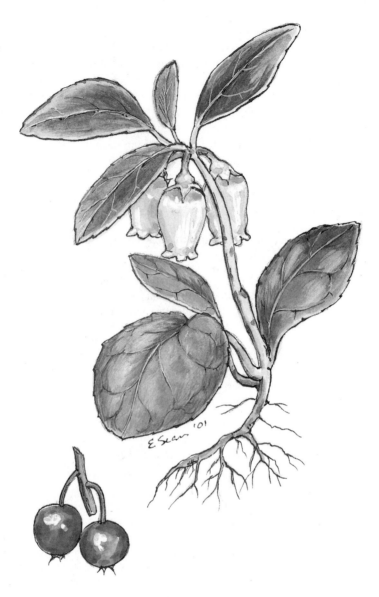

Gaultheria procumbens

Wintergreen

- **LATIN NAME:** *Gaultheria procumbens*

- **FAMILY:** Ericaceae

- **COMMON NAMES:** Wintergreen, teaberry, checkerberry, creeping wintergreen, boxberry, mountain tea, deerberry, spiceberry, ground holly, grouse berry, dewberry, redberry, hillberry

- **HEALTH PATTERN:** Mobility

- **PLANT DESCRIPTION:**
Wintergreen is a small evergreen shrub with slender stems that creep along the ground. Erect branches rise from the stems that bear oval, leathery leaves with toothed margins. The leaves are a glossy, bright green above and pale green below. The plant grows 5 to 6 inches (12.5 to 15 cm) tall and is often found under other evergreens. It likes to grow in large patches on sandy and barren soils, especially in mountainous areas. The plant produces solitary, drooping pink-white flowers from the base of the leaves from June to October, followed by fleshy red berries that have a sweet taste. The odor of the leaves is characteristically aromatic because of the volatile oil contained in them. Wintergreen oil, usually about 0.5% to 0.8% from wintergreen leaves, is obtained by steam distillation of the leaves by a carefully controlled process that yields methyl salicylate (Leung & Foster, 1996). More often today, methyl salicylate is made commercially by distilling a mixture of salicylic acid and methyl alcohol (DeSmet, 1992), instead of being derived directly from wintergreen leaf. Wintergreen is native to the United States, growing from Maine to Florida, and from Pennsylvania to Kentucky.

- **PLANT PARTS USED:** Leaf, berry, and oil

- **TRADITIONAL EVIDENCE:**
Cultural Use

    North American Indian. North American Indians use the berries for food, picking them off the plant even in the snow. They smoke and chew the leaves after drying them slowly over a fire without allowing them to burn. Algonquins chew the leaves to improve their breathing during hunting. They also have applied a poultice of the whole plant to the chest as a cold remedy. They use an infusion of the leaves as a tonic for overeating, for headaches, and general discomfort. The Delaware and many other tribes use the plant internally and externally for rheumatism (Hutchens, 1992; Moerman, 1998). Quebec Indians roll the leaves around teeth that ache (Duke, 1985). The Hoh tribe use *Gaultheria ovatifolia* as a source of fruits that are stewed and made into a sauce or jelly (Moerman, 1998).

North American Indians make wintergreen berry tea by steeping the entire plant in water. The Mi'kmaq tribe uses wintergreen berry as a heart attack preventative and also gives it to people who are recovering from heart attacks. It is used by those with blood clotting disorders and those who have had strokes. The plant is believed to thin and regulate the blood, similar to the action of aspirin, thus preventing the formation of blood clots. (http://www.caribou.bc.ca@psd:nursing/Native_Healing/sld042.htm).

East Indian. *Gaultheria fragrantissima* is found growing freely in Burma and Ceylon, from Nepal to Bhutan, and in Assam. The English refer to it as Indian wintergreen. The Hindustani, Javanese, and Bengali refer to it as *gandapuro*. The native people use the leaf of the plant, sometimes distilling the oil for medicinal use. The oil is considered aromatic, stimulating, carminative, and antiseptic (Nadkarni, 1976).

In the Indian literature, oil of wintergreen is given orally in doses beginning at 10 drops in capsules, gradually increasing the dose as needed. This dose is not recommended in most botanical and essential oil literature (see Oral Use and Cautions). The oil is used to treat acute rheumatism, sciatica, and neuralgia. It also is used externally by itself or in liniments and ointments for the same ailments. It is rare for Ayurvedic physicians not to use this oil to treat cases of decreased mobility due to joint and muscular aches and pains (Nadkarni, 1976).

Culinary Use

Wintergreen oil is used to flavor various foods. To prevent toxicity reactions, the highest level used is about 0.04%, or 405 parts per million (ppm), in candy and other foods. In very small amounts, it is used as a flavoring agent for candies, soft drinks, dental preparations, cough drops, and chewing gum. The berries are very tasty and can be used to make pie (DeSmet, 1992) if enough can be found. The berries also can be steeped in brandy to make a bitter tonic (Grieve, 1971). The dried leaves are added to tea as a flavoring agent (Leung & Foster, 1996). One of my favorite historic restaurants in Maine, called the Goldenrod (any herbalist would love a name like that!), still makes a wintergreen-flavored ice cream called checkerberry chip that is pink and has chocolate chips in it.

Use in Herbalism

Wintergreen tea has been used internally as an antirheumatic, anti-inflammatory, and diuretic agent. Wintergreen oil is readily absorbed by the skin and is more commonly used topically in the form of an ointment or liniment for rheumatism, sprains, sciatica, muscular pain, and neuralgia (Felter & Lloyd, 1983; Wren, 1988). The whole plant tea is used medicinally as an antiseptic, carminative, diuretic, and nervine and to stimulate the onset of delayed menses and to promote breast milk production. It is used as a gargle for sore throats, a douche for leukorrhea, an eyewash in cases of conjunctivitis, and for diarrhea. The tea has been used internally for many years by various cultures, but the distilled and concentrated oil of wintergreen is not used internally because of its potential toxicity. Topical application of wintergreen oil was used in the early twentieth century to relieve the pain of toothache (Felter & Lloyd, 1983). Some have children chew the roots each spring to help prevent tooth decay.

BIOMEDICAL EVIDENCE:

An exhaustive search of the published literature provided no reports of clinical research on the use of wintergreen or wintergreen oil even though there are numerous over-the-counter preparations (many of which are made with synthetic wintergreen oil).

Studies Related to Mobility

No data are available at this time.

Studies Related to Other Health Patterns

No data are available at this time.

Mechanism of Action

The leaves of wintergreen are the source of an essential oil made up almost entirely of methyl salicylate. Salicin-containing plants, such as wintergreen, have been used for hundreds of years for medicinal purposes. They have been used primarily to reduce fevers, as mild analgesics, and for their anti-inflammatory properties (McGuffin et al., 1997). Extensive research has been done on the ability of salicylates to suppress the synthesis of prostaglandins, hormones that are believed to play a central role in pain, fever, and inflammation (McGuffin et al., 1997); however, wintergreen and methyl salicylates are not the same thing.

Wintergreen oil contains not less than 98% ester (a compound formed by the combination of an organic acid with an alcohol) known as methyl salicylate (Leung & Foster, 1996). The alcohol and ester create the characteristic odor of the oil. Wintergreen oil contains methyl salicylate as its chief constituent, but it also contains arbutin, ericolin, gallic acid and gaultheric acid, mucilage, tannin, wax, and others (DeSmet, 1992). Methyl salicylate's mode of action is similar to that of other salicylates taken internally, but wintergreen oil is not to be taken internally. It is used for topical administration in the form of salves, liniments, and other preparations. The absorption of methyl salicylates from the gastrointestinal tract is slower and more erratic than skin absorption (Levine & Caplan, 1984 as reported in DeSmet, 1992).

Because of its potential toxicity and because salicylates are distributed in breast milk, wintergreen oil should be avoided by pregnant and lactating women. Salicylates have been shown to be teratogenic and embryocidal in animal studies. In human studies, the result of chronic maternal salicylate ingestion has been associated with decreased fetal birth weight, increased incidence of stillbirth, neonatal mortality, postpartum maternal hemorrhage, complicated deliveries, prolonged gestation, and spontaneous labor (DeSmet, 1992).

Herbal Caveat—Pregnancy or Lactation

Some herbs are contraindicated in pregnancy because of a risk of the herb or one of its constituents stimulating the uterus and therefore possibly promoting fetal loss. Many herbal practitioners do not recommend herbal remedies, in particular oral doses of herbs, during the first trimester of pregnancy and seek an alternative. However, herbs are successfully used during pregnancy, especially to prepare the body for the birth. Herbs are relatively unstudied in pregnancy and lactation, so patients need to be made aware through education of the potential benefits and risks of using herbs for health conditions that arise during pregnancy or lactation. The use of herbal remedies during pregnancy often warrants a referral to a knowledgeable herbal practitioner.

USE FOR CHILDREN:

Although the essence (alcoholic solution of a volatile oil) of wintergreen is carminative and was used in small doses for flatulent colic of infants in the early twentieth century in the United States (Felter & Lloyd, 1983), wintergreen oil is contraindicated in children. As little as less than a teaspoon (4 ml) of wintergreen oil has caused fatality in infants. Another case cites an instance in which a 21-month-old child ingested 1½ teaspoons (7.5 ml) of oil of wintergreen that was intended for use as a candy flavoring. The child presented with symptoms of acute salicylate toxicity (Howrie et al., 1985 as reported in DeSmet, 1992). The lethal dose of wintergreen oil for a 3-year-old is 1 teaspoon (5 ml) (Buckle, 1997). The United States Poison Prevention Packaging Act of 1970 requires that liquid preparations containing more than 1 teaspoon (5 ml) of methyl salicylate by weight be packaged in child-resistant containers (DeSmet, 1992).

Herbal Caveat—Children

Children have special needs in regard to herbal therapies. They require lesser amounts of herbs and often respond well to mild teas and topical applications such as compresses and baths. The lowest dose of oral preparations should be tried first before increasing the amount given children. Caregivers should observe children closely for responses to herbal remedies. Younger children, particularly infants, have traditionally been given herbs either through their mother's breast milk or in the form of a homeopathic remedy because of their sensitivity to medicines and treatments and

---

the immaturity of their liver. It is recommended that a person knowledgeable in the herbal treatment of children be consulted before the offering of
any herb to a child for the first time.

CAUTIONS:

Wintergreen leaf tea can be consumed safely if used correctly
(McGuffin et al., 1997). The methyl salicylate content of the leaves is
5445 to 7920 ppm (www.ars-grin.gov/cgi-bin/duke/highchem.pl).
One drop of the essential oil is a highly concentrated package of
methyl salicylates (98% according to Leung & Foster, 1996). Oil of
wintergreen is considered toxic in oral doses. The lethal dose for a
70-kg man is between 1 and 6 teaspoons (5 ml to 30 ml) (DeSmet,
1992). Therefore it is best not to use wintergreen oil internally.
Death due to stomach inflammation has resulted from large, frequent oral doses of the oil. Signs of salicylic acid toxicity include tinnitus, nausea, and vomiting (Duke, 1985). The symptoms of oil of
wintergreen poisoning are similar to salicylate poisoning. These include acid-base imbalance, altered glucose metabolism, and central
nervous system toxicity. The severity of the symptoms depends on
the dose of the salicylate consumed, the age of the person, and
whether the ingested dose was acute or chronic. Mild chronic
salicylate toxicity includes headache, dizziness, tinnitus, problems
with hearing, decreased visual acuity, mental confusion, lassitude,
and sleepiness. More severe toxic reactions are characterized by disturbances of the central nervous system that may include seizures
and coma. Fever is usually a prominent characteristic in children.
The severity of symptoms is especially pronounced in children under
five years of age. Acute salicylate toxicity may present with neurologic signs and symptoms such as disorientation, irritability, lethargy, coma, hallucinations, stupor, and seizures (DeSmet, 1992).
Simple gastric irritation caused by smaller doses of salicylates may
cause nausea and vomiting, hyperventilation, and gastrointestinal
fluid loss that lead to mild dehydration. Fluid loss may contribute to
hypokalemia and systemic alkalosis (DeSmet,1992).

People who have an intolerance to analgesics and acetylsalicylic
acid (aspirin) may exhibit sensitivity to the methyl salicylate from the
wintergreen plant and should avoid exposure. There are documented
cases of people who have experienced urticaria, acute pustular psoriasis, and angioedema after contact with the constituents of wintergreen leaves (DeSmet 1992). It is believed that the true wintergreen oil
is much more likely to cause adverse skin reactions if used topically
than the synthetic product (Nadkarni,1976). Essential oil of wintergreen contains beta-asarone and therefore may interact with cytochrome P450 mechanisms; however, this is unlikely because of the
small amounts used in aromatherapy (Buckle, 1997).

Historical Nursing Use

Wintergreen oil has been used topically for its antiseptic, analgesic, and stimulant properties (Harmer & Henderson, 1955).

Potential Nursing Applications

Because the leaves of wintergreen contain an essential oil that is made up almost entirely of methyl salicylate, and the risk of toxic reaction to the oil is high, the oil is rarely if ever used medicinally. However, teas from salicin-containing plants, such as wintergreen, have been used for hundreds of years for medicinal purposes for rheumatic complaints, nausea, or fever. Nurses may want to research further the use of salicylate-containing herbs such as wintergreen and compare the benefits and risks of their use with the benefits and risks of the oral use of nonsteroidal anti-inflammatory drugs (NSAIDs). Because there are so many potential and actual adverse effects to long-term use of NSAIDs, wintergreen leaf might be a welcome and viable alternative, especially in the care of patients with chronic health conditions related to joint pain and stiffness.

Integrative Insight

Nurses have administered salicylate medications since the invention of aspirin. These medications have potential adverse effects as do all medications. As nurses begin to reevaluate the risks and benefits to patients of the anti-inflammatory medications they administer, alternatives are being sought and reviewed. Wintergreen leaf, with its history of safe use and because it contains a small amount of methyl salicylate, has the potential to provide benefit to those with joint pain and stiffness without the adverse effects of a pharmaceutical. The comparison studies have not been conducted as far as I know.

Wintergreen and wintergreen oil have all but gone out of use in nursing practice. Although the oil may be toxic when ingested, this does not mean that the use of the leaf or the topical use of the oil should be overlooked. This is one herb whose clinical potential is not fully understood and that needs further investigation, especially for its use in the care of those with mobility and pain-related complaints.

● **THERAPEUTIC APPLICATIONS:**

Oral

Because of its toxicity, oil of wintergreen should not be taken internally. Wintergreen leaf can be infused or small amounts of the leaf can be added to flavor beverage teas.

Topical

Topical preparations of wintergreen oil containing 2% to 55% methyl salicylate that can be used for joint pain and stiffness are currently sold in the United States.

Environmental

Wintergreen oil (no more than 5 drops) or whole herb (put in a cotton bag) can be added to a bath or steam cabinet. The body should only be submerged to the waist during a wintergreen bath. The shoulders can be sponge-bathed if they are sore. The bath can be taken twice a week (Hutchens, 1992).

The aroma of wintergreen leaf is very soothing and pleasant. Wintergreen oil is rarely used in aromatherapy; birch is a more common, safer substitute.

Herbal Caveat—Therapeutic Applications

In traditional and conventional herbal medicine, amounts of herbs given to patients are based on individual needs. The amounts or "doses" recorded here are provided so that the health practitioner has a general idea of the amounts recommended for an adult patient. Dosing in herbalism not only refers to amount of plant used but also includes when, where, and how to take a plant medicine. These dosages should not be used as guidelines for indiscriminate intervention without proper assessment, critical thinking, and patient education on the part of the practitioner.

Note: Please see chapter 5 for detailed descriptions of how to prepare various applications.

PATIENT INTERACTION:

Use of wintergreen leaf is very different from the use of the essential oil of wintergreen. The herb can be used for muscle and joint aches and pains in bath or liniment form, for example. The leaves of the plant, which can be taken as tea, contain small amounts of methyl salicylate, a substance also found in aspirin. Check with a knowledgeable practitioner about the therapeutic use of wintergreen if you already take a daily aspirin or have reactions of any kind to aspirin. The oil of wintergreen is commonly used in salves and other topical applications created for over-the-counter use; however, synthetic oil is often used. Do not take wintergreen essential oil internally.

Herbal Caveat—Patient Interaction

Patients considering the use of an herb or formula of herbs in self-care benefit from education about the plant itself and the use of the plant in healing. This education can come through many sources, including local herbalists; plant specialists such as botanists; health practitioners such as nurses, nutritionists, naturopaths, and other physicians; and various written references including the scientific literature. Patients need to remember that their unique health care needs are not necessarily represented in any literature they may encounter. Therefore, it is recommended that a knowledgeable mentor be consulted before initiating self-care with any herb being used for the first time.

Note: You may want to keep a journal of your experiences with the herb.

How is wintergreen used where you live? Go to a local pharmacy and see if you can find out. Wintergreen is often used in topical salves for joint and muscle pain. Other remedies that use the flavor are available for digestive complaints. Try the leaf as a tea. Take a look at some of the topical over-the-counter products you find. See if the wintergreen oil used in the products you find is synthetic or natural. If you find a salve with wintergreen in it, consider giving it a try on sore muscles and joints. Record your experience.

CHAPTER 17

Lifestyle Choices

INTRODUCTION

NURSES OBSERVE THE GREAT DIVERSITY OF HUMAN nature in their work. The will to live, for example, is part of human nature, but how that will is expressed is as unique as the individual in whom it resides. Every day, people make choices about how they will live life. How a person creates and expresses these choices in life is their style, their lifestyle. Some life decisions are made in full awareness through deep reflection, and other decisions are habitual, routine, and even unconscious. This chapter is about plants that influence the effects of lifestyle choices, be they conscious or habitual.

The use of medicinal plants, like the choice to use any healing modality, is a lifestyle choice. People choose to use medicinal plants for many reasons. They may use the plant in healing because everyone in their family has used a particular plant for a particular health concern for generations. People may choose to use plant medicines because they have heard of their medicinal benefits. People use plants not only for producing sensations of contentment, comfort, stimulation, and healing, but also when seeking euphoria and inebriation. Plants are used deliberately to alter consciousness and change the state of the mind and soul. Some plants have a unique quality of providing people with the altering experiences they desire. Man has been unable to synthetically manufacture any chemical that satisfies people's euphoric cravings (Lewin, 1998) as do certain plants. Plants such as tobacco with its mentally stimulating action and plant substances such as alcohol and opiates have played a role in the lives of people since they began to seek pleasure when they no longer only had to be concerned with their day-to-day survival.

What causes people to seek pleasure from plants? For some, curiosity is their motivation because they have heard that certain plants can induce different mental states. In addition to seeking out the health benefits of a particular plant, people also use plants to produce a change in their state of mind. For example, they may choose a plant to induce relaxation of the mind and give a temporary surcease from life stressors. Motivations for using plants in this way, as well as reactions to the plants, vary for the individual. For example, it is not exactly understood why one person readily becomes addicted to alcohol while another can easily drink alcoholic beverages in moderation without ever having a hint of craving. Is it the fermented plant beverage that is the cause?

Some plants are known to easily cause habituation, a state whereby the user *adapts* to the effects of the plant. In developing a habitual response to a plant, "the subjective manifestation of the senses, the response to the influence exercised, slowly disappears" (Lewin, 1998, p. 11). Lewin (1998) writes that every person has their "toxic equation" or the "greater or lesser sensibility of the body or its organs to the effects of various chemical substances" (p. 8). As a part of the normal course of daily life, the body seeks to adapt to stressors from the environment. Plants such as opiates challenge the body in such a way as to create a new level of equilibrium, or adaptation, whereby the stressor, the opiate, is no longer a stressor. The new level of equilibrium is only challenged when the plant substance is not present in certain amounts in the body. Because the body quickly adapts to a certain level of tolerance for having the plant substance in the body as part of the internal environment, the internal ecosystem becomes unbalanced when the substance is withdrawn. The body then craves the substance as it seeks to regain balance.

The question still remains whether or not it is only the plant substance or chemical constituents that cause habituation and addiction. "As a matter of course, the cause which produces the phenomenon of habit cannot at the same time be the reason of the habit itself: this must be sought for in the individual concerned" (Lewin, 1998, p. 15). Genetic predisposition, personal choice, and environmental factors are involved in the etiology of substance abuse. Three major substances—tobacco, marijuana, and alcohol—are identified in this chapter as plants and plant substances that have been targeted as causative agents in habituation and addiction. Also included in this chapter are plants that have been shown to have a healing effect on the body that has become habituated or addicted to certain substances. Milk thistle and kudzu are included for this reason.

This chapter discusses both the medicinal and recreational use of the plants profiled. Plants continue to play a major role in the lifestyle choices of people, communities, and countries. While one country may ban the use of a particular plant or plant product for recreational and/or medicinal use because of its mind-altering properties, other countries exert no controls. Often nurses are involved in the health problems their patients may experience with the recreational use of plant substances.

The generally held view that the use of certain plant substances is a moral and social concern rather than a health concern has kept some plants from being accepted and used for health care reasons, even in light of the scientific evidence of their therapeutic benefits (Mack & Joy, 2000). The use of substances, particularly marijuana, has been a cause of addiction difficulties for some people, but not for all people. Nevertheless, decisions regarding their use for any reason have been based on social policy and laws directed by a culture's value orientation and not necessarily by medical and empiric science. Some countries hold the belief that substances that pose a problem for some people should be prohibited for all people (Sullivan, 1995). The problematic use of certain plant substances has been viewed as a bad behavior and moral failing on the part of the individual user that can be corrected by society taking away the substance. And because all too often health care professionals ignore alcohol and substance abuse issues and addiction as health care problems, decisions regarding any use of these substances have been shifted into the hands of publicly employed administrators who determine and legislate the laws governing their use (Murphy-Parker & Martinez, 2000).

Expensive and disturbing social problems are directly due to plant and plant product substance dependence. Studies show that 40% to 60% of people treated for alcohol and drug abuse issues do return to active substance abuse within a year following treatment. It is speculated that an implication of this disappointing result confirms the fact that health care professionals, including nurses, do not believe addiction is a medical illness that can be significantly and positively helped by interventions in health care (McLellan, Lewis, O'Brien, & Kleber, 2000).

It is very important that nurses understand the difference between addiction, what causes addiction, and how the use of substances that may cause addiction also can have beneficial effects in persons who have certain health concerns. It is also important that nurses know that treatment is available for a disease that may have begun as a simple curiosity or a lifestyle choice and that the treatment may include medicinal herbs. Effective medications are available today for treating the significant and lasting changes neurobiologically caused by the excessive use of nicotine, alcohol, and opiates. In the United States, the Physicians' Leadership on National Drug Policy

(1998) states that addiction to alcohol and illicit drugs can be treated with as much success as illnesses like asthma, hypertension, and diabetes. Nurses need to include in their perspective on plant substance use as a lifestyle choice, the fact that many of the plants and plant substances that people use have been used in cultural rituals of all kinds for centuries without leading to dependence and habituation. Plants are often part of spirit-seeking behavior.

Alcoholic beverages are called "spirits." Red wine, for example, continues to be used as part of Christian sacramental ritual. Plants, including psychoactive plants, have been used in the facilitation of spiritual experience for centuries throughout the world. Shamanic traditions "involve non-ordinary states of consciousness induced by a variety of methods including ingesting hallucinogenic plants, drumming, fasting, wilderness vision questing, use of sweat lodges and others" (Metzner, 1998, p. 333). Opiates, tobacco, and marijuana are smoked. Burning plants such as the resin, frankincense, as incense and making smoke have been used in many spiritual rituals as a way of connecting with spirit. Perhaps those who smoke are, at some level of their beings, trying to connect with a higher spirit.

People also engage in the use of tobacco, marijuana, and alcohol as part of social rituals. These plant substances are used as a way of connecting with others. People talk together while they smoke or share a bottle of wine. One common ritual in families is the making of wine. Wine has a history of use that began between 5400 and 5000 B.C. (Soleas et al., 1997). My New Englander mother made dandelion wine that was extraordinary. I remember the yellow flower heads floating as they fermented in the big tub in the basement and then having a small glass of this unique wine on special occasions.

The family of my Hispanic friend from Colorado makes choke cherry wine as part of their family tradition. Years ago my friend's grandmother made the wine to sell because they didn't have much money. Every August they picked the cherries, using their horses to haul the cherries home. At one point, someone reported the grandmother for illegally making wine. A man arrived at their home one day to investigate exactly how the wine was being made. The investigator watched the process and then decided that the wine was fine and dropped the case. The recipe for that special wine is included here.

Choke Cherry Wine

Wash the fruit and remove stems. Use equal amounts of choke cherries and water. It is best to use warm water. Place the fruit and water in a crock or large container that has a cover. Add sugar, using one half the amount of fruit. Add a pinch of dry yeast. Stir well and cover the batch.

Stir the batter *each day* and let sit. The batter will get frothy and remain so for approximately one week. The wine is "working" as long as it is frothy or active (bubbles come from the bottom of the bottle). In approximately one week, you will notice that it is no longer frothing. At this point, you should begin breaking down the cherries with your hands. This is a tiresome job, squishing and squeezing the cherries, but you want the flavor and the rich color of the choke cherries in the wine. After the cherries have been squeezed, use a colander to strain out the liquid. You may add a little water to ensure you get as much flavor from the fruit as possible.

Strain all of the batter and discard the solids such as the seeds and skins. Taste the wine for flavor. You may wish to add a small amount of sugar to suit your taste. Strain the liquid through a cheesecloth and place the wine in jugs or in the original container used. The wine will continue working (bubbling) for days. You will note that sediment collects on the bottom of the container. This will strain out through the cheesecloth.

Strain the wine at least every three days. Again, taste the wine and check the flavor. When no more sediment is on the bottom of the container, your wine may be placed in wine bottles. We recommend loosely placing the corks or tops of the bottles because the wine will continue working for several weeks, and pressure will build inside the bottle. Once there is no sediment, the wine is ready for you to enjoy. This recipe can be used to make other flavors of wine, such as grape, strawberry, or apricot.

From our home to yours, we hope that you will enjoy this delicious wine, and we ask that alcohol be used in a responsible manner.
(Used with permission of Mrs. Cleo Martinez, 2000.)

In an ideal world, people would always use plant substances responsibly or not at all. Responsible use is not just determined by the plant and whether or not its constituents are addicting or whether or not the user is susceptible to addiction. Habituation and addiction as illness are also a result of personal behavior and disposition. The way in which a plant is used, misused, or abused depends on the nature or constitution, personality, and spirit of the user and the motivation for use. In sum, the role of a plant in the lifestyle choices of individual people is an expression of the relationship between the person and the plant.

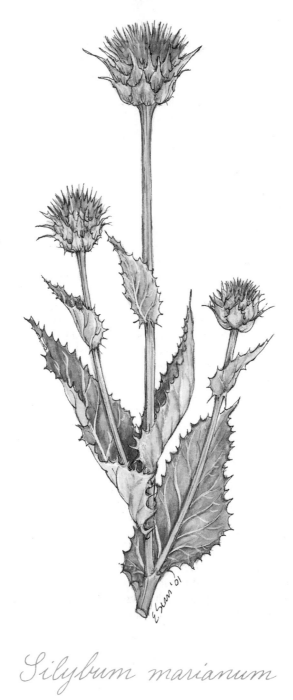

Silybum marianum

Milk Thistle

🍃 **LATIN NAME:** *Silybum marianum* (Its former name, *Carduus marianus L.,* is still used on some products.)

🍃 **FAMILY:** Asteraceae

🍃 **COMMON NAMES:** Milk thistle, holy thistle, Mary thistle, St. Mary's thistle, Marian thistle, lady's thistle
  Note: Do not confuse this plant with blessed thistle, *Cnicus benedictus.*

🍃 **HEALTH PATTERN:** Lifestyle choices

🍃 **PLANT DESCRIPTION:**
Milk thistle has one or more prickly green stalks 3 to 6 feet (1 to 2 meters) high, with stiff wavy leaves that have spines at the margins. The leaves are a deep, glossy green with milk-white veins. The top of the stalk bears a thistlelike head, or flower, consisting of many prickles and purple, threadlike petals. The flowers appear in July and August, and the seeds mature soon after. The plant has numerous tiny seeds, glossy brown to black, with a cocoalike odor and an oily taste. Milk thistle is often found on waste ground, especially by buildings and ditches, old pastures, and roadsides. Milk thistle is indigenous to the Mediterranean area and southwestern Europe. It has been cultivated for centuries as a food and traditional medicine. It is naturalized in North America, especially in California (Leung & Foster, 1996).

🍃 **PLANT PARTS USED:**
The fruit, known as "achenes," which are commonly, but mistakenly, called "seeds," are used medicinally. (Note to reader: This text uses the vernacular and refers to milk thistle fruit as seed.) The leaf is used also, but some ethnobotanists do not consider it to be as effective medicinally (Foster & Tyler, 1999).

🍃 **TRADITIONAL EVIDENCE:**
Cultural Use
  European. Although milk thistle seed is not readily extracted in water, Germany has licensed milk thistle seed infusion for use in digestive disorders, especially for functional disturbances of the biliary system. It has been widely used in Germany for chronic hepatitis and for fatty liver (cirrhosis) that is often associated with alcoholism (Blumenthal, Goldberg, & Brinckman, 2000). European use of milk thistle includes supportive treatment for chronic inflammatory liver disorders, including chronic hepatitis and liver damage due to alcoholism, pharmaceutical drugs, and chemical pollutants. Whereas an infusion of milk thistle is used in Europe in supportive treatment of *Amanita*

mushroom poisoning (Leung & Foster, 1996), many practitioners choose to recommend injectable preparations or oral standardized extracts of milk thistle.

Culinary Use

Historically, milk thistle was grown in Europe as a food source. The roots can be eaten after being soaked overnight to remove the bitterness. The seeds are roasted and used as a coffee substitute (Leung & Foster, 1996) or mixed with sea salt for use as a condiment. Milk thistle seed is high in protein and linoleic acid. The stalks of the milk thistle plant can be peeled and eaten raw or cooked. The young tender leaves can be eaten in salads or steamed and eaten as a vegetable after the spines on the edges of the leaf are cut off. The heads of the milk thistle can be boiled and eaten like artichokes.

Use in Herbalism

Traditionally, the milk-white veins in the leaves of the milk thistle are said to have been created when the milk of the Virgin Mary fell upon the plant. For this reason, milk thistle is sometimes called "Our Lady's thistle" (Grieve, 1971) and the plant is used in promoting production of breast milk in nursing mothers. Milk thistle leaves have been used since the time of the Romans to treat various ailments, including liver problems. Some people use milk thistle preparations from leaf or seed as an alterative to restore the function of the liver and support its ongoing detoxification/blood filtering processes. During the latter nineteenth and early twentieth centuries in the United States, American Eclectic physicians used milk thistle for liver, spleen, and kidney disorders.

Other traditional uses of the plant include jaundice, pleurisy, edema of the lower extremities, melancholia, hydrophobia, and the plague. More recently, milk thistle has been used in the treatment of hepatitis B and C. Externally, milk thistle has been used as an application for cancerous lesions. Some herbalists use the extract as an accessory in chemotherapy to help offset the hepatotoxic effects of the chemotherapeutic agents (Blumenthal et al., 2000). Milk thistle is useful for treating a wide variety of inflammatory conditions of the skin including psoriasis (Pedersen, 1998). The young tender shoots have been eaten boiled as a springtime blood "cleanser" (Grieve, 1971).

Some evidence indicates that the level of silymarin, a physiologically active constituent of milk thistle, necessary to survive contact with digestive juices and be able to enter the bloodstream via the intestinal wall is not achieved by taking teas made from the milk thistle seed. Because silymarin is not very soluble in water and is poorly absorbed from the gastrointestinal tract, a concentrated, standardized extract or injectable form of the plant (mostly available in Europe) often is used to provide the desired effects (Blumenthal et al., 2000; Foster & Tyler, 1999). The commercial preparations usually are standardized to a 70% or 80% concentration of silymarin. Milk thistle standardized extract has been used extensively in people who have liver disease as a result of viruses, exposure to toxic chemicals, or consuming too much alcohol, ibuprofen, or acetaminophen.

Cosmetic Use. Silymarin is being researched for use in dermatology and cosmetics to reduce superficial inflammation of the skin and promote hydration and elasticity in aging skin (Bombardelli, Spelta, Della Loggia, Sosa, & Tubaro, 1990).

🍃 BIOMEDICAL EVIDENCE:

Milk thistle, primarily silmarin in standardized extract form, has been studied extensively. Studies show that milk thistle can normalize liver enzyme levels and regenerate the liver while improving discomfort related to liver diseases such as cirrhosis and hepatitis. Most studies have been done on the standardized extract form of milk thistle. Reviews of the clinical data on milk thistle conclude that while the traditional use of milk thistle in the care of those with liver-related illness seems to be supported by some biomedical studies, there are some limitations to the conclusions that can be drawn because some of the studies had small samples, different types and severities of liver diseases presented in a single study, inconsistencies in control groups, and/or variable end points in the studies (Flora, Hahn, Rosen, & Benner, 1998). Another limitation of the studies evaluating milk thistle for use in alcoholism is that the investigators did not necessarily control alcohol use by participants during the studies and therefore the outcomes of the studies (often milk thistle found ineffective) are suspect. All in all, studies have shown that milk thistle (primarily silymarin) can be effective in the care of those with both acute and chronic viral-, drug-, and toxin-induced and alcoholic hepatitis (Flora et al., 1998).

Studies Related to Lifestyle Choices

In a double-blind, placebo-controlled trial, the mortality of 46 patients with alcoholic cirrhosis ($N = 170$), was markedly reduced in those who received 140 mg of oral silymarin three times a day for about two years. No side effects were reported. Although there were no significant differences in demographic and disease-related characteristics between placebo and treatment groups, the results of the study may have been influenced by the fact that the patients in the placebo group were considered sicker as demonstrated by higher bilirubin levels and higher severity score upon admission to the study. Another significant factor is that some of the subjects continued to drink alcohol while participating in the study (Ferenci et al., 1989). In a conflicting study of 125 patients in which 57 received silymarin, 150 mg three times per day for alcoholic cirrhosis, the data suggested that silymarin has no effect on survival rates or clinical course in alcoholics as compared with placebo. The participants in this study were advised to stop drinking alcohol but were not required to do so (Pares et al., 1998).

One German double-blind study of subjects who suffered from alcohol-induced liver disease found that 31 of 66 subjects who received 420 mg per day of a standardized preparation of silymarin had serum glutamic-oxalacetic transaminase (SGOT), serum glutamic-pyruvic transaminase (SGPT), and gamma-GT levels that returned to normal more quickly than controls (Fintelmann & Albert as reported in Blumenthal et al., 2000).

Studies Related to Other Health Patterns

Restoration. Death from poisoning due to mushroom ingestion is most often related to the *Amanita phalloides* species. More than 150 case reports have recorded the efficacy of silybin, a constituent of silymarin, as infusion therapy in significantly lowering death rates in patients with *Amanita* poisoning (Schulz, Hansel, & Tyler, 1998).

In vitro studies have shown that silymarin, a constituent of milk thistle, has demonstrated hepatoprotective activities against drug toxicity, such as acetaminophen-induced toxicity (Shear et al., 1995). Oral silymarin, 800 mg per day, significantly reduced the lipoperoxidative hepatic damage that occurs as a result of treatment with butyrophenones or phenothiazines, in those participants who received the herbal constituent for ninety days during a double-blind, placebo-controlled trial of 60 participants (Palasciano et al., 1994).

Immune Response. Hepatitis C virus infection has been estimated to be the most common cause of chronic liver disease, cirrhosis, and liver cancer in Western countries (Di Bisceglie et al., 1991). Silymarin has been used as a supportive therapy in the treatment of hepatitis C for years. One double-blind, placebo-controlled study demonstrated that silymarin (Legalon), 420 mg per day, in 77 patients, significantly reduced the normalization time of the liver after being diagnosed with acute viral hepatitis (forty-three days in placebo group and twenty-nine days in treatment group) as measured by biologic tests such as SGPT, SGOT, and bilirubin. Recuperation time was significantly faster and shorter in the treatment group. The frequency of rebounds in participants' SGPT levels was diminished when silymarin was taken (Plomteux, Albert, & Heusgehm, 1977).

Another randomized study of the effect of IdB 1016 (Silipide) in the treatment of 60 participants with viral and alcoholic hepatitis, who were divided into three groups and given different doses of Silipide, found significant decreases in mean serum activity of aspartate aminotransferase ($p < .001$) and total bilirubin ($p < .05$ to .001) at all dose levels of 80 mg twice a day, 120 mg twice a day, and 120 mg three times a day. The two higher doses also resulted in decreases in alanine aminotransferase and gamma-glutamyl transpeptidase, thus leading to the conclusion that IdB 1016 may be significantly beneficial in the treatment of viral and alcoholic hepatitis (Vailati et al., 1993).

An earlier study (Bode, Schmidt, & Durr, 1977) found no significant effects of silymarin (Legalon), two 70 mg tablets three times daily for a total of 420 mg per day in participants with viral hepatitis ($N = 151$), but this study has since been discredited as having serious methodological flaws (Magliulo, Gagliardi, & Fiori, 1978). Magliulo et al. (1978) demonstrated that oral doses of 420 mg of silymarin did reduce bilirubin, SGOT, and SGPT levels in 28 patients ($N = 57$) with acute viral hepatitis.

Hormone Balance. In a randomized, controlled trial, the mean daily blood glucose levels and mean daily insulin requirements decreased significantly in those of 30 noninsulin-dependent diabetic patients with alcoholic liver cirrhosis who received silymarin therapy along with their standard treatment, including insulin, as compared with the nontreatment group of 30 patients who received standard therapy alone. The treatment group received a standardized extract of silymarin, 200 mg, orally three times a day for 12 months, in addition to standard therapy. SGOT and SGPT levels also decreased significantly in the treatment group ($p < .01$) (Velussi et al., 1997).

Skin Care. In vitro studies have shown that silymarin may be effective in the prevention and treatment of skin cancer (Zi & Agarwal, 1999).

Mechanism of Action

The hepatoprotective and other health benefits of milk thistle primarily have been identified as resulting from silymarin, one constituent in milk thistle, and silybin, silydianin, and silychristin constituents in silymarin. Silymarin has two main methods of action: (1) its antioxidant action is thought to alter the structure of the cell membranes of hepatocytes to prevent entrance of the liver toxin into the cells, and (2) it stimulates the liver's regenerative ability and the formation of new hepatocytes by stimulating protein synthesis (Blumenthal et al., 2000; Brinker, 1998; Foster & Tyler, 1999).

Silymarin has been shown to increase the glutathione content of the liver by more than 35% in healthy volunteers. Glutathione is the compound responsible for detoxifying a wide range of toxic chemicals, pesticides, and heavy metals, including mercury, lead, cadmium, and arsenic (Werbach & Murray, 1994). Silymarin has strong free-radical scavenging (antioxidant) activity, ten times stronger than vitamin E (Leung & Foster, 1996). In one study, it was found by measuring participants' SGTP levels that approximately 60% of patients with alcoholic cirrhosis still consumed significant (although varying) quantities of alcohol during the trial; data suggest that the effect of the silymarin is most likely due to the prevention of toxic or metabolic effects of alcohol on the liver rather than to some antabuse-type property (Ferenci et al., 1989).

Milk thistle has been shown to lower cholesterol and decrease fat deposits in the liver of animals (Wren, 1988). The anticarcinogenic activities of the milk thistle constituent silymarin have been found in human cell in vitro studies to be due to the silybinin component of silymarin (Bhatia, Zhao, Wolf, & Agarwal, 1999).

USE IN PREGNANCY OR LACTATION:

One source considers milk thistle safe for use in pregnancy (McGuffin, Hobbs, Upton, & Goldberg, 1997). Because of the ability of milk thistle to facilitate the onset of menstruation, Brinker reports that it is not recommended during pregnancy. However, in one study, silymarin was safely used by six pregnant women with intrahepatic cholestasis. The standardized extract was taken at a dosage of 210 mg three times daily for fifteen days with no ill effects (Brinker, 1998, p. 181). There are no known contraindications to the use of milk thistle during lactation (Blumenthal et al., 2000), and the plant has a long history of use by breastfeeding women to promote lactation.

Herbal Caveat—Pregnancy or Lactation

Some herbs are contraindicated in pregnancy because of a risk of the herb or one of its constituents stimulating the uterus and therefore possibly promoting fetal loss. Many herbal practitioners do not recommend herbal remedies, in particular oral doses of herbs, during the first trimester of pregnancy and seek an alternative. However, herbs are successfully used during pregnancy, especially to prepare the body for the birth. Herbs are relatively unstudied in pregnancy and lactation, so patients need to be made aware through education of the potential benefits and risks of using herbs for health conditions that arise during pregnancy or lactation. The use of herbal remedies during pregnancy often warrants a referral to a knowledgeable herbal practitioner.

USE FOR CHILDREN:

Other than historical data showing that Dioscorides recommended milk thistle seed tea for infants whose "sinews [tendons] were drawn together" (Grieve, 1971, p. 797), there seems to be little evidence of the use of milk thistle in children. Because children, like adults, are exposed to toxic pollutants, alcohol, and pharmaceuticals, it might be beneficial to study the long-term effects of hepatoprotective milk thistle in health promotion in young people. In the meantime, if there are no milk thistles around, children can be introduced to the flavonoids and lignans that may be responsible for the hepatoprotective effects of milk thistle by eating artichokes *(Cynara cardunculus subsp. Cardunculus)*. Artichokes are a relative of milk thistle and are very similar. Some children really like them and can learn a lot about herbs and plants from eating them leaf by leaf. I was a child who loved to eat artichokes. My grandmother used to love to tell the story that on my third birthday we went to a restaurant where the waiter asked what I wanted for dinner. My answer was artichokes. Children, given a little milk to drink after eating an artichoke, are surprised by how sweet the milk tastes!

CAUTIONS:

There are no known cautions for the use of milk thistle. The medicinal components are excreted quickly from the body. One study found that silybin, the main component of silymarin found in milk thistle, given orally 140 mg three times a day, was fully excreted from the body within 72 hours (Lorenz, Mennicke, Behrendt, 1982). A mild laxative effect has occasionally been noticed with the use of milk thistle extracts standardized to 70% to 80% silymarin (Blumenthal et al., 2000), presumably because of its stimulating effects on bile secretion. This herb can lower blood sugar, so diabetics taking this herb are cautioned to watch their blood sugar levels closely.

Although milk thistle has been shown to be a natural regenerator of liver tissue, nurses must advise patients that its use is not a substitute for lifestyle changes, such as alcohol abstinence or alcohol consumption reduction, that are necessary to promote healthy liver function. Inappropriate use of milk thistle includes the use of the plant to rationalize drinking alcohol to excess.

NURSING EVIDENCE:

Historical Nursing Use

No data are available at this time.

Potential Nursing Applications

Nurses who work in substance abuse programs and in occupational and public health settings might want to consider integrating the use of milk thistle seed standardized extract into health promotion programs for patients whose livers may be compromised from exposure to excessive amounts of alcohol and/or environmental toxins. If the cost of the standardized extract is prohibitive, consider milk thistle tea. Analyses of milk thistle tea have found about 10% of the original levels of silymarin in the milk thistle seed (Blumenthal et al, 2000).

Integrative Insight

Nurses work with patients with diseased livers. Whether their illness is caused by alcoholism or hepatitis, these patients are very sick, and often nurses can feel that there is little help or hope. Traditional and biomedical evidence supports the use of liquid alcohol extracts and standardized extracts of milk thistle in the care of these patients. Milk thistle is able to regenerate the liver, and the herb is readily excreted from the body and has not been shown to be toxic. So why aren't more people with serious diseases such as alcoholism and hepatitis informed about the potential benefits of milk thistle? Nurses need to ask these types of questions and find creative ways to integrate the use of milk thistle into health promotion, substance abuse treatment, and public health programs.

Nurses are becoming more aware of the importance that a healthy environment has on the health and well-being of people. Because of the identification of increasing numbers of chemicals in people's bodies, which are not endogenously produced, questions are being raised as to the health effects of the numerous synthetic chemicals found in the environment. Nurses might want to consider exploring, with interdisciplinary research teams, the ability of plants, such as milk thistle, to assist in the detoxification of harmful chemicals from the body.

THERAPEUTIC APPLICATIONS:

Oral

Infusion. Infuse 3.5 g of seeds in 5 oz (150 ml) boiled water for ten to fifteen minutes. Drink three to four times daily one-half hour before meals. (Medicinal components of milk thistle are not easily extracted in water.)

Standardized Extract. Take 1 capsule of milk thistle seed standardized extract containing 100 to 200 mg of silymarin twice daily, or 1 capsule of milk thistle with 140 mg of silymarin two to three times daily. Must be taken with plenty of water.

Tincture. 15 to 25 drops four to five times daily or $\frac{1}{4}$ teaspoon (1 to 2 ml) three times daily (Blumenthal et al., 2000)

Topical

Specific Therapy for *Amanita* Mushroom Poisoning. "The recommended regimen is infusion therapy with a silybin derivative [brand name Legalon SIL sold in the United States as Thisilyn]. The manufacturer recommends a total dose of 20 mg silybin per kg body weight over a 24-hr period, divided into 4 infusions, each administered over a 2-hr period" (Schulz, 1998, p. 218).

Environmental

No data are available at this time.

Herbal Caveat—Therapeutic Applications

In traditional and conventional herbal medicine, amounts of herbs given to patients are based on individual needs. The amounts or "doses" recorded here are provided so that the health practitioner has a general idea of the amounts recommended for an adult patient. Dosing in herbalism not only refers to amount of plant used but also includes when, where, and how to take a plant medicine. These dosages should not be used as guidelines for indiscriminate intervention without proper assessment, critical thinking, and patient education on the part of the practitioner.

Note: Please see chapter 5 for detailed descriptions of how to prepare various applications.

PATIENT INTERACTION:

Milk thistle fruit (seed) has significantly more silymarin, the active constituent in the plant, than the leaves. Milk thistle immature flowers or buds have a long history of use as a food (like an artichoke) and as a medicinal plant often used for regenerating liver tissue that has been harmed by diseases such as hepatitis and cirrhosis and by industrial and environmental toxins. It also has been shown to be helpful for alcoholics with liver impairment but has not been shown to decrease the desire for alcohol. Milk thistle seeds are not extracted very easily into water, so this remedy often is taken as a liquid alcohol extract or as a standardized extract in capsule or tablet form. Some countries in Europe have health care providers who give milk thistle in injectable form. There is no known toxicity with this herb, but it can lower blood sugar, so diabetics taking this herb are cautioned to watch their blood sugar levels closely.

Herbal Caveat—Patient Interaction

Patients considering the use of an herb or formula of herbs in self-care benefit from education about the plant itself and the use of the plant in healing. This education can come through many sources, including local herbalists; plant specialists such as botanists; health practitioners such as nurses, nutritionists, naturopaths, and other physicians; and various written references including the scientific literature. Patients need to remember that their unique health care needs are not necessarily represented in any literature they may encounter. Therefore, it is recommended that a knowledgeable mentor be consulted before initiating self-care with any herb being used for the first time.

NURTURING THE NURSE-PLANT RELATIONSHIP:

Note: You may want to keep a journal of your experiences with the herb.

Nurses are often exposed to toxic substances and environments. They may be exposed to toxic chemicals, such as disinfecting solutions, chemotherapeutic agents, and blood and body fluids that carry hepatitis. A healthy liver is very important to a long, healthy life. Nurses can consider caring for their livers by taking milk thistle on occasion to support the body's natural ability to regenerate. Try a liquid alcohol extract or a standardized extract of milk thistle the next time you are exposed to hepatitis, encounter sick building syndrome, or are exposed to a heavy dose of chemicals.

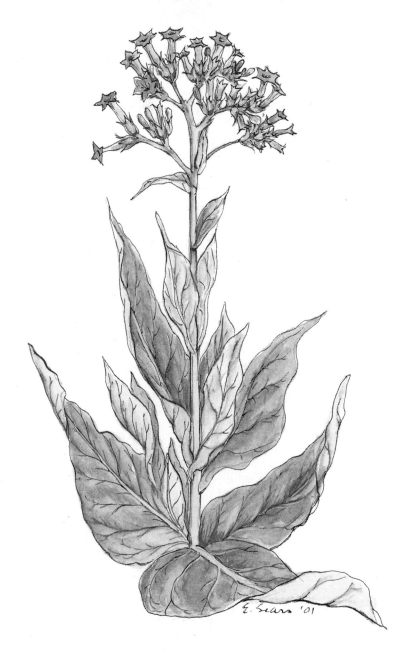

Nicotiana tabacum

Tobacco

🌿 **LATIN NAME:** *Nicotiana tabacum*

🌿 **FAMILY:** Solanaceae

🌿 **COMMON NAMES:** Tobacco, leaf tobacco, tabaci folia
Note: Do not confuse this plant with Indian tobacco or wild tobacco *(Lobelia inflata).*

🌿 **HEALTH PATTERN:** Lifestyle choices

🌿 **PLANT DESCRIPTION:**
Tobacco *(Nicotiana)* is named after Jean Nicot (1530-1600), a Portuguese who introduced the plant to France (Grieve, 1971). Tobacco is an annual with a long, fibrous root. The leaves are pale green, alternate, ovate, and pointed, and are 1 to 2 feet long ($\frac{1}{2}$ meter) and 6 inches (15 cm) across. An erect, round, hairy, 4 to 6 foot (1 to 2 meters) stem protrudes from the center of the plant and produces a rose colored flower. English tobacco produces a greenish yellow flower (Culpeper, 1990). The leaves have a bitter, acrid taste. There are several variations of this plant. Those cultivated for smoking are *N. attenuata, N. rustica,* and *N. tabacum.* Plants with darker leaves are stronger and more powerful than those with light colored leaves. The strongest and most common type is raised in the United States in Virginia, but the Cuban leaf is preferred by some smokers (Felter & Lloyd, 1983).

🌿 **PLANT PART USED:** Cured and dried leaf

🌿 **TRADITIONAL EVIDENCE:**
Cultural Use

North American Indian. Tobacco is used primarily for ceremonial purposes such as smoking of the peace pipe and to ward off evil influences (DeSmet, 1997; Vogel, 1970). Tobacco also has been used in gift giving.

Hispanic. Tobacco is known as "picietl," "hierba yetl," and "tabaco." The fresh leaves of tobacco are inhaled to cure stuffy nose. The leaves are mixed with sheep fat to treat *dolor de ardo,* heat pain. Tobacco is placed in a newborn's navel after the cord falls off (Kay, 1996).

The Mestizo shamans of South America heal with perfume. They sometimes perform *florecer* (meaning to blossom or make whole), in which they take perfume in their mouth, inhale tobacco smoke, and then spray both out on the patient. The shaman's breath is considered sacred (Lawless, 1998). The Aztecs used tobacco in combination with other herbs as a remedy for diarrhea and as an abdominal purge. The Mayans used it for asthma, bites and stings, bowel problems, chills and fever, convulsions, nervous complaints, sore eyes, skin diseases, and urinary ailments.

African. Tobacco is smoked (usually in a pipe) but also is chewed, sniffed (solid form or liquefied) and snuffed (pinch between the lower lip and gum). *N. rustica* has higher levels of nicotine and is popular with Africans. Tobacco has important cultural significance with some tribes. The Tabwa people use it in marriage proposal negotiations, and it is used as a mourning gift. Other groups use it for ceremonial functions and festive occasions (DeSmet, 1997).

East Indian. Tobacco is known as "tambaku" or "tamaku" in Hindi. It is used in the form of cigars, cigarettes, veedees beedies, and cheroots for smoking. It also is used as snuff and is chewed or mixed with molasses to form "tamak." A paste of tobacco powder or snuff with castor oil is applied externally to an infant's navel to relieve colic. Tobacco decoction is applied externally to swollen joints to relieve pain. A poultice of the leaves is applied to the spine of patients with tetanus. Because Indians have observed that no snakes pass through tobacco fields, they use the plant to induce vomiting in people with snake bites (Nadkarni, 1976).

European. The Spaniards brought tobacco to Europe when they returned from America in 1492 (Felter & Lloyd, 1983). Sir Walter Raleigh introduced tobacco in England in 1586 and was initially met with violent opposition. Because it was used as a cure for a variety of ailments, 300 years later, in 1885, the leaves were officially included in the British *Pharmacopeia* (Grieve, 1971).

In Anthroposophical medicine, tobacco has been used safely in homeopathic form where it is chemically undetectable. Homeopathic tobacco is used for its energetic qualities of influencing the musculature of the vascular and respiratory systems, facilitating exhalation, and regulating the activity of the astral body (Husemann & Wolff, 1982).

Culinary Use

Tobacco has no culinary use.

Use in Herbalism

Tobacco leaf has been used medicinally. It is chewed, smoked, snuffed, used topically, and injected either as a smoke or an "infusion" into the rectum (like an enema). Chewing tobacco was the major form of tobacco consumption before the invention of matches. The development of a convenient source of flame in the late 1800s also contributed to the spread of the use of tobacco cigarettes as part of people's daily lifestyle rather than their just using it occasionally as medicine (Slade, 1992). Medicinally, tobacco has been used as a sedative narcotic, diuretic, expectorant, emetic, and antiseptic (Felter & Lloyd, 1983; Grieve, 1971). A tobacco wine has been used for habitual constipation, obstinate hiccough, and tetanus. Tobacco enemas were used historically for impacted cecum, intussusception, and strangulated hernia. Asthmatics and emphysemics smoked tobacco on occasion to relieve the spasms associated with their diseases (Bartholow, 1878).

Externally, a tobacco infusion or ointment has been used for scabies, tinea, and other skin infections. Tobacco smoke blown into the ear is used for earache and headache. Tobacco leaf, either used directly on the skin or as a salve, continues to be used by the people in the Appalachian mountains for insect bites and stings (Crellin & Pilpott, 1990). Although tobacco has a history of medicinal use, even as the "most effective remedy" for illness such as tetanus (Bartholow, 1878, p. 419), few if any herbalists recommend its use. Although tobacco products are one of the leading plant products on the market, herbal texts rarely include tobacco in their materia medica. This is because, over the years, tobacco has been replaced by other safer and more effective plant remedies.

BIOMEDICAL EVIDENCE:

Biomedical research has focused on the study of tobacco products such as cigarettes. Tobacco products may contain a number of chemicals that are additives to the product and not necessarily part of the plant. These additives also have significant effects on the health of the user and must be taken into account when studying the effects of tobacco products. Most of the biomedical evidence has supported the clinical findings that the risks of using tobacco and tobacco products significantly outweigh the benefits associated with tobacco and nicotine use. The data presented here are the results of those epidemiologic studies. No human clinical trials were found that explored the traditional uses of tobacco in healing.

Recently, tobacco has been appearing in the biomedical literature for a new reason. The tobacco plant is being studied for its ability to replace expensive bacterial hosts in the production of designer monoclonal antibodies through genetic alteration of the plant. "The expanding field of genetic engineering is putting tobacco into service to humanity" (Lewis, 1996, p. 122).

Studies Related to Lifestyle Choice

Tobacco products, including cigarettes, cigars, and loose tobacco for pipe smoking and chewing, have been used for decades. The evidence that the recreational, as opposed to medicinal, smoking of tobacco is medically harmful "has been accumulating for 200 years" (Doll, 1999, p. 90). Tobacco cigarette smoking has been positively associated with almost forty diseases or causes of death and is negatively associated with eight more (Doll, 1999). These diseases include cancer, heart disease, chronic bronchitis, asthma, arteriosclerosis, and pneumonia. Some diseases statistically occur less often than expected and may be prevented in smokers because of some of the constituents in tobacco. These include Parkinson's disease, ulcerative colitis, allergic alveolitis, fibroids, nausea and vomiting during pregnancy, and preeclampsia (Doll, 1999). In a retrospective study of over 100,000 registered nurses, respondents smoking 1 to 24 cigarettes per day had twice the risk, and those smoking 25 or more cigarettes per day had four times the risk of depression and committing suicide (Hemenway, Solnick, & Colditz, 1993).

Some evidence indicates that the nicotine in tobacco improves cognitive function and may reduce symptoms of Tourette's syndrome and attention deficit hyperactivity disorder (ADHD) (Shytle, Silver, & Sanberg, 1996). However, smoking and nicotine do not improve general learning (Report of the U.S. Surgeon General, 1988).

What does research say about the reasons people smoke tobacco habitually? In the United States for example, "the habitual use of tobacco is related primarily to psychological and social drives, reinforced and perpetuated by the pharmacological actions of nicotine on the central nervous system. Nicotine-free tobacco or other plant materials do not satisfy the needs of those who acquire the tobacco habit" (1964 Surgeon General Report). Tobacco is a vehicle for the administration of nicotine, the plant constituent identified as the primary cause of addiction.

People like to smoke tobacco. The U.S. Surgeon General's Report (1988) identified some reasons why people may smoke despite the risks of disease and despite the fact that nicotine is addicting. The report states that people who smoke weigh less than nonsmokers (on average 7 pounds less) and those who stop smoking often gain weight. Those who smoke often have high stress levels and experience relief from smoking. Nicotine causes skeletal muscles to relax and has cardiovascular and hormonal effects. Although most people experience an unpleasant sensation when they first use tobacco products, tolerance develops and the unpleasant association is no longer perceived.

Data from both industrialized and low-income countries, when taken together, demonstrate that tobacco is estimated to be responsible for an "average of about 3 million deaths a year, with a range of uncertainty of perhaps 2-4 million" (Doll, 1999, p. 97). Tobacco use is the chief avoidable cause of death in the United States (Report of the U.S. Surgeon General, 1988). Yet people continue to smoke and not just cigarettes. Production of cigars in the United States in 1997 was at its highest level since the 1980s (U.S. Centers for Disease Control and Prevention, 1997). Smokeless tobacco also is used extensively. One study found, in a survey of 11,057 adolescents in the southeastern United States, 3726 adolescents reported having tried smokeless tobacco and 17% of those who had tried it reported that they were addicted to it (Riley, Barenie, Woodard, & Mabe, 1996).

Numerous people are affected indirectly by tobacco. Second-hand tobacco smoke, or passive smoking, poses serious health risks, especially to infants, children, and the infirm. Ten epidemiologic studies have identified a 30% increase in the risk of death from ischemic heart disease in nonsmokers who live with smokers (Glantz & Parmley, 1991). Passive smoking decreases the oxygen-carrying capacity of the blood and increases the amount of lactate in venous blood. Animal studies have shown increases in free radical damage to body tissues as a result of second-hand smoke. While the body of the smoker exhibits an adaptive mechanism in regard to free radical damage due to cigarette smoke, the same cannot be said for the nonsmoker. "Chronic exposure to cigarette smoke appears to increase the free radical scavenging systems in smokers, a 'benefit' that nonsmokers would not have when breathing someone else's smoke" (Glantz & Parmley, 1995, p. 149). Passive smoking is the third leading preventable cause of death in the United States after smoking and alcohol (Glantz & Parmley, 1991).

Studies Related to Other Health Patterns

No data are available at this time.

Mechanism of Action

Nicotine, a dominant alkaloid found in tobacco leaf, is a volatile, colorless liquid that has narcotic properties. It affects both central and peripheral nerves. Nicotine diffuses quickly into the bloodstream and can produce depression of the heart and lungs. Stimulants have been used to counteract these effects (Felter & Lloyd, 1983; Nadkarni, 1976). Tobacco vapor is known to cause illness. Its action may be related to the fact that it contains "numerous basic substances of the picolinic series, and cedes to caustic potash, hydrocyanic acid, sulfuretted hydrogen, several volatile fatty acids, phenol, and creosote" (Bartholow, 1878, p. 417).

One study shows a 40% decrease in the level of monoamine oxidase B (MAO B) in the brains of smokers (Fowler et al., 1996). MAO B inhibition is associated with the enhanced activity of dopamine. MAO B reduction is thought to synergize with nicotine to produce the behavioral effects of smoking, such as its performance enhancing properties. This also may explain why cigarettes are a gateway drug and are used by many patients with mental illness and why cigarette smoking is associated with decreased risk of Parkinson's disease (Fowler et al., 1996). Nicotine has been found to stimulate neurons to release dopamine, norepinephrine, and serotonin. Antidepressants have similar actions on the brain, which might explain the high correlation between depression and smoking and the dysphoria experienced when someone attempts to quit using nicotine (Cinciripini, Hecht, Henningfield, Manley, & Kramer, 1997). Antidepressants have proven to be useful for patients who decide to quit smoking whether or not the person is currently depressed (Benowitz, 1997).

USE IN PREGNANCY OR LACTATION:

Use of tobacco in pregnancy is not recommended because of the possibility of lower birth weight and size in neonates. Pregnant women who smoke have a higher risk of miscarriage, and their offspring have a higher risk of prematurity and neurologic impairment (Brinker, 1998). Tobacco is not recommended for nursing mothers because of diminished breast milk production, and excretion of nicotine and by-products in breast milk causes immediate changes in infant respiration and oxygen saturation (Brinker, 1998; Mitchell, Sobel, & Alexander, 1999).

Herbal Caveat—Pregnancy or Lactation
Some herbs are contraindicated in pregnancy because of a risk of the herb or one of its constituents stimulating the uterus and therefore possibly promoting fetal loss. Many herbal practitioners do not recommend herbal remedies, in particular oral doses of herbs, during the first trimester of pregnancy and seek an alternative. However, herbs are successfully used during pregnancy, especially to prepare the body for the birth. Herbs are relatively unstudied in pregnancy and lactation, so patients need to be made aware through education of the potential benefits and risks of using herbs for health conditions that arise during pregnancy or lactation. The use of herbal remedies during pregnancy often warrants a referral to a knowledgeable herbal practitioner.

USE FOR CHILDREN:

Recreational smoking and second-hand smoke, as well as medicinal use of tobacco, are not recommended for children because of the risk of developing cardiovascular conditions, the potential for addiction, and acute nicotine toxicity (Brinker, 1998). Tobacco use prevention programs can be implemented in schools in an effort to reduce the risk to children (U.S. Centers for Disease Control and Prevention, 1994).

Herbal Caveat—Children
Children have special needs in regard to herbal therapies. They require lesser amounts of herbs and often respond well to mild teas and topical applications such as compresses and baths. The lowest dose of oral preparations should be tried first before increasing the amount given children. Caregivers should observe children closely for responses to herbal remedies. Younger children, particularly infants, have traditionally been given herbs either through their mother's breast milk or in the form of a homeopathic remedy because of their sensitivity to medicines and treatments and the immaturity of their liver. It is recommended that a person knowledgeable in the herbal treatment of children be consulted before the offering of any herb to a child for the first time.

CAUTIONS:

Tobacco has a very powerful personality in that it has captured the interest of so many people and become an integral part of their daily life. "It [tobacco] must have properties peculiarly adapted to the propensities of our nature, to have thus surmounted the first repugnance to its odour and taste, and to have become the passion of so many millions" (Wood & Bache, 1839, p. 669). A lethal dose of nicotine, an active constituent in tobacco, is 40 to 100 mg, but this toxic level is greater for individuals who are regular users. Approximately 1 to 2 mg of nicotine is inhaled with each cigarette. Symptoms of acute poisoning include dizziness, salivation, vomiting, diarrhea, trembling of the hands, and a feeling of weakness in the legs. With high dosages, the person may become unconscious and have respiratory and/or cardiac failure. Regular use of tobacco is associated with cancer of the lung, mouth, pharynx, larynx, esophagus, bladder, and pancreas (Brinker, 1998; Mitchell et al., 1999; Wynder, 1988.) Tobacco smoking can exacerbate existing conditions such as ulcers, high blood pressure, diabetes, osteoporosis, blood clots in the legs, glaucoma, heart disease, emphysema, and bronchitis (Brinker, 1998) and also can cause staining of the teeth and loss of taste sensation. Tobacco is easily absorbed through the skin, potentially causing tobacco poisoning (Wren, 1988).

The addictive properties of nicotine in tobacco are well established. The tobacco industry, at least in the United States, also manipulates nicotine levels in cigarettes and adulterates tobacco products with chemicals like ammonia and letulic acid for the sole purpose of creating and sustaining nicotine and cigarette addiction (Cinciripini, 1997). In 1997, the attorneys general of thirty-nine states in the United States settled their claims against the tobacco industry that were related to treating tobacco-related illness (Seffrin, 1998). Billions of dollars were involved in the out-of-court settlement.

Smokeless tobacco is associated with oral cancer, precancerous lesions of the mouth, and cardiovascular disease. People who use smokeless tobacco often have comparable nicotine serum levels to smokers; this should be considered when a patient attempts to cease use of smokeless tobacco (Riley et al., 1996).

Second-hand smoke is defined as a combination of both the smoke from the burning end of a cigarette, cigar, or pipe and the exhaled smoke of the smoker. Breathing second-hand smoke has been linked to numerous diseases, including lung cancer. Children exposed to second-hand smoke are sick more often with illnesses such as asthma, colds, and ear infections. Children are twice as likely to become smokers if one or both of their parents smoke. Babies are harmed by smoke while they are in utero and after they are born. Newborns of smoking mothers are often small for gestational age. Nicotine stays in the breast milk of a nursing mother for up to five hours after she smokes. Tobacco products also pose serious safety hazards to children and adults. Each year in the United States, hundreds of people are killed in fires caused by tobacco smoking (American Academy of Otolaryngology-Head and Neck Surgery Foundation).

NURSING EVIDENCE:

Historical Nursing Use

Family nurses in the early nineteenth century used tobacco ointment to soothe skin conditions such as irritable ulcers and scald-head (Child, 1997).

Potential Nursing Applications

Nurses are often well informed of the health risks of using tobacco; however, nicotine is often the focus of the information given to patients. Nicotine is an invisible constituent in tobacco. People who make the lifestyle choice to use or abuse tobacco often have little or no understanding of the plant or how they can become addicted to it. They have no understanding that the plant was given as a gift and used ceremonially at one time. Although the plant is not treated as sacred, several societal and behavioral rituals surrounding the activity of smoking tobacco still exist.

This profile has been provided to present information about the plant behind this extensive public health issue. Nurses are well positioned to caution people who use tobacco, either medicinally or recreationally, of the health risks known to be associated with the plant. It is especially important that patients who smoke tobacco cigarettes for recreational and sedative effects understand the actual nature of tobacco and tobacco products. Nurses can provide this information.

Nurses also can provide education and support groups for those who wish to quit smoking. One safe approach to quitting involves gradual withdrawal from nicotine by using nicotine gum or the transdermal nicotine patch. In some countries, several nonprescription nicotine replacement agents have been shown to be very effective. "Active patch subjects were more than twice as likely to quit smoking as individuals wearing a placebo patch, and this effect was present at both high and low intensities of counseling" (Fiore, Smith, Jorenby, & Baker, 1994, p. 1940). Antianxiety interventions (deep breathing and relaxation), recommended as part of many stop-smoking programs, have proven helpful to some people. Often the smoker is more relaxed by the deep breathing they perform as part of the smoking ritual than by the chemical constituents of the tobacco itself. The smoker doesn't have to give up their deep breathing moments when they give up the cigarette, pipe, or cigar.

Smoking behavior has an impact on the amount of nicotine absorbed by the body. Cigarettes usually deliver 1 mg of nicotine to the bloodstream of the smoker, but the difference in intake per cigarette (ranging from 0.3 to 3.2 mg per cigarette) in large part depends on the way in which the cigarette is smoked. "When the number of cigarettes available to an individual smoker is reduced from an average of 38 to 5 per day, the intake of nicotine per cigarette increases an average of threefold, a figure consistent with the maximal absolute bioavailability cited, 40 percent" (Benowitz & Henningfield, 1994, p. 124). This is important data for nurses who routinely ask, "How many cigarettes do you smoke in a day?" but do not ask, "How deeply do you inhale?" or "How many puffs do you take on one cigarette?" To thoroughly assess an individual's level of addiction to the tobacco plant, a full behavioral assessment is advised.

Integrative Insight

Although tobacco's medicinal properties were demonstrated for over 150 years, the risk of its use is now thought to outweigh its benefits. With all the plant and pharmaceutical remedies known today, tobacco is not a remedy of choice by health practitioners because of its potentially toxic and addictive nature. What concerns health practitioners is how the use of one plant can cause such extensive damage to a society. The tobacco industry can only sell to those who wish to buy. Despite the fact that the devastating health effects of tobacco use are known, global consumption of tobacco products is on the rise. Even though biomedical science and herbalism concur that tobacco is not a recommended health treatment, the plant is more prevalent in the lives of people than any other herb. Health practitioners have a different challenge with tobacco—how to help people change their behavior and their lifestyle choices. Practitioners who would assist the healing of society's tobacco addiction must first look at their own behaviors.

Many nurses also continue to smoke tobacco. The International Council of Nurses' (ICN) Position Statement on tobacco use and health encourages the integration of information about tobacco and smoking into all nursing curriculae (International Council of Nurses, November, 2000). Nurses need to support each other in the quest to quit. Perhaps the first place to start is to ensure that every nurse is rewarded with a break during the workday to go outside and deep breathe. Often the only nurses exercising this healthy right are those who smoke. Nurses can replace smoking on breaks with deep breathing, relaxation, and socializing with colleagues.

THERAPEUTIC APPLICATIONS:

Note: The therapeutic applications of tobacco presented here are for the most part historical uses.

Oral

The ashes of the burnt herb (English tobacco) can cleanse the gums and make the teeth white (Culpeper, 1990). The leaf of tobacco is smoked as part of a religious ceremony in some cultures.

Topical

Plaster. A wet tobacco leaf applied to piles for 3 to 4 hours provides relief (Felter & Lloyd, 1983).

Environmental

Tobacco is smoked. Tobacco powder is an effective insecticide and molluscicide (Kay, 1996; Grieve, 1971).

Herbal Caveat—Therapeutic Applications

In traditional and conventional herbal medicine, amounts of herbs given to patients are based on individual needs. The amounts or "doses" recorded here are provided so that the health practitioner has a general idea of the amounts recommended for an adult patient. Dosing in herbalism not only refers to amount of plant used but also includes when, where, and how to take a plant medicine. These dosages should not be used as guidelines for indiscriminate intervention without proper assessment, critical thinking, and patient education on the part of the practitioner.

Note: Please see chapter 5 for detailed descriptions of how to prepare various applications.

PATIENT INTERACTION:

Tobacco is used ceremonially in some cultures. Although tobacco was used medicinally for almost two centuries, the risks of using tobacco therapeutically outweigh the benefits. It is not considered the remedy of choice today when numerous other plant medicines or pharmaceutical alternatives are as or more effective with less toxicity. Many people are familiar with this plant because they have been exposed to the recreational use of this plant in the form of cigarettes, cigars, and chewing tobacco. Most people who smoke do so for the sedative effect. Unfortunately, tobacco contains a highly addictive constituent called "nicotine" that has numerous potentially deadly side effects. Other forms of relaxation are recommended. Nurses can provide information and resources for those who wish to stop smoking tobacco. They also can provide education in relaxation techniques that can be used as an alternative to the sedative effects of smoking.

Herbal Caveat—Patient Interaction

Patients considering the use of an herb or formula of herbs in self-care benefit from education about the plant itself and the use of the plant in healing. This education can come through many sources, including local herbalists; plant specialists such as botanists; health practitioners such as nurses, nutritionists, naturopaths, and other physicians; and various written references including the scientific literature. Patients need to remember that their unique health care needs are not necessarily represented in any literature they may encounter. Therefore, it is recommended that a knowledgeable mentor be consulted before initiating self-care with any herb being used for the first time.

NURTURING THE NURSE-PLANT RELATIONSHIP:

Note: You may want to keep a journal of your experiences with the herb.

Tobacco is a plant with enormous power and control over the lives of many people whether or not they smoke. One way to get to know this plant is to smoke it, but since it is highly addictive, something less direct is recommended. One way to build a positive relationship with this plant is to volunteer to facilitate smoking cessation programs. Long-term users of tobacco products have an intimate understanding of the effects of a relationship with this plant.

Nurses who use tobacco on a daily basis may want to consider finding the plant and smoking the leaf. Without the flavor enhancers manufactured by the tobacco industry to make cigarettes taste pleasant, it is possible that the real leaf and its vile odor may provide a stimulus for starting the process of quitting.

In addition to using a nicotine patch, participating in a smoking cessation program, and creating a negative stimulus to smoking tobacco by smoking the actual leaf, consider creating a positive stimulus for quitting smoking, too. Try adding up all the time spent smoking each day and allocating that time to breathing healing plant fragrances. For example, if you smoke a total of 2 hours per day and that time is now available after deciding to quit, *reward* yourself with a pleasant experience during those two hours. Take a walk in the woods where you can breathe in some new stimulating aromas like juniper, pine, and spruce. Or take those two hours and go to a botanical garden and smell the flowers and herbs in season. Do not take the time you have spent smoking and create a disincentive for quitting by filling that time with more work or an unpleasant experience!

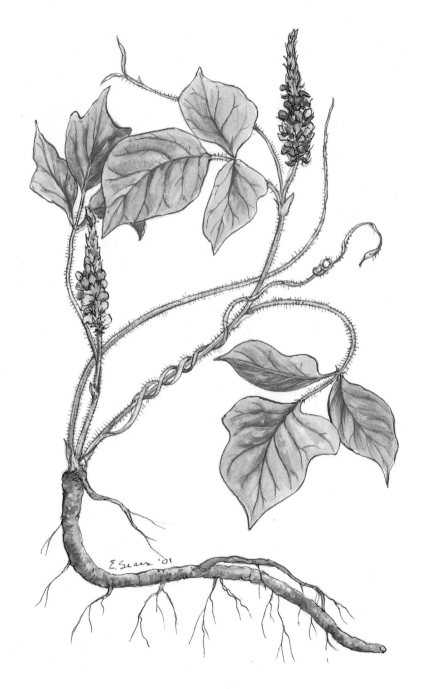

Pueraria lobata

Kudzu

- **LATIN NAME:** *Pueraria montana subsp. var. lobata*

- **FAMILY:** Fabaceae

- **COMMON NAMES:** Kudzu, kudzu root, kudsu, pueraria, pueraria root, kuzu

- **HEALTH PATTERN:** Lifestyle choices

- **PLANT DESCRIPTION:**
Kudzu is a twining, hairy perennial vine that grows quickly and can cover large areas of ground and trees. The leaves are up to 8 inches (20 cm) long and are alternate, pinnately three-divided. The leaves are hairy on the lower surface and the leaf stalks are short. The flowers are reddish purple and are about 1 inch (2.5 cm) long. The flowers appear in August and September and the fragrance is grapelike (Foster & Chongxi, 1992). The stems are woody and the roots are tuberous and up to 24 inches (60 cm) long and 18 inches (45 cm) in diameter. The plant is native to eastern Asia and was introduced in the United States over 100 years ago. It proliferates in the southeastern United States. The root is harvested from the fall to early spring. The tuber is washed, peeled of bark, and sliced into pieces before being dried in the sun or an oven.

- **PLANT PARTS USED:** Root and leaf

- **TRADITIONAL EVIDENCE:**
Cultural Use
   Asian. Chinese physicians have used kudzu, known as "ge gen," for over 2,000 years as a cure for alcoholism. The tea, called "xing-jiu-ling," means "sober up." The root is also pulverized to obtain twelve shot glasses full of the juice and then given to the intoxicated patient (Foster & Chongxi, 1992). Kudzu tonics have been effective for controlling and suppressing the craving for alcohol without adverse effects. Kudzu has been said to reduce the desire for alcohol within one week.
   Kudzu has been used in traditional Chinese medicine and Japanese Kampo for purposes of relaxing the muscles and clearing heat from the body. In Japan, kudzu is called "kakkon." It is used for fevers, headaches, and tension in the upper back and neck. Kudzu encourages the body to retain fluids and alleviates thirst. It also helps the body recover from measles by hastening the eruption of the rash. Kudzu is used in traditional Chinese medicine for diarrhea, hypertension with accompanying paresthesias, dizziness, angina, and tinnitus (Bensky & Gamble, 1993).

In Japan, the kudzu vine is used as both food and medicine in both raw and roasted forms. Raw kudzu powders are used to treat fevers and infections, while roasted kudzu is used for diarrhea (Rister, 1999). The primary use of kudzu is to release tightness in muscles that occurs in the early stages of infection. It is believed that kudzu has the ability to open certain energetic pathways in the body to allow the release of trapped, pathologic influences from tight muscles (Rister, 1999). Kudzu has the ability to clear the heat that can cause headache and stiffness in the upper back and neck. The Japanese recognize kudzu's ability to nourish the fluids in the body and thereby alleviate thirst. The herb also works to stop diarrhea and ease symptoms of high blood pressure such as headache, dizziness, ringing in the ears, and tingling sensations in the body. It is used to strengthen those with general tiredness and decreased vitality. It is useful for intestinal troubles such as diarrhea, cholera, and dysentery. Kudzu is nourishing in cases of chronic illness, colds, fevers, and for those who cannot eat solid foods (Kushi, 1993). In China, the leaf also has been used as a poultice to stop bleeding associated with knife wounds (Foster & Chongxi, 1992).

East Indian. In Ayurvedic medicine, kudzu roots are peeled and mashed into a poultice and applied to joints to reduce swelling. It is taken internally as a demulcent and to reduce fevers. In Nepal it is used to induce vomiting, taken as a tonic, and used internally to promote breast milk production (Nadkarni, 1976).

Culinary Use

Kudzu is often used in Asian cooking to thicken soups, sauces, and stews, and is used in pastries and puddings (Leung & Foster, 1996). It is also used in making noodles and may be cut into slices and slowly cooked for hours with tangerine peel, meat, and other ingredients. Kudzu root powder, the starch that dissolves out from the root and is then hardened, can be purchased from health food stores. It is a very concentrated starch that contains more calories per unit of weight than honey. It is metabolized more slowly by the body than honey (Kushi, 1993).

Use in Herbalism

Kudzu has been used for thousands of years in the treatment of alcoholism. The root and root starch are used to treat alcohol poisoning with unconsciousness and hangover (Leung & Foster, 1996). Recent clinical uses of kudzu include the treatment of hypertension, angina pectoris, migraine, diabetes, traumatic injuries, sinusitis, psoriasis, pruritus, sudden deafness, and itching rashes. It is often used in formulation to treat a symptom pattern that includes stiff neck and upper back with fever and chills without sweating. This formula contains kudzu, cinnamon, ephedra, fresh ginger, jujube fruit, licorice, and peony. The kudzu in this formula relieves tightness in the neck and back, and the other herbs increase circulation and induce sweating. The kudzu formula is used in the early stages of herpes virus infection. The formula does not kill the virus directly or activate the body's immune system. Instead, it is thought to act by blocking the tissue-damaging effects of the virus (Rister, 1999).

Other medical problems that have been treated with kudzu include nasal allergies and colds that are accompanied by a stiff neck and upper back, diarrhea in children, inner ear infection, and sinusitis. It also has been used to treat brain inflammation, hives, polio, and inflammation of the muscles in the neck. It is believed that kudzu decoction will protect eczema-inflamed skin from the damaging effects of herpes infections (Rister, 1999). The isoflavones in kudzu also are found in soy. Kudzu also can be used with conditions related to hormone balance, such as menopause.

BIOMEDICAL EVIDENCE:

There are few published human clinical trials of kudzu. Animal studies seem to support the use of kudzu in the treatment of alcoholism, but one recent human clinical trial has not. More research is needed.

Studies Related to Lifestyle Choices

Early unpublished animal studies in China demonstrate that feeding inebriated mice kudzu extract or an extract of the kudzu constituent, daidzein, shortened alcohol-induced sleep time, and it was therefore hypothesized that kudzu might accelerate alcohol clearance from the blood. The researchers found that daidzein shortened alcohol sleep time by delaying stomach emptying of alcohol (Xie et al., 1994). Numerous controlled animal studies have shown that crude kudzu extract reduced ethanol intake in hamsters and rats that were trained or genetically bred to consume large amounts of alcohol (Keung & Vallee, 1998; Lin & Li, 1998; Lin et al., 1996).

One human study has not supported the successful traditional use of kudzu in chronic alcoholism. Thirty-eight patients who met *Diagnostic and Statistical Manual-IV (DSM-IV)* criteria for chronic alcoholism were given either 1.2 g of kudzu root extract twice a day or placebo. After four months, there was no significant difference between treatment and placebo groups in regard to reduction of alcohol craving or increased sobriety. Limitations of the study are the small sample size and the accuracy of self-report of the subjects (Shebeck & Rindone, 2000). It is also possible that people of Asian ancestry have a genetically lower tolerance for alcohol because 80% of the population lacks the enzyme that processes acetaldehyde, and therefore they may have better results with the use of kudzu (Rister, 1999). The study by Shebeck and Rindone (2000) identified participants as American veterans but did not specify their race.

Studies Related to Other Health Patterns

Mobility. Bensky & Gamble (1993), mention a number of studies on the effect of kudzu on hypertension and related neck stiffness and pain. Although citations and particulars of the studies are not given, the results of the studies are reported as kudzu having no effect on hypertension but significant reduction in subjective symptoms of neck pain and stiffness.

Mechanism of Action

Kudzu decreases the desire for alcohol by causing acetaldehyde to accumulate in the blood faster so that hangover symptoms are experienced while drinking (Duke, 1997). The reversal of alcohol preference by oral doses of kudzu extract or its constituent, daidzein, in animals trained or genetically bred to consume large amounts of alcohol is thought to be mediated via the central nervous system (Lin et al., 1996). The daidzein in kudzu has phytoestrogenic activity enabling it to compete for estrogen receptors. Daidzein's ability to shorten alcohol sleep time may be related to its antioxidant activity. Daidzein has a weaker antioxidant activity and is less potent in dealing with alcohol intoxication (Xie et al., 1994). Puerarin, another constituent in kudzu, has 100 times the antioxidant activity of vitamin E, helps to prevent cancer and heart disease, and has been shown to reduce blood pressure in animals (Duke, 1997). Kudzu improves coronary circulation and decreases the heart's oxygen requirement. It relaxes the muscles in the heart and lowers the heart rate (Rister, 1999).

USE IN PREGNANCY OR LACTATION:

Some sources recommend caution when using kudzu during pregnancy (Bensky & Gamble, 1993). Isoflavones such as daidzein and genistein found in many legumes such as kudzu do have known phytoestrogenic activity and could be "serious if taken by women of childbearing age" (Kaufman, Duke, Brielmann, Boik, & Hoyt, 1997, p. 8).

Herbal Caveat—Pregnancy or Lactation

Some herbs are contraindicated in pregnancy because of a risk of the herb or one of its constituents stimulating the uterus and therefore possibly promoting fetal loss. Many herbal practitioners do not recommend herbal remedies, in particular oral doses of herbs, during the first trimester of pregnancy and seek an alternative. However, herbs are successfully used during pregnancy, especially to prepare the body for the birth. Herbs are relatively unstudied in pregnancy and lactation, so patients need to be made aware through education of the potential benefits and risks of using herbs for health conditions that arise during pregnancy or lactation. The use of herbal remedies during pregnancy often warrants a referral to a knowledgeable herbal practitioner.

USE FOR CHILDREN:

Kudzu pudding or drink can be used to relieve the discomfort of diarrhea in children. See therapeutic applications for how to prepare.

Herbal Caveat—Children

Children have special needs in regard to herbal therapies. They require lesser amounts of herbs and often respond well to mild teas and topical applications such as compresses and baths. The lowest dose of oral preparations should be tried first before increasing the amount given children. Caregivers should observe children closely for responses to herbal remedies. Younger children, particularly infants, have traditionally been given herbs either through their mother's breast milk or in the form of a homeopathic remedy because of their sensitivity to medicines and treatments and the immaturity of their liver. It is recommended that a person knowledgeable in the herbal treatment of children be consulted before the offering of any herb to a child for the first time.

CAUTIONS:

Take care when purchasing kudzu root to be sure that you properly identify it. When buying it in whole dried root form, there are other herbs that look quite similar, such as trichosanthis root *(Trichosanthes kirilowii Maxim.)*. Otherwise, no specific cautions are associated with the use of kudzu (McGuffin et al., 1997).

NURSING EVIDENCE:

Historical Nursing Use

Nurses working in clinics and hospitals where macrobiotic diets are prescribed provide kudzu pudding or drinks for patients. I worked in such a clinic where the nurses had a protocol for kudzu applications.

Potential Nursing Applications

Because kudzu potentially decreases the desire for alcohol, at least in Asians, nurses who work with alcoholic patients may want to consider adding kudzu to the plan of care. More clinical research also is needed. Nurses in outpatient health offices might want to include a warm kudzu drink in their protocols for children or adults with diarrhea or other gastrointestinal upset.

Integrative Insight

Researchers have been interested in the potential of kudzu as a remedy for excessive alcohol consumption and desire because of its successful traditional use in Asian patients with alcoholism. The desire for alcohol is complex and involves both physiologic and psychologic symptoms. As alcoholism is better understood scientifically, perhaps the mechanism of action for kudzu's success in the treatment of alcoholism in Asia will be better understood as well. Alcoholism is a huge public health issue in many countries around the world. Kudzu offers hope for those who perpetually struggle with the debilitating effects of this illness. In the meantime, kudzu could be added to the patient's diet, either in food or supplement form, on a regular basis. Nurses can design rating scales that some patients who are stable could use to monitor their desire for alcohol to see if kudzu has any affect.

THERAPEUTIC APPLICATIONS:

Oral

Decoction from Whole Dried Root. In traditional Chinese medicine, if kudzu is recommended as part of a patient's formula, the kudzu is often taken separately. This is because the cut kudzu root, when decocted, has a somewhat thick, sweet, chalky taste.

Tea from the Extracted Starch Powder. Dissolve 2 heaping teaspoons of powdered kudzu in 1 cup (240 ml) of warm water. Drink it without straining it. Ingesting as much as 3 ounces (90 ml) at one time has no known adverse effects. Or dissolve 1 teaspoon of the powder in a cup (up to 240 ml) of cold water. Then add 1 cup (240 ml) of boiling water. Stir well. A pinch of sea salt or soy sauce may be added (Kushi, 1993).

Kudzu Cream. Dissolve 1 heaping teaspoon of the powder in a little cold water. Add 1 cup (240 ml) of water to this mixture then bring it to a slow boil. Simmer until transparent. Add a pinch of sea salt or soy sauce (Kushi, 1993).

Kudzu Pudding. One heaping teaspoon of the powder is stirred into cold water. A cup (240 ml) of cold water is added and brought to a boil until it is translucent, at which time other ingredients can be added:

For a salty taste add some tamari or sea salt.

For a salty/sour taste add a half a teaspoon of Japanese *ume boshi* plum paste little by little because it will just be suspended in the pudding and won't dissolve. The ume plum paste is more astringent and is helpful if the patient is losing a lot of fluid from diarrhea.

For a sweet taste add chopped apple.

Decrease the Desire for Alcohol. Take 1 to 2 capsules of dried kudzu with the first drink (Duke, 1997). Grind kudzu and fill capsules or purchase as dietary supplement.

Topical

Poultice. Mash fresh root and place on the affected joint. The leaves can be used as a poultice.

Environmental

Kudzu has no environmental uses.

Herbal Caveat—Therapeutic Applications

In traditional and conventional herbal medicine, amounts of herbs given to patients are based on individual needs. The amounts or "doses" recorded here are provided so that the health practitioner has a general idea of the amounts recommended for an adult patient. Dosing in herbalism not only refers to amount of plant used but also includes when, where, and how to take a plant medicine. These dosages should not be used as guidelines for indiscriminate intervention without proper assessment, critical thinking, and patient education on the part of the practitioner.

Note: Please see chapter 5 for detailed descriptions of how to prepare various applications.

PATIENT INTERACTION:

There is a long history of use of kudzu root in squelching the desire for alcohol, especially in Asians. The kudzu is best taken with the first drink so that the drinking experience will become associated with feeling ill rather than pleasantly relaxed. Kudzu can be taken in capsules and also is sold in whole dried herb form. Many people find the processed root powder to be the easiest to use in making remedies. The kudzu starch is removed from the fibers of the root and dried. It can be used just like cornstarch or other dry thickening agents. Kudzu is used as a home remedy for diarrhea, nausea, and symptoms related to sinus infection. Learning how to use kudzu is important in improving the palatability of the herb.

Herbal Caveat—Patient Interaction

Patients considering the use of an herb or formula of herbs in self-care benefit from education about the plant itself and the use of the plant in healing. This education can come through many sources, including local herbalists; plant specialists such as botanists; health practitioners such as nurses, nutritionists, naturopaths, and other physicians; and various written references including the scientific literature. Patients need to remember that their unique health care needs are not necessarily represented in any literature they may encounter. Therefore, it is recommended that a knowledgeable mentor be consulted before initiating self-care with any herb being used for the first time.

NURTURING THE NURSE-PLANT RELATIONSHIP:

Note: You may want to keep a journal of your experiences with the herb.

Kudzu can be very soothing to the gastrointestinal tract. Try making some warm kudzu pudding, either sweet or salty, when you're having gastrointestinal discomfort. Closely follow the instructions previously given, making sure that the pudding is fully cooked. Record your experience.

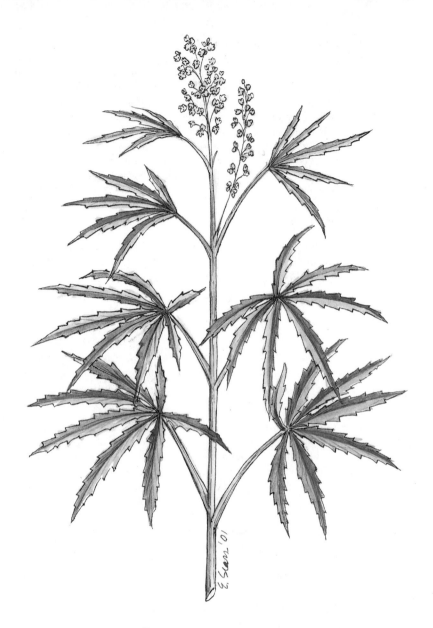

Canabis sativa

CHAPTER 17

Marijuana

- **LATIN NAME:** *Cannabis sativa*

- **FAMILY:** Cannabaceae

- **COMMON NAMES:** Marijuana, hemp, marihuana, Indian hemp
  Slang names include pot, reefer, mary jane, and weed.
  Note: Even though some of the common names for various species of marijuana are often used interchangeably, this profile is about *C. sativa* only.

- **HEALTH PATTERN:** Lifestyle choices

- **PLANT DESCRIPTION:**
  Marijuana is an annual with stems that grow from 3 to 10 feet (1 to 3.5 meters) in height. The leaves are palmate with five to seven leaflets that are linear and lanceolate. The small flowers are pale yellow and downy. The fruit is small and smooth and brown-gray in color. Marijuana is native in Northern India and Southern Siberia and is cultivated in Russia. The resin that oozes from the stem and leaf of the plant is known as hashish. Hashish is usually derived from *Cannabis indica* because of the higher resin content.

  Hemp is *Cannabis sativa,* but a different strain than marijuana, and is very low in tetrahydrocannabinol (THC), a major psychoactive constituent. The THC in marijuana is produced mostly in the female flowers. Marijuana and hemp seeds contain no THC, but when processed, trace amounts of THC from the leaf or flower can stick to the outer husk of the seed to where the THC is identified on analysis (www.rella.com/hempinfo.html).

- **PLANT PARTS USED:** Seed, leaf, and resin

- **TRADITIONAL EVIDENCE:**
  Cultural Use

  Asian. The seed of marijuana is used medicinally in Asia and is called *huo ma ren* in China and *mashinin* in Japan. It has been recorded for use in China since 6000 B.C. According to legend, the ancient emperor Shen Nung, patron deity of agriculture (2700 B.C.) had a transparent abdomen, which allowed him to see the effects of medicines passing through his body. He is credited with the discovery of marijuana as a therapeutic agent (as well as ephedra and ginseng). Shen Nung's pharmacopoeia lists more than 100 ailments treated with marijuana, including female weakness, gout, rheumatism, malaria, beriberi, boils, constipation, and absent-mindedness. Marijuana has been used as an antiemetic, antibiotic, antihelmintic, and to treat leprosy and stop hemorrhage. Marijuana is used to circulate blood and to moisten the gastrointestinal tract. Marijuana seed is a mild purgative that stimulates the intestinal mucous membrane, which increases secretions and movement within the bowel. Ancient Japanese herbalists prescribed Marijuana seed for inflammation of the large intestine with stagnant stools, painful urination, or red urine with fever. Marijuana seed also has been used to lower high blood pressure (Rister, 1999).

North American Indian. The Iroquois use marijuana as a psychologic aid for people who recover after illness but do not think they are well (Moerman, 1998). The Indian hemp *(Apocynum cannabinum)* used medicinally and for fiber by North American Indians should not be confused with *C. sativa* (Vogel, 1970). Marijuana is the most widely used illicit drug among American Indian adolescents (Novins & Mitchell, 1998).

Hispanic. Marijuana is used by Mexican Americans and Maya as a topical lotion or bath for rheumatism, and the Paipai use it for colic and to decrease milk production during lactation (Kay, 1996). It is also mixed with lard and used for healing open wounds.

East Indian. Marijuana is called "vijaya," "siddhapatri," "ganjika," "bhanga," and "hursini" in Sanskrit (Nadkarni, 1976). Marijuana has been associated with magical, medical, religious, and social customs in India for thousands of years. The *Atharva Veda* (1400 B.C.), an ancient Indian text on healing, mentions marijuana as one of five sacred plants used for freedom from distress and states that a "guardian angel resides in the leaves" (Touw, 1981, p. 25). It ordains the practice of throwing hemp boughs into a fire during a magical rite to overcome enemies or evil forces. Sushruta, the most renowned physician of ancient India, recommended it as an antiphlegmatic (dries mucous membranes) and to relieve congestion and regulate bodily fluids. It is also a remedy for catarrh accompanied by diarrhea and is an ingredient for fever cures. Marijuana is said in East Indian medicine to be helpful as a soporific (sleep medication), an excitant, appetite stimulant and digestive aid, an analgesic, and an aphrodisiac. *Raja Valabha,* a seventeenth-century Ayurvedic text, says that marijuana was sent to humans by compassionate gods and is referred to as the "penicillin of Ayurvedic medicine" because of its use in the treatment of numerous infectious diseases (Touw, 1981, p. 28).

Several types and forms of marijuana are used in India. "Bhang" is considered a milder form and "ganja" and "charas" are more potent (Morningstar, 1985). The Indian Hemp Drugs Commission (1893-1894) heard testimony from hundreds of native and Western doctors about the therapeutic uses of marijuana in the treatment of cramps, spasms, convulsions, headache, hysteria, neuralgia, sciatica, tetanus, hydrophobia, cholera, dysentery, leprosy, brain fever, gonorrhea, hay fever, asthma, bronchitis, catarrh, tuberculosis, piles, flatulence, dyspepsia, diabetes, delirium tremens, and impotence; as a sedative and analgesic for toothache, tooth extraction, and many other acute or chronic pains; as an anesthetic for minor surgery including circumcision; as a diuretic, tonic, digestive aid, and disinfectant; and as a means to alleviate hunger and provide freedom from distress. Marijuana leaf powder applied to wounds promotes granulation of tissue, and poultices are applied topically for hemorrhoids, neuralgia, to the eyes in photophobia, and to local inflammations (Nadkarni, 1976).

Marijuana is not universally approved by all Hindus in India and attitudes about its use are very diverse. The Indian government at one time had agreed to full prohibition against marijuana by 1989, but because of its extensive use both medicinally and recreationally and because it grows everywhere in India, the Indian States individually may or may not exercise enforcement of prohibition (Morningstar, 1985). Indians regard marijuana as "sattvik nasha" or "peaceful intoxication." They say that a drunk will fight when provoked but a person using marijuana will walk away. Marijuana is believed to motivate love and peace in people (Morningstar, 1985).

In India, marijuana powder is mixed with equal parts black pepper, dried rose petals, poppy seeds, almonds, cardamoms, cucumber, and melon seeds. Sugar, milk, and water are added to make an intoxicating drink ("thandai") the effects of which last about three hours without hangover (Nadkarni, 1976). *Bhang,* a type of marijuana, is considered an aphrodisiac and helpful for bowel and nervous system complaints.

Middle Eastern. Marijuana is said to have been an incense and an intoxicant in the Old Testament and its Aramaic translation (Touw, 1981).

Russian/Baltic. Russians use marijuana seed medicinally (Touw, 1981).

Culinary Use

Marijuana and hemp have been used in food since ancient times. The seed contains a significant amount of protein (Touw, 1981). Hemp seed is 31% protein after husk removal and is a rich source of vitamins and minerals, including essential fatty acids. The seed is used extensively in food products such as oil and butter. Because the husk is not removed before pressing the oil, there is a greater possibility of THC contamination with the oil than with other food products for which the husk is removed. Hemp food producers often engage in independent lab analysis of their products so that they can ensure their customers that no THC is in their product(www.rella.com/hempinfo.html). The seed used in commercial products is sterilized before entering some countries, such as the United States, to ensure that it cannot be grown. If it is not sterilized, it can be sprouted such as other seeds and also used in foods.

According to Mahayana Buddhist tradition, Gautama Buddha subsisted on one hemp seed daily for six years preceding his enlightenment. Many countries around the world have their own established local recipes that include hemp. The most common way to use the seeds was to grind them into a porridge called "gruel." Still, in parts of China, freshly toasted hemp seeds are sold like popcorn outside movie theatres. In the Ukraine's hemp-growing regions, ancient hemp seed recipes are still shared. The Japanese use ground hemp seeds as a condiment. Some Polish cooks continue to bake them into holiday sweets.

Use in Herbalism

Although marijuana continues to be used medicinally in many cultures, because of its intoxicating nature when smoked and its illegal status in many places, herbalists do not often recommend marijuana. Marijuana is used for easing pain and promoting sleep. It calms the nervous system and is used to relieve symptoms related to gout, rheumatism, neuralgia, high blood pressure, glaucoma, and delirium tremens. Marijuana tincture is used to help promote labor, for gonorrhea, menorrhagia, and chronic cystitis (Grieve, 1971). Marijuana is often smoked and produces intoxication often with hallucinations. Marijuana juice, dropped in the ear, is used for the relieving the pain of earache (Kay, 1996). People with cancer smoke marijuana to relieve the nausea associated with chemotherapy treatment.

🍃 BIOMEDICAL EVIDENCE:

The studies presented here focus on the effects of marijuana plant on lifestyle issues such as alteration of consciousness or attitude. The extensive medicinal benefits of the marijuana plant traditionally identified have not been studied extensively. Studies on the drug Marinol, a drug containing THC, have not been included here unless there is a comparison made to the use of marijuana as a whole plant.

Studies Related to Lifestyle Choice

One small study in airline pilots showed significant impairment of flight simulator performance up to twenty-four hours later in nine pilots who smoked one marijuana cigarette (20 mg of the active ingredient delta 9 THC), even though the pilots reported "no subjective experience" (Leirer, Yesavage, & Morrow, 1991).

Although smoked marijuana is an intoxicant, epidemiologic studies have not demonstrated that smoking marijuana leaf alone increases the risk of culpability for traffic accidents (fatalities or injuries). Smoking marijuana may actually reduce the risk of accidents. Some scientists interpret the evidence to show that drivers who are marijuana intoxicated modify their driving behavior and do not take risks or drive at speeds likely to result in crashes. The possibility also has not been excluded (Bates & Blakely, 1999).

One study reported that performance (memory recall, associative ability, and psychomotor skills) was impaired in 12 healthy male participants for up to twenty-four hours after smoking one marijuana cigarette containing either 1.3% or 2.7% THC, which they were taught to smoke in a particular manner. Only the 2.7% cigarettes significantly impaired recall compared with placebo. Smoking topography demonstrated that participants adjusted their smoking of the marijuana according to THC content. The smokers of the higher potency cigarettes took puffs of smaller volume and shorter duration (Heishman, Stitzer, & Yingling, 1990).

In a study of 10 subjects who smoked one marijuana cigarette with either 1.8% or 3.6% delta-THC, the experience of subjective effects of being high—increased heart rate and pupillary constriction amplitude—were reduced. The subjects also demonstrated reduced smooth pursuit velocity of eye movement. Although this was significant, the subjects did not demonstrate impaired performance on any other cognitive or psychomotor test either at the times tested around the acute smoking phase or on the day after smoking the plant (Fant, Heishman, Bunker, & Pickworth, 1998).

A study of 144 marijuana users and 72 nonusers demonstrated that chronic use is correlated with changes in performance in certain testing conditions but not in overall performance. Heavy marijuana use (using marijuana seven or more times weekly) is associated with impairments in mathematics and verbal expression and in memory retrieval processes. Light use (one to four times weekly) and intermediate use (five to six times weekly) were not associated with deficits. Intermediate use was associated with superior performance in one concept formation test (Block & Ghoneim, 1993).

In a study of 18 young adult marijuana users (frequently used marijuana for less than 5 years) and 13 comparable nonusers who met specific inclusion criteria, there were no significant brain abnormalities or changes in brain tissue volumes as measured by magnetic resonance imaging (MRI). The investigators identified limitations of the study, such as that the marijuana users had been using for less than five years and that smoking marijuana may produce changes undetectable with MRI. This study did not define "frequent use" (Block, O'Leary, Ehrhardt, Augustinack, Ghoneim, Arndt, & Hall, 2000). In another study, PET scans found cerebellar hypoactivity in frequent users (used marijuana greater than or equal to 7 times per week), which can affect cognitive functions, decrease resilience in some areas of the brain, and increase resilience in others for processing information, leading potentially to behavioral changes (Block, O'Leary, Hichwa, Augustinack, Boles Ponto, Ghoneim, Arndt, Ehrhardt, Hurtig, Watkins, Hall, Nathan, & Andreasson, 2000).

The gateway theory proposes that children who smoke marijuana may be at higher risk for using other drugs such as cocaine. Although not definitive of causality, a study of 2871 high school seniors does show an association between marijuana use and other drug use. Seniors using marijuana before the age of 14 were 7.4 times more likely to have used other drugs even when other risk factors were considered (Merrill, Kleber, Schwartz, Liu, & Lewis, 1999).

Studies Related to Other Health Patterns

Emotions and Adaptation. During a six-month study period, schizophrenic patients ($N = 137$) who smoked marijuana had a significantly higher degree of hallucinatory and delusional activity and a greater number of visits to the hospital than schizophrenic patients who did not smoke marijuana (Negrete, Knapp, Douglas, & Smith, 1983). Also, marijuana abuse has been associated with significantly more and earlier psychotic relapses in schizophrenic patients ($N = 24$), and in 23 patients, marijuana abuse preceded the onset of the first psychotic symptoms (Linszen, Dingemans, & Lenior, 1994). In a Swedish longitudinal study that included evaluating 730 high consumers of marijuana, the risk for high abusers of marijuana to develop schizophrenia was 6.0 (95% confidence interval). Nonanonymous questionnaires were used in the survey, so the statistics may be low because people are not as inclined to divulge substance misuse history unless given anonymity. It was concluded that high marijuana use can increase the risk of schizophrenia but is not necessarily linked to causation (Andreasson, Engstrom, Allebeck, & Rydberg, 1987).

Restoration. A small study of 15 healthy young men demonstrated that intraocular pressure drops significantly (2.1 mm at eighty minutes) after smoking a marijuana cigarette containing 12 mg THC as compared with placebo (0.6 mm at thirty minutes). Intraocular pressure decreased only in those who used marijuana moderately and experienced a substantial "high" from the experimental dose (Flom, Adams, & Jones, 1975).

THC began being used effectively to control nausea and vomiting during chemotherapy in the 1970s (Vincent, McQuiston, Einhorn, Nagy, & Brames, 1983). In a study in New Mexico involving 169 cancer patients who received oral delta-9-THC or smoked marijuana to reduce nausea and vomiting from chemotherapy, it was found that both forms were effective, with the inhaled form being superior for vomiting only. The severity of chemotherapy was a significant predictor of improvement and patients on mild or moderate nausea/emetic provoking chemotherapy improved more than those on severe chemotherapy. Prior use of marijuana did not predict improvement. Euphoria was not associated with efficacy. Prior use and mild or moderate chemotherapy were marginally associated with continuation. Mean cannabinoid use on the program was 735 mg per forty-nine 15 mg doses or six two-day treatments (Pierson, 1983).

An anonymous survey conducted in 1990 of 2430 members of the American Society of Clinical Oncology (Doblin & Kleiman, 1991) reported a 43% response rate and results that stated that 44% had recommended marijuana use to at least one cancer patient and 48% would prescribe it if it were legal. Respondents considered inhaled marijuana to be somewhat more effective than oral synthetic pharmaceuticals and "roughly" as safe.

Mechanism of Action

Approximately sixty cannabinoids have been identified in marijuana, but delta-THC is considered the main psychoactive constituent. Smoking marijuana has been reported in several studies to produce paradoxical effects of sedation and stimulation. This type of paradoxical mood effect is not typical of central nervous system depressants or stimulants but is consistent with the effects of psychedelic drugs such as lysergic acid diethylamide (LSD) (Block, Erwin, Farinpour, & Braverman, 1998). THC also has potent anti-inflammatory activity and is a lens aldose reductase inhibitor, which is thought to explain the effect of marijuana on the eye, such as the decrease in intraocular pressure (Wren, 1988).

Positron emission tomography (PET) scans show that frequent marijuana users have substantially lower blood flow to the brain in a large part of the posterior cerebellum and paralimbic and anterior cingulated regions (Block et al., 2000b; O'Leary et al., 2000). Magnetic resonance imaging (MRI) studies of 18 frequent users of marijuana showed no evidence of cerebral atrophy or global or regional changes in brain tissue volume. Ventricular cerebral spinal fluid volume levels were found to be lower in the 18 participants (Block et al., 2000a). The hippocampus has one of the highest densities of cannabinoid receptors in the brain (as reported in Block et al., 2000a).

Prolonged breath holding during the smoking of marijuana increases the subjective "high" experience of users as compared with placebo (Block et al., 1998).

Because cannabinol oxidizes rapidly, drugs made of this constituent are best kept in sealed containers (Grieve, 1971).

USE IN PREGNANCY OR LACTATION:

One multicenter prospective study of 7470 multiethnic pregnant women showed that smoking marijuana was not related to low birth weight, preterm delivery, or abruptio placentae. Eleven percent of the women in the study used marijuana during pregnancy (Shiono et al., 1995). An infusion made from the seed of marijuana is helpful in discomfort related to childbirth after pain and also in cases of prolapse of the uterus (Grieve, 1971). Some women use marijuana during labor to reduce tension or emotional stress. Smoking the plant or taking it in tincture is often the preferred form for use, as compared to tea. Smoking is thought to provide more control over dosage and the effects are more immediate (Weed, 1986).

Following delivery, marijuana tincture has been used in combination with hemostatic herbs such as witch hazel or lady's mantle to slow a postpartum hemorrhage caused by uterine atrophy (Weed, 1986). Marijuana seed is eaten to decrease milk production during lactation (Kay, 1996).

Herbal Caveat—Pregnancy or Lactation

Some herbs are contraindicated in pregnancy because of a risk of the herb or one of its constituents stimulating the uterus and therefore possibly promoting fetal loss. Many herbal practitioners do not recommend herbal remedies, in particular oral doses of herbs, during the first trimester of pregnancy and seek an alternative. However, herbs are successfully used during pregnancy, especially to prepare the body for the birth. Herbs are relatively unstudied in pregnancy and lactation, so patients need to be made aware through education of the potential benefits and risks of using herbs for health conditions that arise during pregnancy or lactation. The use of herbal remedies during pregnancy often warrants a referral to a knowledgeable herbal practitioner.

USE FOR CHILDREN:

Social marijuana use needs to be discouraged in children and adolescents. While there is no definitive causal evidence, research has supported the gateway theory that there seems to be a specific progression or sequence in drug use beginning with alcohol and tobacco, then to marijuana and then on to other illicit drugs (Merrill et al., 1999).

Herbal Caveat—Children

Children have special needs in regard to herbal therapies. They require lesser amounts of herbs and often respond well to mild teas and topical applications such as compresses and baths. The lowest dose of oral preparations should be tried first before increasing the amount given children. Caregivers should observe children closely for responses to herbal remedies. Younger children, particularly infants, have traditionally been given herbs either through their mother's breast milk or in the form of a homeopathic remedy because of their sensitivity to medicines and treatments and the immaturity of their liver. It is recommended that a person knowledgeable in the herbal treatment of children be consulted before the offering of any herb to a child for the first time.

CAUTIONS:

Symptoms of overdose of marijuana seed include nausea, vomiting, diarrhea, numbness of the extremities, irritability, vaginal discharge, spermatorrhea, and even coma and death. Treatment for overdose is fluids, gastric lavage, and symptomatic therapies (Bensky & Gamble, 1993).

Excessive smoking of marijuana may cause alterations in cognition, resting brain function, and memory-related and attention-related brain function (Solowij, 1999). Effects of long-term or excessive smoking of marijuana may include pulmonary infections, respiratory cancer, acute and chronic bronchitis, extensive microscopic abnormalities of the lining of the bronchial passages, overexpression of molecular markers of progression to lung cancer in bronchial tissue, abnormally increased accumulation of inflammatory cells, and impairment in the function of alveolar macrophages reducing their ability to kill microorganisms and tumor cells (Tashkin et al., 1987). Lung infections are more likely to occur in marijuana users because of smoking-related damage to the ciliated cells in the bronchial passages.

Although smoking marijuana has been demonstrated to lower intraocular pressure, continued use at a rate necessary to control elevated intraocular pressure related to glaucoma (approximately 2920 to 3650 marijuana cigarettes per year) could lead to significant pathological changes (Green, 1998).

Although the DSM-IV of the American Psychiatric Association does not recognize withdrawal from marijuana as clinically significant, there are reports of withdrawal symptoms from marijuana, especially among frequent users and those who have concomitant psychiatric symptoms. Withdrawal symptoms include irritability, restlessness, sleep difficulties, decreased appetite, uncooperativeness, fatigue, and depressed mood (Budney, Novy, & Hughes, 1999).

Because there is a possibility of THC adhering to sticky seeds during processing, people eating hemp foods or using marijuana seed (no THC) medicinally can potentially have positive drug screenings.

NURSING EVIDENCE:

Historical Nursing Use

No data are available at this time.

Potential Nursing Applications

Depending on the legal status of the plant and the availability of other medicinal plant alternatives, nurses may want to consider the possibility of researching topical use of marijuana leaf powder for healing wounds and promoting granulation of tissue. Nurses may want to explore the traditional use of inhaled marijuana to increase uterine contractions during labor. This might prove to be a welcome alternative to intravenous Pitocin. Postpartum nurses may want to explore the possibility of using marijuana seed tea with women who decide not to breastfeed or whose breasts become engorged.

Integrative Insight

As more research is done to explore the traditional medicinal uses of marijuana for health and healing, nurses will continue to be challenged with the sociocultural and legal questions being raised about the use of marijuana as a medicinal plant. Because the legalization of marijuana potentially has far reaching consequences in any society, nurses need to be as informed as possible about the issue and the risks and benefits of controlling a population's access to marijuana or any herb.

Although many may suggest that the marijuana plant is not dangerous, the way it may be used or misused can be. Historically, this herb has been misused. Yet, as is discussed throughout this book, the effects on the individual person from any plant are related to the person-plant relationship. Society's relationship with marijuana is complex. Records of medicinal use for which the plant has not been used as an intoxicant span decades; however, use of the plant as an intoxicant has a lengthy history as well. Marijuana causes sedating and stimulating effects in the body but also may be addictive.

Because of the legal and sociobehavioral issues regarding the use of marijuana, it is understandable that some nurses may not want to explore the medicinal benefits of the plant. Public health nurses may want to focus on being part of a solution that includes controlling the use of the plant. On the other hand, nurses may want to consider advocating for the *appropriate* medicinal use of marijuana just the way they might any other herb. Careful consideration based on sociocultural and most importantly legal issues regarding medicinal use for marijuana must be taken. Teaming with clinical herbalists can be helpful in identifying appropriate medicinal use of the plant and potential alternatives to marijuana from the huge medicine chest of plants that are not illegal.

🍃 THERAPEUTIC APPLICATIONS:

Oral

Tincture. 5 to 15 drops
Fluid Extract. 1 to 3 drops (Grieve, 1971)
For postpartum hemorrhage, the usual dose is 10 drops of the herb tincture under the tongue and repeated as necessary (Weed, 1986). Seed can be decocted as tea.

Topical

The resin can be added to ointments or oils and used topically for discomfort related to inflammation and neuralgic complaints (Grieve, 1971).

Leaf powder is sprinkled on wounds to promote granulation of tissue.

Environmental

Although smoking has been found to be a very effective method of delivery, smoking does deliver potentially carcinogenic tars and particulates to the bronchial tree, and hence is viewed by many as an undesirable method of drug delivery for a prescription product. Research is underway in the United Kingdom regarding the development of marijuana delivery methods (other than smoking) that produce rapid absorption via the respiratory tract and oral mucosa. The methods currently under investigation include inhalers of various types and sublingual formulations.

Herbal Caveat—Therapeutic Applications

In traditional and conventional herbal medicine, amounts of herbs given to patients are based on individual needs. The amounts or "doses" recorded here are provided so that the health practitioner has a general idea of the amounts recommended for an adult patient. Dosing in herbalism not only refers to amount of plant used but also includes when, where, and how to take a plant medicine. These dosages should not be used as guidelines for indiscriminate intervention without proper assessment, critical thinking, and patient education on the part of the practitioner.

Note: Please see chapter 5 for detailed descriptions of how to prepare various applications.

🍃 PATIENT INTERACTION:

Marijuana leaf, seed, and/or resin has been eaten and smoked for recreational and medicinal purposes for centuries. This plant also has caused extensive controversy in many societies related to its recreational use and misuse. Some researchers report dependence and withdrawal symptoms related to excessive or long-term use of marijuana. Marijuana is clearly a medicinal plant, yet there seems to be something attractive and possibly even addictive about this plant's personality that encourages the use of this plant for recreation. Perhaps it is the quality of peace and calm that this plant gives to its user that is so often sought out by those who feel that the stresses of daily life are too great.

Some scientists speculate that the effect of marijuana use on the neurotransmitters in the brain is similar to tobacco and other addictive substances. Because of the social momentum of using this plant for recreational use and the extensive abuse that has occurred in some countries, the fact that marijuana may be illegal, and because there may be a risk for dependence, caution should be taken when considering using marijuana for medicinal reasons. A knowledgeable herb practitioner can offer alternatives of which you may have had no previous knowledge simply because most plants do not ever receive any media attention, let alone the amount of attention marijuana gets because of its social status. It is important to understand the development of herbal medicine as a body of medical and sociocultural science. Marijuana has proven to be a very powerful plant with its ability to calm and heal, and it continues to bring more and more people, young and old, to consider its use. There are many other ways of creating peace and calm in the body, such as meditation, that do not include smoking marijuana. The seed of hemp, a subspecies of the same plant that is used as smokeable marijuana, and marijuana seeds, used traditionally as medicinal tea, do not contain THC, the psychoactive constituent that can produce a high. The seed is nutritious and is used in food production. However, seeds are sticky and during processing can adhere to other parts of the plant that do have THC. Food manufacturers often test for the presence of THC in their foods and can be asked for reports by consumers who need assurance that they will not be ingesting THC. Workplace job testing can detect trace amounts of THC in the body. The benefits and risks of the use of this plant must be weighed carefully before use.

Herbal Caveat—Patient Interaction

Patients considering the use of an herb or formula of herbs in self-care benefit from education about the plant itself and the use of the plant in healing. This education can come through many sources, including local herbalists; plant specialists such as botanists; health practitioners such as nurses, nutritionists, naturopaths, and other physicians; and various written references including the scientific literature. Patients need to remember that their unique health care needs are not necessarily represented in any literature they may encounter. Therefore, it is recommended that a knowledgeable mentor be consulted before initiating self-care with any herb being used for the first time.

NURTURING THE NURSE-PLANT RELATIONSHIP:

Note: You may want to keep a journal of your experiences with the herb.

Because this plant is illegal in many countries, it is not recommended that you try smoking or eating marijuana yourself; however, since marijuana is a welcome member of so many societies, you may want to explore what role marijuana plays in your community. Is it part of any cultural traditions? Who routinely uses marijuana where you live? How do they use it and do they tell others that they use it? What are the legal issues regarding the medicinal use of marijuana in your town, city, and country?

CHAPTER 18

Restoration

INTRODUCTION

THIS CHAPTER ON THE HEALTH PATTERN RESTORATION is about herbs that have the uncanny ability to support the renewal of the body. In herbalism, herbs with this action are called "alteratives." Throughout life, people may experience times when the body or parts of the body stop functioning as before. This is most pronounced during the senior years when a person may think, "Am I sick or am I just getting old?" Is aging a disease the cause of which must be discovered and cured? Or is aging a part of life and therefore something that can be lived with and mastered each day? All people, not just the seniors of a community, seek restoration and renewal. Everybody has days when they feel run down or not up to par and they decide to find ways to experience greater health or wellness.

Wellness is a process. Wellness is the patient's perception of optimal well-being related to personal growth and development. Restoration is renewal, and it is a process that can take a person to a new level of wellness. The meaning of restoration in this chapter is not that the body is brought back to an identical former state because, in as much as normal growth and development are evolutionary processes, a person can never fully return to a previous level in his or her personal health history. What is meant by restoration here is that through the use of the herb, a patient may experience a renewed and improved condition and that the renewal and improvement occurs as part of the process of healing. This healing is observed in patients as an increase in vitality.

The herbs in this chapter—red clover, reishi, turmeric, mistletoe, greater celandine, ginkgo, and bilberry—all have an ability to support the body's restorative activities. Although it may be that all herbs have the potential to restore the body in some way, the herbs in this chapter have demonstrated a particular connection with this health pattern. In particular, these herbs have the following characteristics related to restoration:

- Promotion of longevity and healthy aging
- Repair of body systems such as vision, hearing, and memory
- Support of the person experiencing illness related to cancerous growth

Herbs have been used historically to promote longevity and healthy aging. One way that they do this is through their antioxidant action. Antioxidants are substances that prevent oxidation, the loss of electrons in an atom. Antioxidant substances scavenge free radicals, molecules that lack an electron. Because the molecule lacks an electron and electrons are normally found in pairs, the state of the molecule is altered and it becomes very reactive. Free radicals in the body try to rebalance themselves by taking an electron from another molecule. Every time a molecule loses an electron it has the potential to damage a healthy molecule in the process. Free radicals can damage enzymatic structures, protein molecules, and whole cells in the body. The term "free radical damage" is often used to describe the aging of the body. Free radicals can cause lipid peroxidation, cell membrane damage, lysosome damage, and cross-linking through which they actually disrupt the deoxyribonucleic acid (DNA) of a cell (Null, 1995).

Free radicals occur as a result of internal and external processes. Environmental pollutants such as nitrogen oxide and nitrogen dioxide and synthetic pesticide and herbicides can generate free radical production. Free radicals also are produced within the body as a result of normal metabolic and biologic processes such as occur during the stress response. Many plants, including those profiled here, contain constituents known to have antioxidant activity in vitro or in vivo.

Some plant medicines also seem to have the ability to repair delicate systems of the body such as vision, hearing, and the brain. The herbs are thought to improve the microcirculation to the structures involved in vision, hearing, and memory, for example, and restore function. This may at least in part be due to the antioxidant properties of the plant that are known to strengthen vessels and improve capillary circulation.

Plant medicines not only contain constituents that act as antioxidants with the potential to repair cells, but some plants also have the ability to destroy cells, a process called "programmed cell death." "Evidence is accumulating that certain phytochemicals present in dietary herbs (nutraceuticals) exert anti-tumourogenic activity by inducing programmed cell death in cancer cells" (Thatte, Bagadey, & Dahanukar, 2000, p. 205). Plants contain constituents that act as their own anticancer force. They have protective mechanisms against infection, infestation, and destruction. Some of these constituents, when used by humans, seem to have a similar effect. "Flavonoids are diphenyl propanoids widely distributed in edible plants. They play a dual role in mutagenesis and carcinogenesis" (Thatte et al., 2000). Not only herbs, but, "the protective effect of fruits and vegetables persists in almost all studies . . . more difficult to pinpoint has been the exact micronutrient that produces this favorable effect on decreasing cancer development" (DeVita, Hellman, & Rosenberg, 1997, p. 574).

It is not known with scientific precision how herbs such as red clover, ginkgo, and turmeric exert their restorative, antioxidant, antiaging, and antitumor action. But both scientists and traditional herbalists know the following three things:

1. All of the health promotion activities that people are involved in, including healthy diet, rest, managing stress, exercise, and so on contribute to the restoration of the body. Restorative herbs alone do not restore the person to greater vitality. They are best used as an adjunct to a wellness program created and individualized for the patient.
2. As plant foods and medicines are studied, it is realized that just as a single herb or food is not solely responsible for the health or illness of a patient, a single constituent in a medicinal plant is not solely responsible for the restorative action of the plant. Epidemiologic studies have difficulty teasing out which compound (micronutrient) in dietary studies is relevant, and this may explain why the protective effects of fruits and vegetables is so consistent while the benefit of individual micronutrients remains less evident. Studies clearly show that combinations of micronutrients are consistently more protective against carcinogen-induced agents than are individual compounds. This is particularly important since fewer side effects are seen if lower doses of two agents can be used instead of a higher dose of one compound (DeVita et al., 1997, p. 576).
3. The restorative action of an herb is intimately linked with its adaptogen action (see chapter 20 for additional information). Herbs help people adapt to internal and external stressors through their antioxidant, antiaging and anticancer properties. But, how the herb acts in the individual patient in large part depends on the amount of herb used, how the herb is used, and the patient's unique constitution and health needs.

This chapter on restoration is presented to highlight some healing plants' unique abilities to promote and support renewal and greater vitality. The herbs presented here do not represent a fountain of youth or miracle cure, nor do they "cure" cancer. They do, however, represent a history of hope—hope for a better quality of life and continued vitality throughout life when integrated into a total health promotion program.

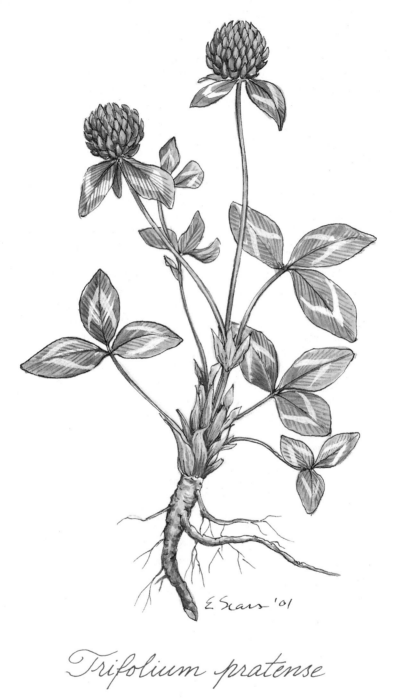

E Sears '01

Trifolium pratense

Red Clover

🍃 **LATIN NAME:** *Trifolium pratense*

🍃 **FAMILY:** Fabaceae

🍃 **COMMON NAMES:** Red clover, pavine clover, meadow clover, cow grass, cow clover, purple clover, cleaver grass, trefoil

🍃 **HEALTH PATTERN:** Restoration

🍃 **PLANT DESCRIPTION:**

Red clover is a biennial or perennial herb native to Europe and temperate parts of Asia and Africa and naturalized in North America. This plant is commonly found growing in fields and meadows. It is a member of the pea family and blooms May through September. Several ascending stems rise from a single root and stand 1 to 2 feet (½ meter) in height. The stems are slightly hairy, bearing noticeable rose-purple fragrant flowers containing 50 to 200 globular florets. The flower is usually about 1 inch (2 cm) wide and about 1 inch (2 cm) long. *Trifolium*, meaning "three leaves," describes the leaf pattern of red clover. The plant has three oval or obovate smooth leaves, which grow on alternate sides of the stems.

🍃 **PLANT PARTS USED:** Flower head, leaf, and root

🍃 **TRADITIONAL EVIDENCE:**

Cultural Use

Asian. The Chinese use a tea made from the flower heads of red clover as an expectorant (Duke, 1985).

North American Indian. Several North American Indian tribes used red clover as a blood purifier, for fever, menopause, and/or cancer. It is used topically as a salve for burns and skin sores and as an eyewash. It also has been shown to be helpful for bronchial spasm, including whooping cough (Hutchens, 1992; Moerman, 1998).

Hispanic. Known as "alfalfon" by some Hispanics, red clover is used for relieving symptoms related to colds, sore throat, arthritis, and for hormonal balance in women.

Australian. In Australia red clover is approved for skin problems, respiratory problems, and as an antispasmodic (McCaleb, Leigh, & Morien, 2000).

Russian/Baltic. In Russia, red clover (called "red clever") infusions are used to restore health in those suffering from anemia, emaciation, asthenia, and diabetes mellitus. It promotes the onset of menstruation, relieves cramps and spasms, and is used to treat uterine hemorrhage. It is also used to treat allergic skin conditions such as eczema. Used externally, red clover relieves inflammation of the ears and eyes. A poultice of the leaf is used to heal wounds and burns. It is recommended to reduce serum cholesterol levels, as prevention for atherosclerosis, and is used as an ingredient in a remedy for tuberculosis (Zevin, 1997).

European. The United Kingdom and Sweden have formally approved red clover to be used in the treatment of skin disorders such as psoriasis, eczema, and rashes and in the treatment of cough, bronchitis, and as an antispasmodic (McCaleb et al., 2000).

Culinary Use

Red clover is a member of the legume family, and the leaves and the flower of the plant are edible. It is used as a flavoring ingredient in nonalcoholic drinks, candy, baked goods, jellies, jams, gravies, and frozen dairy desserts (Leung & Foster, 1996). Red clover has two-thirds more digestible protein than alfalfa (Duke, 1985). The Council of Europe lists red clover as a category N2, indicating small amounts may be added to food for flavor without bringing out the therapeutic effect of the active ingredients (Newall, Anderson, & Phillipson, 1996).

Use in Herbalism

Red clover is used orally as a diuretic, an antispasmodic, a blood purifier for venereal disease, an antitussive, and to treat sore eyes. Red clover tea also has been used for many years both internally and externally to treat and prevent cancer and to relieve symptoms related to malignant ulcers, scrofula, indolent sores, burns, whooping cough, spasms, bronchial conditions, renal conditions, sore throat, and for vaginal and rectal irritation (Felter & Lloyd, 1983; Hutchens, 1992; Leung & Foster, 1996). Poultices of the herb are used for cancerous growths on the skin and for symptoms related to ailments such as psoriasis or eczema. It is often used as an escharotic salve or ointment, or as an enema and/or douche in the treatment of breast and ovarian cancer. Red clover is normally used over a period of time because its therapeutic action takes time (Naiman, 1999). Red clover is used to treat complications of menopause, including cardiovascular disease (McCaleb et al., 2000). Red clover was listed in *The United States Pharmacopoeia* until 1946 as a treatment for skin diseases. It is the main ingredient of Harry Hoxsey's cancer therapy, which is still in use in some Mexican cancer clinics (McCaleb et al., 2000).

BIOMEDICAL EVIDENCE:

A recent systematic review of the literature revealed no published clinical trials supporting the traditional use of red clover or Flor-Essence, an herbal formula containing red clover, in the care of those with cancer. No known human studies support the use of red clover for symptoms related to anemia, blood purification, or any other conditions identified in traditional use. Much of the research has focused on the phytoestrogens in red clover; however, the phytoestrogens are not the same as the whole plant, and red clover blossoms are traditionally taken as whole herb.

Studies Related to Restoration

An in vivo study found that phytoestrogens, or plant estrogens found in plants such as red clover, cause an increase in the bioavailability of estrogen receptor-binding components without causing concurrent elevation in estradiol. These phytoestrogens occupy the estrogen receptor site, preventing human estrogen from binding to the site and stimulating tumor growth (Zava, Dollbaum, & Blen, 1998).

Studies Related to Other Health Patterns

Hormone Balance. Red clover contains plant constituents called isoflavones that when ingested are known to increase estrogen levels in women. Cardiovascular function after menopause improved significantly in a small study of 14 women who consumed 80 mg per day of isoflavones derived from red clover (Novogen). The lack of estrogen produced after menopause contributes to decreased arterial compliance, leading to hypertension and increased left ventricular workload. This double-blind, placebo-controlled study found arterial compliance to be improved within weeks of ingesting isoflavones from red clover (Nestel et al., 1998).

Mechanism of Action

Much of the health benefit of red clover has been attributed to phytoestrogens, which also are called "isoflavones." The isoflavones in red clover are formononetin, biochanin A, pratensein, trifoside, daidzein, and genistein (Leung & Foster, 1996). Genistein is a compound with an antiangiogenic effect in vitro. Red clover may have the potential to stop the formation of new blood vessels from growing in tumors, thereby starving the tumor (Fotsis, Pepper, Adlercreutz, Hase, Montesano, & Schweigerer, 1995). Genistein also has been shown to have powerful antioxidant activity (Tamayo, Richardson, Diamond, & Skoda, 2000). In vitro studies suggest that both genistein and daidzein inhibit the growth of both estrogen receptor negative and positive breast cancer cell lines. These phytoestrogens bind at estrogen receptor sites and tend to normalize estrogen and progesterone (Zava et al., 1998). In vitro studies have shown biochanin A to inhibit carcinogen activation (benzopyrenes, the carcinogens found in barbecued foods) in cell cultures (Cassady et al., 1988). Red clover is active against several bacteria, including *Mycobacterium tuberculosis* (Fitzpatrick, 1954).

USE IN PREGNANCY OR LACTATION:

Because this plant has been known to cause abortion in cows grazing on it and contains 1% to 2.5% isoflavones (Duke, 1997), it is not to be used in pregnancy (McGuffin, Hobbs, Upton, & Goldberg, 1997).

Ewes grazing daily on red clover rich in the phytoestrogen, fomononetin, have demonstrated increased levels of infertility if grazed for prolonged periods of time. The formononetin content has been found to be reduced when the clover is field dried (Kelly, Hay, & Shackell, 1979). Humans, however, do not take enough clover to be concerned about infertility (Duke, 1997).

Some herbalists recommend red clover tea for supporting the reproductive cycle in women. It not only assists in balancing hormones and nourishing the uterus, but also the calcium and magnesium found in the plant help regulate the impact of stressors on the nervous system, and it is thought to balance the acid/alkaline level in the vagina and uterus in favor of conception (Weed, 1986).

Herbal Caveat—Pregnancy or Lactation

Some herbs are contraindicated in pregnancy because of a risk of the herb or one of its constituents stimulating the uterus and therefore possibly promoting fetal loss. Many herbal practitioners do not recommend herbal remedies, in particular oral doses of herbs, during the first trimester of pregnancy and seek an alternative. However, herbs are successfully used during pregnancy, especially to prepare the body for the birth. Herbs are relatively unstudied in pregnancy and lactation, so patients need to be made aware through education of the potential benefits and risks of using herbs for health conditions that arise during pregnancy or lactation. The use of herbal remedies during pregnancy often warrants a referral to a knowledgeable herbal practitioner.

USE FOR CHILDREN:

In Russia, children are given red clover as tea, a decoction, or with vodka for restoring health when they are weak and for treating shortness of breath related to anemia and respiratory problems (Hutchens, 1992).

Herbal Caveat—Children

Children have special needs in regard to herbal therapies. They require lesser amounts of herbs and often respond well to mild teas and topical applications such as compresses and baths. The lowest dose of oral preparations should be tried first before increasing the amount given children. Caregivers should observe children closely for responses to herbal remedies. Younger children, particularly infants, have traditionally been given herbs either through their mother's breast milk or in the form of a homeopathic remedy because of their sensitivity to medicines and treatments and the immaturity of their liver. It is recommended that a person knowledgeable in the herbal treatment of children be consulted before the offering of any herb to a child for the first time.

⚘ CAUTIONS:

Red clover contains significant amounts of plant constituents known as "coumarins" that have a tendency to affect the blood clotting process in the body. Coumarins may thin the blood. Although there is no supporting research for this recommendation, those who are having surgical procedures of any kind may want to choose to refrain from taking red clover in any form for two weeks before and after the surgery to avoid the possibility of excessive bleeding.

Red clover should be used with caution by patients with known estrogen positive receptor cancer cells such as breast cancer. In vitro studies have shown red clover to have agonist activity on estrogen positive receptor cells when bound to the cell (Zava et al., 1998). Plant therapies should be used under the guidance of a knowledgeable practitioner when the person using the plant is undergoing chemotherapy and/or radiation therapy.

⚘ NURSING EVIDENCE:

Historical Nursing Use

In the 1920s, Rene Caisse, a Canadian nurse who noted the combination of several herbs formulated by an Ojibwa healer to have cured a woman's breast cancer, named this formula Essiac. Caisse opened a clinic offering this treatment by both injection and tea. She experimented with this formula for over 40 years with hundreds of cancer patients while keeping the formula's recipe secret. Essiac is believed by some to have positive effects on the immune system, the appetite, and on pain; decreasing volume of cancer burden; prolonging cancer survival; and improving overall quality of life (Kaegi, 1998).

Canada's Cancer Commission reviewed Essiac in 1938 under the Cancer Remedies Act of Ontario and submitted a report declaring limited evidence for approving Essiac as a cancer treatment. Between 1959 and 1978 while working with Dr. Charles Brusch, Caisse added red clover as one of four herbs to the formula originally containing four main herbal ingredients. They believed red clover, watercress, blessed thistle, and kelp potentiated the effects of burdock root, Indian rhubarb, slippery elm bark, and sheep sorrel as well as adding flavor (Kaegi, 1998). In 1977, the formula was given to Resperin, a Toronto corporation, for testing and marketing. In 1982 the Department of Health and Welfare placed restrictions on the product being promoted as a cancer treatment. Today Essiac is available through Health Canada's Compassionate Use Drug Program or from the manufacturer in health food stores under the brand name Essiac (Kaegi, 1998).

The widely available eight-herb recipe is being manufactured in Canada as Flor-Essence and is promoted as a health-enhancing herbal tea. Advocates of this herbal therapy believe Flor-Essence to be compatible with other cancer treatments such as chemotherapy and radiation therapy without serious side effects noted. A study is being conducted in Canada to determine the effect of Flor-Essence on the quality of life of cancer patients (Tamayo et al., 2000).

Potential Nursing Applications

Potential opportunities for nursing research are plentiful. The integration of herbal therapy along the cancer care continuum and for other chronic illnesses must be researched to establish practice guidelines. Nursing research has the potential to validate the credibility of these therapies, making them more available in many practice settings. Nurses believe that human beings can experience healing and even periods of "health" while experiencing various states of disease and impending death. Although historic research on red clover has not proven that it promotes a complete tumor response or prolongs life by standards of Western biomedical measurement, nursing research, using a combination of quantitative and qualitative methods may find support for the use of red clover as a beneficial intervention for people experiencing biomedical cancer treatment.

Nurses also may consider the clinical use of red clover tea in women experiencing discomfort related to menopause. Nurses can explore the effects of external use of a red clover poultice and compresses in the restorative care of wounds and burns. Because of the antiangiogenic effect of one constituent in red clover, chewing red clover buds may be helpful in the prevention of tumors of the mouth and tongue of former chewing tobacco addicts (Duke, 1997). Addiction nurses may want to consider the use of red clover buds in those who chew tobacco.

Integrative Insight

For many years, red clover has been known to cleanse the blood. Although the vernacular use of this term may refer to the healing of venereal disease, many herbalists have used red clover as a cleanser or purifier for the blood, and it has been used extensively in the healing of those with cancer. Cancer is an illness, not just a disease. The disease process is scientifically understood as wild cell growth, as in the development of tumors. Scientific evidence has shown that red clover seems to address this by closing off the blood flow to the tumor, thereby starving it. Red clover, from a traditional standpoint, has other benefits that have been recorded over the years but may not be as easy to measure or prove at first.

Red clover traditionally has been used in conjunction with a detoxification program. In traditional healing, cancer is the poisoning of the body through chronic autointoxication, constipation, and inactivity of the organs of elimination (Kloss, 1939). The poisons are said to accumulate around the organs that have been weakened through injury or toxic exposure, for example. Red clover, along with a program including balanced diet, fresh air, massage, water therapy, and proper elimination has been used for years to address the illness associated with the disease of cancer. People who are detoxifying require more than the cure of the disease; they also need the removal of the tumor or the cause of the disease.

Oncology nurses witness the toxic effects of the diseases manifested in their patients. They also recognize the toxic effects of the treatments they give that can be lifesaving in terms of tumor growth. Nurses know that the chronic illness that follows biomedical treatment can sometimes be devastating for an individual. Thinking in terms of primary prevention, even those people who are not diseased and are not undergoing cancer treatment need to help their bodies detoxify on a regular basis. Proper nutrition helps minimize the ingestion of toxins and carcinogens and proper elimination helps move out that which can potentially make the body sick.

Herbs such as red clover have been used to facilitate the detoxification process. They seem to have a shielding, protecting, and balancing effect that is not clearly understood from a scientific perspective, but that will come. For example, we are beginning to understand that phytoestrogens in plants such as red clover have the ability to help regulate hormone balance. Hormones have been identified as being involved in some cancers and other diseases. Integration of the evidence seems to suggest that the use of whole herb red clover in those needing detoxification, such as those with cancer, be explored more fully. But the nurse also learns from the traditional evidence that many herbs are not used alone. All of the lifestyle management and nutrition skills the nurse has to offer a patient will be needed to create an integrated program that includes the use of herbs such as red clover that can build the blood and detoxify the body.

THERAPEUTIC APPLICATIONS:

Oral

> **Tea.** 1 cup of tea three to four times per day
> **Tincture.** 15 to 30 drops one to four times per day
> **Liquid Extract.** 1:1 (g/ml) $\frac{1}{2}$ teaspoon (1.5 to 3 ml) three times per day
> **Standardized Extract.** Take 1 to 2 tablets per day. Tablets should contain 40 mg of total isoflavones.
> Can also be taken as a syrup.

Topical

Red clover can be used as a salve or poultice for malignant and indolent ulcers, wounds, and burns.

Environmental

Rickets can be treated by bathing the affected part in a tea (Hutchens, 1992).

PATIENT INTERACTION:

Traditional data have shown that red clover can be effective in restoring strength and health after illnesses such as anemia and cancer. Used externally, red clover has been found to stop the growth of cancerous lesions. It also contains plant constituents known as isoflavones that may assist in estrogen balance in women, which can be especially helpful during menopause and perimenopause. Red clover has traditionally been integrated with health promotion and detoxification programs that include balanced diet, proper elimination, massage, water therapies, and proper rest. Because of the plant constituents known as coumarins present in red clover, this herb should not be taken as part of self-care practices at the same time as other blood-thinning medicines or within two weeks of surgery when there is a risk related to excessive bleeding.

NURTURING THE NURSE-PLANT RELATIONSHIP:

Note: You may want to keep a journal of your experiences with the herb.

Try taking a walk in a field of sweet-smelling clover. Remove some plump florets from the flower head and suck gently on the inner part to taste the nectar of the flower.

Red clover makes a very pleasant tasting tea. This plant is a virtual storehouse of vitamins, minerals, and protein and is known for its ability to strengthen a weakened, depleted body. Try replacing your cup of coffee with a cup of red clover tea for one week and see how you feel.

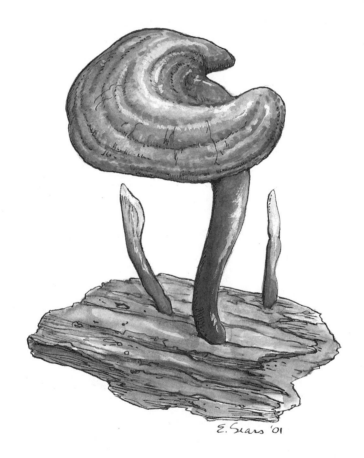

E. Sears '01

Ganoderma lucidum

Reishi

🍃 **LATIN NAME:** *Ganoderma lucidum*

🍃 **FAMILY:** Polyporaceae

🍃 **COMMON NAMES:** Reishi, lingzhicao, lingchih, spiritual vegetable meat, ten thousand year mushroom, phantom mushroom

🍃 **HEALTH PATTERN:** Restoration

🍃 **PLANT DESCRIPTION:**
Wild reishi fungi are found growing on old Japanese plum trees at the ratio of 10 fungi to 100,000 trees (Rister, 1999). Reishi also grow at stumps of oak and decaying conifers along coastal areas of China, Japan, Korea, and North America (Leung & Foster, 1996). Some say that Reishi fungi look like human hands. Japanese farmers grow reishi indoors, using a method that takes two years to culture spores on plum-tree sawdust. The fungi are collected in the fall and then are washed and dried.

The cap is corklike, the shape of a kidney, and has a firm surface on top. The coloring of the reishi graduates from yellow to reddish brown to purple. The cap sizes vary from 1.4×1.2 inches (4×3 cm) to 8×4 inches (20×10 cm) and up to 1 inch (0.5 to 2 cm) in thickness. The stalk grows upright to 7.6 inches (19 cm) in height and up to 1 inch (0.5 to 2.5 cm) thick. The fungus is dark and shiny with purple, brown, and black hues.

🍃 **PLANT PARTS USED:** Fruiting body and mycelium

🍃 **TRADITIONAL EVIDENCE:**
Cultural Use
Asian. Reishi, called "ling zhi" in China and "reishi" in Japan, has been used in China and Japan for over 4000 years to increase longevity and to treat liver disease including hepatitis. Reishi also is used to clear alcohol or fatty food toxicity of the liver and for altitude sickness. Reishi is used to nourish and tonify the body and remove toxins. Different types of reishi have different tastes and therefore affect different organs. Reishi has been used in Japan to treat cancer, chronic bronchitis, heart disease, hypertension, joint inflammation, and ulcers (Hobbs, 1996).

Russian/Baltic. Reishi has been used in a research center in Moscow for treating cancer patients (Hobbs, 1996).

Culinary Use
Hydroalcoholic extracts of reishi are used as a flavoring and aroma agent in soups and herbal drinks (Leung & Foster, 1996).

Use in Herbalism

Reishi is known as the "mushroom of immortality" and is thought to "release trapped emotional energy from the liver so that an individual can turn to higher, more spiritual pursuits" (Rister, 1999, p. 104). Reishi also is said to mend the heart by improving coronary blood flow and relieving chest pain. Reishi has been used extensively for deafness; asthma; insomnia; strengthening tendons and bones; improving the complexion; as an antihistamine; to decrease inflammation of uterine fibroids; and to stimulate the differentiation of macrophages, the white blood cells necessary for controlling infectious bacteria and yeast. Reishi also is said to be effective in treating discomfort associated with yeast infection, leukemia, atherosclerosis, myotonia dystrophica, chronic hepatitis, pyelonephritis, mushroom poisoning, and altitude sickness. Reishi also is used topically and internally to reverse signs of aging such as removing wrinkles and age spots (Rister, 1999) and has been shown to protect against ionizing radiation when given before and after treatment (as reported in Hobbs, 1996).

BIOMEDICAL EVIDENCE:

Although Reishi has been used traditionally for hundreds of years and has been studied (animal, in vitro, and some human trials), the clinical effectiveness of reishi in a wide range of disorders "is still largely unsubstantiated by *modern* internationally-recognized scientific standards, but is currently being used in clinics and tested extensively throughout Asia and other parts of the world" (Hobbs, 1996, p. 101).

Studies Related to Restoration

In a large Chinese clinical study of more than 2000 patients with chronic bronchitis given a tablet form of reishi syrup, 60% to 90% had significant improvement within 2 weeks (Chang & But as reported in Hobbs, 1996).

Animal studies of reishi show that reishi extract corrected the mutations in mouse white blood cells that cause sarcoma 180 leukemia. Under the influence of reishi, the mutated white blood cells matured and cycled normally (Lieu, Lee, & Wang, 1992). Another animal study of freeze-dried extract of reishi demonstrated no protective effects against test mutagens (Chiu, Wang, Leung, & Moore, 2000).

Studies Related to Other Health Patterns

Mobility. Patients with myotonia dystrophica given 400 mg/day of intramuscular water-soluble reishi spores showed significant improvement in muscle strength, walking, speech, sleeping and eating patterns, and weight gain within 1 to 2 weeks (Fu & Wang as reported in Hobbs, 1996).

Mechanism of Action

The antitumor effects of reishi are due to polysaccharides and triterpenoids. The antihistaminic effects are due to ganoderic acids C and D (Leung & Foster, 1996). Reishi is a liver detoxifying agent. It protects against liver damage induced by carbon tetrachloride and demonstrates activity to extract fat-soluble materials. The hypolipemic, hypercholesterolemic effects are from ganoderic acid derivatives. The hypoglycemic effects are due to polysaccharides. Central nervous system sedative, analgesic, and anticonvulsive effects are due to adenosine. Hypertensive, hypotensive, and improved blood flow through the coronary arteries related to reishi intake are due to triterpenoids (Leung & Foster, 1996).

Reishi induces the maturation process of macrophages (Rister, 1999). Macrophages are large mononucleated cells of the reticuloendothelial system that have the ability to ingest and destroy infectious bacteria, protozoa, cells, cell debris, dust particles, colloids, and yeast. They are found in loose connective tissues and multiple organs of the body. These organs include the Kupffer's cells of the liver, splenocytes of the spleen, dust cells of the lung, microglia of the spinal cord and brain, Langerhans' cells of the skin, and cells in breast and placental tissue and in serous cavities. Macrophages play an important immune function by recognizing and ingesting foreign antigens through receptors on their cell membranes. Macrophages clear the blood of abnormal and old cells and process antigens by attracting T-cells and releasing immune-mediating substances (Thomas, 1997). Reishi at 300 mg/kg significantly prolongs the lethal time in mice given strychnine (Kasahara & Hikino, 1987).

Reishi contains significant amounts of germanium (Ge), a metal known to have antimutagenic, antioxidant, and antitumor effects; an ability to stimulate the immune system; and to be of little risk to humans, which may explain some of reishi's restorative properties (Chiu et al., 2000). One in vitro study also has identified that reishi contains at least two antiviral substances with low cytotoxicity to host cells and that these natural substances could be developed as antiviral agents (Eo, Kim, Lee, & Han, 1999). Reishi stabilizes immunoglobulin levels such as IgE, IgM, IgA, and IgG. In animals, reishi inhibits the release of histamine (as reported in Hobbs, 1996).

USE IN PREGNANCY OR LACTATION:

No data are available at this time.

Herbal Caveat—Pregnancy or Lactation

Some herbs are contraindicated in pregnancy because of a risk of the herb or one of its constituents stimulating the uterus and therefore possibly promoting fetal loss. Many herbal practitioners do not recommend herbal remedies, in particular oral doses of herbs, during the first trimester of pregnancy and seek an alternative. However, herbs are successfully used during pregnancy, especially to prepare the body for the birth. Herbs are relatively unstudied in pregnancy and lactation, so patients need to be made aware through education of the potential benefits and risks of using herbs for health conditions that arise during pregnancy or lactation. The use of herbal remedies during pregnancy often warrants a referral to a knowledgeable herbal practitioner.

Restoration

No data are available at this time.

Herbal Caveat—Children

Children have special needs in regard to herbal therapies. They require lesser amounts of herbs and often respond well to mild teas and topical applications such as compresses and baths. The lowest dose of oral preparations should be tried first before increasing the amount given children. Caregivers should observe children closely for responses to herbal remedies. Younger children, particularly infants, have traditionally been given herbs either through their mother's breast milk or in the form of a homeopathic remedy because of their sensitivity to medicines and treatments and the immaturity of their liver. It is recommended that a person knowledgeable in the herbal treatment of children be consulted before the offering of any herb to a child for the first time.

⚘ CAUTIONS:

There is little data on the long-term effects of using reishi (Hobbs, 1996). Rare side effects of reishi that have been documented after three to six months of use include xerostomia and dry throat, urticaria, nausea, epistaxis, and bloody stools (McGuffin et al., 1997). There is one documented case of someone developing a skin rash after drinking reishi wine and one reported case of anaphylactic shock after an intramuscular injection (McGuffin et al., 1997). When purchasing reishi as a supplement, either as a single substance or in formulation, ensure that the reishi, especially if imported from China, does not contain heavy metals of any kind. Check the label or ask the shop owner for a complete list of ingredients. Shop owners who sell Chinese herbs as patent medicines (e.g., tablet or capsules) are aware of this concern and usually buy from importers that perform chemical testing of products to ensure safety.

In animal studies, a water extract of reishi did antagonize the central nervous system stimulant effects of caffeine and reduced hexobarbital-induced sleeping time (Kasahara & Hikino, 1987).

⚘ NURSING EVIDENCE:

Historical Nursing Use

No data are available at this time.

Potential Nursing Applications

Reishi can be considered as an adjunctive therapy for the promotion of the body's own restorative and immunoprotective powers. Scientists at the Institute for Medicinal Plant Development near Beijing, China, in the department of medicinal fungi have developed an injectable "immunostimulant drug from reishi that can be used as an adjunctive therapy for cancer patients undergoing chemotherapy" (Foster & Chongxi, 1992, p. 9). Many countries have highly developed medical means of dealing with chronic diseases, including cancer, but few developments are recorded that address the concerns of patients who are weakened by the course of medical treatment itself. Nurses can advocate for the restorative needs of patients. Nurses can demonstrate their commitment to addressing the restorative needs of patients in many ways. One way might be to consider adding reishi to the diet of patients to promote higher energy levels and immune function when they are experiencing fatigue related to disease or biomedical treatments.

Many pharmaceuticals stimulate histamine release. Nurses may want to consider the effects of the integration of medicinal substances such as reishi into the treatment plan of a patient to serve as an agent that might prevent side effects of drugs known to cause histamine release. Nurses also may want to explore the effects of reishi tea in patients with chest pain.

Integrative Insight

Reishi is known for its ability to promote longevity and stimulate the immune system. As mentioned above, the Chinese are developing an injectable form of the fungus to be used as an adjunctive therapy to chemotherapy. Many patients have used diet, herbs, and other lifestyle changes in combination with their biomedical treatments to help them heal. Patients involved in integrative care sometimes take or undergo more than one modality at a time. Sometimes they undergo only one modality. Nurses have much to offer in the process of integrative care. Do patients receiving injectable reishi with their chemotherapy suffer fewer adverse effects? This is just one of many questions that can be asked. Integrative care demands excellent observation skills and individualization of care. If a patient chooses to use reishi when receiving chemotherapy or radiation therapy, the patient must be monitored closely during the time when myelosuppression is likely to occur and thrombocytopenia may result. Nurses sharing their integrative care experiences through publications and paper presentations can add to the knowledge base of the discipline. Reishi not only has potential to support those who are ill but also can be integrated into the health promotion strategies of well patients.

THERAPEUTIC APPLICATIONS:

Oral

Tea. Use 3 to 6 teaspoons of dried reishi per cup (240 ml) of boiling water or two 1-g tea bags per cup of tea.

Topical

Reishi extracts can be found in skin care products and are known traditionally to hydrate and nourish the complexion.

Environmental

No data are available at this time.

Herbal Caveat—Therapeutic Applications

In traditional and conventional herbal medicine, amounts of herbs given to patients are based on individual needs. The amounts or "doses" recorded here are provided so that the health practitioner has a general idea of the amounts recommended for an adult patient. Dosing in herbalism not only refers to amount of plant used but also includes when, where, and how to take a plant medicine. These dosages should not be used as guidelines for indiscriminate intervention without proper assessment, critical thinking, and patient education on the part of the practitioner.

Note: Please see chapter 5 for detailed descriptions of how to prepare various applications.

PATIENT INTERACTION:

Reishi is an edible fungus effectively used for centuries in Asia for the promotion of health and longevity and the ability to restore a person to health after a difficult and debilitating illness. It has been used traditionally for cancer, arrhythmias, asthma, altitude sickness, anemia, joint stiffness, calming the spirit, and in symptoms related to aging. Reishi can be eaten or taken as tea and has rarely been associated with side effects.

Herbal Caveat—Patient Interaction

Patients considering the use of an herb or formula of herbs in self-care benefit from education about the plant itself and the use of the plant in healing. This education can come through many sources, including local herbalists; plant specialists such as botanists; health practitioners such as nurses, nutritionists, naturopaths, and other physicians; and various written references including the scientific literature. Patients need to remember that their unique health care needs are not necessarily represented in any literature they may encounter. Therefore, it is recommended that a knowledgeable mentor be consulted before initiating self-care with any herb being used for the first time.

NURTURING THE NURSE-PLANT RELATIONSHIP:

Note: You may want to keep a journal of your experiences with the herb.

Living a long, healthy life is a foundational part of Asian culture, where reishi is well known. Reishi has been used in Asia for centuries to promote longevity and the restoration of body and spirit. Chinese emperors developed whole health care systems around the concept of longevity and balance. Eating herbs and foods such as reishi as a way to restore the body's life force or "qi" is only one part of the emperors' plan for healthy and long life. Qian Long, the emperor who reigned from 1736 to 1796, left behind a list of fourteen things he believed led to his ability to live a long and healthy life. To nurture your relationship with reishi and improve your everyday health, try eating some reishi and implementing the fourteen keys of Qian Long (Flaws, 1994).

1. Rise early and breathe in pure air and exhale stale air.
2. Use herbs and foods that restore *qi*.
3. Click the teeth together.
4. Swallow the saliva.
5. Massage the ears.
6. Rub the nose.
7. Roll the eyes.
8. Knead the feet.
9. Stretch the limbs.
10. Raise the anus.
11. Do not speak while eating.
12. Do not chat while lying down.
13. Do not drink excessively.
14. Do not indulge in sex.

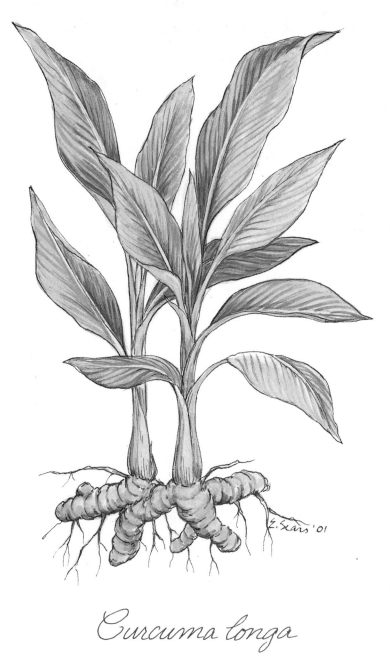

Curcuma longa

Turmeric

- **LATIN NAMES:** *Curcuma longa L., Curcuma aromatica Salisbury, Curcuma domestica Valet*

- **FAMILY:** Zingiberaceae

- **COMMON NAMES:** Turmeric, Indian saffron, curcuma, yellow ginger (Note: Do not confuse turmeric with goldenseal, which is sometimes referred to as "turmeric root.")

- **HEALTH PATTERN:** Restoration

- **PLANT DESCRIPTION:**

A relative of ginger, turmeric is a perennial plant grown in tropical and subtropical areas of south and southeast Asia. It grows mainly in India, China, Indonesia, Malaysia, and Jamaica. The rhizome of the plant is harvested in the winter when the aerial parts of the plant have shriveled. The leaves are attached to the stem by slender stalks with pairs of leaves that are lance shaped and grow on alternate sides of the stem. The turmeric plant grows to 3 feet (1 meter) tall with pale yellow flowers on each shoot. The rhizome is fleshy and branched with a deep yellow-orange color inside. Once dried, the tubers are 2 to 3 inches (5 to 7.5 cm) long, 1 inch (2.5 cm) in diameter, and pointed at the end.

- **PLANT PARTS USED:** Rhizome and tuber

- **TRADITIONAL EVIDENCE:**

Cultural Use

Asian. Turmeric is known in Chinese as *jiang huang* (rhizome) or *yu jin* (tuber), in Korean as *kanghwang,* and in Japanese as *kyoo.* In Chinese herbal medicine, turmeric root is used to move the blood and *qi,* especially in the abdomen and shoulders. It has been used in Japanese Kampo medicine since the mid-seventh century A.D. It is used as a treatment for inflammation, dysmenorrhea, liver damage, gall bladder stagnation and stones, jaundice, to stimulate the flow of energy through the shoulders, to relieve pain and swelling caused by traumatic injury, and in wound management. Turmeric is contraindicated in people who do not have symptoms of stagnant blood and *qi* and who do have blood deficiency. The Chinese *Materia Medica* lists turmeric as a useful antiseptic for both gram-positive and gram-negative organisms, an antiparasitic, and an antifungal (Bensky & Gamble, 1993).

Pacific Islander. Turmeric is known as *olena* in the Hawaiian Islands and is well known to traditional healers. In the Cook Islands the plant is known as *renga* and in the Marquesas the plant is called *ena* or *eka*. The juice from the root of the turmeric plant is obtained by pounding the root. The juice is strained through a cloth and is traditionally used for earache, sinus congestion, and colds. Hawaiians use fresh turmeric root to treat symptoms related to fungal infections (Naiman, 1999). Turmeric also is used for the treatment of symptoms related to cancer, diabetes, hypertension, and other heart problems. In Samoa, Tonga, and Futuna, a salve of the root is used for sores in the mouth and for rashes such as shingles. *Olena* is combined with seawater and sprinkled on people as part of purification ceremonies (Judd, 1997).

African. Turmeric is known as "shambala," "kitambwe," "Swahili," "mandano," and "kilunga kuku" in Africa. It is used as an ointment for skin disorders and smallpox lesions. It is also used to treat parasitic intestinal worms, conjunctivitis, headache, and as a uterine stimulant (Iwa, 1993).

East Indian. In India, turmeric is known by the names, "rajani," "gauri," "varnavat," "haridra," and "nisha." It is the most prevalent taste and smell in curry powder. It is used medicinally as a powder, paste, ointment, oil, lotion, and inhalant. Turmeric is used as a treatment for liver diseases, such as jaundice; urologic problems; and dyspepsia. Juice from the root is used in salves, and poultices are used to treat inflammation, sprains, arthralgias, wounds, and skin disorders. Turmeric mixed with slaked lime is also a home remedy used for the pain and swelling associated with sprains and injuries (Ammon & Wahl, 1990). Ghee (clarified butter) is mixed with turmeric and given to relieve cough. A thin paste of turmeric is applied to chicken pox vesicles to promote healing (Nadkarni, 1976).

European. Turmeric is approved in Germany for the treatment of dyspepsia. Turmeric tea is a recognized treatment for digestive system complaints, including symptoms related to gall bladder problems (Blumenthal, Goldberg, & Brinckman, 2000).

Culinary Use

Turmeric is used as a spice and is a main ingredient in curry powder. It is drunk as a beverage tea. Other culinary uses include use as a coloring agent for prepared mustards and as a food preservative.

Use in Herbalism

Turmeric has not always been used medicinally in some countries. It is now being researched and used increasingly for its restorative qualities and its ability to prevent cancerous growth. Turmeric has been used topically for skin ulcers, wounds, scabies, acne, and eczema. It calms the skin and is added to escharotics to lessen scarring and infection. It is taken internally and applied as an ointment after treatment to reduce scar tissue (Naiman, 1999). Turmeric is considered for its powerful antioxidant properties and hepatoprotection ability especially when a patient is exposed to carcinogens and medicines that are known to cause liver damage.

BIOMEDICAL EVIDENCE:

When reading the literature on turmeric, it is important for the reader to be clear as to whether the studies conducted used whole herb turmeric or only a constituent of the plant, such as curcumin.

Studies Related to Restoration

The restorative potential of turmeric is significant. A review article on diet and cancer reports that either from animal, in vivo, or in vitro studies, turmeric and its constituents—curcumin and turmerin—have demonstrated strong antioxidant activity. Turmeric and curcumin have demonstrated cytotoxic properties as well (Soudamini & Kuttan and Srinivas et al., as reported in Krishnaswamy & Polasa, 1995).

Turmeric, given in 1.5 g doses orally each day for thirty days in a human study of 16 chronic smokers, significantly reduced the urinary excretion of mutagens as compared with controls. It is hypothesized that an active constituent in turmeric, curcumin, may have detoxified the tobacco mutagens normally found in significant levels in the urine of smokers (Polasa, Raghuram, Krishna, & Krishnaswamy, 1992).

In a study of 62 patients with symptoms of itching, exudate, pain, and foul smell related to cancerous skin lesions, turmeric (10 g powder extracted overnight in 200 ml of ethanol or curcumin ointment) applied three times a day was shown to reduce clinical symptoms of smell (90%), itching (percent not reported), and exudate (70%). For example, itching was reduced in women with cancer of the vulva and foul smell was reduced in women with ulcerated breast cancer lesions. Pain was reduced but could have been a result of the analgesics the patients received concomitantly. The patients in the study did not receive any other cancer treatments or antibiotics during the study (Kuttan, Sudheeran, & Josph, 1987).

In a review article, the pharmacologic action of dietary turmeric was found to demonstrate "adjuvant chemoprotection in experimental forestomach and oral cancer models of Swiss mice and Syrian golden hamsters" (Azuire & Bhide as reported in Eigner & Scholz, 1999). Another animal study demonstrated that turmeric and curcumin increase the survival rate of animals with lymphoma (Kuttan, Bhanumathy, Nirmala, & George, 1985).

The isolation of curcuminoids from turmeric in a study conducted by Roth et al. (1998) (as reported in Blumenthal et al., 2000) showed enzyme inhibition activity of topoisomerase I and II. Studies are currently underway to investigate the antioxidant activity of turmeric. Some evidence exists that indicates that both turmeric's rhizome and active ingredient, curcumin, protect DNA breakage caused by singlet oxygen. Genotoxicity and mutagenic activity are associated with singlet oxygen (Blumenthal et al., 2000).

Curcumin has been shown to prevent the damage attributed to aflatoxin exposure (Blumenthal et al., 2000). Aflatoxins are produced by aspergillus species of molds. They are found in high concentrations in groundnuts and corn in Africa, Southeast Asia, China, and the United States. Epidemiologic studies have shown a strong connection between the degree of aflatoxin exposure and the risk of development of primary liver cancer (DeVita et al., 1997).

A number of animal and in vitro studies have demonstrated the various ways turmeric and/or curcumin protects against cancer itself or the side effects of cancer treatment. Curcumins from turmeric have a demonstrated anticarcinogenic activity against a number of potent mouse stomach and skin carcinogens (Nagabhushan & Bhide, 1992). In mice, preexposure application of curcumin protects the skin from the effects of ultraviolet-A light, which can lead to skin cancer (Ishizaki et al., 1996). Oral doses of curcumin (200 μmol/kg) also have been shown to protect rats against the side effects of radiation treatment for cancer (Thresiamma, George, & Kuttan, 1996) and (at 200 mg/kg in 1% gum acacia) prevent lung damage in rats caused by the chemotherapeutic agent cyclophosphamide (Venkatesan & Chandrakasan, 1995).

Studies Related to Other Health Patterns

Skin. In a study of the use of a paste made from turmeric root (half the length of the index finger) and a handful of neem leaves spread all over the body for the treatment of scabies, 97.9% of 824 people with scabies showed complete cure after treatment for three to fifteen days. Preliminary treatment of scrub baths and boiling of fomites was also critical to the positive results. No side effects were noted, such as occurred with the use of topical benzyl benzoate (Charles & Charles, 1992).

Turmeric powder applied to septic and antiseptic wounds in rats and rabbits is reported to accelerate the healing process but no supporting data are given (Eigner & Scholz, 1999).

Comfort and Pain Relief. In a study using objective and subjective measures for pain relief and comfort, curcumin, 400 mg capsules three times a day for five days, given to 45 male patients after inguinal hernia and/or hydrocele repair, was shown to significantly reduce inflammation, cord edema, and tenderness as compared with placebo and phenylbutazone, but not operative site pain and tenderness (Satoskar, Shah, & Shenoy, 1986).

Mechanism of Action

The compound curcumin in turmeric inhibits prostaglandins in the body, which is probably how turmeric came to be known for its ability to ease pain and inflammation. At high doses, curcumin stimulates the adrenal glands to release the body's own natural cortisone (Duke,

1997). Curcumin "exerts its potent antiplatelet activity through inhibition of COX [Cyclooxygenase] activity and the blockade of calcium signaling" (Shah et al., 1999, p.1169). One study reports that the antitumor effects of turmeric are due to the interaction with arachidonate metabolism (Roe et al., as reported in Blumenthal et al., 2000). Turmeric has choleretic and cholecystokinetic properties in addition to its anti-inflammatory properties (Schulz, Hansel, & Tyler 1998).

🌿 USE IN PREGNANCY OR LACTATION:

While one source reports that turmeric is an emmenagogue and uterine stimulant and should not be used during pregnancy (McGuffin et al., 1997), this must be clarified. The whole fresh or dried root is contraindicated in pregnancy, but in India for example, turmeric powder (aged turmeric) used in curries is eaten liberally by pregnant women (Personal communication, Usha Varma, MD, May 2001).

Herbal Caveat—Pregnancy or Lactation
Some herbs are contraindicated in pregnancy because of a risk of the herb or one of its constituents stimulating the uterus and therefore possibly promoting fetal loss. Many herbal practitioners do not recommend herbal remedies, in particular oral doses of herbs, during the first trimester of pregnancy and seek an alternative. However, herbs are successfully used during pregnancy, especially to prepare the body for the birth. Herbs are relatively unstudied in pregnancy and lactation, so patients need to be made aware through education of the potential benefits and risks of using herbs for health conditions that arise during pregnancy or lactation. The use of herbal remedies during pregnancy often warrants a referral to a knowledgeable herbal practitioner.

🌿 USE FOR CHILDREN:

No data are available on the internal use of turmeric in therapeutic quantities.

Herbal Caveat—Children
Children have special needs in regard to herbal therapies. They require lesser amounts of herbs and often respond well to mild teas and topical applications such as compresses and baths. The lowest dose of oral preparations should be tried first before increasing the amount given children. Caregivers should observe children closely for responses to herbal remedies. Younger children, particularly infants, have traditionally been given herbs either through their mother's breast milk or in the form of a homeopathic remedy because of their sensitivity to medicines and treatments and the immaturity of their liver. It is recommended that a person knowledgeable in the herbal treatment of children be consulted before the offering of any herb to a child for the first time.

🌿 CAUTIONS:

Turmeric is contraindicated in therapeutic quantities for people with bile duct obstruction or cholelithiasis and should not be given to people with gastric ulcers or hyperacidity (McGuffin et al., 1997). Turmeric is an emmenagogue and uterine stimulant and therefore may be contraindicated for women experiencing pelvic inflammatory disease or excessive bleeding during menstruation (McGuffin et al., 1997).

The use of turmeric should be avoided with congestive heart failure of unknown etiology. This condition has been attributed to overactivity of the p53 gene leading to weakening of the heart. Curcumin protects p53 and through this action may augment destruction of heart tissue (Rister, 1999).

Because one study of the anti-inflammatory effects of curcumin in animals demonstrated that much higher oral doses were necessary to achieve an anti-inflammatory effect than when given intraperitoneally, and because after oral application, only traces of curcumin were found in the blood, some researchers speculate that curcumin is poorly absorbed through the gastrointestinal tract and may be better given by an alternate route (Ammon & Whal, 1991). The shelf life of volatile oil content is lost at 0.5% per year and should be calculated into dosing (Blumenthal et al., 2000).

NURSING EVIDENCE:

Historical Nursing Use

No data are available at this time.

Potential Nursing Applications

Nurses may want to consider including turmeric as one of the spices to be used in a healthy diet, especially for those patients who smoke tobacco. Nurses might consider the use of turmeric paste or ointment in the care of patients with wounds and skin disorders such as scabies. Further research is needed on the ability of turmeric and/or curcumin to protect the skin of patients undergoing radiation therapy. Nurses also may want to consider employing turmeric's anti-inflammatory activity, especially in patients with shoulder pain.

Integrative Insight

Turmeric can be found in many people's kitchens, however, many people do not know of the traditional or scientific evidence regarding the medicinal use of turmeric. The scientific literature, though primarily animal studies, provides some support for the traditional topical applications of turmeric to skin conditions and to joint pain. Turmeric seems to restore balance under very challenging situations such as exposure to ultraviolet light. Turmeric taken internally may improve the ability to overcome illness due to cancer. Turmeric reminds us that some very good medicines are right at our fingertips. They are inexpensive and science and technology show that they have potential to be effective and preventive. Turmeric not only tastes good in curry and relieves a stomachache, but also it has powerful anti-inflammatory, antioxidant, and antitumor activity.

THERAPEUTIC APPLICATIONS:

Oral

1 teaspoon ground rhizome in water or juice three to four times daily (Hoppe, 2000)

Standardized Extract. 400 to 600 mg curcumin three times daily (typically standardized to 95% curcuminoids) (Hoppe, 2000)

Note: Combining curcumin with bromelain enhances absorption and activity (Werbach & Murray, 1994).

Topical

Turmeric can be made into a poultice, paste, oil, salve, ointment, or lotion for topical use.

Environmental

No data are available at this time.

Herbal Caveat—Therapeutic Applications

In traditional and conventional herbal medicine, amounts of herbs given to patients are based on individual needs. The amounts or "doses" recorded here are provided so that the health practitioner has a general idea of the amounts recommended for an adult patient. Dosing in herbalism not only refers to amount of plant used but also includes when, where, and how to take a plant medicine. These dosages should not be used as guidelines for indiscriminate intervention without proper assessment, critical thinking, and patient education on the part of the practitioner.

Note: Please see chapter 5 for detailed descriptions of how to prepare various applications.

PATIENT INTERACTION:

Turmeric, a well-known spice and ingredient in curry powder, also can be used medicinally. Numerous animal and in vitro studies have demonstrated the anticancer benefits of turmeric and one of its constituents, curcumin. Turmeric also has anti-inflammatory properties, is helpful in healing wounds, and can be used for a number of skin conditions, such as eczema and scabies, when applied topically. Turmeric is contraindicated in therapeutic quantities for people with bile duct obstruction or gallstones, and should not be eaten by people with gastric ulcers or hyperacidity. Turmeric is an emmenagogue and uterine stimulant and may be contraindicated for women experiencing pelvic inflammatory disease or excessive bleeding during menstruation.

Herbal Caveat—Patient Interaction

Patients considering the use of an herb or formula of herbs in self-care benefit from education about the plant itself and the use of the plant in healing. This education can come through many sources, including local herbalists; plant specialists such as botanists; health practitioners such as nurses, nutritionists, naturopaths, and other physicians; and various written references including the scientific literature. Patients need to remember that their unique health care needs are not necessarily represented in

---

any literature they may encounter. Therefore, it is recommended that a knowledgeable mentor be consulted before initiating self-care with any herb being used for the first time.

🌿 NURTURING THE NURSE-PLANT RELATIONSHIP:

Note: You may want to keep a journal of your experiences with the herb.

Try experiencing turmeric as a spice, one of the ingredients of a fragrant curry. You can give yourself a break from cooking and try a nearby Indian or Nepali restaurant or you can make a pot of *dal* for yourself and your family. *Dal* is a spiced lentil dish that is eaten with rice and *chapati* (flat bread). Here is a recipe that has about 0.5 to 1.5 g of turmeric per serving (adapted from Eigner & Scholz, 1999): Wash and soak 2 cups (454 g) of lentils for 15 minutes. Add to 5 cups (1200 ml) boiling water with 2 teaspoons of turmeric and a pinch of salt and cook on low fire until lentils are plump and soft. Finely chop one large onion and 6 teaspoons fresh ginger and sauté in ½ cup ghee (clarified butter) until brown. Add 1 teaspoon black cumin seed and sauté for 1 minute. When the lentils are nearly cooked, add the onion mixture and 2 teaspoons chopped coriander leaf, 2 green chilies, and 1 teaspoon black pepper and cook for 5 minutes. The *dal* should have the consistency of a stovetop casserole. If available, add 5 drops of asafoetida water before serving to help digestion of the lentils. Breathe in the aroma of the turmeric, taste, and enjoy!

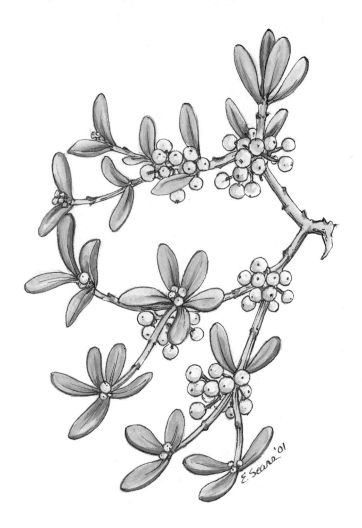

Viscum album

Mistletoe

🍃 **LATIN NAME:** *Viscum album*

🍃 **FAMILY:** Viscaceae

Note: Approximately 1400 plant species are called mistletoe. The species discussed here is *Viscum album* or white berry mistletoe.

🍃 **COMMON NAMES:** Mistletoe, white berry mistletoe, bird lime, European mistletoe, Devil's fuge, herbe de la Croix, mystyldene

🍃 **HEALTH PATTERN:** Restoration

🍃 **PLANT DESCRIPTION:**

Mistletoe is a succulent evergreen parasite that grows on the branches of host trees. Mistletoe grows on fruit trees, hardwood, elms, oaks, hickory, pines, and poplars and contains slightly different properties because its nutrients are obtained from the host. Mistletoe grows throughout Europe and is naturalized in one county in California (Leung & Foster, 1996). It is uniformly branched with lance-shaped, yellow-green, leathery leaves that grow in pairs and are 1-3 inches (2 to 8 cm) long. The stems are jointed and grow up to 40 inches (100 cm) long. The flower has four petals that bloom in early spring and turn into a sticky white globular berry in the winter. All parts of the plant contain viscin, commonly called "bird glue," a resinous, adhesive substance that is insoluble in water and slightly soluble in alcohol (Felter & Lloyd, 1983).

🍃 **PLANT PARTS USED:** Leaves and berry

🍃 **TRADITIONAL EVIDENCE:**

Cultural Use

Asian. In Asia, mistletoe has been used as a medicinal tea in the treatment of symptoms related to lumbago, hypertension, and tumors (Park, Hyun, & Shin, 1999).

North American Indian. The mistletoe used by North American Indians is *Phoradendron* (Kay, 1996) not *Viscum.*

Hispanic. The mistletoe used by Mexican Americans is *Phoradendron* (Kay, 1996) not *Viscum.*

East Indian. In Hindi, mistletoe is known as "banda." *V. album* is used to decrease liver and spleen hypertrophy, decrease edema, and to control hemorrhage and excessive menstrual bleeding. It also is used in decreasing heart palpitations, as an antispasmodic, to calm hysteria, and to control epilepsy. It is used topically for abscesses (Nadkarni, 1976).

European. The use of mistletoe dates back to Hippocrates (460–370 B.C.) when it was used to treat disorders of the spleen (Kienle,

1999). During the Renaissance, mistletoe was used to counteract phlegm (Kay, 1996). Mistletoe was the sacred plant of the Druids who believed that the plant protected the person who possessed the plant from evil and that the oak trees upon which the mistletoe grew were respected as a source of many cures. Many Druid rituals involved the use of mistletoe, including the announcing of the new year with a sprig of the plant, a ritual similar to today's decoration with mistletoe during the Christmas season. The writings of Pliny the Elder explain that the Druidic ritual included the cutting of the mistletoe from the oak with a sickle on the "sixth day of the moon," followed by the sacrifice of two white bulls (Ellis, 1994, p. 139). The Celts use mistletoe not only for fertility but also as an "antidote for all poisons" (Ellis, 1994, p. 139).

The white berry of mistletoe is used in an Anthroposophical medicine preparation called "Iscador." Iscador is a cancer treatment that has been used in Germany, Switzerland, and Austria for almost 80 years. Iscador (WELEDA) is the best known Anthroposophical preparation; others are Helixor, Abnoba Viscum, and Iscucin (by WALA). The difference between the Anthroposophical product and other mistletoe products is the complicated pharmaceutical process used in mixing the whole plant extract and the fact that the mistletoe is harvested specifically during the winter and summer. Other German commercial non-Anthroposophical preparations like Lektinol and Eurixor use a standardization process standardizing to the constituent, mistletoe lectin 1 (ML-1). The theoretical foundation for cancer treatment with mistletoe is based upon the work of Rudolf Steiner. Anthroposophical medicine practitioners use mistletoe to activate the "individual configurative vital forces of patients in the tumor area" (Gorter, 1998). They use mistletoe to purposefully stimulate the body's immune system. Because mistletoe contains very potent cytostatics, high dosages of the extract are never given. Mistletoe preparations are used in near-homeopathic dilutions. The purpose of the mistletoe treatment is to help the patient's immune system to cytologically detect the foreign properties of the cancer cells. "Up to two thirds of cancer patients in Germany and Austria receive alternative therapies, primarily mistletoe treatments" (Kienle, 1999, p. 34).

Studies with Iscador are described in the Biomedical Evidence section. Mistletoe treatment is fully covered by medical insurance in parts of Europe such as Germany (personal communication, Matthias Seidel, MD, May 2001).

Culinary Use

Although the Council of Europe lists mistletoe berry and branches as sources of food flavoring (Newall et al., 1996), this plant is not generally used in food.

Use in Herbalism

Mistletoe is used as a nervine, narcotic, sedative, an antispasmodic, diaphoretic, and tonic. It has been used usually in the form of fluid extract or powdered leaf, to treat epilepsy, hysteria, insanity, paralysis, and chorea (Felter & Lloyd, 1983; Grieve, 1971). Mistletoe is used to treat several cardiovascular problems including lowering of blood pressure, depressing cardiac activity, treating cardiac hypertrophy, valvular insufficiency, weak pulse edema, dyspnea, and to counteract the cardiac effects of typhoid fever (Felter & Lloyd, 1983). Mistletoe is used to treat undelivered placenta or heavy bleeding after labor, dysmenorrhea, and amenorrhea (Felter & Lloyd, 1983; Weed, 1986).

BIOMEDICAL EVIDENCE:

Many of the clinical studies on mistletoe have been conducted on the injectable preparation, Iscador. In 1983, the American Cancer Society released a statement in *CA-A Cancer Journal for Clinicians* stating that because they have no evidence that Iscador "results in objective benefit in the treatment of cancer in human beings," they "strongly urge individuals afflicted with cancer not to participate in treatment with Iscador" (p. 186). The extensive data reviewed by the Society was from the Lukas Clinic in Switzerland and included 17 chemical and clinical papers dealing with the effect of mistletoe on humans and a summary review of 25 publications and 14 unpublished manuscripts on the subject. Since 1983, health practitioners at the Lukas clinic, an Anthroposophical medicine clinic, have continued to treat patients with Iscador and to publish their results. The interpretation of the results of the research on Iscador continues to be controversial. Many question the validity of the studies because so few are randomized, "due primarily to ethical concerns about randomization among Anthroposophical physicians as well as strong patient preference" (Kienle, 1999, p. 34). The German Cancer Society supports the unlimited use of Mistletoe preparations in palliative situations because there is evidence that the preterminal patient treated with mistletoe is more active (higher Karnovsky index), has less pain, and has markedly fewer prescriptions of analgesic medication (personal communication, Matthias Seidel, MD, May 2001).

The American Cancer Society's present conclusion on the literature is that there are "no controlled clinical human trials that have shown mistletoe to have any significant anti-tumor activity and most of the studies that have shown positive results from mistletoe extract in the treatment and prevention of cancer are not considered scientifically dependable" (personal communication, Information Specialist, American Cancer Society, October 24, 2000). Another review of the literature raises questions about the validity and reliability of some of the Iscador research; however, it points out that Iscador does not have the side effects of biomedical cytotoxic agents and, "In spite of its relatively weak anti-tumor effects it may be a preparation that could usefully be used in the long term treatment of cancer patients alongside surgery and radiotherapy and not be reserved for the more limited role of the majority of current chemotherapeutic agents due to their relative non-specificity and toxicity" (Evans & Preece, 1974, p. 19).

Studies Related to Restoration

Measurable effects of immunomodulation were observed in breast cancer patients after a single intravenous infusion of the Iscador preparation, Iscador M 2%, 0.21 to 0.38 mg/kg in 250 ml saline over three hours. Evaluation of peripheral blood showed neutrophilia, juvenile neutrophilia, increased granulocyte phagocytic activity, natural killer cell activity, antibody-dependent cell-mediated cytotoxicity, and increased levels of large granular lymphocytes. The natural killer cell and antibody-dependent cell-mediated cytotoxicity activity was noted to be similar in kinetic pattern to alpha-interferon. Fever increased by 2.3 to 2.4 degrees centigrade in all patients receiving the infusion. Stimulating the immune system of these patients caused mild side effects during the first few hours, including chills, nausea, or headache (Hajto, 1986). Fever is considered a sign of an active healthy immune system by Anthroposophical medicine practitioners.

Intravenous infusions of Iscador were administered to 20 breast cancer patients at the Lukas Clinic in Arlesheim, Switzerland. Patients were noted to experience a febrile reaction with increased neutrophil granulocytes. Lymphocytes initially decrease then increase to include natural killer cells and antibody dependent killer cells (Gorter, 1998).

A study of 14 breast cancer patients showed that Iscador seems to increase DNA repair attributed to the stimulation of enzymes by lymphokines or cytokines whose function is to repair. An ongoing Iscador study for cervical dysplasia showed a 77% response rate after six months of treatment. At the time of publication, it was planned to have the 100 women involved in the study be followed for two years to see if Iscador might prevent cervical malignancy from developing (Gorter, 1998).

One case study reported that a 59-year-old male with small cell lung carcinoma who refused chemotherapy lived five years and seven months after being treated with Iscador injections for five days followed by oral Iscador, homeopathic remedies, and radiation therapy two years later. Patients with this diagnosis typically live six to seventeen weeks without treatment and three years with chemotherapy treatment (Bradley & Clover, 1989).

Iscador may inhibit the progression of human immunodeficiency virus (HIV) disease. A study of Iscador treatment in which subcutaneous doses of 0.01 to 10 mg were self-administered two times a week in gradually increasing doses for two to seventeen weeks by HIV-positive patients showed Iscador to have immunomodulating effects and to be safely administered by HIV-positive patients without severe side effects. In this study of 32 HIV patients and 9 healthy subjects, a favorable response was noted to include an improvement in physical well-being; an increase in appetite, body weight, sleep, mental strength, and physical strength; and a decrease in pain. It also was noted that people tolerated chemotherapy and radiation therapy better while on Iscador (Gorter, Van Wely, Reiff, & Stoss, 1999).

Studies Related to Other Health Patterns

Immune Response. One placebo-controlled study was performed with Iscador on 30 children with recurrent acute respiratory infections after nuclear radiation exposure in Chernobyl. The children had increased cytotoxic activity of natural killer cells and a significant improvement in the degree of tiredness, sweating, headaches, muscle and joint pain, and emotional lability. The children experienced slight pain locally when the highest dose was injected and 3 children had hyperemia of (1 to 4 cm) at the injection site that disappeared gradually before the next injection (Chernyshov et al., 1997).

Mechanism of Action

Mistletoe's immunostimulating activities are thought to be due to both polysaccharides and lectins (Gorter, 1998; Schulz et al., 1998). The polysaccharides in mistletoe have been found in in vitro studies to stimulate and activate the complement system (Schulz, 1998). In vitro studies using human leukemia cells and animal sarcoma cells in culture show cytotoxic activity attributed to two toxic proteins isolated from mistletoe. The first protein is mistletoe lectin, which interferes with protein synthesis intracellularly, preventing the cell from dividing. The second protein is the toxic viscotoxin, which lyses the cell membrane (Gorter, 1998). Viscumin is the lectin, a complex protein-sugar compound with the ability to bind to the surfaces of cells. This is believed to interfere with cellular protein synthesis, leading to the manufacture of cytokines, motivating the manufacture and mobilization of leukocytes. This lectin may have an affect on both the process of metastasis and apoptosis (Stirpe, Sandvig, Olsnes, & Pihl, 1982; Thatte, Bagadey, & Dahanukar, 2000). Viscotoxin, also a lectin, is thought to be more cytotoxic than vicumin. The cytotoxicity leads to cellular necrosis (Kaegi, 1998; Thatte et al., 2000). Mistletoe also contains alkaloids with biologic activity. The clinical significance has yet to be determined (Kaegi, 1998).

Some Iscador preparations have been shown in studies of human tissue samples to induce an activation of CD4+ and CD8+ lymphocytes (Gorter, Van Wely, Stoss, & Wollina, 1998). In vitro, mistletoe extracts appear to increase DNA stability and inhibit growth (Kaegi, 1998; Thatte, 2000).

USE IN PREGNANCY OR LACTATION:

Some state that Mistletoe has been used as an abortifacient (Leung & Foster, 1996) and is contraindicated in pregnancy, perhaps because Mistletoe contains tyramine, which has been shown in animal studies to be a uterine stimulant (Brinker, 1998). However, the injectable form (e.g., Iscador) used in Europe has been given successfully during pregnancy and lactation. Anthroposophical physicians report that mistletoe preparations assist the placenta in adhering better to the uterus (personal communication, Matthias Seidel, MD, May, 2001). Pregnant women with breast cancer in Europe have been treated successfully with intravenous and subcutaneous mistletoe preparations without complication.

Herbal Caveat—Pregnancy or Lactation

Some herbs are contraindicated in pregnancy because of a risk of the herb or one of its constituents stimulating the uterus and therefore possibly promoting fetal loss. Many herbal practitioners do not recommend herbal remedies, in particular oral doses of herbs, during the first trimester of pregnancy and seek an alternative. However, herbs are successfully used during pregnancy, especially to prepare the body for the birth. Herbs are relatively unstudied in pregnancy and lactation, so patients need to be made aware through education of the potential benefits and risks of using herbs for health conditions that arise during pregnancy or lactation. The use of herbal remedies during pregnancy often warrants a referral to a knowledgeable herbal practitioner.

USE FOR CHILDREN:

No reported severe side effects were found with the Chernobyl children studied who received Iscador (Gorter, 1998).

Herbal Caveat—Children

Children have special needs in regard to herbal therapies. They require lesser amounts of herbs and often respond well to mild teas and topical applications such as compresses and baths. The lowest dose of oral preparations should be tried first before increasing the amount given children. Caregivers should observe children closely for responses to herbal remedies. Younger children, particularly infants, have traditionally been given herbs either through their mother's breast milk or in the form of a homeopathic remedy because of their sensitivity to medicines and treatments and the immaturity of their liver. It is recommended that a person knowledgeable in the herbal treatment of children be consulted before the offering of any herb to a child for the first time.

CAUTIONS:

This plant is often regarded as poisonous, which is what I was taught as I was growing up. Although "an analysis of more than 300 reported mistletoe ingestion cases in the United States found that a majority of patients were asymptomatic and no fatalities occurred" (Leung & Foster, 1996, p. 373), there is still a higher potential for toxicity with mistletoe use because of the lectins in the plant. Self-medication with this herb is not advisable. This herb should be used under the guidance of a knowledgeable practitioner. When taken as a tea, blood pressure should be monitored. Mistletoe is contraindicated in protein hypersensitivity and chronic progressive infections such as acquired immunodeficiency syndrome (AIDS) and tuberculosis (McGuffin et al., 1997). Reported adverse reactions include flulike syndrome, hypersensitivity reactions, contact dermatitis, fever, headache, and chest pain (Gorter et al., 1999; Leung & Foster, 1996). Studies have shown Iscador injections to cause a local reaction (56%) that slowly subsides over 10 hours. The local reaction is followed by induration, itching, swelling, pain, and hyperthermia. Use of steroids or antihistamines to suppress these symptoms is not recommended because the reaction is used to determine optimal dose. The size of this reaction should not exceed 1 to 2 inches (3 to 5 cm) (Gorter, 1998). Side effects of Iscador have been found to be similar to commonly prescribed biologic response modifiers such as recombinant interleukin-2 (IL-2), IL-3, and human IL-6 (Gorter, 1999).

A study conducted by Park et al. (1999) showed mistletoe's cytotoxicity to be reduced considerably in vitro by heat. This should be taken into consideration when teas or infusions are made with boiling water. Mistletoe lectin is a protein that can be destroyed or denatured by gastric acid, which is one reason why it is best used in injectable form (personal communication, Matthias Seidel, MD, May, 2001). People who are taking monoamine oxidase (MAO) inhibitors should not take tyramine. Mistletoe contains tyramine and may be contraindicated (Kay, 1996).

NURSING EVIDENCE:

Historical Nursing Use
No data are available at this time.

Potential Nursing Applications
Oncology nurses may find that increasing numbers of patients are aware of the use of mistletoe preparations in the treatment of cancer. Nurses can read and evaluate the extensive European literature, especially on Iscador, to be better informed to provide guidance for patients considering their options. Nurses who have knowledge of qualitative research methods and the integration of quantitative and qualitative research methods can assist in researching the use of mistletoe preparations such as Iscador in the treatment of cancer patients.

Integrative Insight
Mistletoe has been used for many years in the care of patients with serious disease such as cancer and heart disease. It is a plant medicine that must be used with care and therefore is often excluded from texts on herbal remedies. It has been included here because many patients and health practitioners are becoming more aware of its extensive use in treating cancer. Nurses need to know about it too. As is the case with herbal remedies in general and mistletoe in particular, the person using the remedy must understand the plant and how to prepare it for use. In the case of mistletoe, this is very important.

Science has helped define that certain plant constituents, such as lectins, can be very toxic to humans. It is also known that lectins can be removed. The lectin found in castor beans is removed during processing into oil (McGuffin et al., 1997). Park et al. (1999) found that the lectins in mistletoe are not as cytotoxic when heated to make tea. This is a good thing if a person is worried about toxicity of the plant, but it is not beneficial if the heat takes away the healing power of the mistletoe, which also happens to be its cytotoxic effect.

The history of mistletoe use in healing is a good demonstration that herbs like mistletoe are best used and developed within the framework of an interdisciplinary approach. Those who use Iscador seem to be using an integrated approach in which different members of the treatment team, including the patient, provide feedback about the remedy and its use. The pharmacists create a remedy that may indeed be safer for use than whole herb because it has gone through a processing phase to identify the level of toxic constituent. Physicians, nurses, and patients determine appropriate dosing and application through observation of patient responses and making adjustments as needed. Traditional healers and botanists are the ones who direct the team to the appropriate plant and source in the first place and raise questions such as, "Is the healing effect of mistletoe taken from elm trees different from that taken from the oak?" Although the research on Iscador is not perfect, important scientific information regarding the use of mistletoe in the care of cancer patients is available for nurses. This includes the scientific importance of the interdisciplinary team and the possibility of the integration of mistletoe into the long-term care of cancer patients.

THERAPEUTIC APPLICATIONS:

Note: Mistletoe herb has a shelf life of approximately one year (Felter & Lloyd, 1983).

Oral

Tea. 2.5 g infused in cold water for ten to twelve hours up to two times a day (McGuffin et al., 1997)

Liquid Extract. 1:1 (g/ml) in 25% alcohol ½ teaspoon (1 to 3 ml) three times per day

Tincture. 1:5 (g/ml) in 45% alcohol (0.5 ml) three times daily

Powder. 2 to 6 g (Wren, 1988)

Topical

Parenteral. The preparation of Iscador is given by subcutaneous injection. One ampule is administered several (usually three) times a week around the cancer site or operation scar, in escalating doses beginning at 0.01 to 20 mg for long-term therapy. Intravenous injections of Iscador are occasionally administered in an inpatient hospital setting and is restricted to physicians familiar with mistletoe treatment and the potential reactions to intravenous administration that can occur. Mistletoe is frequently used in formula preparations, and dosage depends on the formula used (Gorter, 1998; personal communication, Matthias Seidel, MD, May 2001).

Environmental

An old pagan custom still used today involves the hanging of mistletoe in the house as a symbol of peace, friendship, and goodwill. Today the ritual of kissing beneath the mistletoe plant at Christmas time for good fortune is still practiced (Grieve, 1971; Lawless, 1998).

Herbal Caveat—Therapeutic Applications

In traditional and conventional herbal medicine, amounts of herbs given to patients are based on individual needs. The amounts or "doses" recorded here are provided so that the health practitioner has a general idea of the amounts recommended for an adult patient. Dosing in herbalism not only refers to amount of plant used but also includes when, where, and how to take a plant medicine. These dosages should not be used as guidelines for indiscriminate intervention without proper assessment, critical thinking, and patient education on the part of the practitioner.

Note: Please see chapter 5 for detailed descriptions of how to prepare various applications.

❧ PATIENT INTERACTION:

Mistletoe contains some constituents that are not only potentially helpful in the treatment of cancer but also can be toxic when the plant is not used correctly. Therefore, mistletoe should only be used under the guidance of a knowledgeable practitioner. Iscador and other mistletoe products have been used in the treatment of cancer, particularly in Anthroposophical medicine clinics and hospitals in Germany, Switzerland, and Austria for 80 years. These treatments are prescribed by physicians and are injected subcutaneously or intravenously. Extensive research has been conducted on mistletoe preparations, but some have questioned the scientific quality of the work. Mistletoe is not recommended in those with protein hypersensitivity and chronic progressive infections such as AIDS and tuberculosis. Reported adverse reactions may include flulike syndrome, hypersensitivity reactions, contact dermatitis, fever, headache, and chest pain.

Herbal Caveat—Patient Interaction

Patients considering the use of an herb or formula of herbs in self-care benefit from education about the plant itself and the use of the plant in healing. This education can come through many sources, including local herbalists; plant specialists such as botanists; health practitioners such as nurses, nutritionists, naturopaths, and other physicians; and various written references including the scientific literature. Patients need to remember that their unique health care needs are not necessarily represented in any literature they may encounter. Therefore, it is recommended that a knowledgeable mentor be consulted before initiating self-care with any herb being used for the first time.

Note: You may want to keep a journal of your experiences with the herb.

When thinking of mistletoe, some people may remember a tradition of kissing underneath the mistletoe during the Christian holiday of Christmas. An old custom still used today involves the hanging of mistletoe in the house as a symbol of peace, friendship, and goodwill. Mistletoe reminds us about the importance of love, intimacy, and peace in the home. Homes need to be places where we can heal and recreate. Get to know mistletoe through this ancient tradition from Europe. Purchase a little sprig for your home. Try hanging it near your front door where you can see it when you come home to remind you to leave the cares of the day outside. Taking off your (nursing) shoes when you enter your house, as is done in countries such as Japan, also can be a symbolic way of reminding yourself to leave the world outside so that your home can be a place to rest and heal.

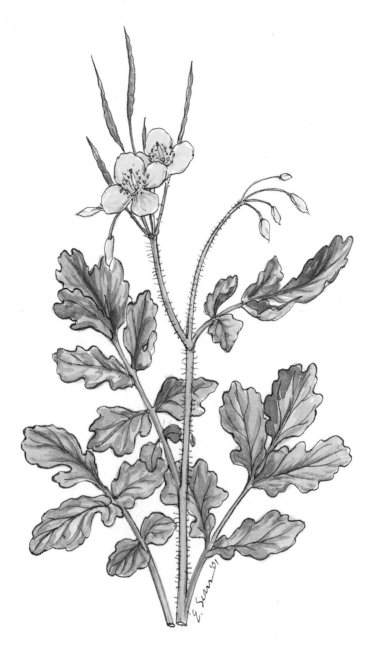

Chelidonium majus

Greater Celandine

🍃 **LATIN NAME:** *Chelidonium majus*

🍃 **FAMILY:** Papaveraceae

🍃 **COMMON NAMES:** Greater celandine, celandine, garden celandine, tetterwort, felonwort, swallow wort
  Note: Although the herb is referred to only as celandine in this profile, it should not be confused with lesser celandine *(Ranunculus ficaria),* also known as pilewort.

🍃 **HEALTH PATTERN:** Restoration

🍃 **PLANT DESCRIPTION:**
Celandine is a perennial plant indigenous to Europe. It is found growing in human habitat areas such as gardens, along walls, hedges, and waste or drainage areas. Celandine blooms from May to October. Celandine is a pale green evergreen that has slightly hairy 1 to 3 foot (up to 1 meter) stems. The leaves are bright greenish-yellow and consist of four small wide petals. The flower stalks spread from a common center followed by thin, black seed-containing pods. The root is thick, fleshy, and reddish-brown. Breaking the stems or leaves releases a bright yellow-orange sap that can have a strong odor and a very pungent, bitter taste.

🍃 **PLANT PARTS USED:** Aerial parts of plant and root

🍃 **TRADITIONAL EVIDENCE:**
Cultural Use

  Asian. Celandine is used in Asia as an analgesic, antitussive, anti-inflammatory, and detoxifying agent. In China, celandine is used for stomach cancer, peptic ulcer, and skin ailments. One source states that clinical studies have been conducted in China on the use of celandine in bronchitis and whooping cough, but no other data, including the species studied, is provided (Wren, 1988).

  Hispanic. Some Hispanic people use celandine for digestion, gall bladder complaints, liver disease, hepatitis, and eczema and other skin disorders.

  Russian/Baltic. Celandine is known as "chistotel bolshoy" in Russian. "Chistotel" means body cleansing. Russia continues to use this plant as an effective treatment for cancer, in particular for malignant "swellings" (Hutchens, 1992). Other approved uses for the orange latex of the stem include wart, freckle, and corn removal and treatment of fungal diseases of the skin. "Dr. V.C. Yagodka, working in the Kiev State Institute for Advanced Medical Training of the Ukraine Health Ministry, found that the herb inhibits cancerous growths of the skin. He applies it to areas where cancerous skin growths have been surgically removed, and the celandine preparation prevents them from recurring" (Zevin, 1997, p. 50).

European. Documentation from the Middle Ages cites celandine as a medicine used to remove film collected on the cornea of the eye. In the fourteenth century, a celandine drink was used to cleanse the blood. Old European alchemists used celandine to cure jaundice (Grieve, 1971). In Germany, celandine, called "Schollkraut," is used for the treatment of gallstone disease and dyspepsia (Benninger et al., 1999).

Culinary Use

Celandine is not used in foods because of the unpleasant bitter flavor of the sap.

Use in Herbalism

Celandine is used as an alterative and a diuretic. It is commonly used to treat jaundice and eczema and as a topical juice or oil applied to ringworm, corns, and warts. Celandine also is used extensively to alleviate the symptoms associated with many different types of cancers. The tincture is used in liver cancer when the patient's urine has a strong odor (Naiman, 1999). Celandine also is used for eye conditions. The word "chelidon" in Greek signifies a swallow, the bird. Swallows are known to use greater celandine to apply to the eyes of their babies whose eyes get pecked. People also use celandine for the restoration of the eyes. Either the sap directly from the stem and leaf or a bright green oil made from the celandine leaf can be applied to the eyelids (not the eye) to relieve and restore aching, tired eyes. I have used the external application of celandine tincture on patients; for example, the tincture was used on a woman who got gasoline in her eyes. Her eyes were pain and infection free by the following morning.

The root, boiled with a few aniseeds in white wine, is used for liver and gall bladder obstruction and "old sores" of the lower limbs. The root is also bruised, covered in chamomile oil, and then applied to a woman's navel to ease abdominal pain. Gargling the herb has been used for toothache (Culpeper, 1990). Celandine is also very effective in wart removal. The outer layer of skin is gently scraped with a scalpel until the blood supply of the wart is exposed. Then the celandine oil is applied and the wart covered. I have seen warts that were still growing after medical treatments with chemotherapeutic agents and cryotherapy disappear after a few days use of topical celandine oil.

BIOMEDICAL EVIDENCE:

Very little clinical research is available supporting the traditional uses of celandine. Some studies have been conducted on a phytopharmaceutical, semisynthetic compound of celandine alkaloids called "Ukrain."

Studies Related to Restoration

In a small study of 2 people with Kaposi's sarcoma, 5 mg of Ukrain was given by injection every other day for ten injections. The Kaposi's lesions decreased in size, lightened in color, and no new lesions appeared during the thirty-day posttreatment period. The patients in the study also exhibited improved immunohematologic status as well (Voltchek, Liepens, Nowicky, & Brozosko, 1996). Preliminary animal (in vitro and in vivo) studies have shown that Ukrain, given intravenously, is effective against the development of malignant tumors (Sotomayor, Rao, Lopez, & Liepins, 1992).

Studies Related to Other Health Patterns

No data are available at this time.

Mechanism of Action

The traditional use of celandine as a remedy for skin disease and wart and tumor growth is supported by in vitro data that identify tertiary benzophenanthridine alkaloids (BPA), chelidonine and coptisine, and quaternary BPAs called "sanguinarine" and "chelerythrine." Studies have shown that these alkaloids in celandine are responsible for the inhibition of cell proliferation by several cellular mechanisms and indirectly affect the cell's ability to metastasize. Human keratinocytes, which proliferate at a fast rate, have been found to be inhibited by the benzophenanthridine alkaloids of celandine (Vavreckova, Gawlik, & Muller, 1996).

In mice with mammary carcinoma, the cytotoxicity of Ukrain is thought to be due to its ability to function as an "up-regulator of the immune system" that restores the cytolytic ability of macrophages (Sotomayor et al., 1992). Ukrain has been found to be highly cytotoxic on sixty cell lines of eight major types of human cancer without being toxic to normal cells in therapeutic doses (study by Liepins et al. as reported in Voltchek et al., 1996).

One of the active constituents of celandine, an alkaloid called chelidonine, acts as a mild antispasmodic and a weak central analgesic. The ability of celandine extract to increase bile flow in animals is thought to be due to choleretic effects (study by Baumann, 1975 as reported in Schulz, Hansel, & Tyler, 1998).

USE IN PREGNANCY OR LACTATION:

Celandine has uterine stimulant properties and therefore is contraindicated in pregnancy (McGuffin et al., 1997; Brinker, 1998). Celandine herb and bruised root "bathed with oil of chamomile" can be applied to the breast to decrease milk production (Culpeper, 1990).

Herbal Caveat—Pregnancy or Lactation
Some herbs are contraindicated in pregnancy because of a risk of the herb or one of its constituents stimulating the uterus and therefore possibly promoting fetal loss. Many herbal practitioners do not recommend herbal

remedies, in particular oral doses of herbs, during the first trimester of pregnancy and seek an alternative. However, herbs are successfully used during pregnancy, especially to prepare the body for the birth. Herbs are relatively unstudied in pregnancy and lactation, so patients need to be made aware through education of the potential benefits and risks of using herbs for health conditions that arise during pregnancy or lactation. The use of herbal remedies during pregnancy often warrants a referral to a knowledgeable herbal practitioner.

USE FOR CHILDREN:

Celandine is not to be used in children because of empiric knowledge of its toxicity potential (Brinker, 1998; McGuffin et al., 1997). No differentiation is made between topical and internal use and some practitioners might opt to recommend topical applications of celandine for the treatment of plantar warts, for example, after weighing the benefits and risks of other treatments. A homeopathic preparation of celandine (potency 3X) is often recommended for jaundice in infants, but the actual plant remedies are not to be given to infants or children (Weed, 1986). Celandine is very stimulating to the liver when taken internally and is therefore not recommended for internal use in children, in particular small children and infants whose livers are not fully developed.

Herbal Caveat—Children

Children have special needs in regard to herbal therapies. They require lesser amounts of herbs and often respond well to mild teas and topical applications such as compresses and baths. The lowest dose of oral preparations should be tried first before increasing the amount given children. Caregivers should observe children closely for responses to herbal remedies. Younger children, particularly infants, have traditionally been given herbs either through their mother's breast milk or in the form of a homeopathic remedy because of their sensitivity to medicines and treatments and the immaturity of their liver. It is recommended that a person knowledgeable in the herbal treatment of children be consulted before the offering of any herb to a child for the first time.

CAUTIONS:

The sap of celandine, if ingested, may cause stomatitis and gastroenteritis (Duke, 1985). Digestive system irritation can occur upon ingestion of fresh juice from celandine, but the dry plant is approved in countries such as Germany for internal use without contraindications (McGuffin et al., 1997). Topically celandine plant juice is caustic, an irritant, a vesicant, and the plant itself can cause dermatitis by direct contact (Duke, 1985). Symptoms of overdose of celandine include stomach pain, intestinal colic, hematuria and urgency, dizziness, and stupor (Schulz et al., 1998). Celandine is capable of inducing acute cholestatic hepatitis (Benninger, Schneider, Schuppan, Kirchner, & Hahn, 1999). Do not confuse greater celandine with lesser celandine, also know as pilewort (Wren, 1988).

Historical Nursing Use

No data are available at this time.

Potential Nursing Applications

Nurses may want to explore the topical application of celandine for skin symptoms related to warts, eczema, and suspicious growths and the possibility of improving eyesight and recovery from eye injury with topical applications.

Integrative Insight

In vitro and animal studies have started to explain the successful traditional use of celandine in the treatment of warts and cancers, especially of the skin. The mechanism of how celandine is able to restore and repair the eye is virtually unknown. Clinical research on celandine needs to begin somewhere. Perhaps it can begin with topical applications. Nurses attend to the skin of patients everyday. Nurses are experts in skin and wound care. Plantar warts are not life threatening, but they can be annoying and difficult to eradicate. Nurses may want to try celandine infused oil on plantar warts as a way of getting to know more about the healing actions of the plant.

     Integrating what is known about the physiology of warts (i.e., they have their own blood supply) with knowledge of the traditional use of celandine for skin disease such as warts can lead to the development of new protocols in caring for the skin of people with plantar warts. For example, rather than instructing patients to try over-the-counter preparations, the nurse might scrape away the top layer of skin over a plantar wart and then apply celandine juice or oil to smother the wart. The scraping is not painful and observing celandine's action over a few days can help the process of understanding how the plant medicine works. Some states might consider the scraping of a wart a surgical technique, so this part might need to be performed by a nurse practitioner. Celandine's healing actions can remind practitioners of the power of topical applications of herbal remedies.

🍃 THERAPEUTIC APPLICATIONS:

Oral

Anyone tasting celandine will be immediately alerted that this herb lets its user know that it should not be taken in large amounts. Because it is harder to control dosage of the alkaloids in celandine when decocting as tea, some recommend taking celandine only as a standardized extract when taking internally.

    Tea. Add 1 teaspoon herb to 1 cup boiled water and steep for thirty minutes. A common dosage is to drink $\frac{1}{2}$ cup at room temperature daily (Zevin, 1997). Standard dose is 600 mg to 5 g per day (McGuffin et al., 1997).

Liquid Extract. Approximately ½ teaspoon (2 to 4 ml) (Wren, 1988)

Topical

Oil. Made from the fresh leaf and soft stems and applied as needed

Poultice. The fresh roots can be put in a food processor to extract the juice. The slurry (chopped up plant material) is then strained and a small amount is applied to the skin no more than three times daily.

Environmental

Celandine is not used in this manner.

Herbal Caveat—Therapeutic Applications
In traditional and conventional herbal medicine, amounts of herbs given to patients are based on individual needs. The amounts or "doses" recorded here are provided so that the health practitioner has a general idea of the amounts recommended for an adult patient. Dosing in herbalism not only refers to amount of plant used but also includes when, where, and how to take a plant medicine. These dosages should not be used as guidelines for indiscriminate intervention without proper assessment, critical thinking, and patient education on the part of the practitioner.

Note: Please see chapter 5 for detailed descriptions of how to prepare various applications.

PATIENT INTERACTION:

Celandine is a powerful herb that is best used under the guidance of a knowledgeable practitioner. The pungent, bitter sap from this plant can be extracted in an oil or tincture and used topically with symptoms related to skin conditions such as eczema, warts, and cancer. Celandine can be taken internally by adults but when taken internally is best taken in the form of dry herb. The fresh herb has been known to cause severe irritation to the digestive system. Celandine is available in some countries as a standardized extract where the dosage of the alkaloid constituent is controlled. Signs and symptoms of celandine overdosage may include gastrointestinal colic, urinary urgency, and hematuria accompanied by central nervous system symptoms.

Herbal Caveat—Patient Interaction
Patients considering the use of an herb or formula of herbs in self-care benefit from education about the plant itself and the use of the plant in healing. This education can come through many sources, including local herbalists; plant specialists such as botanists; health practitioners such as nurses, nutritionists, naturopaths, and other physicians; and various written references including the scientific literature. Patients need to remember that their unique health care needs are not necessarily represented in any literature they may encounter. Therefore, it is recommended that a knowledgeable mentor be consulted before initiating self-care with any herb being used for the first time.

Note: You may want to keep a journal of your experiences with the herb.

After a hard day at work, our eyes are often weary and sore. Cool or warm moist compresses to the eyes are often helpful, but a small drop of celandine juice, oil, or tincture applied to the eyelid (not the eye) is amazingly refreshing. If you ever have the opportunity to be formally introduced to celandine by someone who knows the plant, break open a stem and be ready for the powerful bitter and pungent flavor you will experience when you touch your tongue to it!

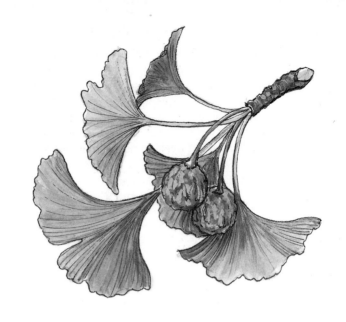

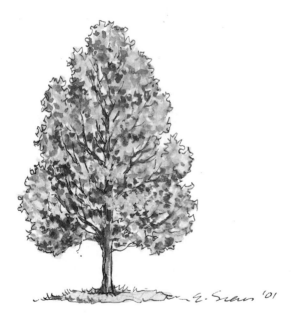

Ginkgo biloba

Ginkgo

🌿 **LATIN NAME:** *Ginkgo biloba*

🌿 **FAMILY:** Ginkgoaceae

🌿 **COMMON NAMES:** Ginkgo, maidenhair tree, ginkyo, ginan, icho, ityo, kew tree, pei-wen, temple balm, yin guo, yinhsing

🌿 **HEALTH PATTERN:** Restoration

🌿 **PLANT DESCRIPTION:**
Ginkgo is the world's oldest tree, existing virtually unchanged from its origins over two hundred million years ago (Blumenthal et al., 2000). It grows up to 100 feet (approximately 33 meters) tall, and its fan-shaped leaves with parallel veins can grow to 5 inches (12 cm) long. Each leaf has two distinct lobes; hence, the species name "bi-loba." Ginkgo is a widely cultivated tree that is often planted as an ornamental because of its high resistance to disease, pollution, and insects. It grows wild on a limited basis in undisturbed forests in China where the seeds and leaves have been traditionally used for many years. The leaves are grown commercially in the United States, France, and China and are harvested in autumn after the leaf has turned yellow.

🌿 **PLANT PARTS USED:** Leaf and seeds

🌿 **TRADITIONAL EVIDENCE:**
Cultural Use

Asian. According to traditional Chinese medicine (TCM), ginkgo leaves are sweet, bitter, and astringent and have been used for symptoms related to lung deficiency, such as asthma. The leaves also have been used for symptoms related to cerebrovascular disease and angina (Bensky & Gamble, 1993). The roasted seeds have been used as an expectorant and for asthma, tuberculosis, excessive urination, and leukorrhea. Ginkgo seed also has been used in cosmetics and soaps and as the base of fine oriental lacquerware. The Japanese use the seeds as a food called "gin-nan" (DeSmet, 1997). The dried bark, burned to ash and mixed with a vegetable oil, has been used in Chinese folk medicine as a topical application for neurodermatitis (Leung & Foster, 1996).

In TCM, ginkgo seed (also called ginkgo nut) affects the kidney and lung channels, or energy systems, of the body. It is used to expel phlegm, stop wheezing and coughing, and decrease copious sputum. Ginkgo seed stops discharges from the body and is used for vaginal discharge and turbid urine, urinary frequency, incontinence, and abnormally frequent spermatorrhea (Bensky & Gamble, 1993). TCM practitioners are aware of the toxic effects of ginkgo seed, particularly when used raw, and are careful not to use it orally for extended periods of time or in large quantities. Symptoms of overdose are headache, fever, tremors, shortness of breath, and irritability (Bensky & Gamble, 1993). The antidote for overdose is 12 teaspoons (60 g) of boiled raw licorice or 5 teaspoons (30 g) of boiled ginkgo shells. It is believed that side effects can be avoided by including the shells and thin lining of the nut when using the seed internally (Bensky & Gamble, 1993).

European. Ginkgo has not been used as a traditional herbal medicine in Europe. It is only currently that the phytopharmaceutical extracts from the leaves have begun to be used to treat cerebral insufficiency and peripheral arterial disease in the elderly (DeSmet, 1997). EGb761, a ginkgo standardized extract developed in 1964, is one of the top five prescriptions in Germany. Over five million prescriptions have been recorded each year in Germany (McGuffin et al., 1997). The German Commission E has approved the use of ginkgo for the treatment of intermittent claudication, vertigo, tinnitus, and organic brain syndrome (Blumenthal et al., 2000).

Culinary Use

In China and Japan, ginkgo seeds are considered a delicacy, but they are edible only after the acrid, foul-smelling pulp surrounding them has been removed. The seeds must be boiled or roasted. They should be eaten sparingly, no more than eight or ten per day. Raw seeds are reported to be toxic and ingestion has caused diarrhea, nausea, stomach pain, convulsions, weak pulse, restlessness, difficulty breathing, and shock. They have been reported to cause death in children. The pulp surrounding the seeds can cause contact dermatitis, so gloves should be worn when harvesting the seeds.

Use in Herbalism

According to traditional herbalism, the longevity of the ginkgo tree and its ability to resist disease and pollution is a signature for its potential uses in humans. Practitioners believe that the characteristics of the tree are transferred to people when using the herb. Ginkgo leaf extract has been used in herbalism for its neuroprotective effects and its regenerative effect on the circulation, in particular, microcirculation. For this reason, ginkgo often is used with elderly patients. More currently, ginkgo has been used to prevent altitude sickness and for erectile dysfunction.

Ginkgo has been used internally for symptoms related to cerebral insufficiency and organic brain syndrome, including memory deficits, dizziness, tinnitus, headache, disturbed concentration, and depression. Ginkgo also is taken internally for symptoms related to intermittent claudication. To restore pain-free walking, ginkgo often is recommended as part of a healing regimen that includes regular physical exercise such as walking. Ginkgo also is used internally to help relieve vertigo and tinnitus that is of vascular origin. Ginkgo has been used in the treatment of symptoms related to Raynaud's disease; acrocyanosis (persistently poor circulation to the hands and feet); and in post-phlebitis syndrome with painful, swollen veins.

BIOMEDICAL EVIDENCE:

The studies presented here were conducted using a ginkgo standardized extract preparation, not the whole herb or liquid extract.

Studies Related to Restoration

In a double-blind, randomized trial of twenty patients with mild-to-moderate dementia of the Alzheimer type, those participants who received ginkgo standardized extract 240 mg per day for three months demonstrated a significant improvement in memory performance and attention when compared with placebo. The participants also demonstrated significant positive effects on the central nervous system as shown by electroencephalogram (Maurer, Ihl, Dierks, & Frolich, 1997).

After six to twelve months, oral doses of 40 mg ginkgo biloba standardized extract three times a day has been shown in a randomized, double-blind, placebo-controlled study of 202 patients to significantly stabilize and/or improve cognitive performance and social functioning of patients with dementia (Le Bars et al., 1997).

In a controlled trial of 44 patients with vertigo, dizziness, or both caused by vascular vestibular disorders, ginkgo oral standardized extract, 80 mg twice daily, significantly improved oculomotor and visuovestibular function in those patients receiving the extract (Cesarani et al., 1998).

One review of the literature on the use of ginkgo for cerebral insufficiency states that of forty controlled trials done on the subject, in which 120 to 160 mg was the oral dose most often given, it was shown that ginkgo needs to be taken for four to six weeks before positive effects are noted. Of the forty trials conducted, the authors of this analysis state that eight of the studies were well-performed and demonstrated that ginkgo standardized extract is effective for the treatment of symptoms related to cerebral insufficiency (Kleijnen & Knipschild, 1992). Another review states that ginkgo also shows promise in the treatment of the neurologic symptoms related to normal aging, tinnitus, stroke, and macular degeneration (Diamond et al., 2000). Although some participants in one study of the effect of ginkgo on symptoms of tinnitus experienced significant relief of symptoms, statistically, ginkgo was not shown to be significant in the treatment of tinnitus (Holgers, Axelsson, & Pringle, 1994).

In a study of 55 patients with acute ischemic stroke, no significant improvement in neurologic deficits were found after administration of ginkgo 240 mg per day, for two and then four weeks as compared with placebo (Garg, Nag, & Agrawal, 1995).

Studies Related to Other Health Patterns

Mobility. Ginkgo standardized extract given orally in a placebo-controlled, double-blind trial of 111 patients, significantly increased pain-free walking distance in patients with intermittent claudication by almost 50% without side effects (Peters, Kieser, & Holscher, 1998).

Mechanism of Action

Although, as with many botanical remedies, ginkgo's mechanism of action is not completely understood, ginkgo's ability to exert protective action on vascular and other tissues is thought to be due to the presence of certain flavonoids. The flavonoids in ginkgo are able to scavenge free radicals that may be created to a higher extent under certain disease conditions such as hypoxia, ischemia, and metabolic disturbances. Free radicals can damage the lining of blood vessels, cause lipid peroxidation, and interfere with many cellular processes. If free radicals are allowed to proliferate, over time they may cause cardiovascular and metabolic disturbances (DeSmet, 1997).

The protective action includes the ability to relax spastic blood vessels but increase the tone of abnormally relaxed vessels, protect against capillary permeability, inhibit platelet aggregation, and exhibit antiedematous and anti-ischemic properties (Blumenthal et al., 2000). The terpenoids are responsible for the antagonism of platelet-activating factor (Braquet et al. as reported in Cesarani et al., 1998).

USE IN PREGNANCY OR LACTATION:

There are no known restrictions for the use of ginkgo leaf in pregnancy (McGuffin et al., 1997). Several unknown ginkgo extracts were investigated for adverse effects. No effects such as carcinogenicity, toxicity to the reproductive process, or genetic mutations were observed. It is not known whether these results can be extended to all ginkgo preparations (Blumenthal et al., 2000). Ginkgo has been used to induce labor in some cultures. It is not known if ginkgo is secreted in the breast milk of nursing mothers (World Health Organization [WHO], 1999).

Herbal Caveat—Pregnancy or Lactation

Some herbs are contraindicated in pregnancy because of a risk of the herb or one of its constituents stimulating the uterus and therefore possibly promoting fetal loss. Many herbal practitioners do not recommend herbal remedies, in particular oral doses of herbs, during the first trimester of pregnancy and seek an alternative. However, herbs are successfully used during pregnancy, especially to prepare the body for the birth. Herbs are relatively unstudied in pregnancy and lactation, so patients need to be made aware through education of the potential benefits and risks of using herbs for health conditions that arise during pregnancy or lactation. The use of herbal remedies during pregnancy often warrants a referral to a knowledgeable herbal practitioner.

● USE FOR CHILDREN:

There are no known restrictions on the use of the leaf in children (McGuffin et al., 1997). The product data information of the leading ginkgo preparation EGb 761 (Tebonin intens 120 mg) suggest that the product should not be used in children under 12 (Blumenthal et al., 2000).

Herbal Caveat—Children

Children have special needs in regard to herbal therapies. They require lesser amounts of herbs and often respond well to mild teas and topical applications such as compresses and baths. The lowest dose of oral preparations should be tried first before increasing the amount given children. Caregivers should observe children closely for responses to herbal remedies. Younger children, particularly infants, have traditionally been given herbs either through their mother's breast milk or in the form of a homeopathic remedy because of their sensitivity to medicines and treatments and the immaturity of their liver. It is recommended that a person knowledgeable in the herbal treatment of children be consulted before the offering of any herb to a child for the first time.

● CAUTIONS:

Rare side effects of stomach and intestinal discomfort, headaches, and allergic skin reactions, irritability, restlessness, diarrhea, and vomiting have been reported with standardized products (Blumenthal et al., 2000). Hypersensitivity to ginkgo preparations has been observed, but is thought to be the result of overdosage (Wren, 1988). It is not common for hypersensitivity or side effects to be reported with the use of the crude leaf and liquid extracts.

Although animal in vitro studies suggest that ginkgo might potentiate the action of MAO inhibitors possibly by the inhibition of serotonin and dopamine (Brinker, 1998), a current study found that ginkgo does not have an inhibitory effect on MAO A or B in human brains as measured by positron emission tomography (PET) scan (Fowler et al., 2000). A few cases of excessive bleeding possibly related to ginkgo leaf standardized extract have been reported in the literature (Matthews, 1998; Rosenblatt & Mindel, 1997). This is not the case with other ginkgo applications such as whole leaf liquid extract or tea.

Ginkgo is known to contain ginkgolides, a constituent that antagonizes platelet aggregating factor and therefore should be used cautiously when taking aspirin (Brinker, 1998). Because ginkgo extracts can reduce the clotting time of the blood, and the interaction between herbal and pharmaceutical anticoagulants is not completely understood, patients must be helped in making an informed choice as to whether to take pharmaceutical anticoagulants or ginkgo standardized extract. The two are best not taken together.

● NURSING EVIDENCE:

Historical Nursing Use

No data are available at this time.

Potential Nursing Applications

Nurses working with the elderly may want to consider the use of ginkgo for improving symptoms related to unhealthy aging such as memory loss. Nurses may want to consider researching the clinical effects of ginkgo oral applications on the behavior of dementia patients.

Integrative Insight

Nurses who work with the elderly may want to consider becoming familiar with ginkgo. This tree is a metaphor for successful aging in that it is the oldest tree on the planet. Elderly patients are at risk for dementia and stroke when their diets are not healthy and balanced and their circulation is compromised. The literature mentions the possibility that heavy metals are involved in the diminishing health of the brain (Christen, 2000). Improving the microcirculation of the brain seems to help with managing the oxidative stress and destruction of brain tissue by heavy metals. With research that says ginkgo standardized extracts improve microcirculation, they could easily be put into the realm of biomedical cures.

Knowledgeable herbalists do not just depend on one herb to work as a "magic bullet." Nurses also know the importance of including the elderly in health promotion programs that include attention to lifestyle, diet, and activity. Nurses must guard against using ginkgo in a rote and standardized way. Making sure that nursing home patients get a healthy diet, plenty of exercise, and social interaction is just as important as the herbs nurses might recommend. When choosing an herb, ginkgo is not the only plant that has the ability to improve microcirculation, memory, or healthy aging. Rosemary or monarda shampoo might be just as, if not more, effective in improving memory and brain function in the elderly because they contain numerous plant substances, (e.g., thymol) that inhibit the breakdown of acetylcholine and are readily absorbed through the skin.

Because of the multiple pathologic and neurochemical deficits found with Alzheimer's disease, some clinicians are calling for increasing research efforts to explore combination therapy in the treatment of early Alzheimer's disease, such as combining pharmaceuticals and ginkgo or other antioxidant supplements in an integrated approach often used for other chronic illness (Doraiswamy & Steffens, 1998). Ginkgo is proved to be a viable option, especially when used in conjunction with a healthy lifestyle.

THERAPEUTIC APPLICATIONS:

Oral

Tea. 3 to 6 g for a 2-day period (Bensky and Gamble, 1993).
Liquid Extract. 1:1 (g/ml) 0.5 ml three times a day (WHO, 1999)
Standardized Extract. Standardized extract should contain 24% ginkgo flavonol glycosides and 6% terpene lactones (Blumenthal et al., 2000). Ginkgo standardized extract has been shown to stimulate the

desired physiologic effects in those with more severe illness more readily than crude leaf preparations of lower concentration. For symptoms of dementia, ginkgo standardized extract in dry or liquid form is recommended at 120 to 240 mg in two or three daily oral doses. A minimum of eight weeks of therapy is recommended for dementia. For symptoms of vertigo, tinnitus, and poor circulation, ginkgo native dry extract at 120 to 160 mg in two or three daily doses is recommended (Blumenthal et al., 2000).

Topical
No data are available at this time.

Environmental
No data are available at this time.

Herbal Caveat—Therapeutic Applications
In traditional and conventional herbal medicine, amounts of herbs given to patients are based on individual needs. The amounts or "doses" recorded here are provided so that the health practitioner has a general idea of the amounts recommended for an adult patient. Dosing in herbalism not only refers to amount of plant used but also includes when, where, and how to take a plant medicine. These dosages should not be used as guidelines for indiscriminate intervention without proper assessment, critical thinking, and patient education on the part of the practitioner.

   Note: Please see chapter 5 for detailed descriptions of how to prepare various applications.

PATIENT INTERACTION:

Standardized extracts of ginkgo leaf have been studied extensively and found to be helpful in improving memory and circulation to the brain, thereby improving brain function. Ginkgo may be especially helpful for the elderly. Do not take ginkgo standardized extract if you are already taking an anticoagulant medication such as aspirin, without discussing your options with a knowledgeable health practitioner. In appropriate doses, along with a healthy, balanced diet rich in essential fatty acids, vitamin B_{12}, and thiamine, ginkgo may be helpful in restoring and promoting a healthy brain.

Herbal Caveat—Patient Interaction
Patients considering the use of an herb or formula of herbs in self-care benefit from education about the plant itself and the use of the plant in healing. This education can come through many sources, including local herbalists; plant specialists such as botanists; health practitioners such as nurses, nutritionists, naturopaths and other physicians; and various written references including the scientific literature. Patients need to remember that their unique health care needs are not necessarily represented in any literature they may encounter. Therefore, it is recommended that a knowledgeable mentor be consulted before initiating self-care with any herb being used for the first time.

Note: You may want to keep a journal of your experiences with the herb.

Trees have a gentle strength that is palpable. If you have a ginkgo tree nearby, make a cup of ginkgo leaf tea and take your tea to the tree. Sit near the tree, touch it, and drink your tea. If you have no ginkgo, try sitting by another type of tree. See what happens to you when you spend time by a tree. Trees have a very special wisdom. "Trees are the teachers of the law. . . . When people come upon an ancient tree, some event occurs that takes them out of themselves and they, for a moment, feel the touch of a greater and much deeper reality" (Buhner, 1996, p. 178). Sometimes the most healing thing nurses can do for themselves or their patients is to reconnect with their spirit. Connecting with a tree such as ginkgo can help us step out of ourselves or our perception of who we are, so that we can reconnect with our inner nature and the life force within that is a source of healing.

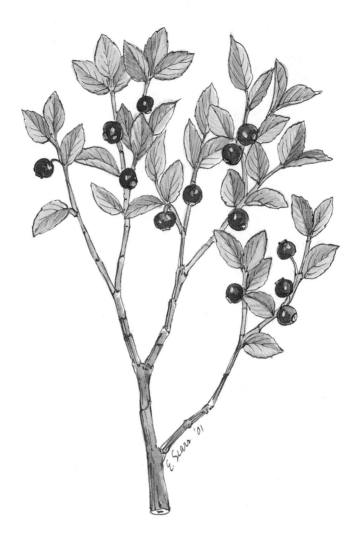

Vaccinium myrtillus

BILBERRY

@ **LATIN NAME:** *Vaccinium myrtillus*

@ **FAMILY:** Ericaceae

@ **COMMON NAMES:** Bilberry, whortleberry, airelle, black whortles, bleaberry, trackleberry, whinberry, huckleberry, dwarf bilberry, European blueberry

@ **HEALTH PATTERN:** Restoration

@ **PLANT DESCRIPTION:**

Bilberry is a shrub with wiry, angular branches that grows up to 14 inches (35 cm) tall. It has pale bluish flowers that appear in March and April and black berries that ripen in July and August. The berries, when ripe, are covered with a delicate gray bloom. Its leaves are leathery and turn red in the autumn. The bush is found in open areas and woodlands in Europe, Asia, and subalpine areas of North America and south into Arizona and New Mexico (Leung & Foster, 1996). Related species include cranberries *(Vaccinium macrocarpon)* and blueberries (*Vaccinium* spp.).

@ **PLANT PARTS USED:** Fruit, leaves, root

@ **TRADITIONAL EVIDENCE:**

Cultural Use

North American Indian. There are about eighteen different species of *Vaccinium* that many North American Indian tribes have used traditionally as food and medicine. For example, the Seminoles use an infusion of the leaves of *Vaccinium* spp. for sun sickness, eye disease, headaches, high fevers, and for diarrhea. The Cree use a decoction of the leafy stems or of the whole plant to induce menstruation; to prevent pregnancy; to cause sweating; and paradoxically, to slow excessive menstrual bleeding. Native Alaskans eat the berries raw or cooked in pies, puddings, and muffins. The berries are valued as a good source of vitamin C. The berries are also frozen or canned for winter use (Moerman, 1998).

The Algonquin of Quebec use an infusion of the leaves for colic in infants and to prevent miscarriage in women, but an infusion of the roots was said to be able to induce labor. The berries are made into preserves, pies, cobblers and cakes, and fruit butters. As a cash crop, the berries were at one time gathered and sold. The Iroquois mash the berries, form them into small cakes, and dry them for future use. The cakes are used as a convenient food to take on hunting trips. This tribe also used *Vaccinium* spp. flowers to make preserves. The Ojibwa dry the berries in the sun and store them for use during the winter, at which time they are cooked with corn, rice, and venison (Moerman, 1998).

Russian/Baltic. In Russia, bilberries are popular as a wild fruits. People commonly harvest the berries during the summer from the forested areas. The berries are cooked and made into preserves that are used during the winter, but they also are used fresh or dried. The fruits are used for treating diarrhea, dysentery, inflammation of the mucous membranes of the gastrointestinal tract, heartburn, and generalized itching. A decoction of bilberry fruit is used to expel intestinal worms and to improve night vision. It also can be used as a gargle for relieving symptoms of tonsillitis (Zevin, 1997).

Russian herbalists also have traditionally recommended the use of bilberry leaves for the treatment of various ailments. The leaves are made into an infusion and used for stomach and intestinal disorders, low stomach acid, inflammation, and diarrhea. It is used for inflammation in the kidneys, bladder, and liver and to reduce high blood sugar. The leaf infusion is used as a vaginal douche for the relief of symptoms of leukorrhea and as an enema to treat bleeding from hemorrhoids. Cold compresses of bilberry leaf infusion can be applied topically to treat skin ulcers, wounds, and eczema (Zevin, 1997).

European. Bilberry fruit has been a traditional European medicine for almost 1000 years. It was used by the twelfth century German mystic, nurse-herbalist Hildegard von Bingen for promotion of menstruation and was later used by sixteenth century herbalist Hieronymos Bock. The leaves have been used to support those with diabetes mellitus and for prevention and treatment of gastrointestinal problems. Additionally, it has been used for urinary tract disorders, arthritis, dermatitis, heart problems, gout, hemorrhoids, and poor circulation. Preparations of the fruit are used for the treatment of diarrhea and for inflammations of the membranes of the mouth and throat.

In Germany, bilberry fruit is approved for internal use to treat diarrhea, especially in children, and for external use to treat inflammation of the mucous membranes of the mouth (Blumenthal et al., 2000). In Italy, bilberry fruit preparations are used to treat disorders of the microcirculation such as varicose veins, atherosclerosis, and venous insufficiency. It seems to have a particular affinity for the eye and so is used for macular degeneration, glaucoma, and cataracts (Blumenthal et al., 2000).

Culinary Use

The bilberry is well known for its food value. It is used to make jams, jellies, conserves, pastries, syrups, and is eaten raw. The fruit also is used to flavor alcoholic and nonalcoholic beverages and to provide a red coloring to wines. The dried fruits are used in beverage teas.

Use in Herbalism

Bilberry has been used for diarrhea, dysentery, to relieve scurvy and painful urination, and to help stop the flow of breast milk (Blumenthal et al., 2000). Bilberry fruit is crushed with the roots and steeped in gin and used internally as a diuretic. This preparation had value for edema of the lower extremities and for kidney stones. The fruit also has been used to "cool the heat of the liver and stomach" and to prevent "vomitings and loathings" (Culpeper, 1990). The bilberry leaves and the bark of the root are used as a topical application to ulcers and inflammations of the mouth and throat (Grieve, 1971). A tea is prepared from the leaves and used to treat diabetes (Grieve, 1971).

Bilberry fruit is used for nonspecific, mild, transient diarrhea and as a mouthwash or gargle for inflammations of the mouth and throat (Schulz et al., 1998). Bilberry fruit and its extracts are becoming more popular, especially among the aging, for their antiaging effects and for their positive effect on night vision. The fruit is used to help restore the ability of the eye to adjust to darkness and to glare. Traditional belief is that a single dose of bilberry can improve night vision within hours. Additional improvements include increased visual acuity during both the night and day, strengthening of connective tissue and prevention of free-radical damage. Bilberry also has been used in the treatment and prevention of glaucoma, macular degeneration, cataracts, retinitis pigmentosa, diabetic retinopathy, and night-blindness (Werbach & Murray, 1994). Bilberry fruit is known for its antioxidant ability to prevent chronic degeneration of tissue; it has been used in the treatment of diseases such as diabetes, rheumatoid arthritis, Raynaud's disease, gout, periodontal disease, and varicose veins (Werbach & Murray, 1994).

BIOMEDICAL EVIDENCE:

Several studies have shown bilberry to be significantly helpful in the restoration of microcirculation, such as in the eye, thereby improving function. The studies are performed with standardized extracts of bilberry containing specific amounts of anthocyanoside, a constituent in bilberry.

Studies Related to Restoration

Ten patients with varying levels of diabetic retinopathy related to diabetes type II demonstrated significant retinal improvement with decrease or disappearance of hemorrhage when given an oral bilberry preparation called Tegens, containing 80 mg of bilberry anthocyanosides per capsule, two capsules three times a day for six months (Orsucci, Rossi, Sabbatini, Menci, & Berni 1983).

After one week of receiving oral doses of two 30 mg tablets per day of bilberry anthocyanosides, 8 patients demonstrated significant improvement in macular recovery time and night vision. Improvement was noted particularly in regards to the reading of optotypes with medium-high angle, between 0.85 and 0.22 degrees ($p < .05$) (Paronzini & Indemini, 1988).

A double-blind, randomized controlled study of 40 patients with diabetic or hypertensive vascular retinopathy, found that 79% of patients given one capsule of Tegens containing 160 mg of bilberry anthocyanosides, two times a day for approximately one month had significant retinal improvement as demonstrated by ophthalmoscopic examination and fluoroangiography (Perossini, Guidi, Chiellini, & Siravo, 1987).

In another study of 40 patients, ages 15 to 75 years, the lungs of patients with asthma and chronic bronchitis who received Tegens, an oral preparation of bilberry anthocyanosides 480 mg in three divided doses for ten to thirty days, demonstrated reduced microcirculation changes induced by cortisone therapy (Carmignani, 1983).

Studies Related to Other Health Patterns

Elimination. In a study of 51 pregnant women, a significant reduction in discomfort related to either venous insufficiency or hemorrhoids was noted when the women were given 160 to 320 mg of bilberry anthocyanosides (Tegens) divided in two to three doses per day for ninety days (Teglio, Mazzanti, Tronconi, & Guerresi 1987).

In a randomized trial, 60 postoperative grade three hemorrhoidectomy patients ages 21 to 52 years, had less postoperative itching and edema according to subjective and objective data when the patients were given 320 mg of bilberry anthocyanosides per day in two divided doses, along with their anti-inflammatory and analgesic medications (Pezzangora, Barina, De Stefani, & Rizzo, 1984).

Mobility. In a controlled study of 54 pregnant women between the ages of 24 and 37 years, significant improvements ($p < .01$) in pain, paresthesias, burning, heaviness, and leg cramps related to venous insufficiency and capillary fragility were observed after the subjects were given 320 mg per day of a bilberry anthocyanosides preparation (Tegens) for 60 to 80 days beginning in their sixth month of pregnancy (Grismondi, 1980).

Significant improvement in symptoms of edema and leg heaviness in 97 patients with various stages of venous disease of the legs was observed in patients given oral daily doses of 480 mg of bilberry anthocyanosides for 6 months (Tori & D'Errico, 1980).

Skin Care. Topical application of a bilberry preparation called Myrtocyan (0.5% to 2% in 0.2 ml once a day for three days) significantly reduced the area of wounded skin in rats as compared with controls treated with prednisone alone. The 2% concentration was the most effective (Cristoni & Magistretti, 1987).

Mechanism of Action

Bitter compounds called anthocyanosides are the blue pigment structurally related to flavonoids that are responsible for the color of the bilberry. Over 15 different anthocyanosides are found in the fruit of bilberry *(V. myrtillus)*. Fresh bilberries contain a 0.1% to 0.25% concentration of anthocyanosides. Concentrated extracts should be standardized to 36% anthocyanosides and capsules to 25% (Duke, 1999).

"The composition of the anthocyanosides from *V. myrtillus* fruits of different geographic areas appears rather constant" (Morazzoni & Bombardelli, 1996, p. 5).

Anthocyanosides are powerful antioxidants. They are thought to inhibit collagen destruction, scavenge free radicals, reduce capillary permeability, and increase blood circulation to the periphery and to the brain.

The positive effects of bilberry on night vision and visual acuity are related to its ability to decrease the breakdown of rhodopsin (retinal purple), a light sensitive pigment located in the rods of the retina. It also has the ability to regenerate rhodopsin (Blumenthal et al., 2000). Bilberry extract may reduce platelet aggregation possibly because of its ability to promote the release of prostacyclin, which has potent blood vessel dilating effects and platelet antiaggregating activity (Werbach & Murray, 1994). The medicinal action of bilberry, including its effects on wound healing, is also attributed to the tannin content (Schulz et al., 1998).

USE IN PREGNANCY OR LACTATION:

There are no known restrictions on the medicinal use of bilberry fruit. Bilberry has been used traditionally in Europe to help stop the flow of breast milk (Blumenthal et al., 2000).

Herbal Caveat—Pregnancy or Lactation
Some herbs are contraindicated in pregnancy because of a risk of the herb or one of its constituents stimulating the uterus and therefore possibly promoting fetal loss. Many herbal practitioners do not recommend herbal remedies, in particular oral doses of herbs, during the first trimester of pregnancy and seek an alternative. However, herbs are successfully used during pregnancy, especially to prepare the body for the birth. Herbs are relatively unstudied in pregnancy and lactation, so patients need to be made aware through education of the potential benefits and risks of using herbs for health conditions that arise during pregnancy or lactation. The use of herbal remedies during pregnancy often warrants a referral to a knowledgeable herbal practitioner.

USE FOR CHILDREN:

A mouthwash of 10% decoction of bilberries has proved effective for oral candidiasis in infants (Schilcher, 1992). A decoction made from dried bilberries is very effective against diarrhea in children and infants. A high-dose water extract must be used to be effective (13 ounces [400 ml] of hot water over 3 heaping tablespoons [30 g] of the dried bilberry fruit used over the course of one day). Do not exceed 3 tablespoons (30 g) of the dried fruit each day (Schilcher, 1992).

Herbal Caveat—Children
Children have special needs in regard to herbal therapies. They require lesser amounts of herbs and often respond well to mild teas and topical applications such as compresses and baths. The lowest dose of oral prepara-

tions should be tried first before increasing the amount given children. Caregivers should observe children closely for responses to herbal remedies. Younger children, particularly infants, have traditionally been given herbs either through their mother's breast milk or in the form of a homeopathic remedy because of their sensitivity to medicines and treatments and the immaturity of their liver. It is recommended that a person knowledgeable in the herbal treatment of children be consulted before the offering of any herb to a child for the first time.

CAUTIONS:

Bilberries are a food as well as a medicinal herb and are often eaten liberally when in season. It is the same with its relatives, blueberry and cranberry. All three berries have antioxidant and other medicinal properties. Bilberry is considered by many to be the most potent and medicinal of the three berries, which may relate to its anthocyanoside content. Many people may look at the cost of a standardized extract of bilberry and reach for the fresh bilberries or blueberries instead, especially if they are fortunate enough to live in an area where the berries grow abundantly. Bilberries and blueberries are not the exact same berries but have similar histories of use. There is something to be said for selecting the herb that grows locally. North Americans who use blueberries may fare just as well as the Europeans who use bilberry. There are no contraindications associated with bilberry or the standardized extract (Blumenthal et al., 2000).

Although bilberry leaf is used throughout Europe, the therapeutic use of the leaves is not recommended (Leung & Foster, 1996). Those diabetic patients who choose to use bilberry leaf while taking insulin need to monitor themselves closely because the combined effect may cause significant reduction in blood sugar levels (Brinker, 1998).

NURSING EVIDENCE:

Historical Nursing Use
No data are available at this time.

Potential Nursing Applications
Although nurses witness the restorative power of the human body almost as a matter of course in biological processes such as wound healing, most have a great desire to provide as much support for the restorative process as possible. Bilberry is one herb that clearly provides support for the restoration of the microcirculation in the eye and other tissues and can be considered as a supplement in those patients who suffer repeated retinal hemorrhage or diabetic retinopathy, for example. Nurses also may want to further explore the potential of the topical use of bilberry for the restoration of skin tissue and the promotion of granulation tissue. Bilberry can be considered for use as a mouthwash to promote healing of sore and ulcerated mouths such as

often occurs in cancer patients undergoing chemotherapy. It can also be considered for use in patients with hemorrhoids.

Integrative Insight

Bilberry has been shown to have tremendous antioxidant and restorative properties and a long tradition of safe use as a food and medicinal plant. How does a plant help the eye or the skin to heal? Is it just a matter of the active constituents such as the anthocyanosides? It is only in the past few decades that science has begun to explain the restorative action of bilberry and more study is welcome. Nurses can add to the body of knowledge of the medicinal use of bilberry by participating in scientific observation of patients who use bilberry. Perhaps ethnographic studies can be done to see if those who have diets that include larger amounts of bilberries and blueberries (because they live where the berries grow) have different health patterns. Do they have better vision perhaps? Science supports traditional use in the case of bilberry. While some scientists continue to research the mechanism of action in bilberry, the next step for nurses may be to consider the integration of the knowledge of the medicinal use of the berry into a health promotion program that includes bilberry as an option for obtaining and maintaining optimal health and promoting healthy aging.

THERAPEUTIC APPLICATIONS:

Oral

Fresh berries can be eaten in season.

Dried Whole Fruit Powder. Take up to 4 to 8 g with water, several times daily.

Decoction. Use 5 to 8 g of the crushed dried whole fruit in 5 ounces (150 ml) of water. Drink this cool decoction several times daily for diarrhea until the problem is gone.

Cold Macerate. Soak 5 to 10 g of the crushed dried fruit in 5 ounces (150 ml) cold water for two hours, allowing the fruit to swell. Strain then drink the liquid cool several times daily.

Standardized Extract. Liquid (standardized) extracts are standardized to 36% anthocyanosides and dry fruit in capsules 25% (Duke, 1999). Use 80 to 160 mg, three times daily.

Liquid Extract. 1:1 (g/ml) $\frac{1}{2}$ to $\frac{3}{4}$ teaspoon (2 to 4 ml) three times daily (Blumenthal et al., 2000)

Topical

Decoction for External Use. Place $\frac{1}{8}$ to $\frac{1}{4}$ ounce (5 to 8 g) of the crushed dried fruit into 5 ounces (150 ml) of water. Bring to a boil for about ten minutes. Strain and use warm for topical applications.

Gargle or Mouthwash. Prepare a 10% decoction. The bilberry leaves can be used as a topical application to ulcers and inflammations of the mouth and throat (Grieve, 1971).

Compress. To make a leaf infusion, pour 1 cup (240 ml) of boiling water over 2 teaspoons (10 g) of the leaves (Zevin, 1997).

Environmental

No data are available at this time.

Herbal Caveat—Therapeutic Applications

In traditional and conventional herbal medicine, amounts of herbs given to patients are based on individual needs. The amounts or "doses" recorded here are provided so that the health practitioner has a general idea of the amounts recommended for an adult patient. Dosing in herbalism not only refers to amount of plant used but also includes when, where, and how to take a plant medicine. These dosages should not be used as guidelines for indiscriminate intervention without proper assessment, critical thinking, and patient education on the part of the practitioner.

Note: Please see chapter 5 for detailed descriptions of how to prepare various applications.

PATIENT INTERACTION:

Although bilberries are a highly nutritious, antioxidant-rich food, they also can be used medicinally. They can be taken as a tea, dried standardized extract, fluid extract, and used topically for a number of medicinal purposes with a very low risk of toxicity other than the standard precautions for taking in any substance for the first time. Cool bilberry tea can be taken for diarrhea and as a mouthwash for sores in the mouth. Bilberry also can be taken orally for visual problems, hemorrhoids, very poor circulation of the legs leading to pain and swelling, and for hard-to-heal wounds. Bilberry has been used safely by children and pregnant women. Traditionally, bilberry has been known to stop the flow of breast milk in lactating women. If you are taking bilberry for diarrhea and the condition persists for more than three to four days, consult a physician because of the danger of electrolyte imbalance. This is especially critical for infants and children.

Herbal Caveat—Patient Interaction

Patients considering the use of an herb or formula of herbs in self-care benefit from education about the plant itself and the use of the plant in healing. This education can come through many sources, including local herbalists; plant specialists such as botanists; health practitioners such as nurses, nutritionists, naturopaths, and other physicians; and various written references including the scientific literature. Patients need to remember that their unique health care needs are not necessarily represented in any literature they may encounter. Therefore, it is recommended that a knowledgeable mentor be consulted before initiating self-care with any herb being used for the first time.

🍃 NURTURING THE NURSE-PLANT RELATIONSHIP:

Note: You may want to keep a journal of your experiences with the herb.

If you live in an area where bilberries or blueberries grow, try harvesting the berries yourself. Picking berries can be very relaxing as well as stimulating to the senses. The berries should be plump and ripe (dark blue) when you pick them. Try eating them plain at first and then add them to fruit salad, breads, or cake. Growing up, I spent the summers in Maine where my Granny used to make the most wonderful blueberry crumb cake with the berries we'd picked. The trick to making pancakes or other baked goods with blueberries or bilberries is to be gentle with them, and coat them lightly with flour before adding them to a batter, so that they appear whole and don't end up as blue food coloring.

Try the standardized extract too if you, like so many caring nurses, are on your feet for long hours, day after day, year after year, and start to develop leg pain and edema. Although support stockings and exercise often help tremendously, adding bilberry fruit may help.

CHAPTER 19

Learning More

EVERY GOOD GUIDE KNOWS THE LIMITS OF THE JOURNEY. If you follow a guide through a large museum, a knowledgeable guide always picks a route for which there is a natural ending for the time allotted and gives ideas for future visits. If you follow a guide through a national forest, the skillful guide never leaves you stranded somewhere in the middle of the dense growth of trees to find your way out alone, but rather leads you to a place of safety, makes sure you have a map, and reminds you of the ways you must be careful in further exploration. This herb guide, too, has a natural ending and a place of safety from which the explorer must be sent on his or her way. The natural ending and safe place for this guide is found in resources for further learning.

The first five chapters of this guide provided a foundation for learning about plants and their historical and present day therapeutic uses. Chapters 6 to 18 provided a foundation for learning about specific healing plants. The purpose of this chapter is to provide a map for further learning. Plant medicine is an ever-changing and expanding field of knowledge. This guide is only a beginning, or introduction, to that body of knowledge. Plant art and science can be absorbing and fascinating. Learning about plants can be a lifetime commitment. If a nurse makes the choice to integrate plant use into his or her practice, then there must be commitment to further learning. Three primary areas for further learning are discussed in this chapter: (1) nature care education, (2) research, and (3) understanding the law.

783

Nurses who are interested in integrating natural remedies such as plant therapies into their practice need to consider the benefits of formal education. Very few schools of nursing offer education in the use of plant therapies any more. As mentioned previously, some schools in Europe that are affiliated with Anthroposophical hospitals offer their students education in plant therapies from the Anthroposophical perspective. In China, some nurses learn herbalism from the perspective of traditional Chinese medicine (TCM). In both of these programs, nurses are still working under the auspices of the physician. There is also the option of creating a place for plant therapies within the current scope of practice of professional nurses that is independent of physician oversight. This is not a new concept.

Historically, long before the institutionalization of nursing, caregivers used herbs in practice independent of college-educated physicians. They may have learned about plants from indigenous healers, as did the American midwives of the 1700s. For example, one midwife known as the widow Benton is thought to have learned about local herbs from Native Americans (Haller, 2000). Nurses and midwives today can continue to learn from traditional herbal healers. They can find ways to integrate traditional knowledge with their biomedically focused practice and to work with traditional herbal healers for the provision of health services. This is what the World Health Organization (WHO) has been proposing as a means to improving health care for all people. It is up to an individual country's nurses and herbal healers to work together to create a plan for how plant therapies might be integrated into the current health care system that, in some cases, has marginalized the use of herbs for centuries. Nurses must be aware of the value in the oral traditions surrounding the use of herbs, the plant wisdom that has been passed through generations of herbal healers. There is also value in systems of formal education regarding the use of herbs that have evolved in many countries, such as in the Ayurvedic and TCM systems, and also in the formal university-based programs that have developed in Exeter, England, for example.

Examples of practitioners who receive formal education in plant therapies include Doctors of Oriental Medicine (DOM), Traditional Chinese Medicine Herbalists (TCMH), Medical Herbalists (MH), and Naturopathic Physicians (ND). Students of naturopathic and Oriental medicine receive education in healing modalities other than plant therapies. The DOM learns acupuncture and cupping and the ND learns homeopathy and hydrotherapies, for example. Nurses also can create study plans that include plant therapies as an integrated part of preparation for professional nursing practice. One university-based nursing program in Australia, for example, has even begun a program through which nurses can obtain a double degree in naturopathy (includes the study of herbs) and nursing (see resources listed at the end of this chapter) (McCabe, 2000). Plant therapies are a natural addition to nursing education, which historically has included the fundamental modalities of touch, environmental interaction, nutrition, communication, and energy as ways of demonstrating care (Libster, 2001).

Nurses in the state of Washington recognized the importance of nurses being involved in patient care using plant therapies and other naturopathic remedies and changed their nurse practice act to reflect that nurses could take orders from naturopathic physicians. This might be helpful in some cases, such as in a clinic where ND's treat specific diseases and nursing care is needed. However, in the overall plan for formal integration of plant therapies in nursing practice, properly educated nurses are capable of independently using plant therapies. If nurses pursue taking orders from naturopaths or other herbal practitioners rather than pursuing their own plant therapies education, the precedent will be established that nurses take orders for herbal remedies, a practice that is not completely congruent with earlier days in the development of nursing practice. There are some herbal uses, such as those outlined in this book, for which nurses would be quite capable of discerning the appropriate use in their patients. Nurses' herb education programs must focus on the use of herbal teas (including liquid extracts) and topical and environmental applications. Nurses already routinely offer patients herbal beverages as a matter of course, even in hospitals. These culinary practices could be expanded to therapeutic use. Increasing education and research could make it so.

Plant therapies education and research must have a strong nursing focus on providing comfort and care to an individual with an illness, as opposed to emphasizing the disease process, which is the domain and expertise of medical colleagues. The focus also must be to help the patient find a greater sense of personal wellness through self-care and nursing care. The focus of the work of integrating plant therapies into nursing practice must include an integration of the biomedical, traditional, and historical nursing perspectives of plant use in health care. Educational programs for nurses that include all three paradigms must be created so that graduates can "walk between the worlds," producing holistic, synergistic plant therapy solutions to include in individualized plans of care. Nurses who receive herbal education from all three perspectives have the foundation for providing integrative care in which that integration is exhibited as a willingness to bring together multiple perspectives for herb use. Integrative care is a diplomatic approach that uses knowledge and wisdom from different perspectives when helping patients make health care choices. This diplomatic approach also must be present when health practitioners engage in defining the focus of practice, which in this case is the use of herbs. The focus in nursing has never been cure. It has been to seek understanding and relationship with a patient and provide interventions that suggest opportunity for greater health and well-being. The focus of herbal education must not be cure. It must be working together with plants in patient care—*nature care.*

SAMPLE NATURE CARE CURRICULUM:

Table 19-1 outlines a sample curriculum for an introductory thirty-two-week course of study for nurses on the integrative use of plant therapies. The goal of this course is to provide an opportunity for the study of and experience with plants and their therapeutic use that is evidence based, culturally and clinically relevant, patient focused, and wellness oriented.

Overall course objectives include the following:

1. Students will verbalize an understanding of various historical theories that guide the use of herbs in healing.
2. Students will demonstrate a beginning understanding of the science and art of medicinal plant use, in particular, when describing the relationship of the modality to conventional nursing practice.
3. Students will identify the ways in which cultural traditions and historical plant use by nurses and biomedicine have added to the body of knowledge of medicinal plant use.
4. Students will verbalize how they can use an integrative approach to the use of herbs in providing nursing care.

Each class must have specific objectives that relate to these general objectives. The suggested outline in Table 19-1 follows the chapters of this book, which can be used as a primary text.

Reasonable Research

After education, nurses need to consider the issue of research and herbal therapies. So often nurses and other health care practitioners suggest that herbs only be used if they can be proven safe and efficacious by randomized clinical trials (RCTs), the gold standard of biomedical science most often used in the testing of pharmaceutical drugs. Some actually dismiss the question of the use of an herb in practice simply because no RCTs justify its use. Is this reasonable? There are some pros and cons to holding herbs to the same standards as pharmaceutical drugs. First of all, herbs do not have the same history as pharmaceutical drugs. Plant therapies often have been used extensively in one culture or another, sometimes for hundreds of years, whereas drugs have not been used at all. Denying the use of drugs that have not been thoroughly studied is reasonable when they have never been used in humans. But is it reasonable to suggest that herbs that have been safely used by humans for hundreds of years should now only be used based on whether or not RCTs have proved that they are helpful and not just executing a placebo effect?

786   CHAPTER 19

Table 19-1

32-WEEK (96-HOUR) CLASS OUTLINE: NATURE CARE FOR NURSES

Weeks 1–3 (9 hours)	The world of healing plants: Introduction to plant therapies, botany, plant taxonomy: Chapter 1 and supplemental readings
Weeks 4–5 (6 hours)	The history and theories of herbalism: Chapter 2 and supplemental readings
Weeks 6–10 (15 hours)	Evidence-based herbalism: The three paradigms of biomedicine, tradition, and nursing: Chapter 3 and supplemental readings
	Cultural traditions and the development of herbal medicine and therapies: Chapter 6 and additional readings
Weeks 11–13 (9 hours)	Carefulness and conservation issues: Chapter 4 and supplemental readings
	Current events in the safety of all medicines and therapeutics and in the status of medicinal plant conservation: Includes the concepts from chapter 19 on reasonable research
Weeks 14–19 (18 hours)	Nursing care and plants: Back to the roots: Plant therapy applications
	Includes workshops in the preparation and nursing care associated with the various applications covered in this text in chapter 5 with supplemental readings and CD-ROM with video version of preparing herbal remedies
Weeks 20–28 (27 hours)	Plant profiles: In-depth lecture and discussion of each herb (chapters 6–18) and workshop experience with the suggestions under the Nurturing the Nurse-Plant Relationship section of each profile; includes discussion of potential areas for further research as well as supplemental reading and World Wide Web studies related to each plant
Weeks 29–30 (6 hours)	Herbs—The environment and the mind: Covers introductory material on horticultural therapy (chapter 5), aromatherapy (chapter 5), Bach flower remedies (chapter 20), and resources for further learning
Weeks 31–32 (6 hours)	The final two sessions can be used for field trips including herb walks with local plant experts, wildcrafting experiences, and visits to botanical gardens. Emphases are on observing medicinal plants in their natural state and increasing understanding of community education programs on plant therapies. Medicinal plants and the law (chapter 19) and the nine steps in communicating with patients about herbal therapies (chapter 20) are covered in this section. A concluding discussion on the vision of the continued integration of herb use in nursing practice and the goal of health care for all is included (chapter 20).

Secondly, the concept of the standard RCT is not acceptable to all cultures. For example, Chinese scientists do not agree philosophically with the concept of using placebo. Is it reasonable to believe that all cultures will honor and value the RCT as the gold standard for good science or good herbal practice? It may seem culturally biased to some to suggest that the RCT is the only truly acceptable measure of the safety and efficacy of an herb.

Questions have been raised within the biomedical community about the feasibility and the effect of holding the RCT as the gold standard for health science in the first place. RCTs are very expensive and logistically challenging. In fact, RCTs have not been carried out for many of the medical treatments in existence. And even when RCTs are available, it is difficult to extrapolate the findings to the individual patient because the entry criteria into the RCTs are usually very stringent and the clinician may never find an RCT that matches the patient seeking treatment. "The ideal of standardized and rigorous process for evaluating treatments seems at odds with everyday clinical practice, in which small sample sizes, even just one case, are frequently enough to convince clinicians and patients that something works . . . the treatment of an individual patient in routine clinical practice can be likened to a therapeutic experiment" (Larson, Ellsworth, & Oas, 1993, p. 2708).

Some have suggested that single patient trials (SPTs), or "n-of-1" studies, may be more feasible and more helpful in directing patient care (Jaeschke, Cook, & Sackett, 1992). The SPT provides research that supports the treatment of the *individual* patient. The goal of the SPT is the determination of the most suitable treatment for a given patient. As with all research methods, there are limitations to SPTs. "The limitations of n-of-1 trials arise from the prerequisites for their execution" (Jaeschke, Cook, & Sackett, 1992, p. 228). To perform an SPT, both the clinician and the patient must agree that there is some doubt about the effectiveness of the treatment under consideration. This doubt can be related to one or more of the following circumstances: (1) The patient is taking a remedy that the clinician feels is worthless. (2) The patient may be experiencing symptoms that may be construed as having adverse effects. (3) The clinician and/or the patient is doubtful about the effectiveness of a particular treatment. (4) The clinician and/or the patient is uncertain about the quantity of medication or therapy to be used. Although SPTs have been considered in terms of pharmaceutical drug studies, it is possible this method may be helpful in working with the individual patient using some form of plant therapy, be it an herbal bath, compress, or tea.

The questions regarding the feasibility of any clinical trial involving plant therapies relate primarily to randomization and blindedness. There have been concerns that many complementary therapies may not best be studied by the clinical trial method. "Alternative medicine therapies may also possess a theoretical basis, may stem from a cultural tradition that is seemingly antithetical to a quantitative, biomedical framework, or may possess little foundation research on which to base a controlled evaluation" (Margolin, Avants, & Kleber, 1998, p. 1626). Often with herbal remedies, the investigator is seeking to understand established therapeutic outcomes. Because the mechanism of action is often unknown, establishing controls for a particular study is difficult. In many cultural traditions, the herbal remedy being studied might preclude the blinding of the practitioner in the study because the relationship between healer, plant, and patient is highly significant and influential in the treatment outcome. For example, if a nurse-investigator wanted to study the effects of aloe vera plasters on second- or third-degree burns, the preparation and application of the plaster (the method) is just as significant as the aloe material itself when considering the therapy as a whole. How the plaster is applied and how the care is demonstrated are as important to nursing practice as the biochemical action of the aloe. These factors also are important in traditional herbalism and, in some cases, are considered more important.

If the way in which care is provided did not matter to nurses, we would not spend time teaching students how to communicate or educate patients. Students would not be taught how to walk into a sick room as discussed by Nightingale, or how to touch a patient therapeutically, or how to respond when one sees a gross malformation such as a gaping wound on a patient for the first time. None of this would matter. But it does matter to nurses, and to patients. How an herb is prepared and applied matters too. "How nurses creatively demonstrate caring is the art of nursing. It is the beauty of nursing. It is also the science of nursing" (Libster, 2001, p. 3). How does one reasonably measure the art of nursing?

This has been an ongoing concern for nurse-scholars. The concern about research in nursing is very similar to the concern about researching complementary therapies such as herbal medicine. Although clinical trials have been done with herbal medicines, especially with standardized extract preparations, is the herbal *therapy* really understood? Can understanding the mechanism of action of a plant or its constituents give a clinician a reasonably good understanding of the safety and efficacy of the plant as a remedy or healing modality? Is it reasonable to ask that herbal practitioners change their scientific and theoretic framework for working with plants and patients to conform to a biomedical standard that does not adequately address the research question at hand?

Several scientific methods might be helpful in adding to the body of plant medicine knowledge. Nursing practice benefits not only from quantitative studies such as the RCT but also from qualitative studies. For example, ethnographic and narrative inquiries could be helpful in understanding traditional uses of herbal remedies that are highly valued by communities. Studies that lead to a greater understanding of the relationship of the plant in the healing rituals of an individual may be just as insightful as the studies that lead to greater understanding of the inner workings of the plant itself.

Nurses can benefit from many types of research relating to plant therapies. Integration of understanding gained from biomedical and traditional research may be the most reasonable approach because the focus of herbal applications is not standardization but meeting of individual patient needs for healing and greater well-being. Nonjudgmentally observing patients' use of herbs in self-care, writing up the results as case studies, and comparing notes on herbal use in individual locations can add to the body of scientific information on herb use in patient care. Although RCTs may be helpful, it is not reasonable to believe that they are forthcoming or necessary in informing nurses' use of plants in patient care or in understanding and supporting patient self-care with herbs.

REPORTING RESEARCH:

Because nurses have a history of supporting and promoting self-care, they often encounter patients who are using plant remedies in self-treatment or treatment of their family members. Nurses are often in a position to provide research and information to patients about the herbal remedies they are using or considering using. The public, although interested in scientific research, is often uninformed regarding the variation of methodologies used to study herbs. It is the ethical responsibility of health practitioners and researchers to clearly report findings and include any limitations of the study's meaning to the consumer as an individual patient. This means that if a large clinical trial on an herb shows favorable, generalizable responses, consumers must not be led to believe that *they* are assured benefit. This also means that just because an RCT shows no benefit in an herb that traditional herbalists or a community has used for hundreds of years, there is *no* health benefit. RCTs are very specific, and the results must be reported regarding the study's inclusion criteria, the herb used, and how it was used. For example, if the RCT involved the use of standardized extract of a particular constituent from an herb such as alliin from garlic *(Allium sativum),* it should not be reported in a way that would leave the consumer with the impression that whole garlic or other garlic products would have the same results.

One example of ethically flawed reporting occurred with the release of results of an in vitro study of four herbs' effect on penetration of *hamster* oocytes and the integrity of donor (presumably human) sperm deoxyribonucleic acid (Ondrizek, Chan, Patton, & King, 1999). The results of the in vitro study were that flooding the oocytes with a "concentrated herbal solution" of each of the four herbs resulted in reduced or zero penetration of oocytes. Exposure of sperm cells to some of the herbs resulted in denaturation of DNA. One well-known American physician appeared on a major national news program and reported to the public that anyone trying to conceive should not take any of the herbs evaluated in the study. He mentioned that many herbs are not "studied" and therefore are suspected to be potentially unsafe. It was never mentioned that the study was on hamster instead of human cells. The physician did mention in passing that the study was an in vitro study, but he did not clarify for the listener what that meant. The essence of the report was that the four herbs have not been studied, they are unsafe, and pose a danger to those trying to conceive. The report was made without consideration of the need for clear, unbiased representation of research findings.

In reporting research findings about herbal remedies it is important to include the following:

1. The exact herb used and the preparation
2. The type of study
3. The subjects involved
4. The results and the limitations of those results

An example of reporting research information to a patient would be, "The randomized, double-blind, placebo-controlled study involved 30 men taking whole garlic *(Allium sativum)* in capsules (amount if known) for 3 months. The study of these men showed that taking the garlic capsules did lower total cholesterol levels in all of the men by ____ (number) points." If speaking to a woman, it might be emphasized that the study only included men. If someone were taking whole garlic in their diet, it might be emphasized that the results of the study were related to the use of capsulated whole garlic. Nurses have a responsibility not only to perform reasonable research but also to reasonably report research findings in a manner that clearly informs the public and does not mislead them to believe strongly in benefits or risks that do not necessarily exist.

Medicinal Plants and the Law

As nurses engage in the exploration of integrating plant therapies into nursing practice, either directly as a caring modality or indirectly in providing patient education and information about herbal therapies, they must consider the laws of their country of residence. Nurses must consider the laws related to their own practice issues, which ultimately protect the public, and the laws created for the protection of plant populations.

Many countries now have guidelines or position statements on the use or integration of complementary therapies into nursing practice. Every nurse considering the use of herbal therapies in practice is best advised to be well informed as to their country's position on the use of plant therapies in practice. Most Western countries consider plant therapies a "complementary therapy." The term "complementary therapy" was created to describe a practice that complements conventional biomedicine. Because professional nurses around the globe have a practice that is very much a part of the biomedical system (many nurses continue to be educated in hospital-based programs), nurses also consider plant or herbal therapies as not inherently part of nursing practice, but as complementary to that practice. This conceptualization of practice also is true for other touch therapies such as massage, reflexology, and therapeutic touch. Until such time as nursing is reconceptualized in terms of the reintegration of historical nursing modalities such as plant therapies, it is important for nurses to consider the position of those bodies governing their practice in regard to complementary therapies.

In Australia, for example, the Royal College of Nursing and the Australian Nursing Federation have policies and several state nursing boards have guidelines for the integration of complementary therapies in nursing practice. The policies all state that nurses must be appropriately qualified in a therapy when using it as a nursing intervention (personal communication, McCabe, February 2001).

In Canada, the national nursing organization has a position statement that defines herbal therapies as complementary and is formulated as follows:

> *The practice of nursing is defined in legislation throughout Canada, and commonly includes promoting, maintaining and restoring health and the assessment and provision of care for health conditions by supportive, preventive, therapeutic, palliative, and rehabilitative means. If a complementary therapy meets these criteria then it falls into the scope of nursing practice . . . nurses practicing complementary therapies must do so in the context of a nursing framework and that there must be evidence of the nursing process of assessment, planning, intervention, and evaluation. (www.cna-nurses.ca/pages/ issuestrends/nrgnow/compl_thrp.htm)*

Nurses in the United Kingdom must ensure that no nursing action is "detrimental to the interests, condition, or safety of patients and clients" (Nazarko, 1995, p. 34). As Nazarko (1995) points out in an article on whether it is prudent for nurses to recommend cranberry juice for symptoms related to urinary tract infection, "the role of the nurse is therefore not to dictate to the patient but to present the evidence and listen to the views and wishes of the patient who makes the decision" (p. 34). With so many patients using plant remedies, it would seem important that, at the very least, nurses have a basic understanding of herbalism and can offer some information and opportunity for referral to medical herbalists if the nurse herself does not have the education to advise the patient (Libster, 1999).

Some of the questions nurses must ask themselves before using plant therapies in their caring practice are as follows:

1. What education is required in my country to include the use of plant therapies in practice?
2. Are there any legal requirements in my country, state, and/or of my nursing regulatory board or agency regarding the use of herbs in caring for patients? Are those requirements specific to any particular use of herbs in practice such as oral remedies?

3. Are there any legal or ethical ramifications of *not* knowing anything about herbal remedies and *not* providing assistance to patients who are making decisions about the use of herbal remedies in self-care?

4. Herbal medicine is a very large scientific field. What herbal education do I want and need to integrate herbal remedies into my present practice?

5. Are my qualifications adequate to address the particular need of an individual patient regarding the use of herbal therapies, or are there other practitioners who are better qualified to address the needs of the patient? For example, I once had a patient who was concerned about a "curse" and was wondering about specific herbs for addressing the physiologic effects of the curse. Because I was not informed of the spiritual and cultural issues associated with the curse and the traditional uses of herbs related to this aspect of my patient's culture, I was not qualified to address the questions even though I have extensive education and experience in the use of herbs. It was better to refer the patient to a traditional healer.

6. Nurses also must clarify their legal role in relation to the use of herbal remedies. Nurses must use the nursing process and not fall into the trap of practicing medicine with herbs. First of all, practicing medicine without education and licensure is illegal. Secondly, the focus of the way nurses have historically used herbs in caring practice has not been to "cure" disease but to allay the symptoms that may be associated with disease or may just be symptoms of discomfort associated with everyday living or with illness, not necessarily disease. For example, pregnancy is not a disease. Nurse-midwives often use herbs in practice to help women cope with the changes in their bodies and to promote the health of the mother and the fetus.

Nurses also must have an understanding of the laws regarding the use of various healing plants in their countries. Some medicinal plants are protected because they are at risk for extinction. Plants can become endangered because their habitats are threatened or because they are overused. This is especially a problem when the root or bark of the plant is the medicinal part sought.

Nurses need to be aware of any restrictions on the use of plants they might be using in practice. Using plant medicine formulations in practice requires another level of understanding and education that nurses may or may not have. When using herbal formulations, such as patent formulas or herbal supplements, the nurse not only is responsible for the knowledge of the individual plants in the formula, but also for understanding the interaction and/or synergy of the herbs in formulation. For example, in TCM, certain herbs in formulation have been found over many years to potentiate or be synergistic with the action of other herbs. Occasionally, certain herbs have been found to be dangerous in formulation together. Nurses who do not understand formulations and use them in practice pose a potential risk to health promotion. In addition, nurses who use these supplements often sell the products to their patients, posing a potential conflict of interest. Nurses must be aware of their legal and ethical responsibilities regarding the provision of herbal formulations as supplements.

Nurses in rural areas who collect the herbs they use in practice also must be aware of legal and ethical wildcrafting practices in their areas. In general, "plants are considered by the public as a product of nature, which may be freely collected by anyone, even on private land" (de Klemm, 1991, p. 259). It is not hard to imagine what can happen if a locally grown plant is discovered to be highly medicinal and the market price skyrockets. People trespass on private properties and have been known to gouge the earth of the plants. Countries in which the culture of respecting medicinal plants has been taught from generation to generation have protected the right to collect what is needed for personal use, not economic gain. For example, in Bavaria in Germany, the right to gather wild plants anywhere is "enshrined in the Constitution" (de Klemm, 1991, p. 260). In many countries such as Austria and Switzerland, the uprooting of plants is prohibited and the amount of the aerial parts that can be wildcrafted is limited to five to twenty flowering stems or branches, depending on the area, and in some cases, the maximum amount that can be harvested is that which can be held in the palm of one hand (de Klemm, 1991). Because nurses who use herbs in practice are not just using that which they would normally use in their own self-care, they must be aware of the impact that wildcrafting the herbs they use in practice will have on plant populations. If wildcrafting is to be done, it is best if a nurse teams up with a local botanist. When I was coordinating the herb program for a group I worked with in a rural community, I regularly checked in with the lead botanist associated with a nearby national forest and went out on herb walks with him to identify the plants in my area. It was fun and educational!

Conservation of medicinal plants is not a simple matter. Legislation protecting endangered species, although necessary, is considered inadequate. Plant habitats also must be protected to sustain the growth of medicinal plant populations. In the 1991 *Proceedings of an International Consultation* on the conservation of medicinal plants, organized by the WHO and others, seven points related to legislation regarding the management of medicinal plants were raised (de Klemm, 1991):

1. Prevention of overcollection
2. Use permits as management instruments
3. Use a management plan
4. Implementation of controls on the trade of medicinal plants
5. Collection of license fees
6. Habitat protection
7. Incentives for artificial propagation

Nurses who use herbs in practice may want to consider propagating their own plants. Ensuring that the herbs used in remedies are of the highest quality is important. When growing plants for nursing use it is recommended that samples of the plants be sent to laboratories for analysis each year. Nurses who use their own herbs in practice must be aware of any laws pertaining to this practice in their location. My experience is that when working in poorer, rural areas, regulatory agencies recognize the expertise and education of the practitioner who uses their own herbs. They often welcome the care provided by an herbalist because the modality is very helpful to patients, is inexpensive, and has few if any side effects.

Integrating herbal therapies into nursing practice involves reflection and creativity. It also involves education. I once worked with a pediatrician who, when patients asked what he knew about herbal medicine, answered honestly and knowledgeably, "I'm sure that there is much to be considered with the use of herbs. . . . I just don't have the time to study it. I am so busy keeping up with the stuff I have to know to run my practice as it is." He clearly demonstrated to patients that he does not take herbal therapies lightly and that education was needed to understand their use. He made referrals instead when the patients wanted more information. This is a wise approach that goes a long way in the protection of patients, practitioners, and plant populations.

Resources for Further Learning

The following are examples of herbal education programs. Nurses might consider taking college level courses, if and when available, and studying both Eastern and Western herbalism.

Note: Other plant therapies resources are located in the appendix. Inclusion in the following list of examples does not represent endorsement of any one particular program.

Courses on Herbs and Resource Centers to Find Courses on Herbs

Integrative Associates, LLC
Courses on Botanical Therapies
www.integrativeassociates.com
contact: Martha Libster, Director

Dr. James Duke's Medical Botany Course
contact: Dr. James Duke, Ethnobotanist
The Herbal Village
8210 Murphy Road
Fulton, Maryland 20759
www.ars-grin.gov/duke/syllabus

American Herbalists Guild

The American Herbalists Guild provides a directory of herbal education programs for $14 (U.S.) and can be contacted at (www.healthy.net/herbalists/Educat.htm).

School of Phytotherapy Registrar
Bucksteep Manor
Bodle Street Green
Hailsham, East Sussex BN27 4RJ
England
Phone: 01323-833812/4
Fax: 01323-833869
medherb@pavilion.co.uk

Herb Research Foundation
1007 Pearl Street, Suite 200
Boulder, CO 80302
Phone: 303-449-2265 (office) 800-748-2617 (voice mail)
Fax: 303-449-7849
www.herbs.org/

The Herb Research Foundation provides research and information services, including lists of educational workshops, programs, and courses available through the foundation and educational institutions in the United States.

American Botanical Council
P.O. Box 144345
Austin, TX 78714-4345
Phone: 512-926-4900
Fax: 512-926-2345
www.herbalgram.org

The American Botanical Council has an excellent catalog of herbal education books.

Rocky Mountain Center for Botanical Studies
Feather Jones
P.O. Box 19254
Boulder, CO 80308-2254
303-442-6861

Sage Mountain Herbs
Rosemary Gladstar
P.O. Box 420
E. Barre, VT 05649
802-476-9825

Tai Sophia Institute-School of Botanical Healing
American City Building
10227 Wincopin Circle, Suite 100
Columbia, MD 21044
410-997-4888 or 800-735-2968
www.tai.edu

The National College of Phytotherapy
3030 Isleta Boulevarde S.W.
Albuquerque, NM 87105
505-452-3468
phyto@swcp.com
   Founded by Amanda McQuade Crawford, the National College of
Phytotherapy offers a three-year bachelor's degree in herbal medicine.

Dominion Herbal College
Contact: Judy Nelson
7527 Kingsway
Burnaby, BC V3N 3C1
604-792-8832

Herbal Therapeutics, Inc.-School of Botanical Medicine
Contact: David Winston
P.O. Box 553
Broadway, NJ 08808
dwherbal@nac.net

Southwest School of Botanical Medicine
Michael Moore
P.O. Box 4565
Bisbee, AZ 85603

Northeast School of Botanical Medicine
7 Song
P.O. Box 6626
Ithaca, NY 14851-6626
607-564-1023

School of Natural Healing (Founded by John R. Christopher)
P.O. Box 412
Springville, UT 84663
800-372-8255
   The School of Natural Healing was founded by John R. Christopher.

Therapeutic Herbalism
Contact: David Hoffmann
2068 Ludwig Avenue
Santa Rosa, CA 95407-6415
707-544-7210

American School of Herbalism
10226 Empire Grade Road
Santa Cruz, CA 95060
408-457-9096 or 408-457-9097
    The American School of Herbalism was founded by Michael Tierra
and Christopher Hobbs.

Institute of Traditional Herbal Medicine and Aromatherapy
54A Gloucester Avenue
London, NW1 8JD
England

Traditional Chinese Herbal Medicine and Japanese Herbalism

Rocky Mountain Herbal Institute
Contact: Roger Wicke, Ph.D.
P.O. Box 579
Hot Springs, MT 59845
406-741-3811

American Academy of Acupuncture & Traditional Chinese Medicine
9100 Parkwest Drive
Houston, TX 77063
713-780-9777

Academy of Chinese Culture & Health Sciences
1601 Clay Street
Oakland, CA 94612
510-763-7787

American College of Traditional Chinese Medicine
455 Arkansas Street, Suite 302
San Francisco, CA 94107
415-282-7600

Colorado School of Traditional Chinese Medicine
1441 York Street, Suite 100
Denver, CO 80206
303-329-6355

International College of Traditional Chinese Medicine
3011847 W. Broadway
Vancouver, BC V6M 461 Canada
604-731-2926

Samra University of Oriental Medicine
600 St. Paul Avenue #100
Los Angeles, CA 90017-2014
213-487-2672
   The Samra University of Oriental Medicine offers a thirty-six-month master of science degree.

Santa Barbara College of Oriental Medicine
1919 State Street, Suite 204
Santa Barbara, CA 93101
805-898-1180
   The Santa Barbara College of Oriental Medicine offers master's degree programs.

Minnesota School of Acupuncture & Herbal Studies
5251 Chicago Avenue South
Minneapolis, MN 55417-1731
612-823-6235

Sun Farm Shoji Co., Ltdl. (Japanese Herb School)
Yutaka Onoe, -13-18 Higashikanda, Chiyoda-Ku
Yokyo 101 Japan
Phone: 03-3866-1712
Fax: 03-3866-2302

Aromatherapy Seminars
Rocky Mountain Center for Botanical Studies
Contact: Mindy Green, M.S.
P.O. Box 19254
Boulder, CO 80308-2254

Aromatherapy for Health Professionals
   Contact Jane Buckle, R.N. (www.rjbuckle.com) for information regarding 250 hours of instruction in aromatherapy.

The Institute of Integrative Aromatherapy
Valerie Cooksley, R.N.
877-363-3422 or 888-282-2002
www.Aroma-RN.com
   Contact Valerie Cooksley for information regarding 225 hours of instruction in aromatherapy.

Tisserand Institute
P.O. Box 746
Hove, East Sussex, BN3 3XA
England
0273-206640

Use of Herbs in Anthroposophical Nursing

The Anthroposophical Nurses Association of America
Contact: President Rise Smythe-Freed, R.N.
1923 Geddes Avenue
Ann Arbor, MI 48104-1797
Phone: 734-994-8303
Fax: 734-761-6617
artemisia@anthroposophy.org

Naturopathic Healing

La Trobe University
Bundoora, Victoria 3083, Australia
Phone: 61 3 9479 5955
Fax: 61 3 9479 5988

La Trobe University offers a double major in nursing and naturopathy. For more information contact Pauline McCabe, senior lecturer in naturopathy, at p.mccabe@Latrobe.edu.au

John Bastyr College
Ron Hobbs
144 N.E. 54th Street
Seattle, WA 98105
206-523-9585

The John Bastyr College has a bachelor of science program in herbalism.

National College of Naturopathic Medicine
11231 S.E. Market Street
Portland, OR 97216
503-255-4860

CHAPTER 20
Staying in Contact with the Garden

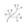

N ATURE IS ALIVE WITH OPPORTUNITIES FOR HEALING. Seeds, nuts, leaves, roots, berries, and bark in addition to flowers of every shape, color, size, smell, and taste bring with them the possibility of greater health and well-being. Whether made into a poultice, compress, or plaster or used cooked, raw, inhaled, or sipped, herbs are Mother Nature's pharmacy. Plants are available to provide their lesson of healing to those who seek connection with the roots of modern medicine. Plant wisdom and knowledge are available for those who would take modern health care into a new era in which the old and the new merge and even transcend present paradigms. Plants have played a large role in the evolution of health care.

Health care has come through a modern period characterized by the development of remarkable technology. However, human beings are not necessarily healed by technology. There are numerous examples of how technology has successfully treated a disease only to find that the patient dies. Healing can occur within the emotional world and consciousness of a patient. People can experience healing during an illness and even as they die. Healing can occur regardless of whether or not the physical body is "fixed."

Healing can manifest when the patient connects with his or her purpose for being and a greater sense of self-awareness emerges. Healing also manifests when patients develop a greater sense of their life as part of the greater web of life. Nurses often witness the changes that emerge in patients, even those who are terminally ill, when the person finds their purpose or meaning in life. Often the patient has an "a-ha" moment, like a light bulb turning on, when they realize the meaning in their life or in their illness. Patients often find that experiencing an illness can be a learning experience. Some patients and nurses do not desire the experience of connecting with the purpose and meaning of life as a part of the quest for greater health. This is a matter of choice. The work of several nurse theorists such as Jean Watson and Margaret Newman have expounded upon finding meaning as part of the healing process. Margaret Newman (1994) discusses the concept of eliciting patients' memories of meaningful moments in their lives as a way of assessing the patient's pattern of health as expanding consciousness. Jean Watson (1999) writes eloquently about the road of human caring as a transpersonal and meaningful experience for patient and caregiver alike.

Exploring meaning and healing is a deeply human experience. What nursing often supports is people experiencing and expressing their humanity in similar and diverse ways. Because nursing is a human science, the laboratory is the person. Because nursing is a human art, the canvas, stage, or score is the person. People do not and cannot exist in isolation. Often in the process of exploring meaning and healing, a person discovers they are not alone. When patients realize they are not alone in their illness, in their work, or in their life and that they are indeed part of a community, even a universe, that includes other human beings, animals, and plant life, they can be relieved of their sense of isolation. They become open to the importance of connection, compassion, and care for self and others in that universe.

In the exploration of meaning and healing, patients often perceive their lives in a new light. Experiencing illness is often a catalyst for new perceptions. Often people will reach for a healing substance or technique that is familiar and comforting and see it in a new way. Herbal remedies are one of those familiar and comforting healing modalities that people reach for. What once was the "bitter tasting tea mom used to give me when I was little" becomes the familiar remedy of an aged and confused adult seeking healing. The family salve becomes a treasured alternative to the new ointments appearing on store shelves every day. Many people in the world have a connection with the healing world of plants because of their family and community relationships. They carry with them an understanding of plants as life forms, not simply alternatives or replacements for pharmaceutical drugs. Others have no awareness of the gifts of healing the plant world offers humans. They may never have had experiences exploring nature or interacted with a family or community member who used herbs in healing. In today's world, many people learn early in childhood how to use the biomedical system in their community, as in how to select an over-the-counter remedy at the pharmacy, but, they may never learn about folk remedies, home remedies, or herbal medicines that they can prepare for themselves. They may have no awareness of the importance of the plant-human relationship.

If a nurse or patient has never used a medicinal plant, the very idea can be threatening. Change of any kind can be disconcerting. To begin thinking and accepting that plants can be healing, someone who has relied on biomedicine their whole life must be able to make a change or a shift in perception that is emotional, intellectual, and physical. A person must be able to explore plants with an open mind without judging the effectiveness of the plant remedies solely in light of how they compare to the biomedical remedies they have used before. To fully appreciate herbal remedies, they must be explored in terms of how the plant remedy may be unique in its effects on emotions, mind, and body. Herbal remedies feel and act differently in the body than drugs even though they may contain chemical constituents found in drugs. Comparing a pharmaceutical drug to an herb is like comparing a bowl of crystallized fructose to an apple. It just is not the same thing, both biologically and energetically.

The concept of energy, especially as it relates to healing, is not new to nursing. Throughout history, nurses have helped patients conserve energy, preserve energy, build up their energy, and restore energy. Florence Nightingale called the patient's energy or strength the "vital power" (Nightingale, 1957, p. 9). "Nurses have been concerned with the preservation of the patient's energy, or vital power, so that he might use his energy for healing" (Libster, 2001, p. 189). Herbs are energetically different from pharmaceutical drugs because they are plant life forms, and therefore, they have a completely different action that transcends the physical biochemistry of the plant's substance.

Plants, like humans, are energy fields, that emit or radiate energy that is measurable through such instrumentation as time-lapse and Kirlian photography, optical pulse recorders, and galvanometers (Tompkins & Bird, 1973). They are affected by energy that surrounds them in the soil, the air, and the light. They actually transform and store energy. "Each day the sun bathes the earth with energy equal to 684 billion tons of coal. Most of this abundance is quickly lost, reflected back into the darkness of outer space. However, the sunlight that falls on chlorophyll-producing plants can be entrapped through photosynthesis and transmuted to more stable forms, holding the energy on earth for a while before it ultimately is released" (Lewis, 1996, p. 5). Plants respond to and interact within the environment just as humans and animals do, although they do it in different ways. When people use plants in healing, they not only receive the plant's chemical constituents but also the life force or energy of the plant.

Sowing the Seeds

Some might say that there is no better way to observe the life force of humans than during the birth process. When a baby is born, it is difficult for people sharing the experience not to shed a tear because of the miraculous way that life takes form and begins to express itself. Planting a seed can cause a similar reaction. Sowing seeds can be a transcendent experience. One tiny carrot seed could easily blow away in the wind, but when placed just a few millimeters under some soil and lightly watered, it produces long soft sprays of greenery and a centimeters-long orange root that can be eaten for supper. What an amazing demonstration of life force. The human who eats the carrot receives not just its vitamin A and other nutrients, but also the life force of the carrot. In Chinese medicine, this energy from food that is then used in creating energy in the human body is called "nutrient qi." Much about the life force or *qi* of plants and plant medicines has yet to be explored.

ADAPTOGEN ACTION:

Within every plant and every human is a seed of potential. Within every baby is a matrix for an adult, and within every acorn is the matrix for the great oak. Humans and plants, although very different in presentation, are very similar conceptually when it comes to energy potential. One manifestation of this energy potential is the ability of plants and humans to adapt to their environment. Humans are marvelous in that they can adapt to changes in the environment by reasoning solutions that ultimately ensure continued evolution of the species. Plants too have been shown to have the ability to adapt to environmental changes. Plants contain signatures for adaptation within an ever-changing environment. They have their own coping mechanisms, such as scent, and movement patterns, such as petal closing at night, that keep predators away.

What happens when humans and plants come together and share their adaptation responses is one of the most fascinating and possibly elusive parts of plant medicine science. Several herbs, such as Siberian ginseng *(Eleutherococcus senticosus),* are known as "adaptogens" or plants that seemingly assist the human body in adapting to environmental stressors. Pharmacognosist Dr. Norman Farnsworth, who has researched the adaptogenic effects of Siberian ginseng in humans, states, "The term adaptogen is used loosely. Some use it to describe a 'tonic' effect and some use the term to describe a stimulant action to the immune system. The adaptogen effect of medicinal plants is related to the secretion of corticosteroids and the anti-stress effect but there are probably other effects as well that are not completely understood" (Farnsworth, personal communication, February, 2001).

This exchange of adaptation potential or adaptation information is not static. Some people who take ginseng *(Panax ginseng)* experience an increase in blood pressure, while others experience a decrease, depending on *their need.* Dr. John Christopher called lobelia *(Lobelia inflata),* an herb used for many health concerns including threatened miscarriage, a "thinking herb." Lobelia also demonstrates its ability to think, an adaptogen action. "Where the baby is strong, the lobelia seems to have the knowledge to assist in healing a tearing and bleeding condition and stopping the bleeding. But if the baby is

dead and should be aborted, the lobelia has the intelligence of directing the abortion" (Christopher, 1987, p. 47). Numerous herbal medicine practitioners, healers, and plant scientists have made observations of this phenomenon. Plant medicine expert Dr. Jim Duke
theorizes that, "All herbs are adaptogenic in giving your homeostatic
body a whole menu of phytochemicals, and exposed to a choice, the
homeostatic human body grabs those it needs, excluding to a degree
those it doesn't need" (personal communication, February, 2001).

Other examples of "thinking" plants with an adaptogen action are
black cohosh *(Cimicifuga racemosa)* and angelica *(Angelica sinensis),*
which contain phytosterols. Clinical experience has demonstrated to me
that these plants affect female reproductive symptoms similarly to exogenous hormone replacement but without the side effects. Because of
the similarity in action, biomedical practitioners understandably question the safety of the use of herbal remedies in the same way they
question the drugs they have used for years. However, what they do not
know is that research has shown that plant phytoestrogens can "think."
"Phytoestrogens are weaker than the body's own estrogen. In premenopausal women, phytoestrogens compete with women's own, more
potent estrogen, reducing the total effects of estrogen. As women's
estrogen production falls, phytoestrogens supplement this hormone.
When women have too much biological estrogen, phytoestrogens lower
the burden; when they have too little, phytoestrogens pinch-hit" (Duke,
1997, p. 323). What seems to be involved in the thinking process during
the human-herb connection is similar to a lock and key phenomenon in
which receptor sites on certain cells seem to be able to determine the effect of the herb needed to help the body adapt or restore balance.

Although the adaptogen action of plant medicines remains somewhat of a mystery, researchers may be opening the door to a new
"world" of science that might be applicable to the adaptogen phenomena. Candace Pert (1997) in her book, *Molecules of Emotion*, describes
her research with ligands, natural or man-made substances that selectively bind to a specific receptor on a cell. Ligands include neurotransmitters, steroids, and peptides. Pert recognized in her research
that drugs that are nearly identical in molecular structure can fit the
same receptor but have opposite effects. "Both agonist and antagonist
were believed to bind to the same opiate receptor, but somehow their
'intrinsic activity'—the effect they had on the cell—was different"
(Pert, 1997, p. 81). Although this is not exactly the same scenario as
with the identical herb causing opposite reactions depending on the
body's need, it does point to the importance of the "receptor."

In nursing practice, it is clearly understood that no two people respond to the same intervention in the same way. Similarly, no one
person responds to the same intervention in the same way at different times. For example, one woman taking a shower after giving birth
might become lightheaded and need assistance to get back to bed,
whereas another woman might not. An individual patient might have

no pain during a dressing change one time and another time find the intervention agonizing. People change constantly, inside and out. We are in constant state of adaptation. One nurse theorist, Sister Callista Roy, describes in her adaptation model of nursing that the person is an "adaptive system" whose behavior is influenced "both by the environment, that is, the world within and around the person, and by the person's abilities to deal with that world" (Andrews & Roy, 1986, p. 7). The individual as a receptor adapts at both the level of a whole being and at the cellular level—the world within. Herbal medicines seem to have an effect on both levels. They may present the body with tens if not hundreds of phytochemicals, but something else happens. The body has to make a choice whether or not it is receptive to those substances. As with the lock and key phenomenon, if there is no lock for the key, then nothing happens, and vice versa.

Nurses who observe patients using herbal remedies are in a strategic place to observe the thinking herb/adaptogen phenomenon. For example, I had been fascinated by the concept of adaptogens in herbal medicine for a number of years when I became the director of the Natural Healthcare Hotline at the Herb Research Foundation. When answering the phones, I started noticing a pattern in people calling for information about *Panax ginseng*. Sometimes they told me that the ginseng lowered their blood pressure and sometimes they told me that their blood pressure stabilized or went up slightly. Of course, conclusions cannot be drawn from these individual's observations, but the experience caused me to connect what I had learned from traditional herbalists about some herbs being thinking herbs. Over a period of observation and data collection of patient responses to herbs, nurses can potentially add to the development of understanding of this phenomenon.

BACH FLOWER REMEDIES:

One scientist and physician who studied the adaptogenic effects of plants, flowers of plants, and trees in particular was English physician Edward Bach (1886–1936). After a career as a noted infectious disease physician in London, in particular as a researcher of intestinal toxemia, Dr. Bach found his purpose in life during a serious illness and took a post at the London Homeopathic Hospital, a hospital that continues to serve patients to this day. He studied the works of the homeopath Samuel Hahnemann and pursued his vision of simple remedies from plants and trees that would heal more than homeopathy. Dr. Bach found a way of potentizing the flowers from thirty-eight plants and trees using the rays of the sun. Through observational research, Dr. Bach discovered an approach of treating not disease, but the patient as a person. Dr. Bach found that "Disease of the body itself is nothing but the result of the disharmony between soul and mind. . . . Any disease, however serious, however long-standing, will be cured by restoring to the patient happiness, and desire to carry on with his work in life" (Howard & Ramsell, 1990, pp. 50–51).

The Bach flowers used at the London Homeopathic Hospital and around the world are a form of plant energy remedies. The dew from the plants, carrying the essence of the plants studied by Bach, is preserved in a small amount of brandy. A few drops of the mother tincture are then placed on 1 to 2 ounces of pure water and taken under the tongue by dropper. The remedies have been shown to assist adaptation by helping the patient move through emotions and mental states that block happiness and fulfillment in carrying out one's purpose in life. "The action of these remedies is to raise our vibrations and open up our channels for the reception of our Spiritual Self, to flood our natures with the particular virtue we need, and wash out from us the fault which is causing harm. They are able like beautiful music . . . to raise our very natures, and bring us nearer to our Souls. . . . They cure not by attacking disease, but by flooding our bodies with the beautiful vibrations of our Higher Nature, in the presence of which disease melts as snow in the sunshine" (Howard & Ramsell, 1990, p. 62).

I have used Bach flower remedies for years with patients and watched with amazement the adaptation that occurs in the life of the individual patient as they take the remedies. For example, Rescue Remedy is a combination of flowers that Bach recommended for trauma and stressful situations. In one holistic group practice, we routinely offered the remedy to patients undergoing stressful procedures. For example, children needing suturing were offered the "flower water." In many instances, I observed that after taking the Rescue Remedy, the child's need for the parents to stand by them and comfort them was still present, but the child would stop screaming and could listen to the parents and nurse helping them through the procedure.

One of the most important things Dr. Bach is said to have done for his patients was to observe and listen to them. Herbalists, in order to choose the best remedy for the patient, also listen to and closely observe the patient. In traditional herbalism, even the slightest symptom of discomfort expressed by the patient is considered when formulating a remedy. The patient's personality and the remedy are matched. Just as Bach matched the personality profile of the patient with the appropriate flower remedy, the herbalist understands the nature of the plant as well as its biochemical constituents and suggests the herbs that match the profile of the patient. To do this takes connection both with plants and with patients.

Nurses may choose to use herbal remedies in their own self-care and they may also choose to educate and provide patients and families access to experiences with plant therapies. Some patients need lots of support and information because the concept of using plant remedies is foreign to them, while other patients may be very familiar with healing plants. In addition to listening and observing patients, nurses need to learn how to talk with patients about the use of herbs.

After seeding comes weeding. Weeding the garden is necessary for the protection and nurturance of plants. Weeds are those plants that are not valued and are thought to be growing in the wrong place, such as crab grass growing in a lawn. The concept of the weed is the value judgment humans place on the plant, usually based on our own needs or the needs of other plants, which ultimately are satisfying our own needs. Weeds are plants for which no medicinal or culinary value as been found. This does not mean that the plant has no inherent value, but humans may just not have found that value.

While some may not necessarily be able to be used for human consumption, all plants have intrinsic worth and have a purpose that is yet to be understood by people. Choosing herbal remedies or helping patients choose herbal remedies involves "weeding," or identifying that which is of value to the individual patient for their healing. It is important to have an awareness of the paradigm and belief system from which we (and the patient) make health decisions. It is important that we understand both patient and plant as fully as possible. We must make time to talk with patients about herbs. To determine whether an herb or herbs are appropriate for a patient or not, the patient must tell his or her story. A complete nursing assessment is very similar to the assessment done in herbalism. Nurses who continue on for further herbal education can compare the similarities between the disciplines. When working with a patient who is considering using herbs in self-care, the nurse can begin the weeding process by asking himself or herself and/or the patient the nine questions discussed in the following section.

TALKING WITH PATIENTS ABOUT HERBS:

Nine Questions and Nursing Interventions

1. **Are we talking about the same plant?**

    Intervention. Be very careful to be sure that you and the patient are clearly discussing the same plant. Have the patient bring in the plant material or the packaging of a plant product. Do not give information without clarifying the genus and species of a plant. Use the discussion as an opportunity to educate about medicinal plants.

2. **What is the traditional, biomedical, and nursing evidence?**

    Intervention. Be knowledgeable of the traditional, biomedical, and nursing evidence that exists regarding the herbal remedy the patient is considering. Be sensitive to the paradigm of the patient. As patients speak about the herbs they are using, they will discuss their knowledge of the plants from one or more of these paradigms. If in the discussion it is clear that you and/or the patient have not collected the evidence, discuss ways in which you both might work together to do this. Patients really like doing this. They often place value on multiple ways of knowing and like having practitioners who do not only refer to one paradigm.

3. **Listen to the history—What is the story of why the patient is using the plant medicine or therapy?**

Intervention. Often patients have important reasons for taking a particular herbal remedy. Demonstrate genuine acceptance of the patient's reasons and thoughts. Do not correct the patient. Think of encouraging the patient to think through their health decision and what they need for healing as you would for any self-care choice the patient might be making. Listening to the patient's story and the way they make a health decision can provide clues as to how to guide the patient in their healing process.

4. **Is the patient undergoing medical treatment, in particular drug or diet therapies?**

Intervention. Nurses are often more familiar with drugs and diet therapies than herbal remedies. It is important to provide the patient with information about these two therapies if they ask for it. Provide the information in the framework of helping them make an informed choice. Often patients know little about these conventional therapies, and determining what they do know about the therapies they are using is a good place to begin. More consideration must be taken with those patients already involved with drug and diet therapies who wish to begin herbal remedies. Consider your own knowledge and comfort level. This patient may best be referred to a clinical herbalist to discuss the options regarding the integration of therapies. It is not ethical to recommend that because a patient is under the care of a biomedical practitioner, the patient's only choice is to pursue the advice of their physician or nurse practitioner. Nurses must help patients consider all of their options, including the possibility of taking a different course of action (e.g., women considering herbal alternatives to synthetic hormone replacement therapy.)

5. **How long is the patient thinking they might be using the plant remedy?**

Intervention. In general, most herbs can be safely taken as self-care measures for less than thirty days. If the patient is preparing to treat a disease or chronic illness with herbal remedies, recommending a clinical herbalist must be a consideration.

6. **What is the plant's history of use for the way the patient is taking it?**

Intervention. Does the patient have any experience in using the herb? What is known about the method or application of the herb for the way the patient is intending to use it? For example, patients may be planning to ingest herbs in capsules that are not meant to be eaten and have historically been decocted or extracted. Being knowledgeable about historical applications can help the nurse provide the patient with options as to how the herb might be taken.

7. **How is the patient using the plant?**

Intervention. It is important to determine how the patient is using the herb. Are they having an occasional cup of beverage tea or taking a standardized extract? How a patient discusses this information can demonstrate the patient's level of understanding of herbalism. Many people in Western countries have no knowledge of herbs that they see in the supermarket or pharmacy and may believe that the only way to take herbs is in pill or capsule form. I have had patients say to me, "Is it okay to just use fresh garlic or ginger that is in the store?" Also, nurses can be alert to misuse of herbal remedies such as the use of *Ephedra sinensis* to get a "natural" rush or high. Determining how the patient is taking the herb also can lead to further discussion, helping the nurse identify education needs.

The last two questions have to do with the approach the nurse may want to use in addressing herbal therapies.

8. **Would this patient benefit from hearing about biomedical evidence?**

Intervention. Nurses often have close relationships with their patients. Building rapport is not always easy. When a patient shares that they are using a plant remedy from a traditional approach, describing the biomedical data about the plant may or may not be appropriate. Information giving on any topic necessitates an assessment of patient readiness to listen and learn. It also means that the nurse needs to be sensitive to cultural and paradigm differences. I have seen patients withdraw immediately from caregivers who respond to their use of herbs in a manner that the patient could interpret as being condescending or disrespectful. For example, questions such as, "What proof is there that the herbs work?" or saying, "There may be some drug interactions with those herbs so you better check with your doctor before taking them," are not necessarily helpful. People know that biomedical practitioners do not routinely have knowledge of herbal remedies, so referring them to their biomedical practitioner may be an inappropriate next step. Instead nurses can best help patients by providing helpful questions that the patient can use in self-monitoring and self-care. Nurses can make statements such as, "I'm not aware of any research on that herb but I'd be happy to get some information," or, "That herb has not been thoroughly evaluated by biomedical standards," rather than, "That herb is ineffective." Think of ways to demonstrate support for the *patient,* regardless of what you may think or believe about herbs.

Whether a nurse approves or disapproves of herbal remedies, the ethical approach is to find a way to support the patient. This is true for any patient scenario. Nurses must respect patient choice and provide information, education, and nursing care. It is sometimes a delicate balance. Preserving the nurse-patient relationship should be a factor in the decision as to whether or not the nurse intervenes in self-care activities.

9. **Does taking this herb help the patient and make them happy?**

Intervention. Assessing the relationship the patient has to their choice of modality in self-care is critical to maintaining the healing relationship. Does the patient have a relationship with the herb they are using for healing and does taking that herb make them happy? Patients' choices must be respected. Even if a patient is experiencing a placebo effect from the herbs they are taking, it may not be worth discussing if the patient then thinks that the nurse is implying that their remedy is really worthless and their choice is somehow insubstantial.

Self-care with herbs makes people happy. Some people like to make their own medicines and remedies. People trust the herbal remedies that have been used by their families for generations. People like to smell and taste the herbs. They like being given a cup of tea to sip when stressed or rubbed with an aromatic oil when being massaged. Herbs make people happy, an emotion so often lacking in a troubled world. Happiness and comfort are part of the healing. Memory of a simpler, less technical world is comforting to many, especially those in the West. Herbal therapies often remind people of simpler times when there was a strong connection with the earth.

Nurses can benefit from reflecting on or "weeding" through their own paradigm about herbal remedies before interacting with patients. Some patients don't mind a little crabgrass in their lawns. Many patients may prefer the herbal remedy with all its imprecision of dose and potential imperfections. Pharmaceutical drugs are like a lawn in many ways. "A lawn, of course is an artificial community of plants, created by people to make their home grounds more beautiful and habitable. Lawns became less and less natural until some were replaced altogether by synthetic turf or green-painted asphalt" (Jenkins, 1994, p. 133). The creation of the perfect lawn free of terrible weeds has become the goal of many communities.

The lawn and gardens at Versailles in France are often viewed as symbols of man's dominance over nature just as pharmaceutical drugs represent man's struggle for dominance over disease and death. The war on disease and the war on weeds have justified the use and subsequent overuse of synthetic chemicals to support the philosophy that there is a perfect lawn and there is a magic bullet. "In 1989, the National Academy of Sciences was quoted as stating that homeowners tend to use up to ten times more chemicals per acre on their lawns than farmers use on agricultural land" (Jenkins, 1994, p. 166). There is nothing "wrong" in using synthetic chemicals for lawns or health. But when it becomes the only socially acceptable choice, something *is* wrong. Lawn doctors and medical doctors may be necessary at times, but the right of people to choose to have their front yard xeroscaped because they can't afford the watering fees or they are chemically sensitive must be respected, just as the right of people to be able to choose herbal remedies must be honored.

Enjoying the Beautiful Harvest

Professional nurses and their patients have enjoyed a relationship of trust and understanding that has endured many years. Nurses provide the education, compassion, and constant support people need not only during a healing crisis but also as they seek improvement in health and daily life. Plant therapies offer an opportunity for reconnection with the roots of medicine and healing, and they represent a new and old modality or tool to be used in nursing care. Hundreds of plants can be considered for use with patients, and opportunities for greater research and clinical use of plants in nursing practice are seemingly endless. Will nurses embrace the opportunities with herbs, or will opportunities for healing with nature's remedies be ignored?

Nature's pharmacy of herbs offers nurses a new modality and a way of thinking about health and healing that keeps us rooted in our original belief, expressed by Nightingale and others: the belief in the power of the vital spirit or energy in nature *and* in human beings to bring regeneration; rejuvenation; and health and harmony of body, mind, and spirit. A nurse's role is to put the patient in the "best condition for nature to act upon them . . . for nature alone cures" (Nightingale, 1957, p. 75). What does Nightingale mean when she says that the surgery removes a bullet but nature heals the wound? She speaks of the curing nature as a creative life force or vital healing essence that is within human beings. It is not the modality that cures. No surgery cures and no plant cures. But we choose herbs in healing because, like humans, plants contain that creative life force or vital essence that is in human beings and in all life forms. Plants have a unique way of expressing that life force. When interacting with plants, such as tending them or using plants in healing, we experience how plants live, adapt, and heal. We also learn more about human life and human healing through interaction with healing plants. When learning and experiencing the science and art of the world of healing plants, we can learn more about what it means to be human as well. Walking in the woods and standing beneath the fragrant pines, or strolling through a garden and stopping to smell the roses, we can learn through our sensory experience more about who and what we are and where and why we exist. As we scan the towering trees of the forest with our eyes, we experience the beauty of nature. Being able to behold beauty is key to healing, for beauty, especially in natural form, instills balance, purpose, and harmony. We find in geometric leaf and flower patterns an expression of harmony, balance, and beauty in nature.

The golden ratio (also known as the golden mean or by its Greek name [and symbol], phi [Φ]), the mathematical proportion numerically approximated 1.618034 . . . ad infinitum, is, as nature demonstrates, the foundation of organic harmony, beauty, and balance. Many artists, philosophers, scientists, mathematicians, and architects consider the golden ratio an essential component of beauty if not life itself. Ancient Egyptians knew the importance of *phi* in nature and built the pyramids that still stand today. Leonardo Fibonacci, a thirteenth century mathematician, found the numerical sequence generated by the golden ratio. The sequence of numbers consists of terms that are the sum of the two preceding terms (1, 1, 2, 3, 5, 8, 13 . . .). The plant *Achillea ptarmica*, also known as sneezewort, has a leaf pattern that conforms exactly to the Fibonacci sequence (Figure 20-1). Cosmos, from the Greek "kosmos" meaning an "orderly, harmonious systematic universe" (Merriam-Webster, 1999) is governed by *phi*. Flowers blossom into pentagonal shapes, exhibiting *phi* angles. Sunflower heads and daisies have two interwoven petal patterns that follow the geometric pattern known as the golden ratio spiral. The golden ratio spiral is found throughout nature, as in the shell of the chambered nautilus and can be found in traditional Chinese medicine as the T'ai chi, or symbol of life. Inanimate forms like snowflakes and crystals are governed by other mathematical principles, but the golden ratio describes with geometry and numbers a universal pattern or formula for growth that is found only in animate forms.

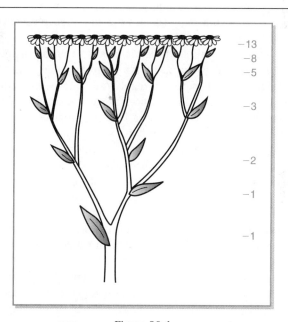

Figure 20-1

The plant *Achillea ptarmica,* also known as sneezewort, has a leaf pattern that conforms exactly to the Fibonacci sequence.

We find in the beauty of design in the plant kingdom and in all of nature a connection among life forms. The shell of the nautilus has the same spiraling design as the inner ear of a human being. Science and mathematics clarify the essence of that common denominator or point of familiarity that people may not really be aware of at conscious levels. Familiarity is important in the healing process. Healing plants contain designs familiar to human genes and human memory. As we look out on the garden, walk in the fields or woods, or swim among the sea vegetation and stop for a moment to consider the harvest, we may find that we remember. We not only remember what herbs are good for a particular ailment, we remember our connection with the Earth, our beautiful home.

Conclusion: Lessons from Lemon Balm and Cues from Cranberry

People who use plants in healing are accessing the energy or life force of the plant. Herbal remedies represent a living, beautiful medicine that people so often seek in a world that can too often engulf one with ugliness, decay, and disharmony. Flowers and leaves, in particular, have represented springtime, growth, and a time of hope and promise of renewed life. Throughout history, people have used flowers as symbolic gestures and expressions of beauty and pleasant emotions and thoughts. Flowers have often served as messengers when words are not enough. It is said that the Victorians, "raised the floral language to its highest level" (Gips, 1990, ix). With the reign of the English Queen Victoria, "flowers gained a regal status. They were thought to have been created by God as the voices of Nature, capable of expressing feelings of friendship and love in a language that uses no written words" (Gips, 1990, p. 5). Herbs and flowers were used in communication.

To conclude this integrative herb guide, I choose to leave you with the thoughts and feelings expressed by two very special plants. When you think of the science and art of plant remedies, therapies, and medicine, think of *cranberry*, which in the language of herbs and flowers, communicates "hardiness and cure for heartache" (Gips, 1990, p. 53) (Figure 20-2). Remember that herbs have been around a long time. They are *hardy* remedies from which we continue to learn more and more every day. Remember that herbal remedies bring many people healing and joy, and they are often a cure for the heartache of the weary. Whenever I talk with nurses about herbs, there is a sense of hope and joy. Nursing work is hard and emotionally challenging at times. Nurses and their patients often encounter the heartache that comes as part of the human experience. Herbs, such as cranberry, not only offer opportunity for relieving infection, they offer a healing process that is alive, hardy, comforting, and joyful.

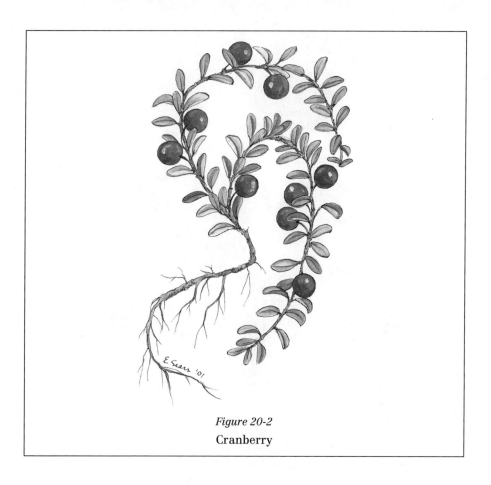

Figure 20-2
Cranberry

The second plant is *lemon balm* (Figure 20-3). The very name of this plant, "balm," suggests a way of healing that is gentle. Herbs are gentle remedies. In the language of herbs and flowers, lemon balm represents "memories" (Gips, 1990, p. 73). "Nurses, through their healing work with patients, not only create healing relationships, they create memory . . . nurses have the opportunity to create powerful memories of a positive healing experience with the patients and for themselves as well" (Libster, 2001, p. 215). Creating remedies, preparing a tea or a compress for patients, and providing that herbal healing experience leaves a lasting impression on patients and their loved ones. When done with full knowledge, wisdom, and harmony, herbal therapies can create a positive memory as part of the healing experience. Lemon balm, in the language of herbs and flowers, also communicates the message, "Don't misuse me" (Gips, 1990, p. 73). Herbs must be used responsibly. Nurses must consider an integrative approach that includes the use of plant therapies within the scope of both traditional herbalism and biomedicine as well as the nursing process.

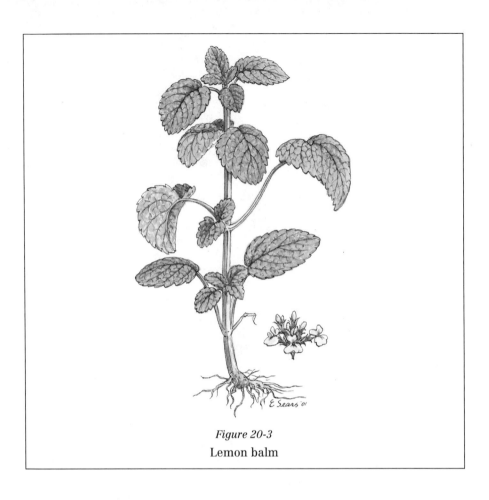

Figure 20-3
Lemon balm

What will be the role of herbs in the professional practice of the nurse? It may be difficult to predict at this time, but one thing is clear. The time is now to make that decision, individually and collectively as a professional discipline, whose roots run deep when it comes to connecting with plants to bring health, healing, and hope to others. So the next time you sit down for a cup of cool water, or bring one to your patient, what about considering making it a cup of herbal tea?

References

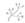

General Reference List (References commonly used in herb profiles)

Bensky, D., & Gamble, A. (1993). *Chinese herbal medicine: Materia medica.* Seattle, WA: Eastland Press.

Blumenthal, M., Goldberg, A., & Brinckman, J. (2000). *Herbal medicine: Expanded Commission E monographs.* Newton, MA: Integrative Medicine Communications.

Bradley, P. (Ed.). (1992). *British herbal compendium.* (Vol. 1). Bournemouth, Dorset: British Herbal Medicine Association.

Brinker, F. (1998). *Herb contraindications and drug interactions.* Sandy, OR: Eclectic Medical Publications.

Buckle, J. (1997). *Clinical aromatherapy in nursing.* London: Arnold, Copublished by Singular.

Castner, J., Timme, S., & Duke, J. (1998). *A field guide to medicinal and useful plants of the upper Amazon.* Gainesville, FL: Feline Press.

Cox, R., & Banack, S. (Eds.) (1991). *Islands, plants, and Polynesians.* Portland, OR: Dioscorides Press.

Culpeper, N. (1990). *Culpeper's complete herbal and English physician enlarged.* Glenwood, IL: Meyerbooks.

DeSmet, P. (Ed.). (1992). *Adverse effects of herbal drugs.* (Vol. 1). Berlin, Germany: Springer-Verlag.

DeSmet, P. (Ed.). (1997). *Adverse effects of herbal drugs.* (Vol. 3). Berlin, Germany: Springer-Verlag.

DeSmet, P. (1999). *Herbs health healers, Africa as ethnopharmacological treasury.* Berg en Dal, Netherlands: Afrika Museum.

Duke, J. (1985). *CRC handbook of medicinal herbs.* Boca Raton, FL: CRC Press.

Duke, J. (1997). *Green pharmacy.* Emmaus, PA: Rodale Press.

Felter, H., & Lloyd, J. U. (1983). *King's American dispensatory.* Sandy, OR: Eclectic Medical Publications.

Foster, S., & Tyler, V. (1999). *Tyler's honest herbal* (4th ed.). New York: Haworth Herbal Press.

Ghazanfar, S. (1994). *Handbook of Arabian medicinal plants.* Boca Raton, FL: CRC Press.

Grieve, M. (1971). *A modern herbal.* New York: Dover Publications.

Gutmanis, J. (1994). *Kahuna La'au Lapa'au.* Honolulu, HI: Island Heritage Publishing.

Husemann, F., & Wolff, O. (1982). *The Anthroposophical approach to medicine.* New York: The Anthroposophic Press.

Hutchens, A. (1992). *A handbook of Native American herbs.* Boston: Shambhala.

Iwu, M. M. (1993). *Handbook of African medicinal plants.* Boca Raton, FL: CRC Press, Inc.

Kay, M. (1996). *Healing with plants in the American and Mexican West.* Tucson, AZ: The University of Arizona Press.

Keville, K., & Green, M. (1995). *Aromatherapy: A complete guide to the healing art.* Freedom, CA: The Crossing Press.

Lassak, E., & McCarthy, T. (1983). *Australian medicinal plants.* Kew Victoria: Reed Books.

Lawless, J. (1998). *Aromatherapy and the mind.* London: Thorsons.

Leung, A., & Foster, S. (1996). *Encyclopedia of common natural ingredients used in food, drugs and cosmetics.* New York: John Wiley & Sons.

McCaleb, R., Leigh, E., & Morien, K. (2000). *The encyclopedia of popular herbs.* Roseville, CA: Prima Health Publishing.

McGuffin, M., Hobbs, C., Upton, R., & Goldberg, A. (1997). *American Herbal Product Association's botanical safety handbook.* Boca Raton, FL: CRC Press.

Moerman, D. (1998). *Native American ethnobotany.* Portland, OR: Timber Press.

Nadkarni, K. (1976). *Indian material medica.* Bombay: Popular Prakashan.

Newall, C., Anderson, L., & Phillipson, J. D. (1996). *Herbal medicines: A guide for healthcare professionals.* London: The Pharmaceutical Press.

Pedersen, M. (1998). *Nutritional herbology: A reference guide to herbs.* Warsaw, IN: Wendell W. Whitman Company.

Rister, R. (1999). *Japanese herbal medicine: The healing art of Kampo.* New York: Avery Publishing Group.

Schilcher, H. (1992). *Phytotherapy in paediatrics.* Stuttgart, Germany: Medpharm Scientific Publishers.

Schulz, V., Hansel, R., & Tyler, V. (1998). *Rational phytotherapy.* Berlin, Germany: Springer-Verlag.

Vogel, V. (1970). *American Indian medicine.* Norman, OK: University of Oklahoma Press.

Weed, S. (1986). *Wise woman herbal for the childbearing years.* New York: Ash Tree Publishing.

Werbach, M., & Murray, M. (1994). *Botanical influences on illness: a sourcebook of clinical research.* Tarzana, CA: Third Line Press.

World Health Organization (1999). *WHO monographs on selected medicinal plants.* (Vol. 1). Geneva, Switzerland: World Health Organization.

Wren, R. (1988). *Potter's new cyclopaedia of botanical drugs and preparations.* Essex, England: The C. W. Daniel Company Limited.

Zevin, I. (1997). *A Russian herbal: Traditional remedies for health and healing.* Rochester, VT: Healing Arts Press.

Introduction

Flanagan, S. (1996). *Secrets of God: Writings of Hildegarde of Bingen.* Boston: Shamballa.

Merriam Webster. (1999). *Merriam-Webster's Collegiate Dictionary* (10th ed.). Springfield, MA: Merriam-Webster, Inc.

Nightingale, F. (1969). *Notes on nursing.* New York: Dover.

Chapter 1. Entering the World of Healing Plants

Bowers, W. (1947). Chlorophyll in wound healing and suppurative disease. *American Journal of Surgery, 73*(1), 37–50.

Buhner, S. (1996). *Sacred plant medicine: Explorations in the practice of indigenous herbalism.* Boulder, CO: Roberts Rinehart Publishers.

Burke, J., & Golden, T. (1958). A clinical evaluation of enzymatic debridement with papain-urea-chlorophyllin ointment. *American Journal of Surgery, 95*(May), 828–842.

Burkhardt, M. (2000). Healing relationships with nature. *Complementary Therapies in Nursing and Midwifery, 6*(1), 35–40.

Cowan, E. (1995). *Plant spirit medicine.* Columbus, NC: Swan-Raven & Co.

Dory, A. (1971). The control of odor in urinary incontinence. *Nursing Homes, 20*(10), 28.

Farnsworth, N., Akerele, O., Bingel, A., Soejarto, D., & Guo, Z. (1985). Medicinal plants in therapy. *Bulletin of the World Health Organization, 63*(6), 965–981.

Farnsworth, N., & Soejarto, D. (1991). Global importance of medicinal plants. In O. Akerele, V. Heywood, & H. Synge (Eds.). *The conservation of medicinal plants* (pp. 25–43). Cambridge: Cambridge University Press.

Golden, T., & Burke, J. (1956). Effective management of offensive odors. *Gastroenterology, 31*(3), 260–265.

Hammel-Dupont, C., & Bessman, S. (1970). The stimulation of hemoglobin synthesis by porphyrins. *Biochemical Medicine, 4*(1), 55–60.

Hughes, J., & Latner, A. (1936). Chlorophyll and haemoglobin regeneration after haemorrhage. *Journal of Physiology, 86,* 388–395.

Hutchinson, J. (1995). On the Amazonian trail of useful plants. *Herbalgram, 33,* 42–43.

Keville, K., & Green, M. (1995). *Aromatherapy: A complete guide to the healing art.* Freedom, CA: The Crossing Press.

McGuffin, M., Hobbs, C., Upton, R., & Goldberg, A. (1997). *American Herbal Product Association's botanical safety handbook.* Boca Raton, FL: CRC Press.

Metzner, R. (1999). *Green psychology: Transforming our relationship to the Earth.* Rochester, VT: Park Street Press.

Merriam Webster. (1999). *Merriam-Webster's Collegiate Dictionary* (10th ed.). Springfield, MA: Merriam-Webster, Inc.

Patek, A. (1936). Chlorophyll and regeneration of the blood. *Archives of Internal Medicine, 57,* 73–84.

Rogers, M. (1992). Nursing science and the space age. *Nursing Science Quarterly, 5*(1), 27–34.

Sarkar, D., Sharma, A., & Talukder, G. (1996) Chlorophyll and chromosome breakage. *Mutation Research, 360*(3), 187–191.

Tompkins, P., & Bird, C. (1973). *The secret life of plants: A fascinating account of the physical, emotional, and spiritual relations between plants and man.* New York: Harper & Row.

Yoshida, A., Yokono, O., & Oda, T. (1980). Therapeutic effect of chlorophyll-a in the treatment of patients with chronic pancreatitis. *Gastroenterologia Japonica, 15*(1), 49–61.

Young, R., & Beregi, J. (1980). Use of chlorophyllin in the care of geriatric patients. *Journal of the American Geriatrics Society, XXVIII*(1), 46–47.

Chapter 2. A History of Healing

Baker, N. B. (1952). *Cyclone in calico: The story of Mary Ann Bickerdyke.* Boston: Little Brown and Company.

Balick, M., & Cox, P. (1996). *Plants, people and culture: The science of ethnobotany.* New York: Scientific American Library.

Brown, J., & Marcy, S. (1991). The use of botanicals for health purposes by members of a prepaid health plan. *Research in Nursing and Health, 14*(5), 339–350.

Caplan, R. (1989). The commodification of American health care. *Social Science and Medicine, 28*(11), 1139–1148.

Ehrenreich, B., & English, D. (1978). *For her own good: 150 years of the expert's advice to women.* New York: Anchor Books.

Eisenberg, D., Davis, R., Ettner, S., Appel, S., Wilkey, S., Van Rompay, M., & Kessler, R. (1998). Trends in alternative medicine use in the United States, 1990–1997: Results of a follow-up national survey. *Journal of the American Medical Association, 280*(18), 1569–1575.

Griggs, B. (1991). *Green pharmacy: The history and evolution of Western herbal medicine.* Rochester, VT: Healing Arts Press.

Haller, J. (1997). *Kindly medicine: Physio-medicalism in America, 1836–1911.* Kent, Ohio: Kent State University Press.

Harmer, B. (1924). *Text-book of the principles and practice of nursing.* New York: The Macmillan Co.

Harmer, B., & Henderson, V. (1955). *Textbook of the principles and practice of nursing.* New York: The Macmillan Company.

Holmstedt, B., & Bruhn, J. (1983). Ethnopharmacology—A challenge. *Journal of Ethnopharmacology, 8*(3), 251–256.

Judd, N. (1997). *Laau Lapaau: A geography of Hawaiian herbal healing.* Doctoral dissertation, University of Hawaii, Honolulu. [unpublished]

Leung, A., & Foster, S. (1996). *Encyclopedia of common natural ingredients used in foods, drugs, and cosmetics.* New York: John Wiley & Sons.

Merriam-Webster. (1999). *Merriam-Webster's Collegiate Dictionary* (10th ed.). Springfield, MA: Merriam-Webster, Inc.

O'Connor, B. (1995). *Healing traditions.* Philadelphia: University of Pennsylvania Press.

Rossi, F., Mangrella, M., Loffreda, A., & Lampa, E. (1994). Wizards and scientists: The pharmacologic experience of the middle ages. *American Journal of Nephrology, 14*(4–6), 384–390.

Schultes, R., & Von Reis, S. (1995). *Ethnobotany: Evolution of a discipline.* Portland, OR: Dioscorides Press.

Snodgrass, M. (1999). *Historical encyclopedia of nursing.* Santa Barbara, CA: ABC-Clio, Inc.

Solecki, R. (1975). Shanidar IV, a Neanderthal flower burial in Northern Iraq. *Science, 190,* 880–881.

Taylor, D. (1996). Herbal medicine at a crossroads. *Environmental Health Perspectives, 104*(9), 924–928.

Tracy, M. (1938). *Nursing an art and a science.* St. Louis: C.V. Mosby Co.

Ulrich, L. T. (1990). *A midwife's tale: The life of Martha Ballard based on her diary, 1785–1812.* New York: Vintage Books.

Vogel, V. (1970). *American Indian medicine.* Norman, OK: University of Oklahoma Press.

Chapter 3. Plants and Paradigms

Baba, S., Akerele, O., & Kawaguchi, Y. (Eds.). (1992). Natural resources and human health—Plants of medicinal and nutritional value. Proceedings of the 1st WHO symposium on plants and health for all: Scientific advancement, Kobe, Japan, 26–28 August 1991. Amsterdam: Elsevier.

Balick, M., & Cox, P. (1996). *Plants, people, and culture: The Science of ethnobotany.* New York: Scientific American Library.

Barnes, D., Eribes, C., Juarbe, T., Nelson, M., Proctor, S., Sawyer, L., Shaul, M., & Meleis, A. I. (1995). Primary health care and primary care: A confusion of philosophies. *Nursing Outlook, 43*(1), 7–16.

Belew, C. (1999). Herbs and the childbearing woman. *Journal of Nurse-Midwifery, 44*(3), 231–252.

Bodeker, G. (1995). Traditional health systems: Policy, biodiversity, and global interdependence. *The Journal of Alternative and Complementary Medicine, 1*(3), 231–243.

Buckle, J. (1999). Clinical aromatherapy and touch: complementary therapies for nursing practice. *Scentsitivity, 9*(3), 12–16.

Bunce, K. (1987). The use of herbs in midwifery. *Journal of Nurse-Midwifery, 32*(4), 255–259.

Burns, E., Blamey, C., Erdder, S., Lloyd, A., & Barnetson, L. (2000). The use of aromatherapy in intrapartum midwifery practice an observational study. *Complementary Therapies in Nursing and Midwifery, 6*(1), 33–34.

Chang, M. (1983). Nursing in China: Three perspectives. *American Journal of Nursing, 83*(3), 389–395.

Davis, R. (1997). Understanding ethnic women's experiences with pharmacopeia. *Health Care for Women International, 18,* 425–437.

Dibgy, A., & Sweet, H. (in press). Western and indigenous medicine: Nurses as culture brokers in twentieth century South Africa. In W. Ernst (Ed.). *Medical pluralism.* England: Routledge.

Duke, J. (1984). (Classical Botanical reprint Number 204). *High pharmaceutical prices call for government-sponsored natural drug research.* Austin, TX: American Botanical Council.

Ehudin-Pagano, E., Paluzzi, P., Ivory, L., & McCartney, M. (1987). The use of herbs in nurse-midwifery practice. *Journal of Nurse Midwifery, 32*(4), 260–262.

Farnsworth, N. (1992). Preclinical assessment of medicinal plants. In S. Baba, O. Akerele, & Y. Kawaguchi (Eds.). *Natural resources and human health. Plants of medicinal and nutritive value* (pp. 87–91). New York: Elsevier.

Farnsworth, N., Akerele, O., Bingel, A., Soejarto, D., & Guo, Z. (1985). Medicinal plants in therapy. *Bulletin of the World Health Organization, 63*(6), 965–981.

Frank, A. (1991). *At the will of the body.* Boston: Houghton Mifflin Co.

Gibson, C., Opalka, P., Moore, C., Brady, R., & Mion, L. (1995). Effectiveness of bran supplement on the bowel management of elderly rehabilitation patients. *Journal of Gerontological Nursing, 21*(10), 21–30.

Griggs, B. (1991). *Green pharmacy.* Rochester, VT: Healing Arts Press.

Hansen, K. (1997). Folk remedies and child abuse: A review with emphasis on caida de mollera and its relationship to shaken baby syndrome. *Child Abuse and Neglect, 22*(2), 117–127.

Hoff, W. (1992). Traditional healers and community health. *World Health Forum, 13*(2–3), 182–187.

Hoff, W., & the WHO Division of Strengthening of Health Services and the Traditional Medicine Programme. (1995). *Guidelines for training traditional health practitioners in primary health care.* Berkeley, CA: International Child Resource Institute.

Houghton, P. (1995). The role of plants in traditional medicine and current therapy. *The Journal of Alternative and Complementary Medicine, 1*(2), 131–143.

Hufford, D. (1997). Integrating complementary and alternative medicine into conventional medical practice. *Alternative Therapies, 3*(3), 81–83.

Ingelfinger, F. (1978). Medicine: Meritorious or meretricious. *Science, 200*(4344), 942–946.

Kenner, D. (1998). Botanical medicine and the clinical paradigm. *Frontier Perspectives, 7*(1), 53–58.

Kincheloe, L. (1997). Herbal medicines can reduce costs in HMO. *Herbalgram, 41,* 49.

Leung, A., & Foster, S. (1996). *Encyclopedia of common natural ingredients used in foods, drugs, and cosmetics.* New York: John Wiley & Sons, Inc.

Lewis, C. (2000). Medical milestones of the last millennium. *FDA Consumer, 34*(2), 8–13.

Libster, M. (2001). *Demonstrating care: The art of integrative nursing.* Albany: Delmar Thomson Learning.

McFarlin, B., Gibson, M., O'Rear, J., & Harman, P. (1999). A national survey of herbal preparation use by nurse-midwives for labor stimulation. *Journal of Nurse-Midwifery, 44*(3), 205–216.

McPartland J., & Pruitt, P. (2000). Benign prostatic hyperplasia treated with saw palmetto: a literature search and experimental case study. *Journal of the American Osteopathic Association, 100*(2), 89–96.

Meleis, A. (1996). Culturally competent scholarship: Substance and rigor. *Advances in Nursing Science, 19*(2), 1–16.

Merriam-Webster. (1999). *Merriam-Webster's Collegiate Dictionary* (10th ed.). Springfield, MA: Merriam-Webster, Inc.

Newall, C., Anderson, L., & Phillipson, J. D. (1996). *Herbal medicines: A guide for healthcare professionals.* London: The Pharmaceutical Press.

Newman, M. (1994). *Health as expanding consciousness.* New York: National League for Nursing Press.

O'Connor, B. (1995). *Healing traditions: Alternative medicine and the health professions.* Philadelphia: University of Pennsylvania Press.

Penn, R. (1986). Adverse reactions to herbal and other unorthodox medicines. In P. D'Arcy & J. Griffin (Eds.). *Iatrogenic diseases* (3rd ed.). Oxford: Oxford University Press.

Roberson, M. (1987). Home remedies: A cultural study. *Home Healthcare Nurse, 5*(1), 35–40.

Rogers, M. (1992). Nursing science and the space age. *Nursing Science Quarterly, 5*(1), 27–34.

Roy, Sr. C., (1984). *Introduction to nursing: An adaptation model.* Englewood Cliffs, NJ: Prentice-Hall.

Sears, B. (1995). *The Zone.* New York: Regan Books/Harper Collins.

Stapleton, H. (1995). The use of herbal medicine in pregnancy and labour. Part 1: an overview of current practice. *Complementary Therapies in Nursing and Midwifery, 1*(5), 148–153.

World Health Organization. (1978). *The promotion and development of traditional medicine: World Health Organization Technical Report Series 622.* Geneva: World Health Organization.

World Health Organization (1996). Fact Sheet N 134: Traditional medicine. (http://www.who.int/inf-fs/en/fact134.html)

Chapter 4. Carefulness and Conservation

Akerele, O. (1993). Summary of the WHO guidelines for the assessment of herbal medicines. *Herbalgram, 28,* 13–16.

Anyinam, C. (1995). Ecology and ethnomedicine: exploring links between current environmental crisis and indigenous medical practices. *Social Sciences and Medicine, 40*(3), 321–329.

Arvigo, R. (1994). *Sastun.* San Francisco: HarperCollins.

Atkinson, T. (2000). Herbal medicine: Yesterday and today. *Herb,* May-June (4), 8–9.

Awang, D. (1997). Feverfew products. *Canadian Medical Association Journal, 157*(5), 510–511.

Bates, E., & Florit, G. (1996). Medication administration and its relationship to meals. *Pharmacy Times, 62*(5), 55–68.

Blumenthal, M., Goldberg, A., & Brinckman, J. (2000). *Herbal medicine: Expanded Commission E monographs.* Newton, MA: Integrative Medicine Communications.

Boyd, M. A., & Nihart, M. A. (1998). *Psychiatric nursing: Contemporary practice.* New York: Lippincott.

Cantox Health Sciences International. (December 19, 2000). *Safety assessment and determination of a tolerable upper limit for ephedra.* Washington DC: Council for Responsible Nutrition.

Chan, T., Chan, A., & Critchley, J. (1992). Hospital admissions die to adverse reactions to Chinese herbal medicines. *Journal of Tropical Medicine and Hygiene, 95*(4), 296–298.

Curtin, M., & Lubkin, I. (1998). What is chronicity? In I. Lubkin (Ed.). *Chronic illness: Impact and interventions.* Sudbury, MA: Jones and Bartlett Publishers.

Davis, R. (1997). Understanding ethnic women's experiences with pharmacopeia. *Health Care for Women International, 18*(5), 425–437.

Day, L. M. (1833). *The improved American family physician, or, sick man's guide to health: Containing a complete theory of the botanic practice of medicine on the Thomsonian and Hygeian system: together with a complete digest on midwifery.* New York: [s. n.]

Diket, A., & Nolan, T. (1997). Anxiety and depression: Diagnosis and treatment during pregnancy. *Obstetrics and Gynecology Clinics of North America, 24*(3), 535–558.

Duke, J. (1992). *Handbook of phytochemical constituents of GRAS herbs and other economic plants.* Boca Raton: CRC Press.

Duke, J. (1997). *The green pharmacy.* Emmaus, PA: Rodale Press.

Duke, J. (1999). *Dr. Duke's essential herbs.* Emmaus, PA: Rodale, Inc.

Duke, J. (January, 2000). Dr. Duke's phytochemical and ethnobotanical databases (www.ars-grin.gov/duke/syllabus/module15.htm).

Ehrenreich, B., & English, D. (1978). *For her own good: 150 years of the experts' advice to women.* New York: Anchor Books.

Farnsworth, N. (1993). Relative safety of herbal medicines. *Herbalgram, 29,* 36A-H.

Farnsworth, N, Akerele, O., Bingel, A., Soejarto, D., & Guo, Z. (1985). Medicinal plants in therapy. *Bulletin of the World Health Organization, 63*(6), 965–981.

Foster, S., & Tyler, V. (1999). *Tyler's honest herbal* (4th ed.). New York: Haworth Herbal Press.

Fuhr, U. (1998). Drug interactions with grapefruit juice. *Drug Safety, 18*(4), 251–272.

Gordon, D., Rosenthal, G., Hart, J., Sirota, R., & Baker, A. (1995). Chaparral ingestion. *Journal of the American Medical Association, 273*(6), 489–490.

Gutmanis, J. (1995). *Kahuna La'au Lapa'au: The practice of Hawaiian herbal medicine.* Aiea, HI: Island Heritage Publishing.

Haller, J. (1997). *Kindly medicine.* Kent, OH: Kent State University Press.

HerbClip. (1994). *CPJ chart on drug-nutrient interactions. Comments on Canadian Pharmaceutical Journal, March.* Austin, TX: American Botanical Council.

Kerns, L. (1986). Treatment of mental disorders during pregnancy: A review of psychotropic drug risks and benefits. *Journal of Nervous and Mental Disease, 174*(11), 652–659.

Kleffel, D. (1996). Environmental paradigms: Moving toward an ecocentric perspective. *Advances in Nursing Science, 18*(4), 1–10.

Klepser, T., & Klepser, M. (1999). Unsafe and potentially safe herbal therapies. *American Journal of Health-System Pharmacy, 56*(2), 125–138.

Kingsbury, J. (1979). The problem of poisonous plants. In Kinghorn, A. (Ed.). *Toxic plants.* New York: Columbia University Press.

Lazarou, J., Pomeranz, B., & Corey, P. (1998). Incidence of adverse drug reactions in hospitalized patients. *Journal of the American Medical Association, 279*(15), 1200–1205.

Leung, A., & Foster, S. (1996). *Encyclopedia of common natural ingredients used in food, drugs, and cosmetics.* New York: John Wiley & Sons, Inc.

Libster, M. (1999). Guidelines for selecting a medical herbalist for consultation and referral: Consulting a medical herbalist. *The Journal of Alternative and Complementary Medicine, 5*(5), 457–462.

Mann, J. (1992). *Murder, magic, and medicine.* Oxford, England: Oxford University Press.

Merriam-Webster. (1999). *Merriam-Webster's Collegiate Dictionary* (10th ed.). Springfield, MA: Merriam-Webster, Inc.

Morbidity and Mortality Report (MMWR). (1992). Chaparral-induced toxic hepatitis—California and Texas, 1992. *MMWR Morbidity and Mortality Report, 41*(43), 812–814.

Morbidity and Mortality Report (MMWR). (1995). Anticholinergic poisoning associated with herbal tea—New York City, 1994. *Morbidity and Mortality Report MMWR, 44*(11), 193–195.

References

Nadkarni, K. (1976). *Indian Materia Medica*. Bombay: Popular Prakashan.

Newall, C., Anderson, L., & Phillipson, J. D. (1996). *Herbal medicines: A guide for health-care professionals*. London: The Pharmaceutical Press.

Pacifici, G., & Nottoli, R. (1995). Placental transfer of drugs administered to the mother. *Clinical Pharmacokinetics, 28*(3), 235–269.

Robinson, G., Stewart, D., & Flak, E. (1986). The rational use of psychotropic drugs in pregnancy and postpartum. *Canadian Journal of Psychiatry, 31*(3), 183–190.

Schiodt, F., Rochling, F., Casey, D., & Lee, W. (1997). Acetaminophen toxicity in an urban county hospital. *New England Journal of Medicine, 337*(16), 1112–1117.

Smart, C., Hogle, H., Vogel, H., Broom, A., & Bartholomew, D. (November, 1970). Clinical experience with nordihydroguaiaretic acid. *Rocky Mountain Medical Journal, 67*(11), 39–43.

Tanne, J. (1998). Food and drugs alter response to anaesthesia. *British Medical Journal, 317*(7166), 1102.

Treasure, J. (Fall, 2000). Herbal pharmacokinetics: A practitioner update with reference to St. John's Wort *(Hypericum perforatum)* herb-drug interactions. *Journal of the American Herbalists Guild, 1*(1), 2–11.

World Health Organization (1991). *The conservation of medicinal plants: proceedings of the International Consultation 1988 Chiang Mai, Thailand*. Cambridge: Cambridge University Press.

World Health Organization (1993). *Guidelines on the conservation of medicinal plants*. Switzerland: World Health Organization.

World Health Organization (1996a). Good manufacturing practices. *WHO Technical Report Series, No. 863*, Annex 8, 109–113.

World Health Organization (1996b). Good manufacturing practices. *WHO Technical Report Series, No. 863*, Annex 11, 178–184.

World Health Organization (1998a). Guidelines for the appropriate use of herbal medicines. *WHO Regional Publications, Western Pacific Series No.23*.

World Health Organization (1998b). *Regulatory situation of herbal medicine: A world-wide review*. Switzerland: World Health Organization.

World Health Organization (1998c). The role of the pharmacist in self-care and self-medication. *Report of the 4th WHO consultative group on the role of the pharmacist*. Switzerland: World Health Organization.

Chapter 5. Nursing Care and Plants: Back to the Roots

Buckle, J. (1997). *Clinical aromatherapy*. London: Arnold Publishers. Copublished by Singular.

Diego, M., Jones, N., Field, T., Hernandez-Reif, M., Schanberg, S., Kuhn, C., McAdam, V., Galamaga, R., & Galamaga, M. (1998). Aromatherapy positively affects mood, EEG patterns of alertness and math computations. *International Journal Neuroscience, 96*(3–4), 217–224.

Duggan, J., & Duggan, S. (1989). *Edgar Cayce's massage, hydrotherapy, and healing oils*. Virginia Beach, VA: Inner Vision Publishing Co.

Flaws, B., & Wolfe, H. (1983). *Prince Wen Hui's cook: Chinese diet therapy*. Brookline, MA: Paradigm Publications.

Friedrich, M. (1999). The arts of healing. *Journal of the American Medical Association, 281*(19), 1779–1781.

Green, J. (1990). *The herbal medicine-maker's handbook*. Forestville, CA: Wildlife & Green Publications.

Glor, B., & Estes, Z. (1970). Moist soaks: A survey of clinical practices. *Nursing Research, 19*(5), 463–465.

Haller, J. (1985). The poultice. *New York State Journal of Medicine, 85*(5), 207–209.

Harmer, B. (1924). *Textbook of the principles and practice of nursing.* New York: Macmillan Co.

Harmer, B., & Henderson, V. (1955). *Textbook of the principles and practice of nursing.* New York: Macmillan Co.

Keville, K., & Green, M. (1995). *Aromatherapy: A complete guide to the healing art.* Freedom, CA: The Crossing Press.

Lad, V., & Frawley, D. (1986). *The yoga of herbs.* Santa Fe, NM: Lotus Press.

Lawless, J. (1998). *Aromatherapy and the mind.* London: Thorsons.

Neergaard, L. (2000, July 19). Herbal tease riles health advocates. *The Denver Post,* p. 4A1.

Nightingale, F. (1957). *Notes on nursing.* Philadelphia, PA: J. B. Lippincott Co.

Nikodem, V., Danziger, D., Gebka, N., Gulmezoglu, A., & Hofmeyr, G. (1993). Do cabbage leaves prevent breast engorgement? A randomized, controlled study. *Birth, 20*(2), 61–64.

Relf, D. (2000). Dynamics of horticulture therapy. Retrieved February 4, 2000, from the World Wide Web: www.hort.vt.edu/human/ht1.html.

Roberts, K. (1995). A comparison of chilled cabbage leaves and chilled gelpaks in reducing breast engorgement. *Journal of Human Lactation, 11*(1), 17–20.

Roberts, K., Reiter, M., & Schuster, D. (1995). A comparison of chilled and room temperature cabbage leaves in treating breast engorgement. *Journal of Human Lactation, 11*(3), 191–194.

Tracy, M. (1938). *Nursing: An art and a science.* St. Louis: C. V. Mosby Co.

van Bentheim, T., Bos, S., de la Houssaye, E., & Visser, W. (1980). *Caring for the sick at home.* New York: Anthroposophic Press.

Vithoulkas, G. (1980). *The science of homeopathy.* New York: Grove Press.

Weeks-Shaw, C. (1914). *A text-book of nursing.* New York: D. Appleton and Co.

Wood, G., & Bache, F. (1839). *The dispensatory of the United States of America.* Philadelphia: Grigg & Elliot.

Chapter 6. Plant Profiles

Browne, E. (1921). *Arabian medicine.* London: Cambridge University Press.

Camazine, S., & Bye, R. (1980). A study of the medical ethnobotany of the Zuni Indians of New Mexico. *Journal of Ethnopharmacology, 2*(4), 365–388.

DeSmet, P. (1999). *Herbs, health and healers.* Berg en Dal, Netherlands: Afrika Museum.

De Waal, M. (1980). *Medicinal herbs in the Bible.* York Beach, ME: Samuel Weiser, Inc.

Flanagan, S. (1996). *Secrets of God: Writings of Hildegard of Bingen.* Boston: Shamballa.

Fleurentin, J., Mazars, G., & Pelt, J. (1983). Cultural background of the medicinal plants of Yemen. *Journal of Ethnopharmacology, 7*(2), 183–203.

Foster, S. (1992). The first herbal from the Americas. *Herbalgram, 27,* 12–17.

Ghai, S., & Ghai, C. (1997). The ancient origin of nursing in India. *The Nursing Journal of India, 88*(6), 131–132.

Grierson, D., & Afolayan, A. (1999). An ethnobotanical study of plants used for the treatment of wounds in the Eastern Cape, South Africa. *Journal of Ethnopharmacology, 67*(3), 327–332.

Gutmanis, J. (1995). *Kahuna La'au Lapa'au: The practice of Hawaiian herbal medicine.* Aiea, HI: Island Heritage Publishing.

Hart, J. (1981). The ethnobotany of the Northern Cheyenne Indians of Montana. *Journal of Ethnopharmacology, 4*(1), 1–55.

Hozeski, B. (1986). *Hildegard von Bingen's mystical visions.* Santa Fe, NM: Bear & Company Publishing.

Iwu, M. (1993). *Handbook of African medicinal plants.* Boca Raton, FL: CRC Press.

Judd, N. (1997). *Laau Lapaau: A geography of Hawaiian herbal healing.* Doctoral dissertation, University of Hawaii, Hawaii. [unpublished]

Kay, M. (1996). *Healing with plants in the American and Mexican West.* Tucson, AZ: The University of Arizona Press.

Lassak, E., & McCarthy, T. (1997). *Australian medicinal plants.* Victoria: Reed Books.

Nadkarni, A. (1976). *Indian Materia Medica.* Bombay: Popular Prakashan.

National Academy of Sciences. (1975). *Herbal pharmacology in the People's Republic of China.* Washington, D. C.: National Academy of Sciences.

Ray, P., & Gupta, H. (1980). *Caraka Samhita: A scientific synopsis* (2nd ed.). New Delhi: History of Sciences in India Publications.

Schilcher, H. (1992). *Phytotherapy in paediatrics.* Stuttgart, Germany: Medpharm Scientific.

Schultes, R. (1994). Amazonian ethnobotany and the search for new drugs. In Derek Chadwick & Joan Marsh (Eds.), *The Ciba Foundation Symposium, Ethnobotany and the search for new drugs* (pp. 106–115). New York: John Wiley & Sons.

Tschanz, D. (1997). The Arab roots of European medicine. Retrieved February 10, 2001, from the World Wide Web: www.users.erols.com/gmqm/euromed1.html.

Vogel, V. (1970). *American Indian medicine.* Norman, OK: University of Oklahoma Press.

Whistler, W. A. (1996). *Samoan herbal medicine.* Honolulu, HI: Isle Botanica.

Wicke, R. (1992). *Clinical handbook of herbal medicine.* (Vol. 1). Hot Springs, MT: Rocky Mountain Herbal Institute Publications.

Zevin, I. (1997). *A Russian herbal: Traditional remedies for health and healing.* Rochester, VT: Healing Arts Press.

Chapter 7. Comfort and Pain Relief

INTRODUCTION:

Lubkin, I. (1998). *Chronic illness: Impact and interventions.* Sudbury, MA: Jones and Bartlett Publishers.

National Institutes of Health. (September, 1998). *Chronic pain: Hope through research.* United States Government Publication # 98–2406. Bethesda, MD: National Institutes of Health.

FEVERFEW:

Anderson, D., Jenkinson, P., Dewdney, R., Blowers, S., Johnson, E., & Kadam, N. (1988). Chromosomal aberrations and sister chromatid exchanges in lymphocytes and urine mutagenicity of migraine patients: A comparison of chronic feverfew users and matched non-users. *Human Toxicology, 7,* 145–152.

Groenewegen, W., Knight, D., & Heptinstall, S. (1992). Progress in the medicinal chemistry of the herb feverfew. *Progress in Medicinal Chemistry, 29,* 217–238.

Heptinstall, S., White, A., Williamson, L., & Mitchell, J. (1985). Extracts of feverfew inhibit granule secretion in blood platelets and polymorphonuclear leucocytes. *The Lancet,* 1(8437), 1071–1074.

Johnson, E., Kadam, N., Hylands, D., & Hylands, P. (1985). Efficacy of feverfew as prophylactic treatment of migraine. *British Medical Journal, 291,* 569–573.

Johnson, E., Kadam, N., Anderson, D., Jenkinson, P., Dewdney, R., & Blowers, S. (1987). Investigation of possible genotoxic effects of feverfew in migraine patients. *Human Toxicology, 6,* 533–534.

Miller, L. (1998). Herbal medicinals: Selected clinical considerations focusing on known or potential drug-herb interactions. *Archives of Internal Medicine, 158,* 2200–2211.

Murphy, J., Heptinstall, S., & Mitchell, J. (1988). Randomized double-blind placebo-controlled trial of feverfew in migraine prevention. *The Lancet, 2*(8604), 189–192.

Palevitch, D., Earon, G., & Carasso, R. (1997). Feverfew *(Tanacetum parthenium)* as a prophylactic treatment for migraine: A double-blind placebo-controlled study. *Phytotherapy Research, 11,* 508–511.

Pattrick, M., Heptinstall, S., & Doherty, M. (1989). Feverfew in rheumatoid arthritis: A double-blind, placebo-controlled study. *Annals of the Rheumatic Diseases, 48,* 547–549.

Rodriguez, E., Epstein, W., & Mitchell, J. (1977). The role of sesquiterpene lactones in contact hypersensitivity to some North and South American species of feverfew *(Parthenium-Compositae). Contact Dermatitis, 3,* 155–162.

Sriramarao, P. & Subba Rao, P. (1993). Allergenic cross-reactivity between *Parthenium* and ragweed pollen allergens. *International Archives of Allergy and Immunology, 100,* 79–85.

LAVENDER:

Blake, C. (1998). The effect of aromatherapy on the anxiety levels of women undergoing mammography screening. Unpublished master's thesis, University of Phoenix, San Diego, California.

Brandao, F. (1986). Occupational allergy to lavender oil. *Contact Dermatitis, 15*(4), 249–250.

Dale, A. & Cornwell, S. (1994). The role of lavender oil in relieving perineal discomfort following childbirth: a blind randomized clinical trial. *Journal of Advanced Nursing, 19,* 89–96.

Hay, I., Jamieson, M., & Ormerod, A. (1998). Randomized trial of aromatherapy. *Archives of Dermatology, 134,* 1349–1352.

Hudson, R. (1995). Use of lavender in a long-term elderly ward. *Nursing Times, 91*(1), 12.

Lis-Balchin, M. & Hart, S. (1999). Studies on the mode of action of the essential oil of lavender (*Lavandul angustifolia* P. Miller). *Phytotherapy Research, 13,* 540–542.

Romine, I., Bush, A., & Geist, C. (1999). Lavender aromatherapy in recovery from exercise. *Perceptual and Motor Skills, 88,* 756–758.

Ziegler, J. (1996). Raloxifene, retinoids, and lavender: "Me too" Tamoxifen alternatives under study. *Journal of the National Cancer Institute, 88*(16), 1100–1102.

PRIMROSE:

Behan, P., Behan, W., & Horrobin, D. (1990). Effect of high doses of essential fatty acids on the postviral fatigue syndrome. *Acta Neurologica Scandinavica, 82,* 209–216.

Berth-Jones, J. & Graham-Brown, R. (1994). Evening primrose oil does not show promise in atopic dermatitis. *British Medical Journal, 309,* 1437.

Budeiri, D., Li Wan Po, A., & Dornan, J. (1996). Is evening primrose oil of value in the treatment of premenstrual syndrome? *Controlled Clinical Trials, 17*(1), 60–68.

Campbell, E., Peterkin, D., O'Grady, K., & Sanson-Fisher, R. (1997). Premenstrual symptoms in general practice patients. Prevalence and treatment. *Journal of Reproductive Medicine, 42*(10), 637–646.

Dove, D. & Johnson, P. (1999). Oral evening primrose oil: Its effect on length of pregnancy and selected intrapartum outcomes in low-risk nulliparous women. *Journal of Nurse-Midwifery, 44*(3), 320–324.

Duke, J. (1999). *Dr. Duke's essential herbs.* Emmaus, PA: Rodale.

Gateley, C., Miers, M., Mansel, R., & Hughes, L. (1992). Drug treatments for mastalgia: 17 years experience in the Cardiff mastalgia clinic. *Journal of the Royal Society of Medicine, 85,* 12–15.

Greenfield, S., Green, A., Teare, J., Jenkins, A., Punchard, N., Ainley, C., & Thompson, R. (1993). A randomized controlled study of evening primrose oil and fish oil in ulcerative colitis. *Alimentary Pharmacology and Therapeutics, 7,* 159–166.

Hederos, C. & Berg, A. (1996). Epogam evening primrose oil treatment in atopic dermatitis and asthma. *Archives of Disease in Childhood, 75,* 494–497.

Humphreys, F., Symons, J., Brown, H., Duff, G., & Hunter, J. (1994). The effects of gamolenic acid on adult atopic eczema and premenstrual exacerbation of eczema. *European Journal of Dermatology, 4,* 598–603.

Jamal, G. & Carmichael, H. (1990). The effect of gamma-linolenic acid on human diabetic peripheral neuropathy: A double-blind placebo controlled trial. *Diabetic Medicine, 7,* 319–323.

Keen, H., Payan, J., Allawi, J., Walker, J., Jamal, G., Weir, A., Henderson, L., Bissessar, E., Watkins, P., Sampson, M., Gale, E., Scarpello, J., Boddie, H., Hardy, K., Thomas, P., Misra, P., & Halonen, J. (1993). Treatment of diabetic neuropathy with gamma-linolenic acid. *Diabetes Care, 16*(1), 8–15.

McFarlin, B., Gibson, M., O'Rear, J., & Harman, P. (1999). A national survey of herbal preparation use by nurse-midwives for labor stimulation. Review of the literature and recommendations for practice. *Journal of Nurse Midwifery, 44*(3), 205–216.

Oliwiecki, S. & Burton, J. (1994). Evening Primrose oil and marine oil in the treatment of psoriasis. *Clinical and Experimental Dermatology, 19,* 127–129.

Pashby, N., Mansel, R., Hughes, L., Hanslip, J., Preece, P. (1981). A clinical trial of evening primrose oil in mastalgia. *British Journal of Surgery, 68,* 801–824.

Pye, J., Mansel, R., & Hughes, L. (1985). Clinical experience of drug treatments for mastalgia. *The Lancet, 2*(8451), 373–377.

Sattar, N., Berry, C., & Greer, I. (1998). Essential fatty acids in relation to pregnancy complications and fetal development. *British Journal of Obstetrics and Gynaecology, 105,* 1248–1255.

Schmidt, M. (1997). *Smart fats: How dietary fats and oils affect mental, physical and emotional intelligence.* Berkeley, CA: Frog, Ltd.

Whitaker, D., Cilliers, J., & de Beer, C. (1996). Evening primrose oil (Epogam) in the treatment of chronic hand dermatitis: Disappointing therapeutic results. *Dermatology, 193,* 115–120.

MUSTARD:

Beach, W. (1843). *The family physician; or the reformed system of medicine: On vegetable or botanical principles.* New York: W. Beach.

Griggs, B. (1991). *Green pharmacy.* Rochester, VT: Healing Arts Press.

Gulbransen, G. & Esernio-Jenssen, D. (1998). Aspiration of black mustard. *Clinical Toxicology, 36*(6), 591–593.

Kirsanov, A. (1982). [Use of mustard plasters. Translated from the Russian]. *Meditsinskala Sestra, 41*(9), 30–32.

Kohl, P. & Frosch, P. (1990). Irritant contact dermatitis induced by a mustard compress. *Contact Dermatitis, 23,* 189–190.

Kunovskii, B. (1982). [Mustard Compresses. Translated from the Russian]. *Fel'dsher I Akusherka, 47*(2), 63–64.

Linder, S., Mele, J., & Harries, T. (1996). Chronic hyperpigmentation from a heated mustard compress burn: A case report. *Journal of Burn Care Rehabilitation, 17,* 351–352.

....

Chapter 8. Hormone Balance

INTRODUCTION:

Beckham, N. (1995). Phyto-oestrogens and compounds that affect oestrogen metabolism. Part I. *Australian Journal of Medical Herbalism, 7*(1), 11–16.

Colditz, G., Hankinson, S., Hunter, D., Willett, W., Manson, J., Stampfer, M., Hennekens, C., Rosner, B., & Speizer, F. (1995). The use of estrogens and progestins and the risk of breast cancer in postmenopausal women. *The New England Journal of Medicine, 332*(24), 1589–1593.

Martin, P., Horwitz, K., Ryan, D., & McGuire, W. (1978). Phytoestrogen interaction with estrogen receptors in human breast cancer cells. *Endocrinology, 103*(5), 1860–1867.

Merriam-Webster. (1999). *Merriam-Webster's collegiate dictionary.* (10th ed.). Springfield, MA: Merriam-Webster, Inc.

WILD YAM:

Burry, K., Patton, P., & Hermsmeyer, K. (1999). Percutaneous absorption of progesterone in postmenopausal women treated with transdermal estrogen. *American Journal of Obstetrics and Gynecology, 180,* 1504–11.

Cooper, A., Slencer, C., Whitehead, M., Ross, D., Barnard, G., & Collins, W. (1998). Systemic absorption of progesterone from Pro-gest cream in postmenopausal women. *The Lancet, 351,* 1255–1256.

Dentali, S. (1994). Hormones and yams, what's the connection? *The American Herb Association Newsletter, 10*(4), 4–5.

Grodstein, F., Stampfer, M., Colditz, G., Willett, W., Manson, J., Joffe, M., Rosner, B., Fuchs, C., Hankinson, S., Hunter, D., Hennekens, C., & Speizer, F. (1997). Postmenopausal hormone therapy and mortality. *New England Journal of Medicine, 336*(25), 1769–1775.

Hudson, T. (1999). *Women's encyclopedia of natural medicine.* Lincolnwood, IL: Keats Publishing.

Ilyia, E., McLure, D., & Farhat, M. (1998). Topical progesterone cream application and overdosing. *Journal of Alternative and Complementary Medicine, 4*(1), 5–6.

Iwu, M., Okunji, C., Ohiaeri, G., Akah, P., Corley, D., & Tempesta, M. (1996). Hypoglycaemic activity of dioscoretine from tubers of *Dioscorea dumetorum* in normal and alloxan diabetic rabbits. *Planta Medica, 56*(3), 264–267.

Keville, K. (1996). Editor's commentary on multi-level yam scam. *The American Herb Association Newsletter, 12*(1), 7.

Lee, J. (1990a). Osteoporosis reversal: The role of progesterone. *International Clinical Nutrition Review, 10*(3), 384–391.

Lee, J. (1990b). Osteoporosis reversal with transdermal progesterone. *The Lancet, 336*(8710), 265–269.

Lee, J. (1991). Is natural progesterone the missing link in osteoporosis prevention and treatment? *Medical Hypothesis, 35*(4), 316–318.

Lee, J. (1998). Use of Pro-gest cream in postmenopausal women: Letter to the editor. *The Lancet, 352,* 905.

MacFarland, S. (1998). Use of Pro-gest cream in postmenopausal women: Letter to the editor. *The Lancet, 352,* 905.

Northrup, C. (1994). *Women's bodies, women's wisdom.* New York: Bantam.

Stevenson, J. & Purdie, D. (1998). Use of Pro-gest cream in postmenopausal women. *The Lancet, 352*(9131), 905–906.

Zava, D., Dollbaum, C., & Blen, M. (1998). Estrogen and progestin bioactivity of foods, herbs, and spices. *Proceedings of the Society for Experimental Biology and Medicine, 217,* 369–378.

FENUGREEK:

Abdo, M. & Al-Kafawi, A. (1969). Experimental studies on the effect of *Trigonella foenumgraecum. Planta Medica, 17*(1), 14–18.

Jensen, R. (1992) Fenugreek—Overlooked but not forgotten. *UCLA Lactation Alumni Association Newsletter, 1,* 2–3.

Madar, Z., Abel, R., Samish, S., & Arad, J. (1988). Glucose-lowering effect of fenugreek in non-insulin dependent diabetics. *European Journal of Clinical Nutrition, 42,* 51–54.

Patil, S., Niphadkar, P., & Bapat, M. (1997). Allergy to fenugreek *(Trigonella foenum graecum). Annals of Allergy, Asthma, and Immunology, 78,* 297–300.

Sauvaire, Y., Petit, P., Broca, C., Manteghetti, M., Baissac, Y., Fernandez-Alvarez, J., Gross, R., Roye, M., Leconte, A., Gomis, R., & Ribes, G. (1998). *Diabetes, 47,* 206–210.

Sewell, A., Mosandl, A., & Bohles, H. (1999). False diagnosis of maple syrup urine disease owing to ingestion of herbal tea. *The New England Journal of Medicine, 341*(10), 769.

Sharma, R., Raghuram, T., & Rao, N. S. (1990). Effect of fenugreek seeds on blood glucose and serum lipids in type I diabetes. *European Journal of Clinical Nutrition, 44,* 301–306.

SOY:

Albertazzi, P., Pansini, F., Bonaccorsi, G., Zanotti, L., Forini, E., & De Aloysio, D. (1998). The effect of dietary soy supplementation on hot flushes. *Obstetrics and Gynecology, 91*(1), 6–11.

Barnes, S. (1998). Evolution of the health benefits of soy isoflavones. *Proceedings of the Society for Experimental Biology and Medicine, 217,* 386–392.

Barnes, S., Peterson, G., Grubbs, C., & Setchell, K. (1994). Potential role of dietary isoflavones in the prevention of cancer. In M. M. Jacobs (Ed.), *Diet and cancer: Markers prevention and treatment* (pp. 135–147). New York: Plenum Press.

Barnes, S., Sfakianos, J., Coward, L., & Kirk, M. (1996). Soy isoflavonoids and cancer prevention. In American Institute for Cancer Research (Ed.), *Dietary phytochemicals in cancer prevention and treatment* (pp. 87–100). New York: Plenum Press.

Brandi, M. (1997). Natural and synthetic isoflavones in the prevention and treatment of chronic diseases. *Calcified Tissue International, 61,* S5–S8.

Cassidy, A., Bingham, S., & Setchell, K. (1994). Biological effects of a diet of soy protein rich in isoflavones on the menstrual cycle of premenopausal women. *American Journal of Clinical Nutrition, 60,* 333–340.

Fukutake, M., Takahashi, M., Ishida, K., Kawamura, H., Sugimura, T., & Wakabayashi, K. (1996). Quantification of genistein and genistin in soybeans and soybean products. *Food and Chemical Toxicology, 34*(5), 457–461.

Gooderham, M., Adlercreutz, H., Ojala, S., Wahala, K., & Holub, B. (1996). A soy protein isolate rich in genistein and daidzein and its effects on plasma isoflavone concentrations, platelet aggregation, blood lipids and fatty acid composition of plasma phospholipid in normal men. *Journal of Nutrition, 126,* 2000–2006.

Horwitz, K., & McGuire, W. (1977). Progesterone and progesterone receptors in experimental breast cancer. *Cancer Research, 37*(6), 1733–1738.

Hudson, T. (1999). *Women's encyclopedia of natural medicine.* Lincolnwood, IL: Keats Publishing.

Ingram, D., Sanders, K., Kolybaba, M., & Lopez, D. (1997). Case-control study of phytooestrogens and breast cancer. *The Lancet, 350,* 990–994.

Kushi, M. (1993). *Macrobiotic home remedies.* Tokyo: Japan Publications.

Kushi, A. & Kushi, M. (1985). *Macrobiotic diet.* Tokyo: Japan Publications.

Liener, I. (1995). Possible adverse effects of soybean anticarcinogens. *Journal of Nutrition, 125*(3 Suppl), 744S–750S.

Lu, L. J., Anderson, K., Grady, J., & Nagamani, M. (1996). Effects of soy consumption for one month on steroid hormones in premenopausal women: Implications for breast cancer risk reduction. *Cancer, Epidemiology, Biomarkers and Prevention, 5,* 63–70.

Messina, M. (1995). Modern applications for an ancient bean: Soybeans and the prevention and treatment of chronic disease. *Journal of Nutrition, 125,* 567S–569S.

Nagata, C., Kabuto, M., Kurisu, Y., & Shimizu, H. (1997). Decreased serum estradiol concentration associated with high dietary intake of soy products in premenopausal Japanese women. *Nutrition and Cancer, 29*(3), 228–233.

Persky, V., & Van Horn, L. (1995). Epidemiology of soy and cancer: Perspectives and directions. *Journal of Nutrition, 125,* 709S–712S.

Potter, S., Baum, J., Teng, H., Stillman, R., Shay, N., & Erdman, J. (1998). Soy protein and isoflavones: their effects on blood lipids and bone density in postmenopausal women. *American Journal of Clinical Nutrition, 68*(6 Suppl), 1375S–1379S.

Slavin, J., Karr, S., Hutchins, A., & Lampe, J. (1998). Influence of soybean processing, habitual diet, and soy dose on urinary isoflavonoid excretion. *American Journal of Clinical Nutrition, 68*(6 Suppl), 1492S–1495S.

Wicke, R. (1992). *Traditional Chinese herbal science,* vol. 2. Hot Springs, MT: Rocky Mountain Herbal Institute Press.

Wicke, R. (2000). *Herbalist Review,* Issue 2000, #4: Health fads from hell: margarine, canola oil, soyfoods, green/black tea. (www.rmhiherbal.org/review/2000-4.html). Hot Springs, MT: Rocky Mountain Herbal Institute.

BLACK COHOSH:

Bruneton, J. (1995). *Pharmacognosy, phytochemistry, and medicinal plants.* Paris: Intercept, Ltd.

Duke, J. (2000). *Dr. Duke's phytochemical and ethnobotanical databases.* (www.ars-grin.gov/cgi-bin/duke/farmacy2.pl). Beltsville, MD: USDA-ARS-NGRL, Beltsville Agricultural Research Center.

Duker, E., Kopanski, L., Jarry, H., & Wuttke, W. (1991). Effects of extracts from *Cimicifuga racemosa* on gonadotropin release in menopausal women and ovariectomized rats. *Planta Medica, 57,* 420–424.

Hare, H. (1892). *A textbook of practical therapeutics, with especial reference to the application of remedial measures to disease and their employment upon a rational basis.* Philadelphia: Lea Brothers & Co.

Liske, E. (1998). Therapeutic efficacy and safety of *Cimicifuga racemosa* for gynecologic disorders. *Advances in Therapy, 15*(1), 45–53.

McFarlin, B., Gibson, M., O'Rear, J., & Harman, P. (1999). A national survey of herbal preparation use by nurse-midwives for labor stimulation. *Journal of Nurse-Midwifery, 44*(3), 205–216.

Northrup, C. (1994). *Women's bodies women's wisdom.* New York: Bantam Books.

Pepping, J. (1999). Black cohosh: *Cimicifuga racemosa. American Journal of Health-System Pharmacy, 56,* 1400–1402.

Wade, C., Kronenberg, F., Kelly, A., & Murphy, P. (1999). Hormone-modulating herbs: Implications for women's health. *Journal of the American Medical Women's Association, 54*(4), 181–183.

ANGELICA:

Foster, S. & Chongxi, Y. (1992). *Herbal emissaries: Bringing Chinese herbs to the West.* Rochester, VT: Healing Arts Press.

Hirata, J., Swiersz, L., Zell, B., Small, R., & Ettinger, B. (1997). Does dong quai have estrogenic effects in postmenopausal women? A double-blind, placebo-controlled trial. *Fertility and Sterility, 68*(6), 981–986.

Page, R. & Lawrence, J. (1999). Potentiation of warfarin by dong quai. *Pharmacotherapy, 19*(7), 870–876.

Qi-Bing, M., Jing-yi, T., & Bo, C. (1991). Advances in the pharmacological studies of radix angelica sinensis (Oliv) diels (Chinese danggui). *Chinese Medical Journal, 104*(9), 776–781.

Zhiping, H., Dazeng, W., Lingyi, S., & Zuqian, W. (1986). Treating amenorrhea in vital energy-deficient patients with angelica sinensis-astragalus membranaceus menstruation-regulating decoction. *Journal of Traditional Chinese Medicine, 6*(3), 187–190.

Zhu, D. (1987). Dong quai. *American Journal of Chinese Medicine, XV*(3–4), 117–125.

KELP:

Fukui, S., Hirayama, T., Nohara, M., Sakagami, Y. (1981). The chemical forms of arsenic in some seafoods and in urine after ingestion of these foods. *Shokuhin Eiseigaku Zasshi, 22*(6), 513–519.

Glatstein, I., Pang, S., & McShane, P. (1997). Successful pregnancies with the use of Laminaria tents before embryo transfer for refractory cervical stenosis. *Fertility and Sterility, 67*(6), 1172–1174.

Guinn, D., Goepfert, A., Christine, M., Owen, J., & Hauth, J. (2000). Extra-amniotic saline, Laminaria, or prostaglandin E2 gel for labor induction with unfavorable cervix: a randomized controlled trial. *Obstetrics and Gynecology, 96,* 106–112.

Konno, N., Makita, H., Yuri, K., Iizuka, N., & Kawasaki, K. (1994). Association between dietary iodine intake and prevalence of subclinical hypothyroidism in the coastal regions of Japan. *Journal of Clinical Endocrinology and Metabolism, 78*(2), 393–397.

Kushi, M. (1993). *Macrobiotic home remedies.* Tokyo: Japan Publications.

Liewendahl, K., & Gordin, A. (1974). Iodine-induced toxic diffuse goitre. *Acta Medica Scandinavica, 196,* 237–239.

Lin, A., Kupferminc, M., & Dooley, S. (1995). A randomized trial of extra-amniotic saline infusion versus Laminaria for cervical ripening. *Obstetrics and Gynecology, 86,* 545–549.

Maruyama, H. & Yamamoto, I. (1992). Suppression of 125I-uptake in mouse thyroid by seaweed feeding: Possible preventative effect of dietary seaweed on internal radiation injury of the thyroid by radioactive iodine. *Kitasato Archives of Experimental Medicine, 65*(4), 209–216.

McMullen, D. (1991). Clinical experience with a calcium alginate dressing. *Dermatology Nursing, 3*(4), 216–219, 270.

Peeples, W., Given, F., & Bakri, Y. (1983). The use of *Laminaria japonica* in intracavitary radiation therapy when anesthesia is contraindicated. *International Journal of Radiation Oncology Biology and Physics, 9,* 1405–1406.

Pitchford, P. (1993). *Healing with whole foods: Oriental traditions and modern nutrition.* Berkeley, CA: North Atlantic Books.

Shilo, S. & Hirsch, H. (1986). Iodine-induced hyperthyroidism in a patient with a normal thyroid gland. *Postgraduate Medical Journal, 62,* 661–662.

Summers, L. (1997). Methods of cervical ripening and labor induction. *Journal of Nurse-Midwifery, 42*(2), 71–85.

Tajiri, J., Higashi, K., Morita, M., Umeda, T., & Sato, T. (1986). Studies of hypothyroidism in patients with high iodine intake. *Journal of Endocrinology and Metabolism, 63*(2), 412–417.

Teas, J. (1983). The dietary intake of *Laminaria,* a brown seaweed, and breast cancer prevention. *Nutrition and Cancer, 4*(3), 217–222.

Yan, X., Nagata, T., & Fan, X. (1998). Antioxidative activities in some common seaweeds. *Plant Foods for Human Nutrition, 52,* 253–262.

Yifeng, G., Zhaojian, H., Meiyu, Q., Fuxing, L., Guang, B., Yixian, M., Xinpei, M., & Fengge, Z. (1991). Suppression of radioactive strontium absorption by sodium alginate in animals and human subjects. *Biomedical and Environmental Sciences, 4,* 273–282.

Chapter 9. Immune Response

INTRODUCTION:

Enby, E., Gosch, P., & Sheehan, M. (1990). *Hidden killers: The Revolutionary medical discoveries of Professor Guenther Enderlein.* Sheehan Communications.

Keville, K., & Green, M. (1995). *Aromatherapy: A complete guide to the healing art.* Freedom, CA: The Crossing Press.

Nightingale, F. (1980). *Notes on nursing.* Edinburgh: Churchill Livingstone.

Pert, C. (1997). *Molecules of emotion.* New York: Scribner.

GOLDENSEAL:

Baker, N. (1952). *Cyclone in calico.* Boston: Little, Brown & Company.

Bergner, P. (1996–1997). Goldenseal and the common cold: The antibiotic myth. *Medical Herbalism, 8*(4), 3–10.

Bruneton, J. (1999). *Pharmacognosy: Phytochemistry medicinal plants.* Paris: Intercept Ltd.

Foster, S. (1997). Goldenseal's bright future. *Better Nutrition,* January, 58–61.

Gupte, S. (1975). Use of berberine in treatment of giardiasis. *American Journal of Diseases in Childhood, 129,* 866.

Howard, J., & Ramsell, J. (1990). *The original writings of Edward Bach.* Bury St. Edmunds, England: C.W. Daniel Co. Ltd.

Khin-Maung-U, Myo-Khin, Nyunt-Nyunt-Wai, Aye-Kyaw, & Tin-U. (1985). Clinical trial of berberine in acute watery diarrhoea. *British Medical Journal, 291*(6509), 1601–1605.

Morgan, J. (1994). Urine tests for drug use: Are they reliable? *Herbalgram, 32,* 46–51, 70.

Murray, M. (1994). *Natural alternatives to over-the-counter and prescription drugs.* New York: William Morrow and Co., Inc.

Rabbani, G., Butler, T., Knight, J., Sanyal, S., & Alam, K. (1987). Randomized controlled trial of berberine sulfate therapy for diarrhea due to enterotoxigenic *Escherichia coli* and *Vibrio cholerae. The Journal of Infectious Diseases, 155*(5), 979–984.

Rehman, J., Dillow, J., Carter, S., Chou, J., Le, B., & Maisel, A. (1999). Increased production of antigen-specific immunoglobulins G and M following in vivo treatment with the medicinal plants *Echinacea angustifolia* and *Hydrastis canadensis. Immunology Letters, 68*(2–3), 391–395.

ECHINACEA:

Awang, D., & Kindack, D. (1991). Echinacea. *Canadian Pharmacy Journal, 124*(11), 512–516.

Barrett, B., Vohmann, M., & Calabrese, C. (1999). Echinacea for upper respiratory infection. *The Journal of Family Practice, 48*(8), 628–635.

Bauer, V., Jurcic, K., Puhlmann, J., & Wagner, H. (1988). [Immunologic in vivo and in vitro studies on Echinacea extracts. Translated from German.]. *Arzneimittelforschung, 38*(2), 276–281.

Bodley, V., & Powers, D. (1997). Long-term treatment of a breastfeeding mother with fluconazole-resolved nipple pain caused by yeast: a case study. *Journal of Human Lactation, 13*(4), 307–311.

Foster, S. (1991). *Echinacea: Nature's immune enhancer.* Rochester, VT: Healing Arts Press.

Gallo, M., Sarkar, M., Au, W., Pietrzak, K., Comas, B., Smith, M., Jaeger, T., Einarson, A., & Koren, G. (2000). Pregnancy outcome following gestational exposure to echinacea: A prospective controlled study. *Archives of Internal Medicine, 160*(20), 3141–3143.

Hoheisal, O., Sandberg, M., Bertram, S., Bulitta, M., & Schafer, M. (1997). Echinagard treatment shortens the course of the common cold: a double-blind, placebo-controlled clinical trial. *European Journal of Clinical Research, 9,* 261–268.

Kindscher, K. (1992). *Medicinal wild plants of the prairie.* Lawrence, KS: University Press of Kansas.

Luettig, B., Steinmuller, C., Gifford, G., Wagner, H., & Lohmann-Matthes, M. (1989). Macrophage activation by the polysaccharide arabinogalactan isolated from plant cell cultures of *Echinacea purpurea. Journal of the National Cancer Institute, 81*(9), 669–675.

Melchart, D., Linde, K., Worku, F., Bauer, R., & Wagner, H. (1994). Immunomodulation with Echinacea—a systematic review of controlled clinical trials. *Phytomedicine, 1,* 245–254.

Melchart, D., Walther, E., Linde, K., Brandmaier, R., & Lersch, C. (1998). Echinacea root extracts for the prevention of upper respiratory tract infections: a double-blind, placebo-controlled randomized trial. *Archives of Family Medicine, 7*(6), 541–545.

Mullins, R. (1998). Echinacea-associated anaphylaxis. *Medical Journal of Australia, 168*(4), 170–171.

Murray, M. (1995). Echinacea: Pharmacology and clinical applications. *The American Journal of Natural Medicine, 2*(1), 18–24.

ELDER:

Brammer, T., Izurieta, H., Fukuda, K., Schmeltz, L., Regnery, H., Hall, H., & Cox, N. (2000). Surveillance for influenza—United States, 1994–95, 1995–96, and 1996–97 seasons. *Morbidity and Mortality Weekly Report CDC Surveillance, 49*(3), 13–28.

Cao, G., & Prior, R. (1999). Anthocyanins are detected in human plasma after oral administration of an elderberry extract. *Clinical Chemistry, 45*(4), 574–576.

Elliman, W. (December, 1994). Elderberry, flu contrary. *Hadassah Magazine,* 40–41.

Zakay-Rones, Z., Varsano, N., Zlotnik, M., Manor, O., Regev, L., Schlesinger, M., Mumcuoglu, M. (1995). Inhibition of several strains of influenza virus in vitro and reduction of symptoms by an elderberry extract *(Sambucus nigra L.)* during an outbreak of influenza B Panama. *Journal of Alternative and Complementary Medicine, 1*(4),361–369.

GARLIC:

American Botanical Council. (June 18, 1998). Confused on garlic products: JAMA study on garlic oil not applicable to most garlic products in U.S. Press Release: American Botanical Council.

Ankri, S., & Mirelman, D. (1999). Antimicrobial properties of allicin from garlic. *Microbes and Infection, 1*(2), 125–129.

Arora, D., & Kaur, J. (1999). Antimicrobial activity of spices. *International Journal of Antimicrobial Agents, 12*(3), 257–262.

Augusti, K. (1996). Therapeutic values of onion *(Allium cepa L.)* and garlic *(Allium sativum L.). Indian Journal of Experimental Biology, 34*(7), 634–640.

Aydin, A., Ersoz, G., Tekesin, O., Akcicek, E., & Tuncyurek, M. (2000). Garlic oil and *Helicobacter pylori* infection. *American Journal of Gastroenterology, 95*(2), 563–564.

Berthold, H., Sudhop, T., & von Bergmann, K. (1998). Effect of a garlic oil preparation on serum lipoproteins and cholesterol metabolism: a randomized controlled trial. *Journal of the American Medical Association, 279*(23), 1900–1902.

Breithaupt-Grogler, K., Ling, M., Boudoulas, H., & Belz, G. (1997). Protective effect of chronic garlic intake on elastic properties of aorta in the elderly. *Circulation, 96*(8), 2649–2655.

Duke, J. (1999). *Dr. Duke's essential herbs.* Emmaus, PA: Rodale Press.

Graham, D., Anderson, S., & Lang, T. (1999). Garlic or jalapeno peppers for treatment of *Helicobacter pylori* infection. *American Journal of Gastroenterology, 94*(5), 1200–1202.

Isaacsohn, J., Moser, M., Stein, E., Dudley, K., Davey, J., Liskov, E., & Black, H. (1998). Garlic powder and plasma lipids and lipoproteins: a multicenter, randomized, placebo-controlled trial. *Archives of Internal Medicine, 158*(11), 1189–1194.

Kiesewetter, H., Jung, F., Jung, E., Mroweitz, C., Koscielny, J., & Wenzel, E. (1993). Effect of garlic on platelet aggregation in patients with increased risk of juvenile ischaemic attack. *European Journal of Clinical Pharmacology, 45*(4), 333–336.

Kushi, M. (1993). *Macrobiotic home remedies.* Tokyo: Japan Publications.

Ledezma, E., DeSousa, L., Jorquera, A., Sanchez, J., Lander, A., Rodriguez, E., Jain, M., & Apitz-Castro, R. (1996). Efficacy of ajoene, an organosulphur derived from garlic, in the short-term therapy of tinea pedis. *Mycoses, 39*(9–10), 393–395.

Mennella, J., Johnson, A., & Beauchamp, G. (1995). Garlic ingestion by pregnant women alters the odor of amniotic fluid. *Chemical Senses, 20*(2), 207–209.

Morioka, N., Sze, L., Morton, D., & Irie, R. (1993). A protein fraction from aged garlic extract enhances cytotoxicity and proliferation of human lymphocytes mediated by interleukin-2 and concanavalin A. *Cancer, Immunology, and Immunotherapy, 37*(5), 316–322.

Sivam, G., Lampe, J., Ulness, B., Swanzy, S., & Potter, J. (1997). *Helicobacter pylori*—in vitro susceptibility to garlic *(Allium sativum)* extract. *Nutrition and Cancer, 27*(2), 118–121.

Superko, H., & Krauss, R. (2000). Garlic powder, effect on plasma lipids, postprandial lipemia, low-density lipoprotein particle size, high-density lipoprotein subclass distribution and lipoprotein(a). *Journal of the American College of Cardiology, 35*(2), 321–326.

Warshafsky, S., Kamer, R., & Sivak, S. (1993). Effect of garlic on total serum cholesterol. A meta-analysis. *Annals of Internal Medicine, 119*(7 Pt 1), 599–605.

SAGE:

Burkhard, P., Burkhardt, K., Haenggeli, C., & Landis, T. (1999). Plant-induced seizures: reappearance of an old problem. *Journal of Neurology, 246*(8), 667–670.

Jalsenjak,V., Peljnjak, S., & Kustrak, D. (1987). Microcapsules of sage oil: Essential oils content and antimicrobial activity. *Pharmazie 42*(6), 419–420.

Ulrich, L. (1990). *A midwife's tale: The life of Martha Ballard.* New York: Vintage Books.

THYME:

Benito, M., Jorro, G., Morales, C., Pelaez, A., & Fernandez, A. (1996). Labiatae allergy: systemic reactions due to ingestion of oregano and thyme. *Annals of Allergy, Asthma, and Immunology, 76*(5), 416–418.

Diamond, J. (1979). *Behavioral kinesiology: The new science for positive health through muscle testing. How to activate your thymus and increase your life energy.* New York: Harper & Row, Publishers.

Dorman, H., & Deans, S. (2000). Antimicrobial agents from plants: antibacterial activity of plant volatile oils. *Journal of Applied Microbiology, 88*(2), 308–316.

Hammer, K., Carson, C., & Riley, T. (1999). Antimicrobial activity of essential oils and other plant extracts. *Journal of Applied Microbiology, 86*(6), 985–990.

Marino, M., Bersani, C., & Comi, G. (1999). Antimicrobial activity of the essential oils of *Thymus vulgaris L.* measured using a bioimpedometric method. *Journal of Food Protection, 62*(9), 1017–1023.

Meeker, H., & Linke, H. (1988). The antibacterial action of eugenol, thyme oil, and related essential oils used in dentistry. *Compendium of Continuing Education in Dentistry, 9*(1), 34–35, 38.

Pearsall, P. (1998). *The Heart's Code.* New York: Broadway Books.

Tabak, M., Armon, R., Potasman, I., & Neeman, I. (1996). In vitro inhibition of *Helicobacter pylori* by extracts of thyme. *Journal of Applied Bacteriology, 80*(6), 667–672.

Taber's Cyclopedic Dictionary. (1997). Philadelphia: F.A. Davis Company.

Veal, L. (1996). The potential effectiveness of essential oils as a treatment for head lice, *Pediculus humanus capitis. Complementary Therapies in Nursing and Midwifery, 2*(4), 97–101.

ONION:

Augusti, K. (1996). Therapeutic values of onion *(Allium cepa L.)* and garlic *(Allium sativum L.). Indian Journal of Experimental Biology, 34*(7), 634–640.

Bordia, T., Mohammed, N., Thomson, M., & Ali, M. (1996). An evaluation of garlic and onion as antithrombotic agents. *Prostaglandins, Leukotrienes, and Essential Fatty Acids, 54*(3), 183–186.

Crellin, J., & Philpott, J., (1990). *Herbal medicine past and present.* Durham, NC: Duke University Press.

Farbman, K., Barnett, E., Bolduc, G., & Klein, J. (1993). Antibacterial activity of garlic and onions: A historical perspective. *The Pediatric Infectious Disease Journal, 12* (7), 613–614.

Guarrera, P. (1999). Traditional antihelmintic, antiparasitic, and repellent uses of plants in Central Italy. *Journal of Ethnopharmacology, 68*(1–3), 183–192.

Kato, T., Michikoshi, K., Minowa, Y., Maeda, Y., & Kikugawa, K. (1998). Mutagenicity of cooked hamburger is reduced by addition of onion to ground beef. *Mutation Research, 420*(1–3), 109–114.

Kim, J-H. (1997). Anti-bacterial action of onion *(Allium cepa L.)* extracts against oral pathogenic bacteria. *Journal of the Nihon University School of Dentistry, 39*(3), 136–141.

Kushi, M. (1993). *Macrobiotic home remedies.* Tokyo: Japan Publications.

Lata, S., Saxena, K., Bhasin, V., Saxena, R., Kumar, A., & Srivastava, V. (1991). Beneficial effects of *Allium sativum, Allium cepa,* and *Commiphora mukul* on experimental hyperlipidemia and atherosclerosis—A comparative evaluation. *Journal of Postgraduate Medicine, 37*(3), 132–135.

Lewis, W., & Elvin-Lewis, P. (1977). *Medical botany: Plants affecting man's health.* New York: John Wiley & Sons.

McAnlis, G., McEneny, J., Pearce, J., & Young, I. (1999). Absorption and antioxidant effects of quercetin from onions in man. *European Journal of Clinical Nutrition, 53*(2), 92–96.

Ulrich, L. (1990). *A midwife's tale: The life of Martha Ballard.* New York: Vintage Books.

Valdivieso, R., Subiza, J., Varela-Losada, S., Subiza, J., Narganes, M., Martinez-Cocera, C., & Cabrera, M. (1994). Bronchial asthma, rhinoconjunctivitis, and contact dermatitis caused by onion. *Journal of Allergy and Clinical Immunology, 94*(5), 928–930.

Whiting, S., & Guinea, M. (1998). Treating stingray wounds with onions. *Medical Journal of Australia, 168*(11), 584.

You, W., Blot, W., Chang, Y., Ershow, A., Yang, Z., An, Q., Henderson, B., Fraumeni, J., & Wang, T. (1989). Allium vegetables and reduced risk of stomach cancer. *Journal of the National Cancer Institute, 81*(2), 162–164.

Zohri, A., Abdel-Gawad, K., & Saber, S. (1995). Antibacterial, anti-dermatophytic and antitoxigenic activities of onion *(Allium cepa L.)* oil. *Microbiological Research, 150*(2), 167–172.

Chapter 10. Skin Care

INTRODUCTION:

Keane, F., Munn, S., du Vivier, A., Taylor, N., & Higgins, E. (1999). Analysis of Chinese herbal creams prescribed for dermatological conditions. *British Medical Journal, 318,* 563–564.

Korting, H., Schafer-Korting, M., Hart, H., Laux, P., & Schmid, M. (1993). Anti-inflammatory activity of hamamelis distillate applied topically to the skin. *European Journal of Clinical Pharmacology, 44*(4), 315–318.

Papantonio, C. (1998). Alternative medicine and wound healing. *Ostomy/Wound Management, 44*(4), 44–55.

CALENDULA:

Boucaud-Maitre, Y., Algernon, O., & Raynaud, J. (1988). Cytotoxic and antitumoral activity of *Calendula officinalis* extracts. *Die Pharmazie, 43*(3), 220–221.

Brown, D., & Dattner, A. (1998). Phytotherapeutic approaches to common dermatologic conditions. *Archives of Dermatology, 134*(11), 1401–1404.

Cook, E. F., & Lawall, C. H. (1926). *Remington's practice of pharmacy.* Philadelphia: J. B. Lippincott Co.

Kalvatchev, Z., Walder, R., & Garzaro, D. (1997). Anti-HIV activity of extracts from *Calendula officinalis* flowers. *Biomedicine and Pharmacotherapy, 51*(4), 176–180.

Kloucek-Popova, E., Popov, A., Pavlova, N., & Krusteva, S. (1982). Influence of the physiological regeneration and epithelization using fractions isolated from *Calendula officinalis. Acta Physiologica et Pharmacologica Bulgarica, 8*(4), 63–67.

Patrick, K., Kumar, S., Edwardson, P., & Hutchinson, J. (1996). Induction of vascularisation by an aqueous extract of the flowers of *Calendula officinalis L.,* the European marigold. *Phytomedicine, 3*(1), 11–18.

Rao, S., Udupa, A., Udupa, S., Rao, P., Rao, G., & Kulkarni, D. (1991). Calendula and hypericum: Two homeopathic drugs promoting wound healing in rats. *Fitoterapia, 52*(6), 508–510.

Treben, M. (1980). *Health through God's pharmacy.* Steyr, Austria: Wilhelm Ennsthaler.

ALOE:

Ardire, L., & Mrowczynski, E. (1997). Necrotizing fasciitis: Case study of a nursing dilemma. *Ostomy/Wound Management, 43*(5), 30–45.

Blitz, J., Smith, J., & Gerard, J. (1963). Aloe vera gel in peptic ulcer therapy: Preliminary report. *Journal of the American Osteopathic Association, 62,* 731–735.

Chithra, P., Sajithlal, G., & Chandrakasan, G. (1998). Influence of *Aloe vera* on collagen characteristics in healing dermal wounds in rats. *Molecular and Cellular Biochemistry, 181*(1–2), 71–76.

Cuzzell, J. (1986). Reader's remedies for pressure sores. *American Journal of Nursing, 86*(8), 923–924.

De Waal, M. (1980). *Medicinal herbs in the Bible.* York Beach, Maine: Samuel Weiser, Inc.

Hayes, S. (1999). Lichen planus—report of successful treatment with aloe vera. *General Dentistry,* May-June, *47*(3), 268–272.

Heggers, J., Pelley, R., & Robson, M. (1993). Beneficial effects of aloe in wound healing. *Phytotherapy Research, 7*(Suppl.), S48–S52.

Hunter, D., & Frumkin, A. (1991). Adverse reactions to vitamin E and aloe vera preparations after dermabrasion and chemical peel. *Cutis, 47*(3), 193–196.

Kaufman, T., Kalderon, N., Ullmann, Y., & Berger, J. (1988). Aloe vera gel hindered wound healing of experimental second-degree burns: A quantitative controlled study. *Journal of Burn Care Rehabilitation, 9*(2), 156–159.

Robson, M., Heggers, J., & Hagstrom, W. (1982). Myth, magic, witchcraft, or fact? Aloe vera revisited. *Journal of Burn Care and Rehabilitation, 3*(2), 157–163.

Sturm, P. (1999). Benefits of aloe vera. *General Dentistry, 47*(3), 269–272.

Syed, T., Ahmed, A., Holt, A., Ahmad, S. A., Ahmad, S. H., & Afzal, M. (1996). Management of psoriasis with aloe vera extract in a hydrophilic cream: a placebo-controlled, double-blind study. *Tropical Medicine and International Health, 1*(4), 505–509.

Trotter, R. (1981). Folk remedies as indicators of common illnesses: Examples from the United States-Mexico border. *Journal of Ethnopharmacology, 4*(2), 207–221.

Visuthikosol, V., Sukwanarat, Y., Chowchuen, B., Sriurairatana, S., & Boonpucknavig, V. (1995). Effect of aloe vera gel to healing of burn wound a clinical and histologic study. *Journal of Medical Association of Thailand, 78* (8), 403–409.

Williams, M., Burk, M., Loprinzi, C., Hill, M., Schomberg, P., Nearhood, K., O'Fallon, J., Laurie, J., Shanahan, T., Moore, R., Urias, R., Kuske, R., Engel, R., & Eggleston, W. (1996). Phase III double-blind evaluation of an aloe vera gel as a prophylactic agent for radiation-induced skin toxicity. *International Journal of Radiation Oncology Biology and Physics, 36*(2), 345–349.

Zawahry, M., Hegazy, R., & Helal, M. (1973). Use of aloe in treating leg ulcers and dermatoses. *International Journal of Dermatology, 12*(1), 68–73.

YARROW:

Chandler, R., Hooper, S., & Harvey, M. (1982a). Ethnobotany and phytochemistry of yarrow, *Achillea millefolium*, Compositae. *Economic Botany, 36*(2), 203–223.

Chandler, R., Hooper, S., Hooper, D., Jamieson, W., Flinn, C., & Safe, L. (1982b). Herbal remedies of the Maritime Indians: Sterols and triterpenes of *Achillea millefolium L.* (yarrow). *Journal of Pharmaceutical Sciences, 71*(6), 690–693.

Coffin, A. (1849). *A treatise on midwifery and the diseases of women and children together with a full description of the herbs, roots, and other preparations prescribed as remedies in the work.* London: British Medico-Botanic Press.

de Laszlo, H., & Henshaw, P. (1954). Plant materials used by primitive peoples to affect fertility. *Science, 119,* May 7, 626–631.

Flanagan, S. (1996). *Secrets of God: Writings of Hildegard of Bingen.* Boston: Shamballa.

Hausen, B., Breuer, J., Weglewski, J., & Rucker, G. (1991). Alpha-peroxyachifolid and other new sensitizing sesquiterpene lactones from yarrow *(Achillea millefolium L., Compositeae). Contact Dermatitis, 24*(4), 274–280.

Montanari, T., de Carvalho, J., & Dolder, H. (1998). Antispermatogenic effect of *Achillea millefolium L.* in mice. *Contraception, 58*(5), 309–313.

Naiman, I. (1999). *Cancer salves.* Santa Fe, New Mexico: Seventh Ray Press.

Treben, M. (1980). *Health through God's pharmacy.* Steyr, Austria: Wilhelm Ennsthaler.

Ulrich, L. T. (1990). *A Midwife's tale: The life of Martha Ballard based on her diary, 1785–1812.* New York: Vintage Books.

ROSE:

Green, M. (1999). The rose. *Aromatic Thymes, 7*(1), 11–15.

Mahmood, N., Piacente, S., Pizza, C., Burke, A., Khan, A., & Hay, A. (1996). The anti-HIV activity and mechanisms of action of pure compounds isolated from *Rosa damascena. Biochemical and Biophysical Research Communications, 229*(1), 73–79.

Maleev, A., Atsev, E., Neshtev, G., Stoianov, S., & Avramova, D. (1971). [Pharmacobiochemical and electrophysiological studies on the Bulgarian rose oil]. [Article in Bulgarian]. *Eksperimentalna Medi K T L Sina I Morfologi K I L A, 10*(3), 149–153.

Maleev, A., Neshev, G., Stoianov, S., & Sheikov, N. (1972). [The ulcer protective and anti-inflammatory effect of Bulgarian rose oil]. [Article in Bulgarian]. *Eksperimentalna Medi K T L Sina I Morfologi K I L A, 11*(2), 55–60.

Wilder, L. B. (1974). *The fragrant garden.* New York: Dover Publications, Inc.

Wood, G., & Bache, F. (1839). *The dispensatory of the United States of America* (4th ed.). Philadelphia: Grigg & Elliot.

WITCH HAZEL:

Beach, W. (1843). *The family physician or the reformed system of medicine: On vegetable or botanical principles.* New York: W. Beach.

Brown, D., & Dattner, A. (1998). Phytotherapeutic approaches to common dermatologic conditions. *Archives of Dermatology, 134*(11), 1401–1404.

Granlund, H. (1994). Contact allergy to witch hazel. *Contact Dermatitis, 31*(3), 195.

Hughes-Formella, B., Bohnsack, K., Rippke, F., Benner, G., Rudolph, M., Tausch, I., & Gassmueller, J. (1998). Anti-inflammatory effect of *Hamamelis* lotion in a UVB erythema test. *Dermatology, 196*(3), 316–322.

Korting, H., Schafer-Korting, M., Hart, H., Laux, P., & Schmid, M. (1993). Anti-inflammatory activity of hamamelis distillate applied topically to the skin. *European Journal of Clinical Pharmacology, 44*(4), 315–318.

Korting, H., Schafer-Korting, Klovekorn, W., Klovekorn, G., Martin, C., & Laux, P. (1995). Comparative efficacy of hamamelis distillate and hydrocortisone cream in atopic eczema. *European Journal of Clinical Pharmacology, 48*(6), 461–465.

Osol, A., & Farrar, G. (Eds.). (1947). *The dispensatory of the United States of America* (24th ed.). Philadelphia: J. B. Lippincott.

Sleep, J., & Grant, A. (1988). Relief of perineal pain following childbirth: A survey of midwifery practice. *Midwifery, 4*(3), 118–122.

Chapter 11. Sleep and Rest

INTRODUCTION:

Wagner, J., Wagner, M., & Hening, W. (1998). Beyond benzodiazepines: alternative pharmacologic agents for the treatment of insomnia. *The Annals of Pharmacotherapy, 32,* 680–691.

Wiley, T., & Formby, B. (2000). *Lights out: sleep, sugar, and survival.* New York: Pocket Books.

VALERIAN:

Houghton, P. (1999). The scientific basis for the reputed activity of Valerian. *Journal of Pharmacy and Pharmacology, 51,* 505–512.

Leathwood, P., Chauffard, F., Heck, E., & Munoz-Box, R. (1982). Aqueous extract of Valerian root *(Valeriana officinalis L.)* improves sleep quality in man. *Pharmacology, Biochemistry and Behavior, 17,* 65–71.

Leathwood, P., & Chauffard, F. (1985). Aqueous extract of valerian reduces latency to fall asleep in man. *Planta Medica, April (2),* 144–148.

Lindahl, O., & Lindwall, L. (1989). Double blind study of a valerian preparation. *Pharmacology, Biochemistry and Behavior, 32,* 1065–1066.

Ottariano, S. (1999). *Medicinal herbal therapy: a pharmacist's viewpoint.* North Hampton, NH: Nicolin Fields Publishing.

Schultz, H., Stolz, C., & Muller, J. (1994). The effect of valerian extract on sleep polygraphy in poor sleepers: a pilot study. *Pharmacopsychiat, 27,* 147–151.

Wagner, J., Wagner, M., & Hening, W. (1998). Beyond benzodiazepines: alternative pharmacologic agents for the treatment of insomnia. *The Annals of Pharmacotherapy, 32*, 680–691.

CHAMOMILE:

Aggag, M., & Yousef, R. (1972). Study of antimicrobial activity of chamomile oil. *Planta Med, 22*(2), 140–144.

Berry, M. (1995). The chamomiles. *The Pharmaceutical Journal, 254*(February 11), 191–193.

Fidler, P., Loprinzi, C., O'Fallon, J., Leitch, J., Lee, J., Hayes, D., Novotny, P., Clemens-Schutjer, D., Bartel, J., & Michalak, J. (1996). Prospective evaluation of a chamomile mouthwash for prevention of 5–FU–induced oral mucositis. *Cancer, 77,* 522–525.

Glowania, H., Raulin, Chr., & Swoboda, M. (1987). The effect of chamomile on wound healing—a controlled clinical-experimental double-blind trial. *Zeitschrift fur Hautkrankheiten, 62*(17), 1262–1271. [In German].

Gould, L., Reddy, R., & Gomprecht, R. (1973). Cardiac effects of chamomile tea. *Journal of Clinical Pharmacology, Nov/Dec,* 475–479.

Harris, B., & Lewis, R. (1994). Chamomile—part 1. *International Journal of Alternative and Complementary Medicine, September,* 12.

Ottariano, S. (1999). *Medicinal herbal therapy: a pharmacist's viewpoint.* North Hampton, NH: Nicolin Fields Publishing.

Pereira, F., Santos, R., & Pereira, A. (1997). Contact dermatitis from chamomile tea. *Contact Dermatitis, 36,* 307.

Safayhi, H., Sabieraj, J., Sailer, E., & Ammon, H. (1994). Chamazulene: an antioxidant-type inhibitor of leukotriene B4 formation. *Planta Medica, 60,* 410–413.

Subiza, J., Subiza, J. L., Alonso, M., Hinojosa, M., Garcia, R., Jerez, M., & Subiza, E. (1990). Allergic conjunctivitis to chamomile tea. *Annals of Allergy, 65*(2), 127–132.

Subiza, J., Subiza, J. L., Hinojosa, M., Garcia, R., Jerez, M., Valdivieso, R., & Subiza, E. (1989). Anaphylactic reaction after the ingestion of chamomile tea: a study of cross-reactivity with other composite pollens. *Journal of Allergy and Clinical Immunology, 84*(3), 353–358.

Weeks-Shaw, C. (1914). *A textbook of nursing.* New York: D. Appleton and Company.

Weizman, Z., Alkrinawi, S., Goldfarb, D., & Bitran, C., (1993). Efficacy of herbal tea preparation in infantile colic. *The Journal of Pediatrics, 122,* 650–652.

HOPS:

Hansel, R., Wohlfart, R., & Schmidt, H. (1982). The sedative-hypnotic principle of hops. *Planta Medica, 45,* 224–228.

Harmer, B. (1924). *Textbook of the principles and practice of nursing.* New York: The MacMillan Company.

Milligan, S. R., Kalita, J. C., Heyerick, A., Rong, H., De Cooman, L., & De Keukeleire, D. (1999). Identification of a potent phytoestrogen in hops *(Humulus lupulus)* and beer. *The Journal of Clinical Endocrinology and Metabolism, 83*(6), 2249–2252.

Salvador, R. (1994). Hops. *Canadian Pharmaceutical Journal, 127,* 203–204, 207.

Weeks-Shaw, C. (1914). *A textbook of nursing.* New York: D. Appleton and Company.

Wohlfart, R., Hansel, R., & Schmidt, H. (1983). The sedative hypnotic principle of hops. *Planta Medica, 48,* 120–123.

LEMON BALM:

Child, L. M. (1997). *The family nurse.* (Reprint of 1837 text.) Bedford, MA: Applewood Books.

Koytchev, R., Alken, R., & Dundarov, S. (1999). Balm mint extract (Lo-701) for topical treatment of recurring *Herpes labialis. Phytomedicine, 6*(4), 225–230.

Perry, E., Pickering, A., Wang, W., Houghton, P., & Perry, N. (1999). Medicinal plants and Alzheimer's disease: from ethnobotany to phytotherapy. *Journal of Pharmacy and Pharmacology, 51,* 527–534.

Wolbling, R., & Leonhardt, K. (1994). Local therapy of herpes simplex with dried extract from *Melissa officinalis. Phytomedicine, 1,* 25–31.

OAT:

Bartram, P., Gerlach, S., Scheppach, W., Keller, F., & Kasper, H. (1992). Effect of a single oat bran cereal breakfast on serum cholesterol, lipoproteins, and apolipoproteins in patients with hyperlipoproteinemia type iia. *Journal of Parenteral and Enteral Nutrition, 16*(6), 533–537.

Bye, C., Fowle, A., Letley, E., & Wilkinson, S. (1974). Lack of effect of *Avena sativa* on cigarette smoking. *Nature, 252* (December 13), 580–581.

Connor, J., Connor, T., Marshall, P., Reid, A., & Turnbull, M. (1975). The pharmacology of *Avena sativa. Journal of Pharmacy and Pharmacology, 27,* 92–98.

He, J., Klag, M., Whelton, P., Mo, J., Chen, J., Qian, M., Mo, P., & He, G. (1995). Oats and buckwheat intakes and cardiovascular disease risk factors in an ethnic minority of China. *American Journal of Clinical Nutrition, 61,* 366–372.

Kumar, P., & Farthing, M. (1995). Oats and celiac disease. *The New England Journal of Medicine, 333,* 1075–1076.

Vogel, H. (1991). *The Nature doctor.* New Canaan, CT: Keats Publishing, Inc.

Chapter 12. Elimination

CRANBERRY:

Avorn, J., Monane, M., Gurwirz, J., Glenn, R., Choodnovskiy, I., & Lipsitz, L. (1994). Reduction of bacteriuria and pyuria after ingestion of cranberry juice. *Journal of the American Medical Association, 271*(10), 751–754.

Blatherwick, N. (1914). The Specific role of foods in relation to the composition of the urine. *Archives of Internal Medicine, 14,* 409–450.

Child, L. M. (1997). *The family nurse.* (Reprint of 1837 text.) Bedford, MA: Applewood Books.

Jackson, B., & Hicks, L. (1997). Effect of cranberry juice on urinary pH in older adults. *Home Healthcare Nurse, 15*(3), 199–202.

Leaver, R. (1996). Cranberry juice. *Professional Nurse, 11*(8), 525–526.

Ofek, I., Goldhar, J., & Sharon, N. (1996). Anti-*Escherichia coli* adhesin activity of cranberry and blueberry juices. *Advances in Experimental Medicine and Biology, 408,* 179–183.

Pedersen, C., Kle, J., Jenkinson, A., Gardner, P., McPhail, D., & Duthie, G. (2000). Effects of blueberry and cranberry juice consumption on the plasma antioxidant capacity of healthy female volunteers. *European Journal of Clinical Nutrition, 54,* 405–408.

Prodromos, P., Brusch, C., & Ceresia, G. (1968). Cranberry juice in the treatment of urinary tract infections. *Southwestern Medicine, 47,* 17.

Schlager, T., Anderson, S., Trudell, J., & Hendley, J. (1999). Effect of cranberry juice on bacteriuria in children with neurogenic bladder receiving intermittent catheterization. *The Journal of Pediatrics, 135*(6), 698–702.

Schultz, A. (1984). Efficacy of cranberry juice and ascorbic acid in acidifying the urine in multiple sclerosis subjects. *Journal of Community Health Nursing, 1*(3), 159–169.

Sobota, A. (1984). Inhibition of bacterial adherence by cranberry juice: Potential use for the treatment of urinary tract infections. *The Journal of Urology, 131,* 1013–1016.

Tsukada, K., Tokunaga, K., Iwama, T., Mishima, Y., Tazawa, K., & Fujimaki, M. (1994). Cranberry juice and its impact on peri-stomal skin conditions for urostomy patients. *Ostomy/Wound Management, 40*(9), 60–67.

Walker, E., Barney, D. P., Mickelsen, J., Walton, R., & Mickelsen, R. (1997). Cranberry concentrate: UTI prophylaxis. *The Journal of Family Practice, 45*(2), 167–168.

Weiss, E., Lev-dor, R., Kashamn, Y., Goldhar, J., Sharon, N., & Ofek, I. (1998). Inhibiting interspecies coaggregation of plaque bacteria with a cranberry juice constituent. *Journal of the American Dental Association, 129*(12), 1719–1723.

Wilson, T., Porcari, J., & Harbin, D. (1998). Cranberry extract inhibits low density lipoprotein oxidation. *Life Sciences, 62*(24), PL 381–386.

Zafriri, D., Ofek, I., Adar, R., Pocino, M., & Sharon, N. (1989). Inhibitory activity of cranberry juice on adherence of type I and type P fimbriated Escherichia coli to eucaryotic cells. *Antimicrobial Agents and Chemotherapy, 33,* 92–98.

PSYLLIUM:

Anderson, J., Allgood, L., Lawrence, A., Altringer, L., Jerdack, G., Hengehold, D., & Morel, J. (2000a). Cholesterol-lowering effects of psyllium intake adjunctive to diet therapy in men and women with hypercholesterolemia: meta-analysis of 8 controlled trials. *American Journal of Clinical Nutrition, 71,* 472–479.

Anderson, J., Davidson, M., Blonde, L., Brown, W. V., Howard, W. J., Ginsberg, H., Allgood, L., & Weingand, K. (2000b). Long-term cholesterol-lowering effects of psyllium as an adjunct to diet therapy in the treatment of hypercholesterolemia. *American Journal of Clinical Nutrition, 71,* 1433–1438.

Ashraf, W., Pfeiffer, R., Park, F., & Quigley, E. (1997). Constipation in Parkinson's Disease: Objective assessment and response to psyllium. *Movement Disorders, 12*(6), 946–951.

Fernandez-Banares, F., Hinojosa, J., Sanchez-Lombrana, J., Navarro, E., Martinez-Salmeron, J., Garcia-Puges, A., Gonzalez-Huix, F., Riera, J., Gonzalez-Lara, V., Dominguez-Abascal, F., Gine, J., Moles, J., Gomollon, F., & Gassull, M. (1999). Randomized clinical trial of *Plantago ovata* seeds (dietary fiber) as compared with mesalamine in maintaining remission in ulcerative colitis. *The American Journal of Gastroenterology, 94*(2), 427–433.

Marlett, J., Li, B. U., Patrow, C., & Bass, P. (1987). Comparative laxation of psyllium with and without senna in an ambulatory constipated population. *The American Journal of Gastroenterology, 82*(4), 333–337.

McRorie, J., Daggy, B., Morel, J., Diersing, P., Miner, P., & Robinson, M. (1998). Psyllium is superior to docusate sodium for treatment of chronic constipation. *Alimentary Pharmacology and Therapeutics, 12,* 491–497.

Washington, N., Harris, M., Mussellwhite, A., & Spiller, R. (1998). Moderation of lactulose-induced diarrhea by psyllium: effects on motility and fermentation. *American Journal of Clinical Nutrition, 67,* 317–321.

CASCARA SAGRADA:

Borkje, B., Pedersen, R., Lund, G. M., Enehaug, J., & Berstad, A. (1991). Effectiveness and acceptability of three bowel cleansing regimens. *Scandinavian Journal of Gastroenterology, 26*(2), 162–166.

deWitte, P., & Lemli, L. (1990). The metabolism of anthranoid laxatives. *Hepato-Gastroenterol, 37,* 601–605.

Hagemann, T. (1998). Gastrointestinal medications and breastfeeding. *Journal of Human Lactation, 14*(3), 259–262.

Hangartner, P., Munch, R., Meier, J., Ammann, R., & Buhler, H. (1989). Comparison of three colon cleansing methods: Evaluation of a randomized clinical trial with 300 ambulatory patients. *Endoscopy, 21,* 272–275.

Petticrew, M., Watt, I., & Sheldon, T. (1997). Systematic review of the effectiveness of laxatives in the elderly. *Health Technology Assessment, 1*(13), iii-iv, 1–52.

SAW PALMETTO:

Bayne, C., Donnelly, F., Ross, M., & Habib, F. (1999). *Serenoa repens* (Permixon®): A 5alpha-reductase types I and II inhibitor—New evidence in a coculture model of BPH. *Prostate, 40,* 232–241.

Boyle, P., Robertson, C., Lowe, F., & Roehrborn, C. (2000). Meta-analysis of clinical trials of permixon in the treatment of symptomatic benign prostatic hyperplasia. *Urology, 55,* 533–539.

Braeckman, J. (1994). The extract of *Serenoa repens* in the treatment of benign prostatic hyperplasia: A multicenter open study. *Current Therapeutic Research, 55*(7), 776–785.

Brinker, F. (1993/1994). An overview of conventional, experimental, and botanical treatments of non-malignant prostate conditions. *British Journal of Phytotherapy, 3*(4), 154–176.

Carraro, J., Raynaud, J., Koch, G., Chisholm, G., Di Silverio, F., Teillac, P., Da Silva, F., Cauquil, J., Chopin, D., Hamdy, F., Hanus, M., Hauri, D., Kalinteris, A., Marencak, J., Perier, A., & Perrin, P. (1996). Comparison of phytotherapy (Permixon®) with finasteride in the treatment of benign prostate hyperplasia: A Randomized international study of 1,098 patients. *The Prostate, 29,* 231–240.

Champault, G., Patel, J., & Bonnard, A. (1984). A double-blind trial of an extract of the plant *Serenoa repens* in benign prostatic hyperplasia. *British Journal of Clinical Pharmacy, 18,* 461–462.

Consumer Reports. (2000). Herbal Rx for prostate problems. *Consumer Reports,* Sept, 60–62.

Di Silverio, F. (1992). Evidence that *Serenoa repens* extract displays an antiestrogenic activity in prostatic tissue of benign prostatic hypertrophy patients. *European Urology, 21,* 309–314.

Gerber, G., Zagaja, G., Bales, G., Chodak, G., & Contreras, B. (1998). Saw Palmetto (*Serenoa repens*) in men with lower urinary tract symptoms: Effects on urodynamic parameters and voiding symptoms. *Urology, 51,* 1003–1007.

Goepel, M., Hecker, U., Krege, S., Rubben, H., & Michel, M. (1999). Saw Palmetto extracts potently noncompetitively inhibit human alpha 1–adrenoceptors in vitro. *Prostate, 38,* 208–215.

Grasso, M., Montesano, A., Buonaguidi, A., Castelli, M., Lania, C., Rigatti, P., Rocco, F., Cesana, B., & Borghi, C. (1995). Comparative effects of alfuzosin versus Serenoa repens in the treatment of symptomatic benign prostatic hyperplasia. *Archivos Espanoles de Urologia, 48*(1), 97–103.

Marks, L., & Tyler, V. (1999). Saw Palmetto extract: Newest (and oldest) treatment alternative for men with symptomatic benign prostatic hyperplasia. *Urology, 53,* 457–461.

McPartland, J., & Pruitt, P. (2000). Benign prostatic hyperplasia treated with saw Palmetto: a literature search and an experimental case study. *Journal of the American Osteopathic Association, 100*(2), 89–96.

NetDoctor (December 20, 1000). Alfuzosin hydrochloride tablets. www.netdoctor.co.uk/medicines/showpreparation.asp?id=4297.

Overmyer, M. (1999). Saw palmetto shown to shrink prostatic epithelium. *Urology Times, 27*(6), 1, 42.

Romics, I., Schmitz, H., & Frang, D. (1993). Experience in treating benign prostatic hypertrophy with *Sabal serrulata* for one year. *International Urology and Nephrology, 25*(6), 565–569.

Winston, D. (1999). *Saw palmetto for men and women.* Pownal, VT: Storey Books.

Chapter 13. Digestion

INTRODUCTION:

Merriam-Webster. (1999). *Merriam-Webster's Collegiate Dictionary* (10th ed.). Springfield, Massachusetts: Merriam-Webster, Inc.

HORSERADISH:

Bentheim, T., Bos, S., de la Houssaye, E., & Visser, W. (1980). *Caring for the sick at home.* New York: Anthroposophic Press.

Child, L. M. (1997). *The family nurse.* (Reprint of 1837 text.) Bedford, MA: Applewood Books.

Crellin, J., & Philpott, J. (1990). *Herbal medicine past and present.* Durham, NC: Duke University Press.

Husemann, F. (1982). *The Anthroposophical approach to medicine.* New York: The Anthroposophic Press.

Pitchford, P. (1993). *Healing with whole foods.* Berkeley, CA: North Atlantic Books.

Rubin, H., & Wu, A. (1988). The bitter herbs of Seder: More on horseradish horrors. *Journal of the American Medical Association, 259*(13), 1943.

Spitzer, D. (1988). Horseradish horrors: Sushi syncope. *Journal of the American Medical Association, 259*(2), 218–219.

Thomson, S. (1841). *The Thomsonian materia medica or botanic family physician* (12th ed.). Albany: J. Munsell.

Vogel, H. (1991). *The nature doctor.* New Canaan, CT: Keats Publishing.

GINGER:

Arfeen, Z., Owen, H., Plummer, J., Ilsley, A., Sorby-Adams, R., & Doecke, C. (1995). A double-blind randomized controlled trial of ginger for the prevention of postoperative nausea and vomiting. *Anaesthesia and Intensive Care, 23*(4), 449–452.

Atal, C., Zutshi, U., & Rao, P. (1981). Scientific evidence on the role of Ayurvedic herbals on bioavailability of drugs. *Journal of Ethnopharmacology, 4*(2), 229–232.

Bone, M., Wilkinson, D., Young, J., McNeil, J., & Charlton, S. (1990). Ginger root—a new antiemetic. The effect of ginger root on postoperative nausea and vomiting after major gynaecological surgery. *Anaesthesia, 45*(8), 669–671.

Fischer-Rasmussen, W., Kjaer, S., Dahl, C., & Asping, U. (1990). Ginger treatment of hyperemesis gravidarum. *European Journal of Obstetrics and Gynecology and Reproductive Biology, 38,* 19–24.

Grontved, A., Brask, T., Kambskard, J., & Hentzer, E. (1988). Ginger root against seasickness. *Acta Otolaryngologica (Stockholm), 105*(1–2), 45–49.

Holtmann, S., Clarke, A., Scherer, H., & Hohn, M. (1989). The anti-motion sickness mechanism of ginger. *Acta Otolaryngologica (Stockholm), 108*(3–4), 168–174.

Kushi, M. (1993). *Macrobiotic home remedies.* Tokyo: Japan Publications.

Lumb, A. (1994). Effect of dried ginger on human platelet function. *Thrombosis and Haemostasis, 71*(1), 110–111.

Meyer, K., Schwartz, J., Crater, D., & Keyes, B. (1995). *Zingiber officinale* (ginger) used to prevent 8–MOP associated nausea. *Dermatology Nursing, 7*(4), 242–244.

Micklefield, G., Redeker, Y., Meister, V., Jung, O., Greving, I., & May, B. (1999). Effects of ginger on gastroduodenal motility. *International Journal of Clinical Pharmacology and Therapeutics, 37*(7), 341–346.

Mowrey, D., & Clayson, D. (1982). Motion sickness, ginger, and psychophysics. *The Lancet, 1*(8273), 655–657.

Mustafa, T., & Srivastava, K. (1990). Ginger *(Zingiber officinale)* in migraine headache. *Journal of Ethnopharmacology, 29*(3), 267–273.

Pancho, L., Kimura, I., Unno, R., Kurono, M., & Kimura, M. (1989). Reversed effects between crude and processed ginger extracts on PGF2 alpha-induced contraction in mouse mesenteric veins. *Japan Journal of Pharmacology, 50*(2), 243–246.

Phillips, S., Hutchinson, S., & Ruggier, R. (1993a). *Zingiber officinale* does not affect gastric emptying rate. *Anaesthesia, 48*(5), 393–395.

Phillips, S., Ruggier, R., & Hutchinson, S. (1993b). *Zingiber officinale* (Ginger)—an antiemetic for day case surgery. *Anaesthesia, 48*(8), 715–717.

Srivastava, K. (1989). Effect of onion and ginger consumption on platelet thromboxane production in humans. *Prostaglandins Leukotrienes and Essential Fatty Acids, 35*(3), 183–185.

Srivastava, K., & Mustafa, T. (1989). Ginger *(Zingiber officinale)* and rheumatic disorders. *Medical Hypotheses, 29*(1), 25–28.

Srivastava, K., & Mustafa, T. (1992). Ginger *(Zingiber officinale)* and rheumatism and musculoskeletal disorders. *Medical Hypotheses, 39*(4), 342–348.

Stewart, J., Wood, M., Wood, C., & Mims, M. (1991). Effects of ginger on motion sickness susceptibility and gastric function. *Pharmacology, 42*(2), 111–120.

Vimala, S., Norhanom, A., & Yadav, M. (1999). Anti-tumour promoter activity in Malaysian ginger rhizobia used in traditional medicine. *British Journal of Cancer, 80*(1/2), 110–116.

Visalyaputra, S., Petchpaisit, N., Somcharaen, K., & Choavaratana, R. (1998). The efficacy of ginger root in the prevention of postoperative nausea and vomiting after outpatient gynaecological laparoscopy. *Anaesthesia, 53*(5), 506–510.

Weeks-Shaw, C. (1914). *A textbook of nursing.* New York: D. Appleton and Company.

LEMON:

Aita, J. F., Aita, J. A., & Aita, V. (1990). 7–Up anti-acid lithiated lemon soda or early medicinal use of lithium. *Nebraska Medical Journal, 75*(10), 277–280.

Bentheim, T., Bos, S., de la Houssaye, E., & Visser, W. (1980). *Caring for the sick at home.* New York: Anthroposophic Press.

Cembrowski, G. (1980). Tempest in a tea cup: The lemon-tea controversy. *New England Journal of Medicine, 302*(6), 352.

Chapel, J., Leonard, M., & Millikan, L. (1983). Lemon juice, sunlight, and tattoos. *International Journal of Dermatology, 22*(7), 434–435.

Christensen, C., & Navazesh, M. (1984). Anticipatory salivary flow to the sight of different foods. *Appetite, 5*(4), 307–315.

Corcoran, D., & Houston, T. (1977). Is the lemon test an index of arousal level? *British Journal of Psychology, 68*(3), 361–364.

Crellin, J., & Philpott, J. (1990). *Herbal medicine past and present.* Durham, NC: Duke University Press.

D'Aquino, M., & Teves, S. (1994). Lemon juice as a natural biocide for disinfecting drinking water. *Bulletin of the Pan American Health Organization, 28*(4), 324–330.

Faschingbauer, C. (1995). [Reduction of antipyretics. A gentler way to reduce fever with lemon compresses along with administration of paracetamol]. [Article in German]. *Pflegezeitschrift, 48*(6), 332–338.

Lad, V., & Frawley, D. (1986). *The yoga of herbs.* Santa Fe, NM: Lotus Press.

Kushi, M. (1993). *Macrobiotic home remedies.* Tokyo: Japan Publications.

Naganuma, M., Hirose, S., Nakayama, Y., Nakajima, K., & Someya, T. (1985). A study of the phototoxicity of lemon oil. *Archives of Dermatological Research, 278*(1), 31–36.

Phillips, M. (1979). Lemon-tea drinkers—A group at risk? *New England Journal of Medicine, 301*(18), 1005–1006.

von Samson, V. E. (1995). [Alternative methods in neurosurgery. Gentle lowering of fever using lemon compresses]. [Article in German]. *Pflegezeitschrift, 48*(5), 252–254.

Warner, L. (1986). Nursing rules: Lemon-glycerine swabs should be used for routine oral care. *Critical Care Nurse, 6*(6), 82–83.

Wiley, S. (1969). Why glycerol and lemon juice? *American Journal of Nursing, 69*(2), 342–344.

Chapter 14. Energy

INTRODUCTION:

Eisenberg, D., Davis, R., Ettner, S., Appel, S., Wilkey, S., Van Rompay, M., & Kessler, R. (1998). Trends in alternative medicine use in the United States, 1990–1997: results of a follow-up national survey. *Journal of the American Medical Association, 280*(18), 1569–1575.

Pearsall, P. (1998). *The heart's code.* New York: Broadway Books.

Pitchford, P. (1993). *Healing with whole foods.* Berkeley, CA: North Atlantic Books.

GINSENG:

Allen, J., McLung, J., Nelson, A., & Welsch, M. (1998). Ginseng supplementation does not enhance healthy young adults' peak aerobic exercise performance. *Journal of the American College of Nutrition, 17*(5), 462–466.

Baldwin, C., Anderson, L., & Phillipson, J. (1986). What pharmacists should know about ginseng. *Pharmaceutical Journal, 237*, 583–586.

Brekhman, I., & Dardymov, I. (1969). New substances of plant origin that increase non-specific resistance. *Annual Review of Pharmacology, 9*, 419–430.

Cai, L., Hui, H., & Yu, L. (1990). Influence of ginseng saponin on the circadian rhythm of brain monoamine neurotransmitters. *Progress in Clinical and Biological Research, 341B*, 135–144.

Chandler, R. (1988). Ginseng—an aphrodisiac? *Canadian Pharmaceutical Journal, 121*(January), 36–38.

D'Angelo, L., Grimaldi, R., Caravaggi, M., Marcoli, M., Perucca, E., Lecchini, S., Frigo, G., & Crema, A. (1986). A double-blind, placebo-controlled clinical study on the effect of a standardized ginseng extract on psychomotor performance in healthy volunteers. *Journal of Ethnopharmacology, 16*(1), 15–22.

Engels, H., & Wirth, J. (1997). No ergogenic effects of ginseng *(Panax ginseng C.A. Meyer)* during graded maximal aerobic exercise. *Journal of the American Dietetic Association, 97*(10), 1110–1115.

Hallstrom, C., Fulder, S., & Carruthers, M. (1982). Effects of ginseng on the performance of nurses on night duty. *Comparative Medicine East and West, 6*(4), 277–282.

Lee, F., Ko, J., Park, J., & Lee, J. (1987). Effects of *Panax ginseng* on blood alcohol clearance in man. *Clinical Experimental Pharmacology & Physiology, 14*(6), 543–546.

LeGal, M., Cathebras, P., & Struby, K. (1996). Pharmaton capsules in the treatment of functional fatigue: a double-blind study versus placebo evaluated by a new methodology. *Phytotherapy Research, 10*, 49–53.

Liberti, L., & Der Marderosian, A. (1978). Evaluation of commercial ginseng products. *Journal of Pharmaceutical Sciences, 67*(10), 1487–1489.

Mitra, S., Chakraborti, A., & Bhattacharya, S. (1996). Neuropharmacological studies on *Panax ginseng. Indian Journal of Experimental Biology, 34*(1), 41–47.

Mizuno, M., Yamada, J., Terai, H., Kozukue, N., Lee, Y., & Tsuchida, H. (1994). Differences in immunomodulating effects between wild and cultured *Panax ginseng. Biochemical and Biophysical Research Communications, 200*(3), 1672–1678.

Salvati, G., Genovesi, G., Marcellini, L., Paolini, P., De Nuccio, I., Pepe, M., & Re, M. (1996). Effects of *Panax ginseng C.A. Meyer* saponins on male fertility. *Panminerva Medicine, 38*(4), 249–254.

Tode, T., Kikuchi, Y., Hirata, J., Kita, T., Nakata, H., & Nagata, I. (1999). Effect of Korean red ginseng on psychological functions in patients with severe climacteric syndromes. *International Journal of Gynaecology and Obstetrics, 67*(3), 169–174.

COFFEE:

Bak, A., & Grobbee, D. (1989). The effect on serum cholesterol levels of coffee brewed by filtering or boiling. *The New England Journal of Medicine, 321*(21), 1432–1437.

Caan, B., Quesenberry, C., & Coates, A. (1998). Differences in fertility associated with caffeinated beverage consumption. *American Journal of Public Health, 88*(2), 270–274.

Joesoef, M., Berel, V., Rolfs, R., Aral, S., & Cramer, D. (1990). Are caffeinated beverages risk factors for delayed conception? *The Lancet, 335*(8682), 136–137.

Kruger A. (1996). Chronic psychiatric patients' use of caffeine: pharmacological effects and mechanisms. *Psychological Reports, 78*(3 Pt 1), 915–923.

LaCroix, A., Mead, L., Liang, K., Thomas, C., & Pearson, T. (1986). Coffee consumption and the incidence of coronary heart disease. *New England Journal of Medicine, 315*(16), 977–982.

Lane, J., Phillips-Bute, B., & Pieper, C. (1998). Caffeine raises blood pressure at work. *Psychosomatic Medicine, 60*(3), 327–330.

Leitzmann, M., Willett, W., Rimm, E., Stampfer, M., Spiegelman, D. Colditz, G., & Giovannucci, E. (1999). A prospective study of coffee consumption and the risk of symptomatic gallstone disease in men. *Journal of the American Medical Association, 281*(22), 2106–2112.

Lesley, M. (1998). The coffee connection: The benefits of memory. *Home Healthcare Nurse, 16*(3), 200.

Miyake, Y., Kono, S., Nishiwaki, M., Hamada, H., Nishikawa, H., Koga, H., & Ogawa, S. (1999). Relationship of coffee consumption with serum lipids and lipoproteins in Japanese men. *Annals of Epidemiology, 9*(2), 121–126.

Quinlan, P., Lane, J., Moore, K., Aspen, J., Rycroft, J., & O'Brien, D. (2000). The acute physiological and mood effects of tea and coffee: the role of caffeine level. *Pharmacology Biochemistry and Behavior, 66*(1), 19–28.

Rao, S., Welcher, K., Zimmerman, B., & Stumbo, P. (1998). Is coffee a colonic stimulant? *European Journal of Gastroenterology and Hepatology, 10*(2), 113–118.

Smith, A., Thomas, M., Perry, K., & Whitney, H. (1997). Caffeine and the common cold. *Journal of Psychopharmacology, 11*(4), 319–324.

Soroko, S., Chang, J., & Barrett-Connor, E. (1996). Reasons for changing caffeinated coffee consumption: the Rancho Bernardo Study. *Journal of the American College of Nutrition, 15*(1), 97–101.

Urgert, R., & Katan, M. (1997). The cholesterol-raising factor from coffee beans. *Annual Reviews of Nutrition, 17,* 305–324.

Vogel, H. (1991). *The nature doctor.* New Canaan, CT: Keats Publishing.

Wakabayashi, K., Kono, S., Shinchi, K., Honjo, S., Todoroki, I., Sakurai, Y., Umeda, T., Imanishi, K., & Yoshizawa, N. (1998). Habitual coffee consumption and blood pressure: A study of self-defense officials in Japan. *European Journal of Epidemiology, 14*(7), 669–673.

Woodward, M., & Tunstall-Pedoe, H. (1999). Coffee and tea consumption in the Scottish Heart Health Study follow-up: conflicting relations with coronary risk factors, coronary disease, and all cause mortality. *Journal of Epidemiology and Community Health, 53*(8), 481–487.

TEA:

August, D., Landau, J., Caputo, D., Hong, J., Lee, M., & Yang, C. (1999). Ingestion of green tea rapidly decreases prostaglandin E2 levels in rectal mucosa in humans. *Cancer Epidemiology, Biomarkers & Prevention, 8*(8), 709–713.

Bingham, S., Vorster, H., Jerling, J., Magee, E., Mulligan, A., Runswick, S., & Cummings, J. (1997). Effect of black tea drinking on blood lipids, blood pressure and aspects of bowel habit. *British Journal of Nutrition, 78*(1), 41–55.

Bunker, M., & McWilliams, M. (1979). Caffeine content of common beverages. *Journal of the American Dietetic Association, 74*(1), 28–32.

Caan, B., Quesenberry, C., & Coates, A. (1998). Differences in fertility associated with caffeinated beverage consumption. *American Journal of Public Health, 88*(2), 270–274.

Dulloo, A., Duret, C., Rohrer, D., Girardier, L., Mensi, N., Fathi, M., Chantre, P., & Vandermander, J. (1999). Efficacy of a green tea extract rich in catechin polyphenols and caffeine in increasing 24–h energy expenditure and fat oxidation in humans. *American Journal of Clinical Nutrition, 70*(6), 1040–1045.

Fujiki, H., Suganuma, M., Okabe, S., Sueoka, E., Suga, K., Imai, K., Nakachi, K., & Kimura, S. (1999). Mechanistic findings of green tea as cancer preventive for humans. *Proceedings of the Society for Experimental Biology and Medicine, 220*(4), 225–228.

Halder, J., & Bhaduri, A. (1998). Protective role of black tea against oxidative damage of human red blood cells. *Biochemical and Biophysical Research Communications, 244*(3), 903–907.

Hindmarch, I., Quinlan, P., Moore, K., & Parkin, C. (1998). The effects of black tea and other beverages on aspects of cognition and psychomotor performance. *Psychopharmacology (Berl), 139*(3), 230–238.

Hindmarch, I., Rogney, U., Stanley, N., Quinlin, P., Rycroft, J., & Lane, J. (2000). A naturalistic investigation of the effects of daylong consumption of tea, coffee, and water on alertness, sleep onset and sleep quality. *Psychopharmacology, 149*(3), 203–216.

Hodgson, J., Puddey, I., Burke, V., Beilin, L., & Jordan, N. (1999). Effects on blood pressure of drinking green and black tea. *Journal of Hypertension, 17*(4), 457–463.

Kaltwasser, J., Werner, E., Schalk, K., Hansen, C., Gottschalk, R., & Seidl, C. (1998). Clinical trial on the effect of regular tea drinking on iron accumulation in genetic haemochromatosis. *Gut, 43*(5), 699–704.

Keenan, J. (1996). The Japanese tea ceremony and stress management. *Holistic Nursing Practice, 10*(2), 30–37.

Leenen, R., Roodenburg, A., Tijburg, L., & Wiseman, S. (2000). A single dose of tea with or without milk increases plasma antioxidant activity in humans. *European Journal of Clinical Nutrition, 54*(1), 87–92.

Mukhtar, H., & Ahmad, N. Green tea in chemoprevention of cancer. *Toxicological Sciences, 52*(Suppl. 2), 111–117.

Rasheed, A., & Haider, M. (1998). Antibacterial activity of *Camellia sinensis* extracts against dental caries. *Archives of Pharmacal Research, 21*(3), 348–352.

Sadakata, S., Fukao, A., & Hisamichi, S. (1992). Mortality among female practitioners of chanoyu (Japanese "tea-ceremony"). *Tohoku Journal of Experimental Medicine, 166*(4), 475–477.

Suganuma, M., Okabe, S., Sueoka, N., Sueoka, E., Matsuyama, S., Imai, K., Nakachi, K., & Fujiki, H. (1999). Green tea and cancer chemoprevention. *Mutation Research, 428*(1–2), 339–344.

Taylor, J., & Wilt, V. (1999). Probable antagonism of warfarin by green tea. *Annals of Pharmacotherapy, 33*(4), 426–428.

Van het Hof, K., Kivits, G., Weststrate, J., & Tijburg, L. (1998). Bioavailability of catechins from tea: the effect of milk. *European Journal of Clinical Nutrition, 52*(5), 356–359.

Weisburger, J. (1999). Tea and health: the underlying mechanisms. *Proceedings of the Society for Experimental Biology and Medicine, 220*(4), 271–275.

Zhao, J., Zhang, Y., Jin, X., Athar, M., Santella, R., Bickers, D., & Wang, Z. Green tea protects against psoralen plus ultraviolet A-induced photochemical damage to skin. *Journal of Investigative Dermatology, 113*(6), 1070–1075.

EPHEDRA:

Astrup, A., Madsen, J., Holst, J., & Christensen, N. (1986). The effect of chronic ephedrine treatment on substrate utilization, the sympathoadrenal activity, and energy expenditure during glucose-induced thermogenesis in man. *Metabolism, 35*(3), 260–265.

Astrup, A., Toubro, S., Cannon, S., Hein, P., & Madsen, J. (1991). Thermogenic synergism between ephedrine and caffeine in healthy volunteers: A double-blind, placebo-controlled study. *Metabolism, 40*(3), 323–329.

Bruneton, J. (1999). *Pharmacognosy: Phytochemistry medicinal plants.* Paris: Intercept Ltd.

Council for Responsible Nutrition. (2000). Ephedra study—Cantox Health Sciences International. www.crnusa.org/crncantoxreportindex.html.

Dickinson, A. (1996). FDA food advisory committee meeting on ephedra-containing dietary supplements. Washington, D.C.: Council for Responsible Nutrition.

Duke, J. (2000). Phytochemical and ethnobotanical databases. www.ars-grin.gov/cgi-bin/duke/farmacy2.pl

Gurley, B., Gardner, S., & Hubbard, M. (2000). Content versus label claims in ephedra-containing dietary supplements. *American Journal of Health-Systems Pharmacists, 57*(10), 963–969.

Gurley, B., Gardner, S., White, L., & Wang, P. L. (1998). Ephedrine pharmacokinetics after the ingestion of nutritional supplements containing *Ephedra sinica* (ma huang). *Therapeutic Drug Monitoring, 20*(4), 439–445.

Haller, C., & Benowitz, N. (2000). Adverse cardiovascular and central nervous system events associated with dietary supplements containing ephedra alkaloids. *New England Journal of Medicine, 343*(25), 1833–1838.

Hikino, H., Konno, C., Takata, H., & Tamada, M. (1980). Antiinflammatory principle of Ephedra herbs. *Chemical and Pharmaceutical Bulletin (Tokyo), 28*(10), 2900–2904.

Liu, Y., Toubro, S., Astrup, A., & Stock, M. (1995). Contribution of beta 3 adrenoceptor activation to ephedrine-induced thermogenesis in humans. *International Journal of Obesity 19*(9), 678–685.

Toubro, S., Astrup, A., Breum, L., & Quaade, F. (1993). Safety and efficacy of long-term treatment with ephedrine, caffeine, and an ephedrine/caffeine mixture. *International Journal of Obesity 17*(Suppl. 1) S69–S72.

White, L., Gardner, S., Gurley, B., Marx, M., Wang, P., & Estes, M. (1997). Pharmacokinetics and cardiovascular effects of ma-huang *(Ephedra sinica)* in normotensive adults. *Journal of Clinical Pharmacology, 37*(2), 116–122.

....

Chapter 15. Emotions and Adaptation

INTRODUCTION:

Lad, V., & Frawley, D. (1986). *The Yoga of herbs: An Ayurvedic guide to herbal medicine.* Santa Fe, NM: Lotus Press.

Pert, C. (1997). *Molecules of emotion: Why you feel the way you feel.* New York: Scribner.

Wicke, R. (1992). *Clinical handbook of herbal medicine.* (Vol. 1). Hot Springs, Montana: Rocky Mountain Herbal Institute Publications.

ST. JOHN'S WORT:

Bergin, A., & Garfield, S. (1994). *Handbook of psychotherapy and behavior change,* 4th ed. New York: John Wiley & Sons, Inc.

Gulick, R., McAuliffe, V., Holden-Wiltse, J., Crumpacker, C., Liebes, L., Stein, D., Meehan, P., Hussey, S., Forcht, J., & Valentine, F. (1999). Phase I studies of hypericin, the active compound in St. John's Wort, as an antiretroviral agent in HIV-infected adults. *Annals of Internal Medicine, 130*(6), 510–514.

Hansgen, K., Vesper, J., & Ploch, M. (1994). Multicenter double-blind study examining the antidepressant effectiveness of the *Hypericum* extract LI 160. *Journal of Geriatric Psychiatry and Neurology, 7*(S1), S15–S18.

Harrer, G., Hubner, W. D., & Podzuweit, H. (1994). Effectiveness and tolerance of the *Hypericum* extract LI 160 compared to maprotiline: A multicenter double-blind study. *Journal of Geriatric Psychiatry and Neurology, 7*(S1), S24–S28.

Hubner, W., Lande, S., & Podzuweit, H. (1994). *Hypericum* treatment of mild depressions with somatic symptoms. *Journal of Geriatric Psychiatry and Neurology, 7*(S1), S12–S14.

Lavie, G., Valentine, F., Levin, B., Mazur, Y., Gallo, G., Lavie, D., Weiner, D., & Meruelo, D. (1989). Studies of the mechanisms of action of the antiretroviral agents hypericin and pseudohypericin. *Proceedings of the National Academy of Science, 86*(15), 5963–5967.

Linde, K., Ramirez, G., Mulrow, C., Pauls, A., Weidenhammer, W., & Melchart, D. (August 3, 1996). St. John's Wort for depression—an overview and meta-analysis of randomized clinical trials. *British Medical Journal, 313,* 253–257.

Martinez, B., Kasper, S., Ruhrmann, S., & Moller, H. (1994). Hypericum in the treatment of seasonal affective disorders. *Journal of Geriatric Psychiatry and Neurology, 7* (Suppl 1), S29–33.

Piscitelli, S., Burstein, A., Chaitt, D., Alfaro, R., & Falloon, J. (2000). Indinavir concentrations and St. John's wort. *Lancet, 355*(9203), 547–548.

Shelton, R., Keller, M., Gelenberg, A., Dunner, D., Hirschfeld, R., Thase, M., Russell, J., Lydiard, R., Crits-Cristoph, P., Gallop, R., Todd, L., Hellerstein, D., Goodnick, P., Keitner, G., Stahl, S., & Halbreich, U. (2001). Effectiveness of St John's wort in major depression: a randomized controlled trial. *JAMA, 285*(15), 1978–86.

Sommer, H., & Harrer, G. (1994). Placebo-controlled double-blind study examining the effectiveness of an *Hypericum* preparation in 105 mildly depressed patients. *Journal of Geriatric Psychiatry and Neurology, 7*(S1), S9–S11.

Steinbeck, K. A., & Wernet, P. (1993). Successful long-term treatment over 40 months of HIV-patients with intravenous hypericin. [Abstract # PO-B26–2012.] *International Conference on AIDS, 9,* 470.

Suzuki, O., Katsumata, M., Oya, M., Bladt, S., & Wagner, H. (1984). Inhibition of monoamine oxidase by hypericin. *Planta Medica, 50*(3), 272–274.

Treasure, J. (Fall 2000). Herbal pharmacokinetics: A practitioner update with reference to St. John's Wort *(Hypericum perforatum)* herb-drug interactions. *Journal of the American Herbalists Guild,* 2–11.

Vitiello, B. (1999). *Hypericum perforatum* extracts as potential antidepressants. *Journal of Pharmacy and Pharmacology, 51,* 513–517.

Vorbach, E., Hubner, W., & Arnoldt, K. (1994). Effectiveness and tolerance of the *Hypericum* extract LI 160 in comparison with imipramine: Randomized double-blind study with 135 outpatients. *Journal of Geriatric Psychiatry and Neurology, 7*(S1), S19–S23.

Wagner, P., Jester, D., LeClair, B., Taylor, T., Woodward, L., & Lambert, J. (1999). Taking the edge off: Why patients choose St. John's wort. *The Journal of Family Practice, 48*(8), 615–619.

Woelk, H., Burkard, G., & Grunwald, J. (1994). Benefits and risks of the *Hypericum* extract LI 160: Drug monitoring study with 3,250 patients. *Journal of Geriatric Psychiatry and Neurology, 7*(Suppl 1), S34–S38.

KAVA:

Almeida, J., & Grimsley, E. (1996). Coma from the health food store: Interaction between kava and alprazolam. *Annals of Internal Medicine, 125*(11), 940–941.

Lebot, V., Merlin, M., & Lindstrom, L. (1997). *Kava: The pacific elixir.* New Haven, CT: Yale University Press.

Jappe, U., Franke, I., Reinhold, D., & Gollnick, H. (1998). Sebotropic drug reaction resulting from kava-kava extract therapy: A new entity? *Journal of the American Academy of Dermatology, 38*(1), 104–106.

Mathews, J., Riley, M., Fejo, L., Munoz, E., Milns, N., Gardner, I., Powers, J., Ganygulpa E., & Gununuwawuy, B. (1988). Effects of the heavy usage of kava on physical health: Summary of a pilot survey in an aboriginal community. *Medical Journal of Australia, 148*(11), 548–555.

Norton, S. (January 1998). Herbal medicines in Hawaii: From tradition to convention. *Hawaii Medical Journal, 57*, 382–386.

Schelosky, L., Raffauf, C., Jendroska, K., & Poewe, W. (1995). Kava and dopamine antagonism. *Journal of Neurology, Neurosurgery, and Psychiatry, 58*(5), 639–640.

Singh, N., & Blumenthal, M. (Spring 1997). Kava: An overview. *Herbalgram, 39*, 33–55.

Singh, N., Ellis, C., & Singh, Y. (1998). A double-blind, placebo controlled study of the effects of kava (Kavatrol) on daily stress and anxiety in adults. *Alternative Therapies in Health and Medicine, 4*(2), 97–98.

Volz, H., & Kieser, M. (1997). Kava-kava extract WS1490 versus placebo in anxiety disorders—a randomized placebo-controlled 25–week outpatient trial. *Pharmacopsychiatry 30*(1), 1–5.

PASSION FLOWER:

Bourin, M., Bougerol, T., Guitton, B., & Broutin, E. (1997). A combination of plant extracts in the treatment of outpatients with adjustment disorder with anxious mood: Controlled study versus placebo. *Fundamentals in Clinical Pharmacology, 11*(2), 127–132.

Fugh-Berman, A., & Cott, J. (1999). Dietary supplements and natural products as psychotherapeutic agents. *Psychosomatic Medicine, 61*(5), 712–728.

Speroni, E., & Minghetti, A. (1988). Neuropharmacological activity of extracts from *Passiflora incarnata. Planta Medica, 54*(6),488–491.

SIBERIAN GINSENG:

Asano, K., Takahashi, T., Miyashita, M., Muramatsu, S., Kuboyama, M., Kugo, H., & Imai, J. (1986). Effect of *Eleutheroccocus senticosus* extract on human physical working capacity. *Planta Medica,* June (3), 175–177.

Brekhman, I. & Dardymov, I. (1969). New substances of plant origin which increase nonspecific resistance. *Annual Review of Pharmacology, 9,* 419–430.

Farnsworth, N., Kinghorn, A. D., Soejarto, D., & Waller, D. (1985). Siberian ginseng *(Eleutherococcus senticosus):* Current status as an adaptogen. In *Economic and Medicinal Plant Research.* (Vol. 1). (pp.155–215). New York: Academic Press.

Foster, S., & Chongxi, Y. *Herbal emissaries: Bringing Chinese herbs to the west.* Rochester, VT: Healing Arts Press.

McRae, S. (1996). Elevated serum digoxin levels in a patient taking digoxin and Siberian ginseng. *Canadian Medical Association Journal, 155*(3), 293–295.

Medon, P. J., Ferguson, P., & Watson, C. F. (1984). Effects of *Eleutherococcus senticosus* extracts on hexobarbital metabolism in vivo and in vitro. *Journal of Ethnopharmacology, 10*(2), 235–241.

Tyler, V. (1993). *The honest herbal.* (3rd ed.). New York: Pharmaceutical Products Press.

Winther, K., Ranlov, C., Rein, E., & Mehlsen, J. (1997). Russian root (Siberian ginseng) improves cognitive functions in middle-aged people, whereas Ginkgo biloba seems effective only in the elderly. *Journal of Neurological Sciences, 150*(Suppl), S90.

Chapter 16. Mobility

INTRODUCTION:

Csikszentmihalyi, M. (1991). *Flow: The psychology of optimal experience.* New York: Harper Perennial.

Todd, M. (1937). *The thinking body.* Pennington, NJ: Princeton Book Co.

CAYENNE:

Bernstein, J. (1992). Capsaicin and substance P. *Clinics in Dermatology, 9*(4), 497–503.

Bjerring, P., & Arendt-Nielsen, L. (1990). Inhibition of histamine skin flare reaction following repeated topical applications of capsaicin. *Allergy, 45*(2), 121–125.

Capsaicin Study Group (1992). Effect of treatment with capsaicin on daily activities of patients with painful diabetic neuropathy. *Diabetes Care, 15*(2), 159–165.

Cichewicz, R., & Thorpe, P. (1996). The antimicrobial properties of chili peppers (*Capsicum* species) and their uses in Mayan medicine. *Journal of Ethnopharmacology, 52*(2), 61–70.

Cruz, F., Guimaraes, M., Silva, C., Rio, M., Coimbra, A., & Reis, M. (1997). Desensitization of bladder sensory fibers by intravesical capsaicin has long lasting clinical and urodynamic effects in patients with hyperactive or hypersensitive bladder dysfunction. *Journal of Urology, 157*(2), 585–589.

Dasgupta, P., & Fowler, C. (1997). Chilies: from antiquity to urology. *British Journal of Urology, 80*(6), 845–852.

Deal, C., Schnitzer, T., Lipstein, E., Seibold, J., Stevens, R., Levy, M., Albert, D., & Renold, F. (1991). Treatment of arthritis with topical capsaicin: a double-blind trial. *Clinical Therapeutics, 13*(3), 383–395.

Harmer, B., & Henderson, V. (1955). *Textbook of the principles and practice of nursing.* New York: The Macmillan Company.

Helme, R., & McKernan, S. (1985). Neurogenic flare responses following topical application of capsaicin in humans. *Annals of Neurology, 18*(4), 505–509.

Henry, C., & Emery, B. (1986). Effect of spiced food on metabolic rate. *Human Nutrition: Clinical Nutrition, 40*(2), 165–168.

Kang, J., Yeoh, K., Chia, H., Lee, H., Chia, Y., Guan, R., & Yap, I. (1995). Chili—protective factor against peptic ulcer? *Digestive Diseases and Sciences, 40*(3), 576–579.

Marks, J. (1989). Treatment of apocrine chromhidrosis with topical capsaicin. *Journal of the American Academy of Dermatology, 21*(2 Pt 2), 418–420.

McCarthy, G., & McCarty, D. (1992). Effect of topical capsaicin in the therapy of painful osteoarthritis of the hands. *The Journal of Rheumatology, 19*(4), 604–607.

McCarty, D., Csuka, M., McCarthy, G., & Trotter, D. (1994). Treatment of pain due to fibromyalgia with topical capsaicin: a pilot study. *Seminars in Arthritis and Rheumatism, 23*(6, S3), 41–47.

Nelson, C. (1994). Heal the burn: pepper and lasers in cancer pain therapy. *Journal of the National Cancer Institute, 86*(18), 1381–1382.

Ottariano, S. (1999). *Medicinal herbal therapy.* Portsmouth, New Hampshire: Nicolin Fields Publishing.

Tominack, R. (1987). Capsicum and capsaicin—a review: case report of the use of hot peppers in child abuse. *Clinical Toxicology, 25*(7), 591–601.

Visudhiphan, S., Poolsuppasit, S., Piboonnukarintr, O., & Tumliang, S. (1982). The relationship between high fibrinolytic activity and daily capsicum ingestion in Thais. *The American Journal of Clinical Nutrition, 35*(6), 1452–1458.

Watson, C., Evans, R., Watt, V., & Birkett, N. (1988). Post-herpetic neuralgia: 208 cases. *Pain, 35*(3), 289–297.

Watson, C., Evans, R., & Watt, V. (1989). The post-mastectomy pain syndrome and the effect of topical capsaicin. *Pain, 38*(2), 177–186.

Weeks-Shaw, C. (1914). *A textbook of nursing.* New York: D. Appleton and Company.

Willard, T. (1991). *The Wild Rose scientific herbal.* Calgary: Wild Rose College of Natural Healing.

Yeoh, K., Kang, J., Yap, I., Guan, R., Tan, C., Wee, A., & Teng, C. (1995). Chili protects against aspirin-induced gastroduodenal mucosal injury in humans. *Digestive Diseases and Sciences, 40*(3), 580–583.

Yoshioka, M., Lim, K., Kikuzato, S., Kiyonaga, A., Tanaka, H., Shindo, M., & Susuki, M. (1995). Effects of red-pepper diet on the energy metabolism in men. *Journal of Nutrition Science and Vitaminology 41*(6), 647–656.

ROSEMARY:

Aruoma, O., Halliwell, B., Aeschbach, R., & Loligers, J. (1992). Antioxidant and prooxidant properties of rosemary constituents: carnosol and carnosic acid. *Xenobiotic, 22*(2), 257–268.

Aqel, M. (1992). A vascular smooth muscle relaxant effect of *Rosmarinus officinalis. International Journal of Pharmacognosy, 30*(4), 281–288.

Burkhard, P., Burkhardt, K., Haenggeli, C., & Landis, T. (1999). Plan-induced seizures: reappearance of an old problem. *Journal of Neurology, 246*(8), 667–670.

De Laszlo, H., & Henshaw, P. (May 7, 1954). Plant materials used by primitive peoples to affect fertility. *Science, 119,* 626–630.

Fernandez, L., Duque, S., Sanchez, I., Quinones, D., Rodriguez, F., & Garcia-Abujeta, J. (1997). Allergic contact dermatitis from rosemary *(Rosmarinus officinalis L.). Contact Dermatitis, 37*(5), 248–249.

Holmes, P. (1998/1999). Rosemary oil. *The International Journal of Aromatherapy, 9*(2), 62–66.

Huang, M. T., Ho, C. T., Wang, Z., Ferraro, T., Lou, Y., Stauber, K., Ma, W., Georgiadis, C., Laskin, J., & Conney, A. (1994). Inhibition of skin tumorigenesis by rosemary and its constituents carnosol and ursolic acid. *Cancer Research, 54*(3), 701–708.

Inatani, R., Nakatani, N., & Fuwa, H. (1983). Antioxidative effect of the constituents of rosemary and their derivatives. *Agricultural and Biological Chemistry, 47*(3), 521–528.

Kovar, K., Gropper, B., Friess, D., & Ammon, H. (1987). Blood levels of 1,8–cineole and locomotor activity of mice after inhalation and oral administration of rosemary oil. *Planta Medica, 53*(4), 315–318.

Lemonica, I., Damasceno, D., & di-Stasi, I. (1996). Study of the embryotoxic effects of an extract of rosemary. *Brazilian Journal of Medical and Biological Research, 29*(2), 223–227.

Singletary, K., MacDonald, C., & Wallig, M. (1996). Inhibition by rosemary and carnosol of 7, 12–dimethylbenz[a]anthracene (DMBA)- induced rat mammary tumorigenesis and in vivo Dmba-Dna adduct formation. *Cancer Letters, 104*(1), 43–48.

ARNICA:

Brinker, F., & Alstat, E. (1995). *Eclectic dispensatory of botanical therapeutics,* v. 2. Sandy, Oregon: Eclectic Medical Publications.

Campbell, A. (1976). Two pilot controlled trials of *Arnica Montana. British Homeopathic Journal, 65,* 154–158.

Ernst, E., & Pittler, M. (1998). Efficacy of homeopathic arnica: a systematic review of placebo-controlled clinical trials. *Archives of Surgery, 133*(11), 1187–1190.

Harmer, B., & Henderson, V. (1955). *Textbook of the principles and practice of nursing.* New York: The Macmillan Company.

Kaziro, G. (1984). Metronidazole (Flagyl) and *Arnica Montana* in the prevention of post-surgical complications, a comparative placebo controlled clinical trial. *British Journal of Oral and Maxillofacial Surgeons, 22*(1), 42–49.

McIvor, E. (1973). *Arnica Montana:* a clinical trial following surgery or trauma. *Journal of the American Institute of Homeopathy, 66*(2), 81–84.

Moore, M. (1993). *Medicinal plants of the pacific west.* Santa Fe: Red Crane Books.

Ottariano, S. (1999). *Medicinal herbal therapy.* Portsmouth, NH: Nicolin Fields Publishing.

Vickers, A., Fisher, P., Smith, C., Wyllie, S., & Rees, R. (1998). Homeopathic arnica 30X is ineffective for muscle soreness after long-distance running: a randomized, double-blind, placebo-controlled trial. *The Clinical Journal of Pain, 14*(3), 227–231.

Willard, T. (1991). *The wild rose scientific herbal.* Calgary: Wild Rose College of Natural Healing.

CINNAMON:

Akira, T., Tanaka, S., & Tabata, M. (1986). Pharmacological studies on the antiulcerogenic activity of Chinese cinnamon. *Planta Medica* (6), 440–443.

Chang, H., & But, P. (Eds.). (1986). *Pharmacology and applications of Chinese materia medica,* v.1. Singapore: World Scientific.

de Waal, M. (1980). *Medicinal herbs in the Bible.* York, Maine: Weiser Books.

Imparl-Radosevich, J., Deas, S., Polansky, M., Baedke, D., Ingebritsen, T., Anderson, R., & Graves, D. (1998). Regulation of PTP-1 and insulin receptor kinase by fractions from cinnamon: implications for cinnamon regulation of signaling of insulin signaling. *Hormone Research, 50*(3), 177–182.

Khan, A., Bryden, N., Polansky, M., & Anderson, R. (1990). Insulin potentiating factor and chromium content of selected foods and spices. *Biological Trace Element Research, 24*(3), 183–188.

Kubo, M., Shiping, M., Wu, J., & Matsuda, H., (1996). Anti-inflammatory activities of 70% methanolic extract from *Cinnamomi* cortex. *Biological and Pharmaceutical Bulletin, 19*(8), 1041–1045.

Lamey, P., Rees, T., & Forsyth, A. (1990). Sensitivity reaction to the cinnamonaldehyde component of toothpaste. *British Dental Journal, 168*(3), 115–118.

Meding, B. (1993). Skin symptoms among workers in a spice factory. *Contact Dermatitis, 29*(4), 202–205.

Pilapil, V. (1989). Toxic manifestation of cinnamon oil ingestion in a child. *Clinical Pediatrics, 28*(6), 276.

Quale, J., Landman, D., Zaman, M., Burney, S., & Sathe, S. (1996). *In vitro* activity of *Cinnamomum zeylanicum* against azole resistant and sensitive *Candida* species and a pilot study of cinnamon for oral candidiasis. *American Journal of Chinese Medicine, xxiv*(2), 103–109.

Rex, J., Rinaldi, M., & Pfaller, M. (1995). Resistance of *Candida* species to fluconazole. *Antimicrobial Agents and Chemotherapy, 39*(1), 1–8.

Schwartz, R. (1990). Cinnamon Oil: Kids use it to get high. *Clinical Pediatrics, 29*(30), 196.

Tanaka, S., Yoon, Y., Fukui, H., Tabata, M., Akira, T., Okano, K., Iwai, M., Iga, Y., & Yokoyama, K. (1989). Antiulcerogenic compounds isolated from Chinese cinnamon. *Planta Medica, 55*(3), 245–248.

Weeks-Shaw, C. (1914). *A textbook of nursing.* New York: D. Appleton and Company.

Westra, W., McMurray, J., Califano, J., Flint, P., & Corio, R. (1998). Squamous cell carcinoma of the tongue associated with cinnamon gum use: a case report. *Head and Neck, 20*(5), 430–433.

WINTERGREEN:

No additional references.

....

Chapter 17. Lifestyle Choices

INTRODUCTION:

Lewin, L. (1998). *Phantastica: A classic survey on the use and abuse of mind-altering plants.* Rochester, VT: Park Street Press.

Mack, A., & Joy, J. (2000). *Marijuana as medicine? The science beyond the controversy.* United States Institute of Medicine. Washington, D.C.: National Academy Press.

McLellan, A., Lewis, D., O'Brien, C., & Kleber, H. (2000). Drug dependence, a chronic medical illness: Implications for treatment, insurance, and outcomes evaluation. *Journal of the American Medical Association, 284*(13), 1689–1695.

Metzner, R. (1998). Hallucinogenic drugs and plants in psychotherapy and shamanism. *Journal of Psychoactive Drugs, 30*(4), 333–341.

Murphy-Parker, D., & Martinez, R. (2000). *The history of treatment of alcohol and drug problems in The United States of America: How is it different from the United Kingdom?* Paper presented at the 16th Annual Conference of the Association of Nurses in Substance Abuse. Manchester, England, April 26, 2000.

Physician Leadership on National Drug Policy. (1998). Physician leadership on national drug policy finds addiction treatment works. *Journal of the American Medical Association, 279*(15), 1149–1150.

Soleas, G., Diamandis, E., & Goldberg, D. (1997). Wine as a biological fluid: History, production, and role in disease prevention. *Journal of Clinical Laboratory Analysis, 11*(5), 287–313.

Sullivan, E. J. (1995). *Nursing care of clients with substance abuse.* St. Louis: Mosby.

MILK THISTLE:

Bhatia, N., Zhao, J., Wolf, D., & Agarwal, R. (1999). Inhibition of human carcinoma cell growth and DNA synthesis by silibinin, an active constituent of milk thistle: comparison with silymarin. *Cancer Letters, 147*(1–2), 77–84.

Bode, J., Schmidt, U., & Durr, H. (1977). Silymarin for the treatment of acute viral hepatitis. [Zur Behandlung der akuten Birushepatitis mit Silymarin.] *Medizinische Klinik, 72*(Nr. 12), 513–518.

Bombardelli, E., Spelta, M., Della Loggia, R., Sosa, S., & Tubaro, A. (1991). Aging skin: Protective effect of silymarin-PHYTOSOME®. *Fitoterapia, LXII*(2), 115–122.

Di Bisceglie, A., Order, S., Klein, J., Waggoner, J., Sjogren, M., Kuo, G., Houghton, M., Choo, Q., & Hoofnagle, J. (1991). The role of chronic viral hepatitis in hepatocellular carcinoma in the United States. *American Journal of Gastroenterology, 86*(3), 335–338.

Ferenci, P., Dragosics, B., Dittrich, H., Frank, H., Benda, L., Lochs, H., Meryn, S., Base, W., & Schneider, B. (1989). Randomized controlled trial of silymarin treatment in patients with cirrhosis of the liver. *Journal of Hepatology, 9*(1), 105–113.

Flora, K., Hahn, M., Rosen, H., & Benner, K. (1998). Milk thistle *(Silybum marianum)* for the therapy of liver disease. *The American Journal of Gastroenterology, 93*(2), 139–143.

Lorenz, D., Mennicke, W., & Behrendt, W. (1982). Elimination of silymarin by cholecystectomied patients. Biliary elimination after multiple oral doses. *Planta Medica, 45*(4), 216–223.

Magliulo, E., Gagliardi, B., & Fiori, G. (1978). The effect of silymarin in the treatment of acute viral hepatitis. [Zur Wirkung von Silymarin bei der Behandlung der akuten Virushepatitis]. *Medizinische Klinik, 73*(Nr. 28/29), 1060–1065.

Palasciano, G., Portincasa, P., Palmieri, V., Ciani, D., Vendemiale, G., & Altomare, E. (1994). The effect of silymarin in plasma levels of malon-dialdehyde in patients receiving long-term treatment with psychotropic drugs. *Current Therapeutic Research, 55*(5), 537–545.

Pares, A., Planas, R., Torres, M., Caballeria, J., Viver, J., Acero, D., Panes, J., Rigau, J., Santos, J., & Rodes, J. (1998). Effects of silymarin in alcoholic patients with cirrhosis of the liver: Results of a controlled, double-blind, randomized and multicenter trial. *Journal of Hepatology, 28*(4), 615–621.

Plomteux, G., Albert, A., & Heusghem, C. (1977). Hepatoprotector action of silymarin in human acute viral hepatitis. *IRCS Medical Science, 5,* 259.

Shear, N., Malkiewicz, I., Klein, D., Koren, G., Randor, S., & Neuman, M. (1995). Acetaminophen-induced toxicity to human epidermoid cell line A431 and hepatoblastoma cell line Hep G2, in vitro, is diminished by silymarin. *Skin Pharmacology, 8*(6), 279–291.

Vailati, A., Aristia, L., Sozze, E., Milani, F., Inglese, V., Galenda, P., Bossolo, P., Ascari, E., Lampertico, M., Comis, S., & Marena, C. (1993). Randomized open study of the dose-effect relationship of a short course of IdB 1016 in patients with viral or alcoholic hepatitis. *Fitoterapia, LXIV*(3), 219–228.

Velussi, M., Cernigoi, A., DeMonte, A., Dapas, F., Caffau, C., & Zilli, M. (1997). Long-term (12 months) treatment with an antioxidant drug (silymarin) is effective on hyperinsulinemia, exogenous insulin need and malondialdehyde levels in cirrhotic diabetic patients. *Journal of Hepatology, 26*(4), 871–879.

Zi, X., & Agarwal, R. (1999). Modulation of mitogen-activated protein kinase activation and cell cycle regulators by the potent skin cancer preventive agent silymarin. *Biochemical and Biophysical Research Communications, 263*(2), 528–536.

TOBACCO:

American Academy of Otolaryngology—Head and Neck Surgery Foundation. *Poisoning our children: The perils of secondhand smoke,* [Video]. Bay Productions.

Bartholow, R. (1878). *A practical treatise on material medica and therapeutics.* New York: Appleton and Company.

Benowitz, N., & Henningfield, J. (1994). Establishing a nicotine threshold for addiction. *The New England Journal of Medicine, 331*(2), 123–1125.

Benowitz, N. (1997). Treating tobacco addiction—nicotine or no nicotine? *The New England Journal of Medicine, 337*(17), 1230–1231.

Child, L. M. (1997). *The family nurse.* (Reprint of 1837 text.) Bedford, MA: Applewood Books.

Cinciripini, P., Hecht, S., Henningfield, J., Manley, M., & Kramer, B. (1997). Tobacco addiction: implication for treatment and cancer prevention. *Journal of the National Cancer Institute, 89*(24), 1852–1867.

Crellin, J., & Pilpott, J. (1990). *Herbal medicine past and present.* Durham, NC: Duke University Press.

Doll, R. (1999). Risk from tobacco and potentials for health gain. *International Journal of Tuberculosis and Lung Disease, 3*(2), 90–99.

Fiore, M., Smith, S., Jorenby, D., & Baker, T. (1994). The effectiveness of the nicotine patch for smoking cessation: A meta-analysis. *Journal of the American Medical Association, 271*(24), 1940–1947.

Fowler, J., Volkow, N., Wang, G., Pappas, N., Logan, J., MacGregor, R., Alexoff, D., Shea, C., Schlyer, D., Wolf, A., Warner, D., Zezulkova, I., & Cilento, R. (1996). Inhibition of monoamine oxidase B in the brains of smokers. *Nature, 379*(6567), 733–736.

Glantz, S., & Parmley, W. (1991). Passive smoking and heart disease. *Circulation, 83*(1), 1–12.

Glantz, S., & Parmley, W. (1995). Passive smoking and heart disease: Mechanisms and risk. *Journal of the American Medical Association, 273*(13), 1047–1053.

Hemenway, D., Solnick, S., & Colditz, G. (1993). Smoking and suicide among nurses. *American Journal of Public Health, 83*(2), 249–251.

International Council of Nurses. Retrieved November, 2000, from the International Council of Nurses website on the World Wide Web: icn.ch/pssmoking99.htm

Lewis, C. (1996). *Green nature human nature: The meaning of plants in our lives.* Chicago: University of Illinois Press.

Mitchell, B., Sobel, H., & Alexander, M. (1999). The adverse health effects of tobacco and tobacco-related products. *Primary Care 26*(3), 463–498.

Report of the U.S. Surgeon General. (1988). The Health Consequences of Smoking: Nicotine Addiction. Retrieved November 2000, from the World Wide Web: www.cdc.gov/tobacco/sgr_1988.htm

Report of the U.S. Surgeon General. (1964). Reducing the Health Consequences of Smoking. Retrieved November 2000, from the World Wide Web: www.cdc.gov/tobacco/sgr/sgr_1964/sgr64.htm

Riley, W., Barenie, J., Woodard, C., & Mabe, P. (1996). Perceived smokeless tobacco addiction among adolescents. *Health Psychology, 15*(4), 289–292.

Seffrin, J. (1998). The politics of addiction: Status of the tobacco settlement. *Cancer Journal for Clinicians, 48*(2), 81–82.

Slade, J. (1992). The tobacco epidemic: Lessons from history. *Journal of Psychoactive Drugs, 24*(2), 99–109.

Shytle, D., Silver, A., & Sanberg, P. (1996). Nicotine, tobacco and addiction: Correspondence. *Nature, 384*(6604), 18–19.

U.S. Centers for Disease Control and Prevention. (1994). Guidelines for school health programs to prevent tobacco use and addiction. *Journal of School Health, 64*(9), 353–360.

U.S. Centers for Disease Control and Prevention. (May 23, 1997). Facts about cigar smoking. Fact Sheet. Retrieved November 2000, from the World Wide Web: www.cdc.gov/od/oc/media/fact/cigars.htm

Wood, G., & Bache, F. (1839). *Dispensatory of the United States of America* (4th ed.). Philadelphia: Grigg & Elliot.

Wynder, E. (1988). Tobacco and health: a review of the history and suggestions for public health. *Public Health Reports, 103*(1), 8–18.

KUDZU:

Foster, S., & Chongxi,Y. (1992). *Herbal emissaries: Bringing Chinese herbs to the West.* Rochester, VT: Healing Arts Press.

Kaufman, P., Duke, J., Brielmann, H., Boik, J., & Hoyt, J. (1997). A comparative survey of leguminous plants as sources of the isoflavones, genistein and daidzein: Implications for human nutrition and health. *Journal of Alternative and Complementary Medicine, 3*(1), 7–12.

Keung, W., & Vallee, B. (1997). Kudzu root: An ancient Chinese source of modern antidipsotropic agents. *Phytochemistry, 47*(4), 499–506.

Kushi, M. (1993). *Macrobiotic home remedies.* Tokyo: Japan Publications.

Lin, R., & Li, T. (1998). Effects of isoflavones on alcohol pharmacokinetics and alcohol-drinking behavior in rats. *American Journal of Clinical Nutrition, 68*(Suppl), 1512S-1515S.

Lin, R., Guthrie, S., Xie, C., Mai, K., Lee, D., Lumeng, L., & Li, T. (1996). Isoflavonoid compounds extracted from *Pueraria lobata* suppress alcohol preference in a pharmacogenetic rat model of alcoholism. *Alcoholism: Clinical and Experimental Research, 20*(4), 659–663.

Shebek, J., & Rindone, J. (2000). A pilot study exploring the effect of Kudzu root on the drinking habits of patients with chronic alcoholism. *The Journal of Alternative and Complementary Medicine, 6*(1), 45–48.

Xie, C., Lin, R., Antony, V., Lumeng, L., Li, T., Mai, K., Liu, C., Wang, Q., Zhao, Z., & Wang, G. (1994). Daidzin, an antioxidant isoflavonoid, decreases blood alcohol levels and shortens sleep time induced by ethanol intoxication. *Alcoholism: Clinical and Experimental Research, 18*(6), 1443–1447.

MARIJUANA:

Andreasson, S., Engstrom, A., Allebeck, P., & Rydberg, U. (1987). Cannabis and schizophrenia. *Lancet, 2*(8574), 1483–1486.

Bates, M., & Blakely, T. (1999). Role of cannabis in motor vehicle crashes. *Epidemiology Review, 21*(2), 222–232.

Block, R., & Ghoneim, M. (1993). Effects of chronic marijuana use in human cognition. *Psychopharmacology, 110*(1–2), 219–228.

Block, R., Erwin, W., Farinpour, R., & Braverman, K. (1998). Sedative, stimulant, and other subjective effects of marijuana: Relationships to smoking techniques. *Pharmacology Biochemistry and Behavior, 59*(2), 405–412.

Block, R., O'Leary, D., Ehrhardt, J., Augustinack, J., Ghoneim, M., Arndt, S., & Hall, J. (2000a). Effects of frequent marijuana use on brain tissue volume and composition. *Neuroreport, 11*(3), 491–496.

Block, R., O'Leary, D., Hichwa, R., Augustinack, J., Ponto, L., Ghoneim, M., Arndt, S., Ehrhardt, J., Hurtig, R., Watkins, G., Hall, J., Nathan, P., & Andreasen, N. (2000b). Cerebellar hypoactivity in frequent marijuana users. *Neuroreport, 11*(4), 749–753.

Budney, A., Novy, P., & Hughes, J. (1999). Marijuana withdrawal among adults seeking treatment for marijuana dependence. *Addiction, 94*(9), 1311–1321.

Doblin, R., & Kleiman, M. (1991). Marijuana as antiemetic medicine: a survey of oncologists' experiences and attitudes. *Journal of Clinical Oncology, 9*(7), 1314–1319

Fant, R., Heishman, S., Bunker, E., & Pickworth, W. (1998). Acute and residual effects of marijuana in humans. *Pharmacology, Biochemistry, and Behavior, 60*(4), 777–784.

Flom, M., Adams, A., & Jones, R. (1975). Marijuana smoking and reduced pressure in human eyes: drug action or epiphenomenon? *Investigative Ophthalmology, 14*(1), 52–55.

Green K. (1998). Marijuana smoking vs cannabinoids for glaucoma therapy. *Archives of Ophthalmology, 116*(11), 1433–1437.

Heishman, S., Stitzer, M., & Yingling, J. (1989). Effects of tetrahydrocannabinol content on marijuana smoking behavior, subjective reports, and performance. *Pharmacology, Biochemistry, and Behavior, 34*(1), 173–179.

Leirer, V., Yesavage, J., & Morrow, D. (1991). Marijuana carry-over effects on aircraft pilot performance. *Aviation, Space, and Environmental Medicine, 62*(3), 221–227.

Linszen, D., Dingemans, P., & Lenior, M. (1994). Cannabis abuse and the course of recent-onset schizophrenic disorders. *Archives of General Psychiatry, 51*(4), 273–279.

Merrill, J., Kleber, H., Schwartz, M., Liu, H., & Lewis, S. (1999). Cigarettes, alcohol, marijuana, other risk behaviors, and American youth. *Drug and Alcohol Dependence, 56*(3), 205–212.

Morningstar, P. (1985). *Thandai and Chilam:* Traditional Hindu beliefs about the proper uses of cannabis. *Journal of Psychoactive Drugs, 17*(3), 141–165.

Negrete, J., Knapp, W., Douglas, D., & Smith, W. B. (1986). Cannabis affects the severity of schizophrenic symptoms: results of a clinical survey. *Psychological Medicine, 16*(3), 515–520.

Novins, D., & Mitchell, C. (1998). Factors associated with marijuana use among American Indian adolescents. *Addiction, 93*(11), 1693–1702.

O'Leary, D., Block, R., Flaum, M., Schultz, S., Boles Ponto, L., Watkins, G., Hurtig, R., Andreasen, N., & Hichwa, R. (2000). Acute marijuana effects on rCBF and cognition: a PET study. *Neuroreport, 11*(17), 3835–3841.

Pierson, L. (1983). The Lynn Pierson Therapeutic Research Program, Behavioral Health Sciences Division, New Mexico State Department of Health. Retrieved November, 2000, from the World Wide Web: www.commongroup.net/olsen/MEDICAL/pierson. html

Shiono, P., Klebanoff, M., Nugent, R., Cotch, M., Wilkins, D., Rollins, D., Carey, J., Behrman, R. (1995). The impact of cocaine and marijuana use on low birth weight and preterm birth: a multicenter study. *American Journal of Obstetrics and Gynecology, 172*(1 Pt 1), 19–27.

Solowij, N. (1999). Long-term effects of cannabis on the central nervous system. In H. Kalant, et al. (Eds.), *The health effects of cannabis* (pp. 193–265). Toronto: Centre for Addiction and Mental Health.

Tashkin, D., Coulson, A., Clark, V., Simmons, M., Bourque, L., Duann, S., Spivey, G., & Gong, H. (1987). Respiratory symptoms and lung function in habitual heavy smokers of marijuana alone, smokers of marijuana and tobacco, smokers of tobacco alone, and nonsmokers. *American Review of Respiratory Disease, 135*(1), 209–216.

Touw, M. (1981). The religious and medicinal uses of cannabis in China, India, and Tibet. *Journal of Psychoactive Drugs 13*(1), 23–24.

Vincent, B., McQuiston, D., Einhorn, L., Nagy, C., & Brames, M. (1983). Review of cannabinoids and their antiemetic effectiveness. *Drugs, 25*(Suppl 1), 52–62.

Chapter 18. Restoration

INTRODUCTION:

DeVita, V., Hellman, S., & Rosenberg, S. (1997). *Cancer principles and practice of oncology* (5th ed.). Philadelphia: Lippincott-Raven.

Null, G. (1995). The Oxygen battlefield. *Townsend Letter for Doctors,* Feb/March, 48–56.

Thatte, U., Bagadey, S., & Dahanukar, S. (2000). Modulation of programmed cell death by medicinal plants. *Cellular and Molecular Biology, 46*(1), 199–214.

RED CLOVER:

Cassady, J., Zennie, T., Chae, Y., Ferin, M., Portuondo, N., & Baird, W. (1988). Use of mammalian cell culture benzo(a)pyrene metabolism assay for the detection of potential anticarcinogens from natural products: Inhibition of metabolism by biochanin A, an isoflavone from *Trifolium pratense L. Cancer Research, 48*(22), 6257–6261.

Fitzpatrick, F. (1954). Plant substances active against *Mycobacterium tuberculosis. Antibiotics and Chemotherapy, 4*(5), 528–536.

Fotsis, T., Pepper, M., Adlercreutz, H., Hase, T., Montesano, R., & Schweigerer, L. (1995). Genistein, a dietary ingested isoflavonoid, inhibits cell proliferation and in vitro angiogenesis. *Journal of Nutrition, 125*(Suppl 3), 790S-797S.

Kaegi, E. (1998). Unconventional therapies for cancer: 1. Essiac. *Canadian Medical Association Journal, 158*(7), 897–902.

Kelly, R., Hay, R., & Shackell, G. (1979). Formononetin content of 'Grasslands Pawera' red clover and its oestrogenic activity to sheep. *New Zealand Journal of Experimental Agriculture, 7,* 131–134.

Kloss, J. (1939). *Back to Eden.* Santa Barbara, CA: Woodbridge Press.

Naiman, I. (1999). *Cancer salves.* Santa Fe, NM: Seventh Ray Press.

Nestel, P., Pomeroy, S., Kay, S., Komesaroff, P., Behrsing, J., Cameron, J., & West, L. (1999). Isoflavones from red clover improve systemic arterial compliance but not plasma lipids in menopausal women. *The Journal of Clinical Endocrinology and Metabolism, 84*(3), 895–898.

Tamayo, C., Richardson, M., Diamond, S., & Skoda, I. (2000). The chemistry and biological activity of herbs used in Flor-essence™ herbal tonic and Essiac™. *Phytotherapy Research, 14*(1), 1–14.

Zava, D., Dollbaum, C., & Blen, M. (1998). Estrogen and progestin bioactivity of foods, herbs, and spices. *Proceedings of the Society for Experimental Biology and Medicine, 217*(3), 369–378.

REISHI:

Chiu, S., Wang, Z., Leung, T., & Moore, D. (2000). Nutritional value of *Ganoderma* extract and assessment of its genotoxicity and anti-genotoxicity using the comet assays of mouse lymphocytes. *Food and Chemical Toxicology, 38*(2–3), 173–178.

Eo, S., Kim, Y., Lee, C., & Han, S. (1999). Antiviral activities of various water and methanol soluble substances isolated from *Ganoderma lucidum. Journal of Ethnopharmacology, 68*(1–3), 129–136.

Flaws, B. (1994). *Imperial secrets of health and longevity.* Boulder, CO: Blue Poppy Press.

Foster, S., & Chongxi, Y. (1992). *Herbal emissaries: Bringing Chinese herbs to the west.* Rochester, VT: Healing Arts Press.

Hobbs, C. (1996). *Medicinal mushrooms: An Exploration of tradition, healing, and culture.* Loveland, CO: Interweave Press.

Kasahara, Y., & Hikino, H. (1987). Central actions of *Ganoderma lucidum. Phytotherapy Research, 1*(1), 17–21.

Lieu, C-W., Lee, S-S., & Wang, S-Y. (1992). The effect of *Ganoderma lucidum* on induction of differentiation in leukemic U937 cells. *Anticancer Research, 12*(4), 1211–1216.

Thomas, C. L. (Ed.). (1997). *Taber's cyclopedic medical dictionary* (18th ed.). Philadelphia: F.A. Davis.

TURMERIC:

Ammon, H., & Wahl, M. (1990). Pharmacology of *Curcuma longa. Planta Medica, 57*, 1–7.

Charles, V., & Charles, S. (1992). The use and efficacy of *Azadirachta indica* ADR('NEEM') and *Curcuma longa* ('turmeric') in scabies. *Tropical and Geographical Medicine, 44*(1–2), 178–181.

DeVita, V., Hellman, S., & Rosenberg, S. (1997). *Cancer principles and practice of oncology* (5th ed.). Philadelphia: Lippincott-Raven.

Eigner, D., & Scholz, D. (1999). *Ferula asa-foetida* and *Curcuma longa* in traditional medical treatment and diet in Nepal. *Journal of Ethnopharmacology, 67*, 1–6.

Hoppe, J. (2000). Turmeric. *Medical Herbalism, 11*(4), 1,3–5.

Ishizaki, C., Oguro, T., Yoshida, T., Wen, C., Sueki, H., & Iijima, M. (1996). Enhancing effect of ultraviolet A on ornithine decarboxylase induction and dermatitis evoked by 12–o-tetradecanoylphorbol-13–acetate and its inhibition by curcumin in mouse skin. *Dermatology, 193*(4), 311–317.

Judd, N. (1997). *Laau lapaau: A geography of Hawaiian herbal healing.* Honolulu, HI: University of Hawaii. [unpublished]

Krishnaswamy, K., & Polasa, K. (1995). Diet, nutrition & cancer—the Indian scenario. *Indian Journal of Medical Research, 102*, 200–209.

Kuttan, R., Bhanumathy, P., Nirmala, K., & George, M. (1985). Potential anticancer activity of turmeric (*Curcuma longa*). *Cancer Letters, 29*(2), 197–203.

Kuttan, R., Sudheeran, P., & Josph, C. (1987). Turmeric and curcumin as topical agents in cancer therapy. *Tumori, 73*(1), 29–31.

Nagabhushan, M., & Bhide, S. (1992). Curcumin as an inhibitor of cancer. *Journal of the American College of Nutrition, 11*(2), 192–198.

Naiman, I. (1999). *Cancer salves.* Santa Fe, NM: Seventh Ray Press.

Polasa, K., Raghuram, T., Krishna, T., & Krishnaswamy, K. (1992). Effect of turmeric on urinary mutagens in smokers. *Mutagenesis, 7*(2), 107–109.

Satoskar, R., Shah, S., & Shenoy, S. (1986). Evaluations of anti-inflammatory property of curcumin (diferuloyl methane) in patients with postoperative inflammation. *International Journal of Clinical Pharmacology, Therapy and Toxicology, 24*(12), 651–654.

Shah, B., Nawaz, Z., Pertani, S., Roomi, A., Mahmood, H., Saeed, S., & Gilani, A. (1999). *Biochemical Pharmacology, 58*(7), 1167–1172.

Thresiamma, K., George, J., & Kuttan, R. (1996). Protective effect of curcumin, ellagic acid and bixin on radiation toxicity. *Indian Journal of Experimental Biology, 34*(9), 845–847.

Venkatesan, N., & Chandrakasan, G. (1995). Modulation of cyclophosphamide-induced early lung injury by curcumin, an anti-inflammatory antioxidant. *Molecular and Cellular Biochemistry, 142*(1), 79–87.

MISTLETOE:

American Cancer Society. (1983). Unproven methods of cancer management: Iscador. *CA: A Cancer Journal for Clinicians, 33*(3), 186–188.

Bradley, G., & Clover, A. (1989). Apparent response of small cell lung cancer to an extract of mistletoe and homeopathic treatment. *Thorax, 44*(12), 1047–1048.

Chernyshov, V., Omelchenko, L., Heusser, P., Slukvin, I., Vodyanik, M., Galazyuk, L., Vykhovanets, E., Pochinok, T., Chernyshov, A., Gumenyuk, M., Schaefermeyer, H., & Schaefermeyer, G. (1997). Immunomodulatory actions of *Viscum album* (Iscador) in children with recurrent respiratory disease as a result of Chernobyl nuclear accident. *Complementary Therapies in Medicine, 5,* 141–146.

Ellis, P. (1994). *The Druids.* Grand Rapids, MI: William B. Eerdmans Publishing Company.

Evans, M., & Preece, A. (1973). *Viscum album*—a possible treatment for cancer? *Bristol Medico-Chirurgical Journal, 88*(325), 17–20.

Gorter, R. W. (1998). *Iscador: Mistletoe preparations used in anthroposophically extended cancer treatment.* Basel, Switzerland: Verlag fur Ganzheits Medizin.

Gorter, R. W., Van Wely, M., Stoss, M., & Wollina, U. (1998). Subcutaneous infiltrates induced by injection of mistletoe extracts (Iscador). *American Journal of Therapeutics, 5*(3), 181–187.

Gorter, R. W., Van Wely, M., Reiff, M., & Stoss, M. (1999). Tolerability of an extract of European mistletoe among immunocompromised and healthy individuals. *Alternative Therapies, 5*(6), 37–48.

Hajto, T. (1986). Immunomodulating effects of Iscador: a *Viscum album* preparation. *Oncology, 43*(Suppl 1), 51–65.

Kaegi, E. (1998). Unconventional therapies for cancer: 3. Iscador. *Canadian Medical Association Journal, 158*(9), 1157–1159.

Kienle, G. S. (1999). The story behind mistletoe: a European remedy from anthroposophical medicine. *Alternative Therapies, 5*(6), 34–36.

Park, J., Hyun, C., & Shin, H. (1999). Cytotoxic effects of the components in heat-treated mistletoe *(Viscum album). Cancer Letters, 139*(2), 207–213.

Stirpe, F., Sandvig, K., Olsnes, S., & Pihl, A. (1982). Action of viscumin, a toxic lectin from mistletoe, on cells in culture. *Journal of Biological Chemistry, 257*(22), 13271–13277.

Thatte, U., Bagadey, S., & Dahanukar, S. (2000). Modulation of programmed cell death by medicinal plants. *Cellular and Molecular Biology, 46*(1), 199–214.

GREATER CELANDINE:

Benninger, J., Schneider, H., Schuppan, D., Kirchner, T., & Hahn, E. (1999). Acute hepatitis induced by greater celandine *(Chelidonium majus). Gastroenterology, 117,* 1234–1237.

Naiman, I. (1999). *Cancer salves.* Santa Fe, NM: Seventh Ray Press.

Sotomayor, E. M., Rao, K., Lopez, D. M., & Liepins A. (1992). Enhancement of macrophage tumourcidal activity by the alkaloid derivative Ukrain: In vitro and in vivo studies. *Drugs Experimental Clinical Research, XVIII*(Suppl.), 5–11.

Vavreckova, C., Gawlik, I., & Muller, K. (1996). Benzophenanthridine alkaloids of Chelidonium majus; II. potent inhibitory action against the growth of human keratinocytes. *Planta Medica, 62*(6), 491–494.

Voltchek, I., Kamyshentsev, M., Lavinsky, Y., Nowicky, J., Medvedev, Y., & Litvinchuk, L. (1996). Comparative study of the cytostatic effects of Oliphen and Ukrain. *Journal of Chemotherapy, 8*(2), 144–146.

Voltchek I., Liepens A., Nowicky, J., & Brozosko, W. J. (1996). Potential therapeutic efficacy of Ukrain (NSC 631570) in AIDS patients with Kaposi's sarcoma. *Drugs Experimental Clinical Research XXII*(3–4–5), 283–286.

GINKGO:

Buhner, S. (1996). *Sacred plant medicine.* Boulder, CO: Roberts Rinehart Publishers.

Cesarani, A., Meloni, F., Alpini, D., Barozzi, S., Verderio, L., & Boscani, P. (1998). Ginkgo biloba (EGb 761) in the treatment of equilibrium disorders. *Advances in Therapy, 15*(5), 291–304.

Christen, Y. (2000). Oxidative stress and Alzheimer disease. *American Journal of Clinical Nutrition, 71*(Suppl), 621S-9S.

Diamond, B., Shiflett, S., Feiwel, N., Matheis, R., Noskin, O., Richards, J., & Schoenberger, N. (2000). Ginkgo biloba extract: Mechanisms and clinical indications. *Archives of Physical Medicine and Rehabilitation, 81*(5), 668–678.

Doraiswamy, P., & Steffens, D. (1998). Combination therapy for early Alzheimer's disease: What are we waiting for? *Journal of the American Geriatric Society, 46*(10), 1322–1324.

Fowler, J., Wang, G., Volkow, N., Logan, J., Franceschi, D., Franceschi, M., MacGregor, R., Shea, C., Garza, V., Liu, N., & Ding, Y. (2000). Evidence that Ginkgo biloba extract does not inhibit MAO A and B in living human brain. *Life Sciences, 66*(9), 141–146.

Garg, R., Nag, D., & Agrawal, A. (1995). A double blind placebo controlled trial of ginkgo biloba extract in acute cerebral ischemia. *Journal of the Association of Physicians in India, 43*(11), 760–763.

Holgers, K., Axelsson, A., & Pringle, I. (1994). Ginkgo biloba extract for the treatment of tinnitus. *Audiology, 33*(2), 85–92.

Kleijnen, J., & Knipschild, P. (1992). Ginkgo biloba for cerebral insufficiency. *British Journal of Clinical Pharmacy, 34*(4), 352–358.

Le Bars, P., Katz, M., Berman, N., Itil, T., Freedman, A., & Schatzberg, A. (1997). A placebo-controlled, double-blind, randomized trial of an extract of ginkgo biloba for dementia. *Journal of the American Medical Association, 278*(16), 1327–1332.

Matthews, M. (1998). Association of ginkgo biloba with intracerebral hemorrhage. *Neurology 50*(6), 1933.

Maurer, K., Ihl, R., Dierks, T., & Frolich, L. (1997). Clinical efficacy of ginkgo biloba special extract EGb 761 in dementia of the Alzheimer type. *Journal of Psychiatric Research, 31*(6), 645–655.

Peters, H., Kieser, M., & Holscher, U. (1998). Demonstration of the efficacy of ginkgo biloba special extract EGb 761 on intermittent claudication—A placebo-controlled, double-blind multicenter trial. *Vasa, 27*(2), 106–110.

Rosenblatt, M., & Mindel, J. (1997). Spontaneous hyphema associated with ingestion of ginkgo biloba extract. *New England Journal of Medicine, 336*(15), 1108.

BILBERRY:

Carmignani, G. (1983). The alteration of microcirculation in cortico-dependent asthmatic patients and their treatment. *Lotta Contro La Tuberc e Malattie Polm Soc, 53*(2–3), 732–736.

Cristoni, A., & Magistretti, M. (1987). Antiulcer and healing activity of *Vaccinium myrtillus* anthocyanosides. *Farmaco, 42*(2), 29–43.

Duke, J. (1999). *Dr. Duke's essential herbs*. Emmaus, PA: Rodale.

Grismondi, G. (1980). Treatment of pregnancy-induced phlebopathies. *Estratto da Minerva Ginecologica, 32,* 1–14.

Morazzoni, P., & Bombardelli, E. (1996). *Vaccinium myrtillus L. Fitoterapia, 57*(1), 3–29.

Orsucci, P., Rossi, M., Sabbatini, G., Menci, S., & Berni, M. (1983). Treatment of diabetic retinopathy with anthocyanosides: a preliminary report. *Clinica Oculistica e Patologia Oculare, 4*(5), 377–381.

Paronzini, S., & Indemini, P. (1988). Modifications of the macular recovery tests in normal subjects after administration of anthocyanosides. *Bollettino di Oculistica, 67*(Suppl. 4), 185–188.

Perossini, M., Guidi, G., Chiellini, S., & Siravo, D. (1987). Diabetic and hypertensive retinopathy therapy with *Vaccinium myrtillus* anthocyanosides (Tegens) double blind placebo-controlled clinical trial. *Annali di Ottalmologia e Clinica Oculistica, CXIII*(12), 1173–1190.

Pezzangora, V., Barina, R., De Stefani, R. & Rizzo, M. (1984). Medical therapy with bilberry anthocyanosides in patients submitted to hemorrhoidectomy. *Gazzetta Medica Italiana—Archivio Scienze Mediche, 143,* 405–409.

Teglio, L., Mazzanti, C., Tronconi, R., & Guerresi (1987). *Vaccinium myrtillus* anthocyanosides (Tegens) in the treatment of venous insufficiency of lower limbs and acute piles in pregnancy. *Quaderni di Clinica Ostetrica e Ginecologica, 42*(May-June), 221–231.

Tori, A., & D'Errico, F. (1980). *Vaccinium myrtillus* anthocyanosides in the treatment of stasis venous diseases of the lower limbs. *Gazzetta Medica Italiana, 139,* 217–224.

Chapter 19. Learning More

Canadian Nurses Association (accessed website January, 2001). (www.cna-nurses.ca/pages/issuestrends/nrgnow/compl_thrp.htm).

De Klemm, C. (1991). Medicinal plants and the law. In Akerele, O., Heywood, V., & Synge, H. (Eds.). *The conservation of medicinal plants* (pp. 259–271). Cambridge: Cambridge University Press.

Haller, J. (2000). *The people's doctors*. Carbondale and Edwardsville, IL: Southern Illinois University Press.

Jaeschke, R., Cook, D., & Sackett, D. (1992). The potential role of single-patient randomized controlled trials (N-of-1 RCTs) in clinical practice. *Journal of the American Board of Family Practice, 5*(2), 227–229.

Larson, E., Ellsworth, A., & Oas, J. (1993). Randomized clinical trials in single patients during a 2–year period. *Journal of the American Medical Association, 270*(22), 2708–2712.

Libster, M. (1999). Guidelines for selecting a medical herbalist for consultation and referral: consulting a medical herbalist. *Journal of Alternative and Complementary Medicine, 5*(5), 457–462.

Libster, M. (2001). *Demonstrating care: The art of integrative nursing*. Albany: Delmar/Thomson Learning.

Margolin, A., Avants, S. K., & Kleber, H. (1998). Investigating alternative medicine therapies in randomized controlled trials. *Journal of the American Medical Association, 280*(18), 1626–1628.

McCabe, P. (2000). Naturopathy, Nightingale, and nature cure: a convergence of interests. *Complementary Therapies in Nursing and Midwifery, 6*(1), 4–8.

Nazarko, L. (1995). The therapeutic uses of cranberry juice. *Nursing Standard, 9*(34), 33–35.

Ondrizek, R., Chan, P., Patton, W., & King, A. (1999). An alternative medicine study of the herbal effects on the penetration of zona-free hamster oocytes and the integrity of sperm deoxyribonucleic acid. *Fertility and Sterility, 71*(3), 517–522.

Chapter 20. Staying in Contact with the Garden

Andrews, H., & Roy, C. (1986). *Essentials of the Roy Adaptation Model.* Norwalk, CT: Appleton-Century-Crofts.

Christopher, J. (1987). *Every woman's herbal.* Springville, UT: Christopher Publications.

Duke, J. (1997). *The green pharmacy.* Emmaus, PA: Rodale Press.

Gips, K. (1990). *Flora's dictionary: The Victorian language of herbs and flowers.* Chagrin Falls, OH: TM Publications.

Howard, J., & Ramsell, J. (1990). *The original writings of Edward Bach.* Essex, England: C.W. Daniel Co.

Jenkins, V. S. (1994). *The lawn: A history of an American obsession.* Washington, D.C.: Smithsonian Institution Press.

Lewis, C. (1996). *Green nature/human nature: The meaning of plants in our lives.* Urbana and Chicago: University of Illinois Press.

Libster, M. (2001). *Demonstrating care: The art of integrative nursing.* Albany: Delmar/Thomson Learning.

Merriam Webster. (1999). *Merriam-Webster's Collegiate Dictionary* (10th ed.). Springfield, MA: Merriam-Webster, Inc.

Newman, M. (1994). *Health as expanding consciousness.* New York: National League for Nursing Press.

Nightingale, F. (1957). *Notes on nursing: What it is, and what it is not.* Philadelphia: Lippincott.

Pert, C. (1997). *Molecules of emotion: Why you feel the way you feel.* New York: Scribner.

Tompkins, P., & Bird, C. (1973). *The secret life of plants: A fascinating account of the physical, emotional, and spiritual relations between plants and man.* New York: Harper & Row Publishers.

Watson, J. (1999). *Postmodern nursing and beyond.* Edinburgh: Churchill Livingstone.

Glossary

Abortifacient   A substance that causes abortion.

Adaptogen   A substance that increases overall, nonspecific resistance to stress.

Aerial   The parts of a plant above the ground.

Alterative   A substance that gradually changes the metabolism and elimination of the body to improve general health. Often referred to as a tonic. Formerly known as blood cleansers.

Annual   A plant that completes its life cycle in one season.

Anthroposophical Medicine   A traditional European system of natural healing based on the spiritual science teachings of Rudolf Steiner.

Antihelminthic   A substance that is antiparasitic.

Aphrodisiac   A substance that increases sexual desire.

Aromatic Bitter   A substance that stimulates appetite through its scent.

Astringent   A substance that causes a contraction of tissue or mucous membranes and reduces the secretion of mucus.

Bitters   A substance (with a bitter taste) used to stimulate appetite and aid the liver in detoxification.

Blood Cleanser   An older term used in herbalism referring to herbs that increase overall vitality of the body and detoxify the blood of impurities due to poor diet, overeating, constipation, improper breathing, and drinking impure water to name a few. The term used today is alterative.

Carminative   A substance that relieves flatulence.

Catarrh   Chronic inflammation of the nose and mucous membranes.

Cathartic   A substance that induces bowel evacuation.

Cholagogue   A substance that promotes flow of bile.

Counterirritant   Remedies which by irritation of the skin affect underlying conditions such as inflammation in organs and tissues.

Cytochrome P450   A protein similar to hemoglobin that is found in liver cells and certain organs and is active in the metabolism of steroid hormones and in the detoxification of chemical substances.

Deficiency (condition)   Terminology used in traditional Chinese medicine to describe a symptom sign pattern that potentially includes fatigue, thin tongue coat, weak pulse, shallow breathing, passive appearance, and quiet voice.

Demulcent   Substances that soothe by providing a protective coating and relieving inflammation of the membranes.

Diaphoretic   A substance that promotes perspiration.

Eclectics   The American botanical physicians of the mid to late nineteenth and early twentieth centuries.

Embrocation A type of calming, rhythmical massage using herbal oil or lotion.

Emetic A substance that causes vomiting.

Emmenagogue Promotes flow of menses.

Escharotic A caustic acid or base substance that causes a chemical reaction with the tissues of the body manifesting as heat, itching, burning, and break down of the tissue involved.

Excess (condition) Term used in traditional Chinese medicine to describe a symptom sign pattern potentially including thick tongue coat, strong pulse, forceful motion, loud speech, outgoing behavior.

Febrifuge A substance that reduces fever.

Five Element Theory One of the earliest theories to develop in traditional Chinese medicine.

Functional Foods Foods to which medicinal herbs or other substances, such as vitamins, have been added to provide an extra nutrition boost. For example, bone-strengthening calcium added to orange juice.

Galactagogue A substance that increases the flow of breast milk.

German Commission E A regulatory agency in Germany that evaluates the therapeutic activities of herbs sold for medicinal purposes.

Ghee Clarified butter used in Ayurveda.

Homeopathy A system of medicine that uses potentized remedies and is based on the Law of Similars, which holds that a substance that produces a set of symptoms in a healthy person can cure that set of symptoms in a sick person.

LD$_{50}$ Median lethal dose. See description in chapter 4.

Macrobiotics Attributed to a Japanese man named George Oshawa, a system of healing that stresses the influence of dietary habits on health and disease.

Materia Medica A description of substances used in preparing medicines.

Meridian Energy pathways related to bodily organs.

Nervine A substance that is healing to the nervous system and relieves nervous tension.

Perennial A plant that comes back yearly.

Pilule A small pill.

Potentize Shaking and dilution of homeopathic remedies.

Rubefacient A substance that is used externally to increase blood supply to the skin.

Soporific A substance that causes sleep.

Tonic A substance that improves overall general health.

Tonify To improve or increase.

Vermifuge A substance that expels parasites from the body.

Vulnerary A substance that promotes wound healing.

Wildcraft To harvest healing plants from their natural habitat.

APPENDIX
Additional
Herb Resources*

Websites

Herb Research Foundation www.herbs.org
American Botanical Council www.herbalgram.org
Medical Herbalism www.medherb.com
Napralert www.cas.org/ONLINE/DBSS/napralertss.html
Bach Flower Remedies: Bach Centre www.bachcentre.com
  Mount Vernon, Bakers Lane, Sotwell, Oxon, OX10 0PZ, UK
  Telephone: +44 (0) 1491 834678 Fax: +44 (0) 1491 825022
Look up herbs at www.wholenurse.com
HealthWorld Online www.healthy.net
Herbal Hall www.herb.com
The Center for World Indigenous Studies www.cwis.org
Edgar Cayce Remedies www.caycecures.com
Horticultural Therapy Links
  www.oznet.ksu.edu/horttherapy/htlinks.htm

Videos

Delmar's Integrative Herb Guide for Nurses CD-ROM
  Albany, NY (© 2002 Delmar)
  www.delmar.com
Herbal Preparations and Natural Therapies by Debra Nuzzi St. Claire
  www.lifebalm.com/bio.html (Click on Christopher Publications and
  at the next page click on "other authors" and scroll to Nuzzi
  St. Claire.)
  Or call 1-800-372-8255, or E-mail publications@snh.cc

*For herb education resources, see chapter 19.

Plant Conservation and Gardening

The Ethnomedicine Preservation Project
44 Rim Road, Boulder, CO 80302
1-800-435-1670
The Findhorn Foundation
The Park
Findhorn, Forres IV36 3TZ, Moray, Scotland
Phone: +44 (0)1309 690311
Fax: +44 (0)1309 691301
www.findhorn.org

Miscellaneous

Sheila Humphrey, BSc (Botany), RN, IBCLC
Herbs and Lactation Consultant
Box 224
Marine on St. Croix, MN 55047
Phone: 651-433-3028
Fax: 651-433-5104
Die Filderklinik (An Anthroposophical medicine hospital)
Träger: Filderklinik Förderverein e.V.
Im Haberschlai 7, 70794 Filderstadt
Phone: 07 11/7 70 30
Fax: 0711/7 70 34 84
The International Federation of Aromatherapists
46 Dalkeith Road
London, England SE 21, 8LS

Index

agonists, 805
AIDS. *See* acquired immunodeficiency
    syndrome
airelle, 773–781. *See* bilberry
air yam, 183–192. *See* wild yam
ajenjibre, 489–500. *See* ginger
ajo, 285–295. *See* garlic
akaakai, 317–325. *See* onion
alcohol, 22, 578
    aldehyde, 21
    cytochrome P-450 and, 74
    decrease in desire and, kudzu and, 696
    diluted, 96
    glyceric, 97
    ketone, 21
    as solvent, 94
alcohol abuse, 664–666
    liver disease and, milk thistle and, 671
alcohol extract, 95–96, 97
    how to make, 95–96
alcoholism
    cayenne and, 611
    evening primrose and, 158
    kudzu and, 692
    milk thistle and, 669
    wild yam and, 185
alcohol poisoning, kudzu and, 692
alcohol tincture, 95–96, 97
    how to make, 95–96
aldehyde alcohols, 21
aldehydes, 22
ale, 411–419. *See* hops
alertness, mental
    coffee and, 528
    mustard and, 172
    rosemary and, 625
alfalfon, 715–723. *See* red clover
algae, brown, 248
algycone molecule, 21
al-Hawi, 124
alkaloids, 20, 21
    belladonna, 71
    pyrrolizidine, 21, 63
    terpenoid, 21
allergies
    ephedra and, 551
    ginger and, 491
    horseradish and, 483
    nasal, kudzu and, 693
    respiratory, passion flower and, 590
    soy for prevention of, 207
    wild yam and, 185
alles zutraut, 405
All-Heal tea, 80
alliin, 790
Allium macrostemon, 317–325. *See* onion
Allium pstulosum L., 317–325. *See* onion
Allium sativum, 285–295, 790–791. *See*
    garlic
All-Union Institute of Herbs and
    Aromatherapy, 125
Alma Ata Declaration of 1978, 55–56
aloe, 21, 22, 55, 124, 126, **338f**, **339–348**
    age spots and, 340
    biomedical evidence, 341–344
    cautions, 345–346
    culinary use of, 340–341
    cultural use of, 339
    digestion, 343
    immune response, 343

    integrative insight, 346
    mechanism of action of, 343–344
    nursing evidence, 346
    nurturing the nurse-plant relationship,
        348
    patient interaction, 348
    plant description, 339
    skin care, **338f, 339–348**
    therapeutic applications, 347
    use for children, 345
    use in herbalism, 341
    use in pregnancy or lactation, 344–345
Aloe Barbadensis Miller, 339–348. *See* aloe
aloe-emodin, 344
Aloe Latex, 347
Aloe perfoliata L. var. *vera*, 339–348. *See*
    aloe
aloes, 339–348. *See* aloe
aloe vera, 339–348. *See* aloe
Aloe vera, 339–348. *See* aloe
aloe vera gel, 342, 378
aloe vera leaf plasters, 103
Aloexylon, 339–348. *See* aloe
aloin, 344
alterative, 711
    elder as, 278
    greater celandine as, 756
    milk thistle as, 670
    red clover as, 716
    in restoration, 711
    in skin care, 329
alternate arrangement of leaves, 17f
altitude, plant growth and, 84
altitude sickness
    ginkgo and, 764
    reishi and, 726
    Siberian ginseng and, 598
alu methi, 195–202. *See* fenugreek
Amanita mushroom poisoning, treatment
    and, milk thistle and, 676
amantilla, 385–395. *See* valerian
amber, 563–575. *See* St. John's wort
ambulation, 605
amebic dysentery, tea and, 540
amenorrhea
    angelica and, 228
    black cohosh and, 218
    mistletoe and, 745
    sage and, 297
    yarrow and, 354
American Academy of Acupuncture &
    Traditional Chinese Medicine, 798
American Botanical Council, 796
American College
    of Nurse Midwives (ACNM), 222–223
    of Traditional Chinese Medicine, 798
American cranberry, 443–449. *See* cranberry
American elderberry, 275–283. *See* elder
American ginseng, 518
American Herbalists Guild, 796
American Museum of Natural History, 25
American Nursing Federation, 792
American Revolutionary War, 5
American School of Herbalism, 798
Amish community, 58
amoebic infections, garlic and, 287
Amoracia rusticana, 14, 481–487. *See*
    horseradish
amsania, 549–558. *See* ephedra
anal fissures, goldenseal and, 254

Raynaud's, bilberry and, 775
rheumatoid. *See* rheumatoid arthritis
artichokes, 674
Arvigo, Rosita, 85
asafetida, emulsion of, 28
asarum, 149
Asclepius, 399
ascorbic acid, 29
Asian ginseng, 517–525. *See* ginseng
Asian use, 116–118
  of aloe, 339
  of angelica, 227–229
  of black cohosh, 217–218
  of cayenne, 609
  of cinnamon, 645–646
  of coffee, 527
  of cranberry, 443
  of elder, 275
  of ephedra, 549–550
  of fenugreek, 195
  of garlic, 285
  of German chamomile, 397
  of ginger, 489–490
  of ginkgo, 763–764
  of ginseng, 517–518
  of greater celandine, 755
  of hops, 411
  of horseradish, 481
  of kelp, 241
  of kudzu, 691–692
  of lavender, 147
  of lemon, 503
  of marijuana, 699–700
  of mistletoe, 743
  of mustard, 168–169
  of onion, 317
  of psyllium, 451
  of red clover, 715
  of reishi, 725
  of rose, 361–362
  of rosemary, 623
  of sage, 297
  of Siberian ginseng, 597
  of soy, 205–206
  of tea, 539
  of turmeric, 733
  of valerian, 385
  of wild yam, 183–184
  of yarrow, 351–352
Asian valerian, 387
aspirin, 37, 49, 80
  medieval, 137–144. *See* feverfew
asthma, 10, 57
  cayenne and, 611
  coffee and, 528
  ephedra and, 551
  evening primrose and, 158
  garlic and, 287
  ginger and, 491
  ginseng and, 519
  lavender and, 149
  passion flower and, 590
  reishi and, 726
  sage and, 300
  saw palmetto and, 468
  soy and, 207
  tobacco and, 681
  wild yam and, 185, 186
astragalus, 92
Astragalus membranicus, 92

astringent, 20
  calendula as, 331
  cayenne as, 611
  cinnamon as, 647
  cranberry as, 443
  rose as, 364
  rosemary as, 623–624
  sage as, 300
  St. John's wort as, 563, 564, 568
  tea as, 540
  witch hazel as, 374
astringent taste, 90
astrologic data, 89
atherosclerosis
  bilberry and, 774
  kelp and, 241
  onion and, 318
  reishi and, 726
athletes, 514
  ephedra and, 551
  Siberian ginseng and, 598
atomizer, essential oil, German chamomile, 406
atony of large intestine, aloe and, 341
atropine, 71
At the Will of the Body, 43
aubergines, 72
Australian use, 121
  of German chamomile, 398
  of kava, 578
  of kelp, 241
  of red clover, 715
  of wild yam, 184
autotrophic nutrition, 14
ava, 577–586. *See* kava
ava pepper, 577–586. *See* kava
Avena sativa, 431–438. *See* oat
avenin, 432
Avicenna, 30, 33, 124, 125, 364
Avogadro's number, 96
awa, 577–586. *See* kava
Ayurveda, 34, 50, 90, 94, 123, 559
Ayurvedic medicine, penicillin of, 699–710.
    See marijuana
Ayurvedic system, 75–76

B
babuna, 397–408. *See* German chamomile
babunag, 397–408. *See* German chamomile
babunaj, 397–408. *See* German chamomile
babunphul, 397–408. *See* German chamomile
Bach, Edward, 806
bachelor's buttons, 137–144. *See* feverfew
Bach flower remedies, 806–807
back
  compress to, German chamomile, 406
  stiff
    black cohosh and, 219
    kudzu and, 692
  tension in, black cohosh and, 219
  tightness in, kudzu and, 693
backache
  cayenne and, 612
  kava and, 578
back pain
  arnica and, 637
  castor oil packs and, 102
  coffee and, 528
  cranberry and, 444
  low. *See* low back pain

bacterial diseases of skin, German
    chamomile and, 400
bacterial dysentery, tea and, 540
bacterial infections
    echinacea and, 265
    garlic and, 287
    hops and, 413
bactericide, lavender as
bad breath, rosemary and, 625
bai jie zi, 169–178. *See* mustard
balance, 91
    traditional Chinese medicine (TCM) and,
    116
baldness, arnica and, 637
Ballard, Martha, 39
balneology, 630
balsam, 420
balsunt, 563–575. *See* St. John's wort
Baltic use. *See* Russian/Baltic use
banda, 743–752. *See* mistletoe
banya, 125
barbaloin, 344
barefoot doctors, 31–32
bark
    cascara sagrada, 463
    cinnamon, 645–653. *See* cinnamon
    decoction of, for topical use, witch hazel,
    378
basil, 90, 92, 477
bassant, 563–575. *See* St. John's wort
bath
    foot. *See* foot bath
    full. *See* full bath
    how to make, 107–108
    sitz. *See* sitz bath
bazaar medicines, 124
bean, calabar, 122
bearberry, 440
Bechamp, Antoine, 250
bed sores
    aloe and, 339
    arnica and, 637
    calendula and, 332, 335
    witch hazel and, 374
bed-wetting, kava and, 579
beech, brown, 645–653. *See* cinnamon
beer, 411–419. *See* hops
beeswax, 105
beet juice, 39
benign tumors, kelp and, 241
belladonna alkaloids, 71
Benton, Mrs., 81
benzene residues, rose absolute and, 365
benzodiazepines
    similar effect, kava and, 580
    withdrawal from, valerian and, 387
benzoin, tincture of, 45, 105
    aloe and, 341
benzophenanthridine alkaloid (BPA), 757
berberine, 256
Berberis vulgaris, 469
bereavement, rose and, 365
bergamot oil, 540
berries, hawthorn, 90
beverage teas, 92
bhang, 699–710. *See* marijuana
bhanga, 699–710. *See* marijuana
bhat, 205–215. *See* soy
Bickerdyke, Mary Ann, 39, 258
biennials, roots of, 15

bier, 411–419. *See* hops
Bifidobacteria, 542
bilberry, **772f, 773–781**
    biomedical evidence, 775–777
    cautions, 778
    culinary use of, 774
    cultural use of, 773–774
    elimination, 776
    integrative insight, 779
    mechanism of action of, 776–777
    mobility, 776
    nursing evidence, 778–779
    nurturing the nurse-plant relationship,
    781
    patient interaction, 780–781
    plant description, 773
    restoration, **772f, 773–781**
    skin care, 776
    therapeutic applications, 779–780
    use for children, 777–778
    use in herbalism, 774–775
    use in pregnancy or lactation, 777
bile, humors and, 33
biliary colic, wild yam and, 184
biliary flow
    cascara sagrada and, 460
    coffee and, 528
bioflavonoids, rosehip and, 364
biomedical evidence, 126–127, 810
    aloe, 341–344
    angelica, 231–232
    arnica, 637–639
    bilberry, 775–777
    black cohosh, 220–221
    calendula, 333–334
    cascara sagrada, 460–461
    cayenne, 612–615
    cinnamon, 648–649
    coffee, 528–529
    cranberry, 444–446
    echinacea, 265–267
    elder, 278–279
    ephedra, 551–552
    evening primrose, 159–161
    of fenugreek, 197–198
    feverfew, 138–140
    garlic, 288–290
    German chamomile, 400–402
    ginger, 492–495
    ginkgo, 765–766
    ginseng, 519
    goldenseal, 255–256
    greater celandine, 756–757
    hops, 413–415
    horseradish, 483
    kava, 579–581
    kelp, 241–244
    kudzu, 693–694
    lavender, 149–151
    lemon, 505–507
    lemon balm, 423–424
    marijuana, 702–705
    milk thistle, 671–674
    mistletoe, 745–747
    mustard, 172
    oat, 433–434
    onion, 319–320
    passion flower, 590–591
    psyllium, 452–454
    red clover, 716–717

blood sugar, elevated
  bilberry and, 774, 778
  fenugreek and, 197, 198
  garlic and, 287
  milk thistle and, 675
  insulin and, 180
blueberries, 773–781
  European, 773–781. *See* bilberry
blue cohosh, 217
blurred vision, black cohosh and, 220
boils
  echinacea and, 265
  fenugreek and, 197
  goldenseal and, 254
  hops and, 413
bone density, decreased, soy and, 207
bone fractures, arnica and, 637
bones, strengthening, reishi and, 726
borage, 158
Boswellia carterii, 106
botany, 11–24
  acids, 20–21
  acid substances, 23
  alkaloids, 21
  carbohydrates, 21
  essential oils, 22
  flowers, 19–20, 19f
  glycosides, 21–22
  growth patterns and plant designs,
    11–20
  latex, 22
  plant constituents and active medicinal
    principles, 20–23
  plant parts, 12–20
  resins, 22
  roots, 14–16, 15f
  seeds, 12–14, 13f
  sensory experience and plant personality,
    23–24
  shoot system, 16–18, 16f, 17f, 18f
  volatile oils, 22
bowel disorders, rose and, 364
bowels, pain in, horseradish and, 482
bowel spasms, wild yam and, 185
boxberry, 655–662. *See* wintergreen
BPA. *See* benzophenanthridine alkaloid
BPH, saw palmetto and, 468
Brahman, 123
brain inflammation, kudzu and, 693
brain injury, St. John's wort and, 565
branches, 16
bran supplement, 54
Brassica alba, 169–178. *See* mustard
Brassica juncea, 169–178. *See* mustard
Brassica nigra, 169–178. *See* mustard
Brassica oleracea L., 103
bread as poultice, 103
breast cancer
  green tea and, 539
  hormone replacement therapy and,
    180
  kelp and, 240, 244
  mistletoe and, 745–746
  red clover and, 716
  rosemary and, 626
  turmeric and, 735
  soy for prevention of, 207
breast milk
  fenugreek and, 83
  herbs benefits through, 83

breast milk inhibition
  bilberry and, 774
  sage and, 300
  tobacco and, 684
breast milk, increasing production
  black cohosh and, 218
  hops and, 415
  kudzu and, 692
  milk thistle and, 675
  wintergreen tea and, 657
breasts
  cancer. *See* breast cancer
  engorged, lactation and, green cabbage
    leaf plasters and, 103
  inflamed, witch hazel and, 374
  saw palmetto and, 468
breath
  bad, rosemary and, 625
  shortness of. *See* shortness of breath
breathing, difficult. *See* difficult breathing
broad-leaf sage, 297–304. *See* sage
bronchial conditions
  onion and, 319
  red clover and, 716
bronchial secretions
  elder and, 278
  onion and, 319
bronchial tubes, fenugreek and, 197
bronchitis
  arnica and, 637
  black cohosh and, 219
  echinacea and, 265
  lemon and, 505
  mustard and, 171
  saw palmetto and, 468
  thymol and, 308
broom of the brain, 147–155. *See* lavender
brown algae, 248
brown beech, 645–653. *See* cinnamon
brown mustard, 169–178. *See* mustard
bruises
  arnica and, 636, 637
  German chamomile and, 400
  hops and, 413
  lavender and, 148
  mustard and, 171
  St. John's wort and, 564, 565
  witch hazel and, 374
Buckle, Jane, 106–107
budshur, 549–558. *See* ephedra
bugbane, 217–225. *See* black cohosh
bugwort, 217–225. *See* black cohosh
Bulgarian rose oil, 5, 364
Bundy, J.H., 460
bunions, onion and, 319
burdock, 16
burn plant, 339–348. *See* aloe
burns
  aloe and, 341
  calendula and, 332, 333
  chamomile and, 402
  echinacea and, 263
  elder and, 278
  fenugreek and, 197
  ginger and, 491
  kelp and, 240
  lavender and, 148, 149
  oat and, 432
  onion and, 319
  red clover and, 716

chamomile, 73, 93, 390, 397–403. *See* German chamomile
  hops and, 413
  passion flower and, 590
  Roman, 399
  valerian and, 387
chamomile essential oil, 399
chamomile salve, 128
chamomile tea, 128, 399
Chamomilla recutita, 397–408. *See* German chamomile
chaparral, 65
charas, 699–710. *See* marijuana
charcoal
  coffee, 528, 533, 534, 535
  for poultice, 103
chaste tree, saw palmetto and, 469
checkerberry, 655–662. *See* wintergreen
chefs, 477
chelerythrine, 757
chelidon, 756
chelidonine, 757
Chelidonium majus, 755–761. *See* greater celandine
che qian zi, 451–457. *See* psyllium
cherry, wild, 39
chest
  arnica and, 637
  lemon compress and, 508–509
  rose and, 364
chest pain, reishi and, 726
chewa, 549–558. *See* ephedra
chewing tobacco, 680
childbirth
  after childbirth
    chamomile and, 398
    cinnamon and, 649
    goldenseal and, 253
    hops and, 415
    oat and, 432
    rosemary and, 627
    witch hazel and, 374
  during childbirth
    arnica and, 636
    black cohosh and, 219, 220
    cinnamon and, 646
    fenugreek and, 195
    sage and, 298
    thyme and, 308
    wild yam and, 185
    yarrow and, 352
children, 79–80, 128–129
  use of aloe and, 345
  use of angelica and, 232–233
  use of arnica and, 639–640
  use of bilberry and, 777–778
  use of black cohosh and, 221–222
  use of calendula and, 335
  use of cascara sagrada and, 462
  use of cayenne and, 616
  use of cinnamon and, 650
  use of coffee and, 532
  use of cranberry and, 447
  use of echinacea and, 268
  use of elder and, 279–280
  use of ephedra and, 553
  use of evening primrose and, 162
  use of fenugreek and, 199
  use of feverfew and, 141
  use of garlic and, 291

use of German chamomile and, 403–404
use of ginger and, 496
use of ginkgo and, 767
use of ginseng and, 522
use of goldenseal and, 257
use of greater celandine and, 758
use of hops and, 415–416
use of horseradish and, 484
use of kava and, 581–582
use of kelp and, 244
use of kudzu and, 694–695
use of lavender and, 151
use of lemon balm and, 425
use of lemon and, 507
use of marijuana and, 706
use of milk thistle and, 674–675
use of mistletoe and, 748
use of mustard and, 173
use of oat and, 435
use of onion and, 321
use of passion flower and, 592
use of psyllium and, 454–455
use of red clover and, 718
use of reishi and, 728
use of rose and, 367
use of rosemary and, 628
use of sage and, 301
use of saw palmetto and, 471–472
use of Siberian ginseng and, 600
use of soy and, 210–211
use of St. John's wort and, 569
use of tea and, 543–544
use of thyme and, 310–311
use of tobacco and, 684
use of turmeric and, 737
use of valerian and, 390
use of wild yam and, 188
use of wintergreen and, 658–659
use of witch hazel and, 376
use of yarrow and, 356
chili
  African, 609–620. *See* cayenne
  Mexican, 609–620. *See* cayenne
chili pepper, 609–620. *See* cayenne
chills
  cranberry and, 444
  mustard and, 172
Chinese angelica, 227–237. *See* angelica
Chinese cinnamon, 645–653. *See* cinnamon
Chinese ginseng, 517–525. *See* ginseng
Chinese herbal medicine, traditional, 798–799
Chinese mustard, 169–178. *See* mustard
Chinese tea, 539–547. *See* tea
chistotel bolshoy, 755–761. *See* greater celandine
chittem bark, 459–465. *See* cascara sagrada
chlorinated soda for poultice, 103
chlorophyll, 7–10, 7f, 45
chlorophyll a, intravenous, 8–9
chlorophyllin, 9
chlorophyllin ointment, 8
choke cherry wine, 666, 667
cholagogue, angelica as, 230
choler, humors and, 33
cholera
  ginger and, 491
  infantile, evening primrose and, 158
  lemon and, 505
  mustard and, 172

douche
  kava as, 584
  red clover as, 716
  wintergreen as, 657
  witch hazel as, 374
Dr. James Duke's Medical Botany Course,
    795
Dremaide Aloe, 342
dribbling, saw palmetto and, 468
dropsies of the heart, coffee and, 528
drowsy intoxication, kava and, 579
drug abuse, 663–665
drug-herb interactions, 74
drug identification number (DIN), 72
drugs, illicit, in urine, masking, goldenseal
    and, 255
dry extract, St. John's wort, 574
dry normalized extract
  containing 30% kavapyrones, 584
  saw palmetto, 474
dry skin, oat and, 432
Duke, Jim, 68, 804–805
dullness, general, rosemary and, 625
duodenum disorders, cascara sagrada and,
    460
dwarf bilberry, 773–781. See bilberry
dysentery
  bilberry and, 774
  evening primrose and, 158
  ginger and, 491
  ginseng and, 519
  goldenseal and, 254
  tea and, 540
  witch hazel and, 374
  yarrow and, 354
dysmenorrhea
  angelica and, 228
  black cohosh and, 218
  calendula and, 331, 333
  mistletoe and, 745
  passion flower and, 590
  sage and, 300
  thyme and, 308
  turmeric and, 733
  wild yam and, 185
dyspepsia
  black cohosh and, 218
  cascara sagrada and, 460
  cayenne and, 611
  evening primrose and, 158
  German chamomile and, 400
dyspnea, mistletoe and, 745
dysuria, kava and, 579

E
ear
  diseases of, black cohosh and, 219
  pain in, rose and, 364
  ringing in, black cohosh and, 220
earache
  cayenne and, 610
  chamomile and, 403
  elder and, 277
  garlic and, 287
  goldenseal and, 254
  hops and, 412
  kava and, 584
  marijuana and, 702
  onion and, 317, 318

passion flower and, 589
tobacco and, 681
turmeric and, 733
Earl Gray tea, 540
ear oil, garlic-mullein flower, 295
East Indian use, 123–124
  of aloe, 340
  of angelica, 229
  of black cohosh, 218
  of calendula, 331
  of cascara sagrada, 459
  of cayenne, 610
  of cinnamon, 646
  of coffee, 527
  of elder, 276
  of ephedra, 550
  of fenugreek, 196
  of garlic, 286
  of German chamomile, 398
  of ginger, 490
  of hops, 412
  of kudzu, 692
  of lavender, 147–148
  of lemon, 503–504
  of lemon balm, 421
  of marijuana, 700–701
  of mistletoe, 743
  of mustard, 169
  of oat, 431
  of onion, 318
  of passion flower, 590
  of psyllium, 452
  of rose, 362
  of sage, 298
  of soy, 206
  of St. John's wort, 564
  of tea, 540
  of thyme, 307
  of tobacco, 680
  of turmeric, 734
  of valerian, 386
  of wild yam, 184
  of wintergreen, 656
  of yarrow, 352
Ebers papyrus, 36, 121–122
echinacea, 262f, 263–272
  antifungal use of, 267, 268
  biomedical evidence, 265–267
  cautions, 268–269
  cosmetic use of, 265
  culinary use of, 264
  cultural use of, 263–264
  goldenseal and, 254
  immune response, 262f, 263–272
  integrative insight, 270
  mechanism of action of, 267
  nursing evidence, 269–270
  nurturing the nurse-plant relationship,
      272
  patient interaction, 271–272
  plant description, 263
  restoration, 266–267
  skin care, 266
  therapeutic applications, 271
  use for children, 268
  use in herbalism, 264–265
  use in pregnancy or lactation, 267–268
Echinacea angustifolia, 263–272. See
    echinacea
Echinacea pallida, 263–272. See echinacea

greater celandine, 124, **754f, 755–761**
  biomedical evidence, 756–757
  cautions, 758–759
  culinary use of, 756
  cultural use of, 755–756
  integrative insight, 759
  mechanism of action of, 757
  nursing evidence, 759
  nurturing the nurse-plant relationship, 761
  patient interaction, 760–761
  plant description, 755
  restoration, **754f, 755–761**
  therapeutic applications, 759–760
  use for children, 758
  use in herbalism, 756
  use in pregnancy or lactation, 757–758
great raisefort, 481–487. *See* horseradish
Great Smokies Diagnostic Laboratory, 166
great wild valerian, 385–395. *See* valerian
Greek clover, 195–202. *See* fenugreek
Greek hay, 195–202. *See* fenugreek
green cabbage leaf plasters for engorged
      breast, lactation and, 103
greenness, 126
green oats, 431–438. *See* oat
greens, white mustard, 174
green tea, 539–547. *See* tea
green tops, 431–438. *See* oat
grenadille, 589–595. *See* passion flower
grief
  lavender and, 153
  rose and, 365
  St. John's wort and, 571
Grifo, Francesca, 25
groats, 431–438. *See* oat
ground holly, 655–662. *See* wintergreen
ground raspberry, 253–261. *See* goldenseal
grouse berry, 655–662. *See* wintergreen
growth patterns and plant designs, 11–20
Gruber, Max, 250
gruel, 702
gudatvak, 645–653. *See* cinnamon
guercetin, 74
gui zhi, 645–653. *See* cinnamon
gum(s), 21
  disease of, rosemary and, 625
  inflammation of, lemon balm and, 423
  pain in, rose and, 364
  sage and, 300
Gymnosperms, 14

H

habituation, 664, 667
Hahnemann, Samuel, 96, 806
hair darkening, sage and, 299, 300
hair loss, yarrow and, 354
hair tonic, arnica as, 637
hai zao, 239–248. *See* kelp
hakugaishi, 169–178. *See* mustard
halitosis, arnica and, 637
Haller, John, 103
hamamelis, 373–379. *See* witch hazel
Hamamelis virginiana, 99, 373–379. *See*
      witch hazel
Hamamelis virginiana L., 90
Hamlet, 625
hands, shaking of, elder and, 277
hangover
  evening primrose and, 158
  kudzu and, 692

rose and, 365
rosemary and, 631
thyme and, 313
hardhay, 563–575. *See* St. John's wort
haridra, 733–740. *See* turmeric
harmony, tea ceremony and, 5
Harpagophytum procumbens, 122
Harry Hoxsey's cancer therapy, red clover
      and, 716
Hawaiian herbal healing, 32, 83, 120–121
hawthorn berries, 90
hazel, witch. *See* witch hazel
headache
  arnica and, 637
  black cohosh and, 219
  cascara sagrada and, 460
  cluster, cayenne and, 612
  congestive, coffee and, 528
  elder and, 277
  feverfew and, 138
  ginger and, 491
  ginkgo and, 764
  hops and, 413
  lavender and, 149
  lemon balm and, 423
  lobelia liniment and, 105
  mustard and, 171
  nervous, lemon balm and, 422
  passion flower and, 590
  rose and, 364, 365
  rosemary and, 626
  sage and, 299
  tea bags and, 540
  tea and, 540
  thyme and, 308
  tobacco and, 681
healer, traditional, 36
healing. *See also* healing plants; herbs
  brief historical perspective of, 30–40
  ethnobotanists and, 32, 36–37
  herbalists and, 32, 33–36
  history of, 25–40
    making medicine, 25–30
    nurses and plant medicines, 27–28
    when food becomes medicine, 28–30
  pharmacognosists and, 37–38
healing foods, oral remedies and, 90–97
healing gardens, 108–109
healing herbs, 114
healing plants, 1-24, 106-109. *See also*
      healing; herbs
  botany and, 11–24
  chlorophyll connection, 7–10, 7f
  individual and international relations,
      4–7, 5f
  plant personalities, 10–24
  relationship of people and plants, 3–10
health
  definition of, 123
  ginseng and, 518
health patterns, 114–115
  comfort and pain relief, 133–178
  digestion, 477–511
  elimination, 439–476
  emotions and adaptation, 559–604
  energy, 513–558
  hormone balance, 179–248
  immune response, 249–325
  lifestyle choices, 663–710
  mobility, 605–662

hyoscyamine, 71
hyperactivity, German chamomile and, 399
hyperbilirubinemia, 128
hypericin, 127, 568
hypericum, 563–575. *See* St. John's wort
Hypericum perforatum, 35, 104, 127,
    563–575. *See* St. John's wort
hypertension. *See* blood pressure, elevated
hypnotic
    chamomile as, 399
    lemon balm as, 423
    passion flower as, 590
    rose as, 366, 368
    valerian as, 386, 389
hypotension, ephedra and, 551
hypothyroidism
    horseradish and, 484
    kelp and, 241
    lemon balm and, 426
    mustard and, 174
hysteria
    hops and, 413
    lavender and, 148
    mistletoe and, 745
    passion flower and, 590
    St. John's wort and, 565

I

Ibn El Beithar, 124
ibuprofen, 80
    overdose of, liver disease and, milk thistle
        and, 671
icho, 763–770. *See* ginkgo
ileostomy, odors related to, chlorophyll
    and, 8
Ilex paraguariensis, 71
illicit drugs in urine, masking, goldenseal
    and, 255
illness, 66
    response to, 116–117
immortality, mushroom of, 726
immune response, 249–325
    aloe, 343
    calendula, 334
    cinnamon, 648
    cranberry, 444
    echinacea, **262f, 263–272**
    elder, **274f, 275–283**
    evening primrose, 160
    garlic, **284f, 285–295**
    ginseng, 518
    goldenseal, **252f, 253–261**
    horseradish, 483
    lavender, 149
    lemon, 506
    lemon balm, 424
    milk thistle, 672–673
    mistletoe, 747
    onion, **316f, 317–325**
    rose, 366
    sage, **296f, 297–304**
    Siberian ginseng, 598
    St. John's wort, 567
    tea, 542
    thyme, **306f, 307–314**, 309
immunity, cayenne, 614
immunoassays, 255
immunostimulating agent, saponins as, 22
impacted cecum, tobacco and, 681
impaired vision from black cohosh, 219

impotence
    cinnamon and, 647
    ginger and, 499
    saw palmetto and, 467
    wild yam and, 185
inadequacy, feelings of, oat and, 432
incense, 106
incensier, 623–632. *See* rosemary
incomplete emptying of bladder, saw
        palmetto and, 469
incontinence
    due to muscular weakness, kava and, 579
    ephedra and, 551
    odors related to, chlorophyll and, 8
    urinary, yarrow and, 354
Indian
    East. *See* East Indian use
    North American. *See* North American
        Indian use
Indian head, 263–272. *See* echinacea
Indian hemp, 699–710. *See* marijuana
Indian licorice, 24
Indian mustard, 169–178. *See* mustard
Indian plant, 253–261. *See* goldenseal
Indian plantago, 451–457. *See* psyllium
Indian saffron, 733–740. *See* turmeric
Indian tobacco, 679
Indian turmeric, 253–261. *See* goldenseal
Indian valerian, 385–395. *See* valerian
Indian wintergreen, 655–662. *See* wintergreen
indigenous people, 6–7
    definition of, 50
indigestion
    cascara sagrada and, 460
    chamomile and, 398
    fenugreek and, 196, 200
    horseradish and, 485
    lemon and, 504
    lemon balm and, 421
    hops and, 413
    rosemary and, 624
    soy and, 211, 214
    wild yam and, 185
indinavir, 575
indolent sores, red clover and, 716
infantile cholera, evening primrose and, 158
infections
    bladder
        cranberry and, 444
        yarrow and, 354
    echinacea and, 264, 265
    garlic and, 287
    hops and, 413
    inner ear, kudzu and, 693
    lavender and, 149
    onion and, 318
    parasitic, ginger and, 491
    resistant to antibiotics, thyme and, 309
    respiratory tract. *See* respiratory tract
        infections
    rose and, 364
    rosehip and, 364
    sinus, thyme and, 309
    skin. *See* skin infections
    turmeric and, 734
    upper respiratory. *See* respiratory tract
        infections
    urinary tract, cranberry and, 444
    yeast. *See* yeast infections
inflamed breasts, witch hazel and, 374

Lousiana long pepper, 609–620. *See* cayenne
low back pain
  cayenne and, 611, 612
  cranberry and, 444
  ginger and, 489
  lemon and, 504
  mustard and, 170
  thyme and, 308
low-bush cranberry, 443–449. *See* cranberry
lower extremities, edema of. *See* edema of
    lower extremities
lower urinary tract discomfort, saw palmetto
    and, 469
lung congestion
  mustard and, 172
  onion and, 319
lung infections, echinacea and, 265
lung problems, angelica and, 230
lung strengthening, thyme and, 308
lupulone, 414
Lycopersicon esculentum, 22
lymph flow, impaired, castor oil packs and,
    102
lymphoma, 43

M
macerate, cold. *See* cold macerate
maceration, 95
Macrocystic pyrifera, 239–248. *See* kelp
macrophages, reishi and, 726
macrotys, 217–225. *See* black cohosh
macular degeneration, bilberry and, 775
ma huang, 549–558. *See* ephedra
maidenhair tree, 763–770. *See* ginkgo
malaria
  coffee and, 528
  echinacea and, 265
  lemon and, 505
  tea and, 540
male fertility, black cohosh and, 220
malignant tumors, kelp and, 241
malignant ulcers, red clover and, 716
mandano, 733–740. *See* turmeric
mandram, 611
manic depression, lavender and, 149
manzanilla, 397–408. *See* German
    chamomile
Mao, 31–32
mao, 549–558. *See* ephedra
MAO B. *See* monoamine oxidase B
maple, 18
maple syrup, 2
maple trees, 2
Marian thistle, 669–677. *See* milk thistle
marigolds, 330
marihuana, 699–710. *See* marijuana
marijuana, 29, 255, 412, 665, 666, **698f,**
    699–710
  biomedical evidence, 702–705
  cautions, 695, 706–707
  culinary use of, 701–702
  cultural use of, 699–701
  emotions and adaptation, 704
  integrative insight, 695–696, 707–708
  lifestyle choice, **698f, 699–710**
  mechanism of action of, 705
  nursing evidence, 695–696
  nurturing the nurse-plant relationship,
      697, 710
  patient interaction, 697, 709–710

  plant description, 699
  restoration, 704
  therapeutic applications, 696–697,
      708–709
  use for children, 694–695, 706
  use in herbalism, 702
  use in pregnancy or lactation, 694,
      705–706
mary jane, 699–710. *See* marijuana
Mary thistle, 669–677. *See* milk thistle
mashinin, 699–710. *See* marijuana
Mashki-kike-winini, 118
masking illicit drugs in urine, 255
massage, 105, 792
  ginger and, 498
  lavender and, 153
  lemon and, 509
  rose and, 369
  rosemary and, 631
  thyme and, 313
  yarrow and, 358
mastalgia, evening primrose and, 158
maté, Paraguay, 71
Materia Medica, Chinese, 116, 117
Matricaria aurea, 397–408. *See* German
    chamomile
Matricaria chamomilla, 390, 397–408. *See*
    German chamomile
Matricaria recutita, 397–408. *See* German
    chamomile
maypop, 589–595. *See* passion flower
maypops, 589–595. *See* passion flower
meadow clover, 715–723. *See* red clover
measles
  black cohosh and, 217
  calendula and, 333
  chamomile and, 403
  echinacea and, 264
  kudzu and, 691
  lemon and, 504
  sage and, 299
  yarrow and, 354
mechanism of action, 127
  of aloe, 343–344
  of angelica, 231–232
  of arnica, 638–639
  of bilberry, 776–777
  of black cohosh, 220–221
  of calendula, 334
  of cascara sagrada, 461
  of cayenne, 614–615
  of cinnamon, 649
  of coffee, 531
  of cranberry, 446
  of echinacea, 267
  of elder, 279
  of ephedra, 552
  of evening primrose, 161
  of fenugreek, 197–198
  of feverfew, 139–140
  of garlic, 290
  of German chamomile, 401–402
  of ginger, 495
  of ginkgo, 766
  of ginseng, 520–521
  of goldenseal, 256
  of greater celandine, 757
  of hops, 414–415
  of horseradish, 483
  of kava, 580–581

goldenseal and, 254
sage and, 299
witch hazel and, 374
mouth ulcers, fenugreek and, 197
mouthwash
arnica, 642
bilberry, 779
calendula, 336
cinnamon as, 647
German chamomile and, 400
lemon balm as, 423
thyme as, 309
thymol as, 308
mucilage, 21
Mucosa, 327
mucosa, oral, inflammation of, coffee and, 528
mucous discharge, excessive, rose and, 364
mucous membranes
bacterial diseases of, German chamomile and, 400
infections of, echinacea and, 265
inflammation of, goldenseal and, 254
irritation of, saw palmetto and, 468
swelling of, ephedra and, 551
mucus discharge, excessive, witch hazel and, 374
mukkopeera, 589–595. *See* passion flower
mullein, 55, 78
mullein flowers, 295
mullein leaf, 107
multiple sclerosis
evening primrose and, 158
oat and, 432
mummification, cinnamon in, 647
muscle fiber spasms, wild yam and, 185
muscle pain, lavender and, 149
muscle relaxant, 72
kava as, 579
muscle spasms
black cohosh and, 219
castor oil packs and, 102
muscle tension, passion flower and, 590
muscular pain
black cohosh and, 219
rosemary and, 626
wintergreen and, 656
muscular tenderness, goldenseal and, 254
mushroom
Amanita, poisoning from, treatment and, milk thistle and, 676
of immortality, 726
phantom, 725–731. *See* reishi
ten thousand year, 725–731. *See* reishi
mushroom poisoning, 77
mustard and, 172
reishi and, 726
Muslims, 124–125
mustard, 23, **168f, 169–178**
biomedical evidence, 172
comfort and pain relief, **168f, 169–178**
culinary use of, 171
cultural use of, 168–169
integrative insight, 176
mechanism of action of, 172
nitrogen, 175
nursing evidence, 175–176
nurturing the nurse-plant relationship, 178
oil of, 171

patient interaction, 177–178
plant description, 169
therapeutic applications, 176–177
use for children, 173
use in herbalism, 171–172
use in pregnancy or lactation, 173
mustard greens, white, 174
mustard seed plaster, 176–177
Mutterkraut (mother herb), 137–144. *See* feverfew
myasthenia gravis, ephedra and, 551
myotonia dystrophica, reishi and, 726
myrrh, 22, 124, 125
mystyldene, 743–752. *See* mistletoe
myth of "no risk," 68–73

N

N. rustica, 680
narcolepsy, ephedra and, 551
narcotic
coffee as, 531
mistletoe as, 744
tobacco as, 680
narcotic poisons, lemon and, 505
Nardostachys jatamansi, 385
nardus, 149
narrow-leaved echinacea, 263–272. *See* echinacea
narrow-leaved purple coneflower, 263–272. *See* echinacea
nasal allergies, kudzu and, 693
nasal congestion
ephedra and, 551
passion flower and, 590
nasal discharge, ginger and, 491
nasal inflammation, goldenseal and, 254
nasal spray, cinnamon as, 647. *See also* sinus spray
National Academy of Sciences, 811
National College
of Naturopathic Medicine, 800
of Phytotherapy, 797
native jing, 514
native medicine, 53
Naturacil, 452
Natural History, 126
natural progesterone cream, 190–191
nature care, 88–109, 783–786
class outline and, 787t
sample curriculum and, 785–786
Naturopathic Healing, 800
Naturopathic Physicians (ND), 784
nausea
from black cohosh, 219
cayenne and, 611
evening primrose and, 158
ginger and, 491
lavender and, 149
marijuana and, 702
rose and, 365
wild yam and, 185
ND. *See* Naturopathic Physicians
neck
stiff
black cohosh and, 219
kudzu and, 692
tension in, black cohosh and, 219
tightness in, kudzu and, 693
neck glands, swollen, cranberry and, 444

Plantago asiatica L., 451–457. *See*
psyllium
Plantago indica L., 451–457. *See* psyllium
Plantago ovata Forssk., 451–457. *See*
psyllium
Plantago psyllium, 451–457. *See* psyllium
Plantago psyllium L., 90, 451–457. *See*
psyllium
plantain seed, 452
plant constituents and active medicinal
principles, 20–23
plant description, 115
plant designs and growth patterns, 11–20
Plant Kingdom Classification System, 13f
plant medicines
history of, 30–40
nurses and, 26–28
plant parts, 12–20, 115
plant potency, 73–84
plant profiles, 111–131, 113t
biomedical evidence, 126–127
cautions, 129
common names, 114
health pattern, 114–115
introduction to, 114–131
Latin name and family, 114
nursing evidence, 130
nurturing the nurse-plant relationship,
131
organization of, 113t
patient interaction, 131
plant description, 115
plant parts used, 115
therapeutic applications, 130–131
traditional evidence, 115–126
use for children, 128–129
use in pregnancy or lactation, 127–128
plants
and biomedical paradigm, 44–49
healing. *See* healing plants
and healing environment, 106–109
and integrative paradigm, 55–61
medicinal, and the law, 791–795
nursing care and, 87–110
and nursing paradigm, 53–55
and paradigms, 41–61
herbal revolution, 48–49
integrative insight, 58–61
interdisciplinary interest, 41–43
plants as potential drugs, 45–46
rigorous testing, 46–47
standardization, 47–48
vision of World Health Organization,
55–58
partnering with, 109–110
personalities of, 10–24
sensory experience and, 23–24
as potential drugs, 45–46
relationship of people with, 3–10
and traditional paradigm, 49–52
plaster, 102–103
cayenne, 619
garlic, for heel, 293
mustard seed, 176–177
tobacco, 687
tofu, 207
platelet aggregation, onion and, 319
Pleomorphism, 250
pleurisy, milk thistle and, 670
Pliny, 412

pneumonia
angelica and, 229
cayenne and, 611
echinacea and, 265
ephedra and, 551
flaxseed and, 27
garlic and, 287
ginger and, 499
goldenseal and, 253
hops and, 412
lemon and, 504
mustard and, 171
poison control centers, 71, 72
poisoning
alcohol, kudzu and, 692
Amanita mushroom, treatment and, milk
thistle and, 676
anticholinergic, 71
black cohosh and, 219
mushroom, 77
mustard and, 172
reishi and, 726
poisons
for arrows, 68
narcotic, lemon and, 505
polar plant, 623–632. *See* rosemary
polio, kudzu and, 693
pollen, 19
polluted water, sickness resulting from
drinking, garlic and, 287
pollution, plant growth and, 85
polycystic ovaries, saw palmetto and, 469
polysaccharides, 21
poppy, opium, 21
poppy flowers, hops and, 413
porphyrins, 8
postanesthesia units, herbal medicines in, 72
postmastectomy pain, cayenne and, 612
postmenopausal vaginal dryness, fenugreek
and, 197
postoperative washing of surgical sites,
echinacea and, 265
postpartum hemorrhage, coffee and, 528
postphlebitis syndrome, ginkgo and, 765
pot, 699–710. *See* marijuana
potatoes, 22, 29, 55, 72
potency, plant, 73–84
potential nursing applications. *See also*
nursing care; nursing evidence
of aloe, 346
of angelica, 233–234
of arnica, 641
of bilberry, 778–779
of black cohosh, 222
of calendula, 335
of cascara sagrada, 463
of cayenne, 617
of cinnamon, 651
of coffee, 533–534
of cranberry, 447–448
of echinacea, 269–270
of elder, 280–281
of ephedra, 555–556
of evening primrose, 163
of fenugreek, 200
of feverfew, 142
of garlic, 292
of German chamomile, 405
of ginger, 497
of ginkgo, 768

smoking
  arnica and, 637
  biomedical evidence, 681–683, 702–705
  cautions, 684–685, 695, 706–707
  culinary use of, 680, 701–702
  cultural use of, 679–680, 699–701
  cytochrome P-450 and, 73–74
  English, 687
  evening primrose and, 158
  integrative insight, 687, 707–708
  lifestyle choice, **678f, 679–689, 698f,
    699–710**
  mechanism of action of, 683, 705
  mountain, 635–643. *See* arnica
  nursing evidence, 686–687, 695–696
  nurturing the nurse-plant relationship,
    689, 697, 710
  patient interaction, 688–689, 697, 709–710
  therapeutic applications, 687–688,
    696–697, 708–709
  use for children, 684, 694–695, 706
  use in herbalism, 680–681, 702
  use in pregnancy or lactation, 684, 694,
    705–706
smoking cessation, arnica and, 637
snakebite
  black cohosh and, 219
  echinacea and, 264
  elder and, 277
snake root, Kansas, 263–272. *See* echinacea
snapping hazel, 373–379. *See* witch hazel
sneezewort, 813f
soapwort, 22
sobering up, coffee and, 528
soda, chlorinated, for poultice, 103
soft native extract, saw palmetto, 473
solanaceous glycoalkaloids, 72
Solanum tuberosum, 22, 29
solid extract, angelica, 235
solvent, alcohol as, 94
soma, 549–558. *See* ephedra
sore eyes, red clover and, 716
sore feet, arnica and, 637
sore joints, sage and, 299
sore muscles, witch hazel and, 374
sore nipples. *See* nipples
sores
  bed
    aloe and, 339
    arnica and, 637
    calendula and, 332
    mustard and, 169
    witch hazel and, 374
  canker. *See* canker sores
  cold, 52
  indolent, red clover and, 716
  lavender and, 149
  of lower limbs, greater celandine and, 756
  mouth. *See* mouth sores
  skin. *See* skin sores
  yarrow and, 354
sore throat
  black cohosh and, 218
  cayenne and, 611, 612
  cranberry and, 444
  elder and, 278
  fenugreek and, 197
  goldenseal and, 254
  mustard and, 172
  red clover and, 716

rosemary and, 626
sage and, 299, 300
thyme and, 308
thymol and, 308
wintergreen and, 657
witch hazel and, 374
yarrow and, 354
soup, 92–93
  miso, 214–215
  onion cress, 325
sour taste, 90
Southwest School of Botanical Medicine, 797
soy, 92–93, **204f, 205–215,** 693
  biomedical evidence, 207–210
  culinary use of, 206–207
  cultural use of, 205–206
  daidzein and, 414
  digestion, 207
  hormone balance, **204f, 205–215**
  integrative insight, 212–213
  mechanism of action of, 209–210
  mobility, 209
  nursing evidence, 211–213
  nurturing the nurse-plant relationship,
    214
  patient interaction, 214
  plant description, 205
  restoration, 209
  therapeutic applications of, 213
  use for children, 210–211
  use in herbalism, 207
  use in pregnancy or lactation, 210
soybean, 205–215. *See* soy
soy lecithin, 205–215. *See* soy
spasms
  associated with chronic cystitis, kava and,
    578
  bladder, cayenne and, 611
  gastrointestinal
    angelica and, 230
    German chamomile and, 400
  lavender and, 149
  red clover and, 716
  sinus, steam inhalation and, German
    chamomile, 406
  thyme and, 308
  wild yam and, 185
  yarrow and, 354
spearmint tea, 80, 84
species, 12
sperma, 12
spiceberry, 655–662. *See* wintergreen
spices, 477–478
spider bites, echinacea and, 264
spikenard, 385
spinach, 8
Spinacia aleracea L., 8
spinal cord injury, St. John's wort and, 565
spine, inflammation of, black cohosh and,
  219
spiny eleutherococc, 597–604. *See* Siberian
  ginseng
Spiraea ulmaria, 49
spirit, science of, 125
"spirits," 666
spiritual vegetable meat, 725–731. *See* reishi
Spiritus fermentae, 30
spleen disorders
  angelica and, 230
  evening primrose and, 158

traditional evidence—cont'd
  tobacco, 679–681
  turmeric, 733–735
  valerian, 385–387
  wild yam, 183–186
  wintergreen, 655–657
  witch hazel, 373–374
  yarrow, 351–354
traditional healer, 36
traditional medicine, definition of, 50
Traditional Medicine Programme, 3,
    55–56, 84
traditional paradigm, 51
  versus biomedical paradigm, 52
tranquility, tea ceremony and, 5
tranquilizer, valerian as, 387
trauma
  arnica and, 637
  kudzu and, 692
tree
  kew, 763–770. See ginkgo
  maidenhair, 763–770. See ginkgo
tree primrose, 157–166. See evening
    primrose
trefoil, 715–723. See red clover
trembling
  of heart, rose and, 364
  sage and, 300
triazolam, interaction of grapefruit juice
    with, 73
Trichosanthes kirilowii Maxim, 695
trichosanthis root, 695
tridosha, 123
Trifolium pratense, 715–723. See red
    clover
trigonella, 195–202. See fenugreek
Trigonella foenum-graecum, 83, 195–202.
    See fenugreek
trikatu, 490
true cinnamon, 645–653. See cinnamon
true ginseng, 517–525. See ginseng
true lavender, 147–154. See lavender
true sage, 297–304. See sage
true wild yam, 183–192. See wild yam
tuber, 15f, 16
tuberculosis
  angelica and, 230
  black cohosh and, 219
  garlic and, 285
  goldenseal and, 253
  hops and, 411
  kava and, 578
  marijuana and, 700
  onion and, 318
  red clover and, 716
  sage and, 299
  saw palmetto and, 468
  soy for prevention of, 207
  witch hazel and, 373
  yarrow and, 352
tumors
  arnica and, 637
  cayenne and, 611
  kelp and, 241
  of mouth, sage and, 300
  skin, onion and, 319
  soy and, 206
  St. John's wort and, 565
  witch hazel and, 374
Turkish culture, 125

turmeric, **732f, 733–740**
  biomedical evidence, 735–737
  cautions, 737–738
  culinary use of, 734
  cultural use of, 733–734
  integrative insight, 738
  mechanism of action of, 736–737
  nursing evidence, 738
  nurturing the nurse-plant relationship,
    740
  patient interaction, 739–740
  plant description, 733
  restoration, **732f, 733–740**
  skin care, 736
  therapeutic applications, 739
  use for children, 737
  use in herbalism, 734–735
  use in pregnancy or lactation, 737
turmeric root, 253–261, 733. See goldenseal
turmerin, 735–736
typhoid fever
  angelica and, 230
  echinacea and, 265
  mistletoe and, 745
  sage and, 299
typhus fever, mustard and, 172
tyrosine, 174

U
Ukrain, 756, 757
ulcers, 66
  aloe and, 341
  cayenne and, 612
  decubitus, chlorophyll and, 8
  gastrointestinal, rose and, 365
  goldenseal and, 254
  leg
    fenugreek and, 197
    soy and, 207
  malignant, red clover and, 716
  mouth
    bilberry and, 775
    fenugreek and, 197
  peptic, 66
  skin. See skin ulcers
  varicose, lavender and, 148
  yarrow and, 354
ultraviolet light, angelica and, 231
Unani, 123
unbalanced nervous system, angelica and,
    231
Undaria, 248
undelivered placenta, mistletoe and, 745
"Understanding Ethnic Women's Experiences
    with Pharmacopeia," 54, 80
unit-dosing system, 26–27
universalism, interpersonal, kava and, 578
upper respiratory tract infections. See
    respiratory tract infections
urea, 8
ureter pain, kava and, 578
urinary incontinence, yarrow and, 354
urinary output
  onion and, 319
  rosehip and, 364
urinary stream, hesitancy in initiation of,
    saw palmetto and, 468
urinary tract infections
  cranberry and, 444
  saw palmetto and, 468

warming joints, ginger and, 491
warming stomach, ginger and, 491
warts, 41
  greater celandine and, 756
  thyme and, 308
wasabi, 481–487. *See* horseradish
wasp stings, echinacea and, 264
wasting, saw palmetto and, 468
water
  Carmelite, 422
  flower, 807
  foam in, saponins and, 22
  rose, 125, 364, 365
    ointment of, 369
  witch hazel, 375
waterly diarrhea, evening primrose and, 158
watermelon, 440
Watson, Jean, 85, 801–802
weakness
  angelica and, 231
  oat and, 432
  rose and, 364
weak pulse edema, mistletoe and, 745
weed, 28, 29, 699–710. *See* marijuana
Weed, Susan, 568, 628
weeding, 808–811
Wegman, Ita, 125
weight, dosage for children based on, 129
weight gain
  cinnamon and, 647
  cranberry juice and, 447
  kelp and, 246
  reishi and, 726
  saw palmetto and, 468
weight loss
  ephedra and, 551
  evening primrose and, 158
  with fatigue, saw palmetto and, 468
Weleeda, 89
wellness, 711
wheezing, feverfew and, 138
whinberry, 773–781. *See* bilberry
white berry mistletoe, 743–752. *See*
  mistletoe
white ginseng, 517–525. *See* ginseng
white mustard, 169–178. *See* mustard
white mustard greens, 174
WHO. *See* World Health Organization
whole body tonic, ginseng as, 518
whole dried root, decoction from, kudzu, 696
whole herb, 79
  ephedra, 556, 557
  garlic, 293
  purgative, 79
whole plant St. John's wort, 127
whole root, cut, kava, 584
whooping cough
  black cohosh and, 219
  coffee and, 528
  evening primrose and, 158
  horseradish and, 482
  red clover and, 716
  saw palmetto and, 468
  thyme and, 308
  thymol and, 308
whorled arrangement of leaves, 17f
whortleberry, 773–781. *See* bilberry
wild chamomile, 397–408. *See* German
  chamomile
wild cherry, 39

wildcraft, 27, 794
wild oats, 431–438. *See* oat
wild passion flower, 589–595. *See* passion
  flower
wild pepper, 597–604. *See* Siberian
  ginseng
wild tobacco, 679
wild yam, **182f, 183–192**
  biomedical evidence, 186–187
  cautions, 188–189
  culinary use of, 184
  cultural use of, 183–184
  hormone balance, **182f, 183–192**
  integrative insight, 189–190
  mechanism of action of, 187
  nursing evidence, 189–190
  nurturing the nurse-plant relationship,
    192
  patient interaction, 191
  plant description, 183
  therapeutic applications, 190–191
  use for children, 188
  use in herbalism, 184–186
  use in pregnancy or lactation, 187–188
wild yam rhizome, 186
willow bark, 124
windmill palm, 467–476. *See* saw palmetto
wine
  choke cherry, 666, 667
  dandelion, 666
  red, 666
Winston, David, 469
winterbloom, 373–379. *See* witch hazel
wintergreen, **654f, 655–662**
  biomedical evidence, 657
  cautions, 659
  culinary use of, 656
  cultural use of, 655–656
  integrative insight, 660
  mechanism of action of, 657
  mobility, **654f, 655–662**
  nursing evidence, 660
  nurturing the nurse-plant relationship,
    661–662
  patient interaction, 661
  plant description, 655
  therapeutic applications, 660–661
  use for children, 658–659
  use in herbalism, 656–657
  use in pregnancy or lactation, 658
wintergreen oil, 655–662. *See*
  wintergreen
wise wimmin, 80
witch hazel, 90, 99, **372f, 373–379**
  biomedical evidence, 374
  cautions, 376–377
  culinary use of, 374
  cultural use of, 373–374
  integrative insight, 377–378
  mechanism of action of, 375
  nursing evidence, 377–378
  nurturing the nurse-plant relationship,
    379
  patient interaction, 379
  plant description, 373
  skin care, **372f, 373–379**
  therapeutic applications, 378–379
  use for children, 376
  use in herbalism, 374
  use in pregnancy or lactation, 375–376